Cyclic Nucleotides in the Nervous System

John Daly

National Institute of Arthritis, Metabolism
and Digestive Diseases
National Institutes of Health
Bethesda, Maryland

PLENUM PRESS · NEW YORK AND LONDON

Library of Congress Cataloging in Publication Data

Daly, John W
  Cyclic nucleotides in the nervous system.

  Bibliography: p.
  Includes index.
  1. Cyclic adenylic acid. 2. Cyclic guanylic acid. 3. Neurochemistry. I. Title.
QP625.A35D34   599'.01'88   76-62999
ISBN 0-306-30971-8

© 1977 Plenum Press, New York
A Division of Plenum Publishing Corporation
227 West 17th Street, New York, N.Y. 10011

Printed in the United States of America

To KATHLEEN

Preface

The elucidation of the cellular and molecular bases underlying the integrated function of the central nervous system, both in disease and in health, must ultimately come from the combined efforts of scientists from many disciplines, including biology, chemistry, histology, pathology, physiology, pharmacology, and psychology. Communication between scientists from these various disciplines—vital to the advancement of our understanding of the function of the nervous system—has become more and more difficult in recent years. Both increasing specialization and the incredible increases in publications pertinent to brain research in a wide spectrum of journals, in symposium volumes, in monographs, in abstracts, and in reviews contribute to the problems of cross-communication and even of communication within a scientific discipline. Research on the significance of cyclic nucleotides to the function of nervous systems is particularly illustrative of the communication problem. Since the initial publications by Sutherland, Rall, and Butcher in the late fifties and early sixties on high levels of adenylate cyclase, phosphodiesterases, and cyclic AMP in brain, the ensuing literature of this field has expanded exponentially. At the present time, from five to ten publications relevant to cyclic nucleotides and the nervous system appear each week. Indeed, these are minimal numbers based mainly on examination of literature titles and key index words. Many articles concerned with some aspect of central function contain, buried within their text, experiments with or related to cyclic nucleotides. Other articles concern studies on agents or manipulations known to affect the formation, degradation, or action of cyclic nucleotides, but in these articles no attempt has been made to relate the results to the cyclic nucleotide systems. For any scientist, to maintain an overview of cyclic nucleotide research as it relates to the function of the nervous system has, thus, become a virtually impossible task. This was quite apparent during the compilation of the literature for this monograph.

The present monograph *attempts,* as concisely and succinctly as possible, to reference, summarize, and place in the context the literature on cyclic nucleotides in the nervous system. The word *attempt* should be stressed since even after considerable effort many references and "buried" literature data on cyclic nucleotides have certainly been missed. Over 1200 references have been cited for the period of 1961 to 1976. In 1961–2 only six references pertained, and only nine papers were published on cyclic nucleotides in the nervous system during the next four years. However, in 1967, twenty-one papers were published followed by increases to twenty-eight in 1969, fifty-four in 1970, ninety-nine in 1971, one hundred forty-three in 1972, one hundred sixty-seven in 1973, one hundred ninety-two in 1974, three hundred seventy-five in 1975, and finally to at least one hundred twenty for the first few months of 1976. The present attempt to cover the literature on cyclic nucleotides in the nervous system illuminated the need for more extensive use of key words designed to facilitate computer-assisted literature searches with computer-assisted elimination of nonrelevant publications through required pairing of key words.

The interrelationships between scientific endeavors, of course, transcend the present artificially imposed limitation to the nervous system. It was, however, not feasible to even attempt to summarize relevant findings from the voluminous literature on cyclic nucleotides in biological preparations from other than the nervous system or even to summarize the literature on cyclic nucleotide systems in innervated tissue intimately associated with neuronal function such as in striated, smooth, and cardiac muscle and in various endocrine glands, especially the adrenal, pituitary, and pineal. Literature on cultured tumor cells derived from neurons or glia has been surveyed and the results fairly adequately outline the advance of knowledge on cyclic nucleotide systems in cultured cells. Similarly, it was not feasible to attempt to summarize and define the possible correlations of the vast literature in other areas of brain research to cyclic nucleotide-dependent mechanisms. In the latter stages of the preparation of the present monograph, the dynamic nature of research and publication on cyclic nucleotides in the nervous systems and on related areas of research further frustrated efforts at completeness. In spite of these various limitations, it is to be hoped that the present volume will be valuable (i) in providing the cyclic nucleotide specialist, burdened by the ever increasing literature, with a fairly comprehensive survey and overview of the literature and directions of research on cyclic nucleotides in the nervous system and (ii) in providing other neuroscientists with a volume through which they may perceive interrelationships of their own research and the field of cyclic nucleotides.

National Institute of Arthritis,
Metabolism and Digestive Diseases   JOHN DALY*
National Institutes of Health
Bethesda, Maryland

*This book was written by the author in his private capacity. No official support nor endorsement is intended nor should be inferred.

Contents

1

Introduction

The complexity of the central nervous system makes investigation and elucidation of the factors involved in the establishment, regulation, and integration of neuronal function a formidable task. However, on the molecular level a variety of evidence indicates that the nucleotides, cyclic AMP and cyclic GMP,* are involved in regulatory roles associated with neuronal function. Cyclic AMP regulates prime functions in many other tissues: gluconeogenesis in liver, lipolysis in fat, secretion in endocrine glands. Definitive roles for cyclic GMP have as yet not been established, but in many tissues cyclic GMP has been proposed to have effects opposing those of cyclic AMP (Goldberg *et al.,* 1973, 1975). These cyclic nucleotides are formed from intracellular ATP and GTP, respectively, by the action of cyclase enzymes. The cyclic nucleotides are degraded by phosphodiesterases to their respective 5'-phosphates. The diverse biological effects of cyclic nucleotides appear to be manifested through activation of protein kinases which specifically phosphorylate enzymes and other functional proteins and thus alter their properties. The specificity and nature of the effects of cyclic nucleotides presumably depend, therefore, not only on the intracellular site of generation of the cyclic nucleotide, but also on the substrate specificity of the activated kinases and the accessibility of endogenous protein substrates. Termination of the physiological effects initiated by the cyclic nucleotides presumably occurs via the action of phosphoprotein phosphatases which hydrolyze the phosphorylated proteins. In certain tissues or cells, levels of cyclic AMP and cyclic GMP appear to be inversely related; increases in one nucleotide are accompanied by decreases in the other, suggesting a functional interrelationship.

---

*For structures of cyclic nucleotides, analogs, and related compounds see Appendix.

The mechanisms involved in the formation and role of cyclic nucleotides in nervous tissue have been investigated on many levels: (1) with cell-free preparations, (2) with incubated brain slices, (3) with cells of neuronal or glial origin, (4) with functional ganglia or discrete central neurons, (5) in intact animals. With cell-free preparations, the levels and properties of cyclases, phosphodiesterases, and cyclic-nucleotide-dependent protein kinases have been investigated. With brain slices from control animals and in animals subjected to prior drug or environmental manipulation, the effects of putative neurotransmitters, other regulatory agents, electrical stimulation, and various drugs on the intracellular accumulation of cyclic nucleotides have been studied. Cultured cells of neuronal or glial origin have provided model intact cell systems for studying the effects of such agents. Regulatory roles for cyclic nucleotides have been investigated *in situ* in ganglia, peripheral neurons, and central neurons. The effect of centrally active drugs on levels of brain cyclic nucleotides and the behavioral effects of administered cyclic AMP and its derivatives have been studied in whole animals. Central to an elucidation of the role(s) of cyclic nucleotides in the nervous system is the correlation of the effects of phosphodiesterase inhibitors and of various agonists and antagonists on formation and levels of cyclic nucleotides and the pharmacological effects of such agents. Additional pharmacological effects of "specific" agents have confounded such correlations. The *O,N*-dibutyryl and *N*-monobutyryl derivatives of cyclic AMP and cyclic GMP have been used extensively. Structures of agonists and antagonists and the nature of their possible interactions with cyclic nucleotide systems are presented in the Appendix.

The present monograph *attempts* to survey the results of investigations on cyclic nucleotides in nervous tissue as of April, 1976, with emphasis on relevance to the functional roles of cyclic AMP and cyclic GMP in the central nervous system. Only selected abstracts have been cited. Many reviews concerned with formation, degradation, and action of cyclic nucleotides in the nervous system have appeared during the past few years (Rall and Gilman, 1970; Drummond and Ma, 1973; Schorderet, 1974; Bloom, 1975; Daly, 1975a,b, 1976; Weiss and Greenberg, 1975). Reviews concerned with more specific topics will be cited in appropriate sections of the present monograph.

2

Enzymatic Formation, Degradation, and Action of Cyclic Nucleotides

2.1 Adenylate Cyclases

The enzyme, adenylate cyclase catalyzes the conversion of ATP to cyclic AMP and pyrophosphate. The enzyme in most cells appears associated with plasma membrane, with its activity regulated by a receptor(s) exposed to extracellular space (cf. review by Perkins, 1973). Receptors include those for the following hormones: catecholamines, histamine, serotonin, and polypeptides. In addition, the activity of adenylate cyclase is dependent on a variety of other control mechanisms. Magnesium ions are required for enzyme activity. Calcium ions stimulate cyclase activity but are inhibitory at high concentrations. High concentrations of fluoride ions markedly enhance cyclase activity in cell-free preparations, but not in intact cells. GTP appears to play an important regulatory role, enhancing cyclase activity in cell-free preparations and potentiating or permitting hormone responses. Adenosine inhibits adenylate cyclase from certain cell types, such as fat cells, and stimulates cyclases from platelets and neuroblastoma cells. Finally, macromolecular factors which activate or inhibit cyclases have been reported. Adenylate cyclase in homogenates is usually assayed in the presence of a phosphodiesterase inhibitor. When radioactive ATP is used as substrate, often a trapping pool of cyclic AMP is added in addition to the phosphodiesterase inhibitor. The activity of cyclase will depend on the concentration of ATP and the ratio of ATP and magnesium ions. Often, low concentrations of ATP are employed along with an ATP-regenerating system.

2.1.1 Regional Distribution of Adenylate Cyclase in Brain

Brain contained high levels of adenylate cyclases which varied considerably in different brain regions. High activity was present in gray matter and low in white matter. Levels of adenylate cyclase have been studied in brain regions of rabbit (Duffy *et al.*, 1975); rat (Weiss and Costa, 1968; Weiss, 1971; Duffy *et al.*, 1975; Weiss and Greenberg, 1975; Nakazawa *et al.*, 1976); mouse (Kuo and Greengard, 1970c); monkey (Williams *et al.*, 1969); human (Williams *et al.*, 1969; Weiss and Strada, 1973; Duffy *et al.*, 1975); sheep (Klainer *et al.*, 1962; Sutherland *et al.*, 1962); calf and steer (Sutherland *et al.*, 1962); cat (Klainer *et al.*, 1962; Krishna *et al.*, 1970); pig (Sutherland *et al.*, 1962); and chicken (Nahorski *et al.*, 1976). Basal levels of adenylate cyclase in rat brain regions are shown in Table 1. A threefold range of fluoride-stimulated adenylate cyclase activity in rat brain was observed, with levels decreasing in the following order: neocortex > olfactory bulb, thalamus, hippocampus, cerebellum, olfactory tubercle > septum-fornix, hypothalamus, caudate nucleus, medulla-pons, spinal cord (Weiss and Costa, 1968). Levels of adenylate cyclase in neuron-enriched fractions from rat brain were as follows: cerebellum > striatum > hypothalamus, cortex, hippocampus, midbrain, brain stem (Palmer, 1973a). Levels in glia-enriched fractions were quite constant for the different brain regions with the exception of the cerebellum where the level was twofold higher than in other regions. In each region, the glial activity was lower than that of the neuronal activity.

TABLE 1. Levels of Cyclases, Phosphodiesterases, and Cyclic Nucleotides in Rat Brain[a]

| Brain region | Adenylate cyclase | Guanylate cyclase | Phosphodiesterase | | Cyclic GMP | Cyclic AMP | Cyclic GMP |
| | | | Cyclic AMP | | | | |
			Low K_m	High K_m			
Cerebral cortex	0.25–0.30	0.03–0.06	4	30–50	25	8–15	0.2–0.5
Cerebellum	0.40–0.60	0.02–0.04	2	5–10	3	10–20	8–12
Hippocampus	0.20	—	7	50	—	8–12	—
Thalamus	0.25	—	3	24	—	14	—
Midbrain	—	0.02–0.05	—	—	5	6–12	—
Striatum (caudate)	0.14	—	4	30	—	6–12	0.5
Hypothalamus	0.15	—	2	20–25	—	7–16	0.5–1.0
Medulla-pons	0.10–0.13	0.01–0.02	1.3	6–10	2.5	4–10	—
Brain stem (spinal cord)	0.18	0.01–0.02	1.3	5–10	2.5	8–18	1.0

[a]Values are from the literature cited in the text and are meant to provide indices of relative levels in different brain regions. Enzyme activities are in nanomoles per milligram of protein per minute and cyclic nucleotide levels are in picomoles per milligram of protein.

2.1.2 *Regional Distribution of Cyclic AMP in Brain*

Levels of cyclic AMP varied considerably in different brain regions and probably reflect both the activity of cyclases and phosphodiesterases and the availability of ATP. For example, total adenylate cyclase activity is relatively high and phosphodiesterase relatively low in cerebellum, and this brain region in rat exhibited the highest basal level of cyclic AMP. Levels of cyclic AMP have been studied in brain regions of rat (Cramer *et al.*, 1971; Ebadi *et al.*, 1971a,b; Schmidt *et al.*, 1971, 1972; Volicer and Gold, 1973; Wellman and Schwabe, 1973; Jones *et al.*, 1974; Mao *et al.*, 1974a; De La Paz *et al.*, 1975); mouse (Steiner *et al.*, 1972; Wellman and Schwabe, 1973); and human (Kodama *et al.*, 1973; Weiss and Strada, 1973). Cyclic AMP levels were in various species high in cerebellum, intermediate in telencephalon and mesencephalon, and low in medulla-pons. For example, levels of cyclic AMP after microwave irradiation of rats were high in cerebellum and brain stem, intermediate in midbrain and hypothalamus, and low in hippocampus and cortex (Schmidt *et al.*, 1971, 1972). Basal levels of cyclic AMP, using liquid nitrogen freezing followed by softening with trichloroacetic acid–acetone and dissection, were highest in rat hypothalamus and septum and nearly the same in whole brain, telediencephalon, cortex, hippocampus, thalamus–midbrain–striatum, brain stem, and cerebellum (De La Paz *et al.*, 1975). In mouse brain, cyclic AMP levels decreased in the following order: striatum, hypothalamus, thalamus, brain stem, cerebral cortex, hippocampus, cerebellum, spinal cord, with striatal levels about fourfold higher than levels in spinal cord (Steiner *et al.*, 1972). Levels of cyclic AMP in rat brain regions are shown in Table 1.

2.1.3 *Postdecapitation Changes in Brain Cyclic AMP*

Measurements of endogenous levels of cyclic AMP in brain are complicated by rapid postdecapitation changes, the magnitude of which depends on the brain region and species (see Section 4.4.1). Postdecapitation increases were most marked in cerebellum (Schmidt *et al.*, 1971). Essentially, four methods have been used for rapid fixation of brain tissue in small animals: (1) immersion of the whole animal in liquid nitrogen, (2) decapitation of the head into liquid nitrogen, (3) expulsion of the brain tissue into liquid nitrogen (freeze blowing), and (4) microwave irradiation. The freeze-blowing technique probably results in the most rapid fixation of brain tissue but is of course unsuitable for regional studies. A comparison of levels of cyclic AMP in whole rat brain fixed by the four methods gave the following values: (1) 1.63 ± 0.16, (2) 2.62 ± 0.17, (3) 1.17 ± 0.13, and (4) 0.73 ± 0.05 nmol/g wet wt (1 nmol/g wet wt $\approx$ 10 pmol/mg protein) (Lust and Passonneau, 1973). Similar results have been reported by others (Schmidt *et al.*, 1971, 1972; Nahorski and Rogers, 1973; Guidotti *et al.*, 1974). Although levels of cyclic AMP were lowest after microwave irradiation, levels of ATP and phosphocreatine were also lowest with this technique. Levels of ATP are known to decrease during the anoxia following sacrifice of animals. Microwave irradiation inactivated most enzymes within 1.5 to 2 sec in rat brain, while only 0.5 sec was required in mouse (Guidotti *et al.*, 1974). Others have compared brain levels of cyclic AMP after decapitation into liquid nitrogen and microwave technique (Jones *et al.*, 1974). Lowest values for cyclic AMP in six rat brain regions were obtained using microwave irradiation.

2.1.4 Morphological Localization of Cyclic AMP in Brain

Immunofluorescent assay of cyclic AMP in rat cerebellar slices revealed pronounced fluorescence in Purkinje neurons and granule neurons (Bloom *et al.*, 1972a; Siggins *et al.*, 1973). The molecular layer, which consists predominantly of Purkinje dendrites and parallel fibers, was weakly fluorescent, while white matter was unreactive. Weak fluorescence in the molecular layer of the cerebellum appeared associated with Purkinje dendrites. Certain large multipolar neurons of the lateral reticular formation were strongly immunofluorescent. Staining of Purkinje cells was primarily in the cytoplasm. The extent of fluorescence in Purkinje neurons increased greatly after decapitation. Prior administration of anesthetics reduced the immunofluorescence of both Purkinje and granule cells. Cyclic AMP levels were not altered in cerebellum of nervous mutant mice in which Purkinje cells are virtually absent (Mao *et al.*, 1975b). Levels of cyclic AMP in mouse cerebellum were slightly higher in the granular layer as compared to the molecular layer (Rubin and Ferrendelli, 1976).

Adenylate cyclase activity has been demonstrated histochemically with adenosine 5'-imidodiphosphate in capillaries and on surface membranes of astrocytes in rat cerebral cortex (Joo *et al.*, 1975b). Only a few synapses contained detectable cyclase activity. The reliability of the histochemical assays for adenylate cyclase based on precipitation of lead phosphate has been questioned (Lemay and Jarett, 1975).

2.1.5 Subcellular Distribution of Adenylate Cyclases and Cyclic AMP

High levels of adenylate cyclase and cyclic AMP have been detected in synaptosomal fractions and synaptic membranes of brain homogenates (De Robertis *et al.*, 1967; Goldberg *et al.*, 1970; Krishna *et al.*, 1970; Weller *et al.*, 1972; Von Hungen and Roberts, 1973b; Middlemiss and Franklin, 1975; Nakazawa *et al.*, 1976). Adenylate cyclases in brain were associated to a limited extent with other membranal fractions including the nucleus. High levels of cyclic AMP were reported by one group (Johnson *et al.*, 1973) to be associated with vesicles isolated from synaptosomal fractions. Other workers (Goldberg *et al.*, 1970) found only low levels of cyclic AMP associated with such vesicles. An adenylate cyclase has been detected in membranes of secretory vesicles from adrenal medulla (Nikodijevic *et al.*, 1976). In contrast to adenylate cyclases from other sources it was inhibited by isoproterenol and epinephrine. Nerve growth factor also inhibited the cyclase. Propranolol blocked the inhibition by catecholamines and growth factor.

2.1.6 Activation and Inhibition of Adenylate Cyclases

Metal Ions

Adenylate cyclase activity in brain homogenates was enhanced by magnesium or manganese ions, while calcium ions were generally stimulatory at low concentrations and inhibitory at high concentrations (Bradham *et al.*, 1970; McCune *et al.*, 1971; Bradham, 1972; Johnson and Sutherland, 1973; Perkins, 1973; Swislocki and Tierney, 1973; Von Hungen and Roberts, 1973a,b; Franks *et al.*, 1974; MacDonald, 1975). Analysis of magnesium ATP and magnesium ion interactions with a detergent-solubilized adenylate cyclase from rat cerebellum was compatible with a kinetic model in which magnesium-ATP was the substrate and magnesium ion a requisite activator, and in which free ATP did not inhibit the enzyme (Garbers and Johnson, 1975). Free ATP has been generally considered to inhibit cyclases perhaps through an allosteric mechanism. The effects of calcium have been extensively studied. In general, inhibition of adenylate cyclase by EGTA was overcome by addition of calcium ions. The metal ion, presumably calcium, removed by EGTA to yield a partially deactivated cyclase was very tightly bound, since it was still present in detergent-dispersed cyclase from rat or bovine brain (Johnson and Sutherland, 1973; MacDonald, 1975). Although both basal and fluoride-stimulated beef brain adenylate cyclase were inhibited by EGTA, the inhibition of the fluoride response by EGTA was not complete (MacDonald, 1975). Interestingly, calcium did not activate cyclases from striatum, while having marked stimulatory effects on cyclases from rat cerebral cortex, hippocampus, and cerebellum (Von Hungen and Roberts, 1974). Very low concentrations (25 μM) of calcium inhibited a partially purified soluble rat brain adenylate cyclase (Swislocki and Tierney, 1973). Lithium ions inhibited basal adenylate cyclase activity in homogenates from cortex, caudate, and hippocampus, but not brain stem and cerebellum (Walker, 1974). The activation of adenylate cyclases by fluoride in homogenates from rodent cerebral cortex was antagonized by lithium ions (Dousa and Hechter, 1970; Forn and Valdecasas, 1971). Lead ions (IC_{50}, 3 μM) were potent inhibitors of rat brain adenylate cyclases (Nathanson and Bloom, 1975). Inhibition by lead was only partially reversible. Lanthanum ions inhibited cerebellar cyclases (Nathanson et al., 1976).

Fluoride Ion

High concentrations of fluoride ions stimulated adenylate cyclases in most cell-free preparations from brain (Drummond et al., 1971; Perkins and Moore, 1971; Johnson and Sutherland, 1973; Katz and Tenenhouse, 1973a; Perkins, 1973; Swislocki and Tierney, 1973; MacDonald, 1974), but had no effect on accumulations of cyclic AMP in whole cells. The stimulation by fluoride was time dependent and relatively irreversible. The apparent K_m for ATP was similar in the presence and absence of fluoride ions. In striatal preparations, fluoride either enhanced cyclase activity (Puri et al., 1975), had no effect (Mishra et al., 1974), or enhanced only in the presence of calcium ions (Clement-Cormier et al., 1975). Fluoride activated cyclases in lyzed neuron and glia fractions from all brain regions (Palmer, 1973a). After freezing, cyclases are usually unaffected by fluoride.

Detergents activated cyclases in brain homogenates and have been used to prepare relatively stable solubilized adenylate cyclases from brain (Johnson and Sutherland, 1973; Swislocki and Tierney, 1973; MacDonald, 1975; Middlemiss and Franklin, 1975; Nakazawa et al., 1976). Fluoride inhibited a detergent-dispersed cyclase from rat brain (Johnson and Sutherland, 1973). The nonionic detergent itself had greatly activated the cyclase. If the detergent was removed from the cyclase, fluoride became stimulatory. In another solubilized brain cyclase preparation fluoride was found to have no effect (MacDonald, 1975), while in a third preparation, solubilized and partially purified from rat brain, fluoride activated the enzyme (Swislocki and Tierney, 1973). Addition of phosphatidylserine was in the latter study cited as increasing the activity of the partially purified enzyme.

Sulfhydryl Reagents and Drugs

With a solubilized adenylate cyclase, dithiothreitol enhanced enzyme activity both in the presence and absence of detergent (Johnson and Sutherland, 1973). Sulfhydryl reagents such as N-ethylmaleimide, ethacrynic acid (IC_{50}, 300 μM), and dithiobisnitrobenzoic acid (IC_{50}, 200 μM) inhibited adenylate cyclases in brain homogenates (Ferendelli et al., 1973a; Izumi et al., 1975b). Cysteine stimulated the cyclase.

Phenothiazines inhibited basal and fluoride-stimulated adenylate cyclases in brain homogenates (Uzunov and Weiss, 1971, 1972b; Palmer and Manian, 1974a,c). Haloperidol and thioxanthenes were also inhibitory. High concentrations (IC_{50}, 1 mM) of adenosine inhibited basal and fluoride-stimulated rat brain adenylate cyclase (McKenzie and Bar, 1973). The inhibition was reversible and appeared noncompetitive with respect to the substrate, ATP. High concentrations of narcotic analgesics such as levorphan, dextrorphan, and *d*- and *l*-methadone inhibited brain adenylate cyclases (Clouet and Iwatsubo, 1974; Clouet *et al.*, 1975). Alloxan (IC_{50}, 5 mM) inhibited brain adenylate cyclases (Cohen and Bitensky, 1969).

Macromolecular Factors

A soluble heat-stable factor was reported to activate membranal adenylate cyclase in brain homogenates (Kauffman *et al.*, 1972). The factor caused an enhancement of activity of particulate adenylate cyclase from rat cerebral cortex similar to that caused by fluoride. Activation of particulate adenylate cyclases from rat cerebellum by supernatant fractions from the same tissue has been reported, but whether or not a macromolecule was responsible was not determined (Weiss and Costa, 1968). A heat-stable factor or factors in supernatant from rat cerebral cortex markedly stimulated synaptosomal adenylate cyclase from the same tissue (Izumi *et al.*, 1975a,b).

The calcium-binding protein which is required for activation of calcium-dependent phosphodiesterases (see Section 2.3.5) has been shown to enhance the activity of brain adenylate cyclase (Brostrom *et al.*, 1975). The activator protein was separated from a detergent-dispersed adenylate cyclase preparation from porcine brain by ECTEOLA-cellulose chromatography (Figure 1). After this procedure, activity of the cyclase was nearly completely dependent on calcium and the activator protein. The activation was reversed by EGTA. Half maximal activation of adenylate cyclase and of calcium-dependent phosphodiesterase occurred at about 0.7 μg of activator/ml. The K_m of calcium for activation of adenylate cyclase was not determined. Similar results have been reported by Cheung *et al.*, (1975a). Thus, an activator protein (mol wt 19,000) isolated from lubrol-solubilized cyclase preparations from bovine and rat brain stimulated, in the presence of calcium, the activator-deficient brain adenylate cyclases and phosphodiesterases. The stimulation was rapid and reversible. Calcium ions appeared necessary for the formation of an activated complex between adenylate cyclase and the activator protein (Lynch *et al.*, 1976).

Ubiquitin, a polypeptide (mol wt 8451) which stimulated adenylate cyclases through interaction with a β-adrenergic receptor, has been proposed to be present in most cells including those of guinea pig brain (Goldstein *et al.*, 1975a; Schlesinger *et al.*, 1975). Agonist properties of this peptide apparently have not as yet been investigated in brain tissue.

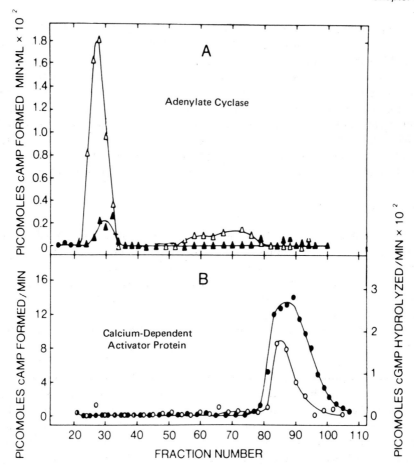

Figure 1. Adenylate cyclase and calcium-dependent activator protein from porcine brain. Detergent-dispersed adenylate cyclase was fractionated on an ECTEOLA-cellulose column. (A) Fractions were assayed in the absence (▲———▲) and presence (△———△) of calcium-dependent activator protein. (B) Boiled fractions were assayed for calcium-dependent activator with adenylate cyclase (○——○) or a cyclic GMP-phosphodiesterase (●——●). (Modified from Brostrom *et al.*, 1975, *Proceedings of the National Academy of Sciences.*)

A polypeptide (mol wt 1000) isolated from liver inhibited hormone responses of adenylate cyclases from a variety of sources (Levey *et al.*, 1975). It apparently has not as yet been investigated specifically in brain tissue. A polypeptide (mol wt 1200) from rat liver has been reported to inhibit brain cyclase activity (Izumi *et al.*, 1975b).

2.1.7 Activation by Putative Neurotransmitters

Adenylate cyclase measured with exogenous ATP in cell-free preparations from brain retains little of the receptor-mediated regulation of activity which is usually seen with cell-free preparations from other tissues. Thus, although significant intracellular accumulations of cyclic AMP can result from incubations of brain slices with biogenic amines, adenosine, or prostaglandins, the cyclases in homogenates from the same tissue often show marginal or no enhancement of activity with the same compounds (Klainer *et al.*, 1962; Burkard and Gey, 1968; Weiss and Costa, 1968; Williams *et al.*, 1969; Krishna *et al.*, 1970; Rall and Gilman, 1970; Sattin and Rall, 1970; Schmidt *et al.*, 1970; Abdulla and McFarlane, 1972; Kodama *et al.*, 1973).

Norepinephrine*

Catecholamines caused activation of cyclases in homogenates and washed particles of cerebral cortex and cerebellum of cat, sheep, and steer (Klainer *et al.*, 1962). In cerebellum, the potencies of the catecholamines were as follows: isoproterenol > epinephrine > norepinephrine. The physiologically inactive *d*-isomers were much less effective. The stimulatory effects of epinephrine on different preparations of cyclase ranged from 10 to 80% with cortex and from 25 to 125% with cerebellum. The reason for this variation was not apparent. These pioneering investigations established that cyclases in brain homogenates could be activated by catecholamines, but the variability discouraged subsequent investigators, many of whom (see above references) saw no consistent response to catecholamines or other agents. The observation that chelating agents could potentiate the response of cyclases to epinephrine (Klainer *et al.*, 1962) foreshadowed later extensive investigations by Von Hungen, Roberts, and co-workers (see below) wherein EGTA was routinely employed in studying amine stimulation of brain cyclases.

Subsequent observations on activation of cyclases by catecholamines in cell-free preparations from rat brain have been rather inconsistent. For example, Burkard and Gey (1968) reported no stimulatory effect of (nor)epinephrine or a monoamine oxidase inhibitor on adenylate cyclase activity in rat brain homogenates. The degree of enhancement of cyclase activity by norepinephrine was marginal in cerebral homogenates of rats (Kohrman, 1973). Norepinephrine had no significant effect on levels or release of cyclic AMP from rat cerebral cortical synaptosomes (De Belleroche *et al.*, 1974). Epinephrine elicited a small increase in cyclase activity in cell-free preparations from rat cerebral cortex (Katz and Tenenhouse,

---

*For structures of noradrenergic agonists and antagonists see Appendix.

1973b). The response was not, however, observed when the cyclase was maximally activated by manganese ions or when calcium ions were absent. Both α- and β-antagonists reduced the responses to epinephrine. A small activation of cyclases in cell-free preparations from rat cerebellum by epinephrine was reported (Drummond *et al.*, 1971). (Nor)epinephrine, dopamine, and isoproterenol were reported to activate adenylate cyclases from rat cerebral cortex about twofold (Van Inwegen *et al.*, 1975). Duffy and Powell (1975) reported activation of rat brain cyclases by norepineph- rine. Very high concentrations of the $D(-)$ isomer of the β-antagonist, nifenalol (IPNEA), but not of the $L(+)$ isomer antagonized a small epineph- rine-elicited activation of rat brain adenylate cyclases (Janiec *et al.*, 1970). Norepinephrine stimulated cyclases from rat occipital cortex nearly two- fold (Racagni and Carenzi, 1976). Dopamine had virtually no effect except at very high concentrations. Norepinephrine, isoproterenol, and dopamine were reported to stimulate cyclases in homogenates of rat cerebral cortex (Palmer *et al.*, 1976b). Remarkably, neither propranolol or phentolamine inhibited the stimulatory effect of norepinephrine. After osmotic disruption of neuronal and glial enriched fractions from different brain regions, norepi- nephrine was found to elicit small increases in cyclase activity from vir- tually all rat neuronal and glial fractions (Palmer, 1973a). The inhibition of adenylate cyclases by a great variety of phenothiazines in rat cortical and hypothalamic homogenates and in lysed rat and rabbit glial and neuronal enriched fractions has been reported (Palmer and Manian, 1974a,b,c). Chlorpromazine, fluphenazine, prochlorperazine, promazine, prometha- zine, and various mono- and di-phenolic derivatives were found to inhibit basal, fluoride-stimulated, and norepinephrine-stimulated cyclases in such cell-free preparations. Haloperidol, phenothiazine itself, and chlorproma- zine sulfoxide were inactive. Very high concentrations of tricyclic antide- pressants were required to inhibit basal or norepinephrine-sensitive cyclases of lysed neuronal or glial fractions from rat cerebral cortex (Pal- mer, 1976). The only exception was 2-hydroxyimipramine which at 100 μM inhibited the neuronal norepinephrine-sensitive cyclase by 50%. The small stimulation of cyclase activity by norepinephrine in homogenates from rat cortex, brain stem, and hippocampus was inhibited by lithium, while the amine response in cerebellum was not inhibited by lithium (Walker, 1974). Norepinephrine inhibited cyclase in homogenates from caudate. Lead ions were stated to inhibit the response of rat brain adenylate cyclase to norepinephrine (Nathanson and Bloom, 1975). Another group reported that norepinephrine significantly enhanced cyclase activity in preparations from rat cortex, hippocampus, or cerebellum (Walker and Walker, 1973b). The degree of activation of cyclases by catecholamines in rat brain preparations depended on the age of the animals (see Section 2.1.8). The reasons for the variable results on catecholamine-sensitive cyclases in cell-free preparations from rat brain have not been resolved. Von Hungen, Roberts, and co-workers (see below) have, however, in EGTA-inhibited rat brain cyclase preparations been able to obtain consistent and informative results.

Species differences in responses of brain cyclases to catecholamines in cell-free preparations have been noted. Adenylate cyclases in homogenates of bovine and rabbit cerebellum were somewhat activated by β-adrenergic agonists, while cyclases from rat cerebellum were not (cf. Robison *et al.*, 1970b). Catecholamines activated brain cyclases from cat, sheep, and steer (Klainer *et al.*, 1962). Lithium ions were stated to inhibit the response of rabbit brain adenylate cyclase to epinephrine (Dousa and Hechter, 1970). In beef brain homogenates, activation of cyclases by epinephrine, but not by epinine, adrenalone, or mono-phenolic analogs of epinephrine was reported (Rigberg *et al.*, 1969). In homogenates of cerebrum, cerebellum, and medulla oblongata from human fetuses adenylate cyclase activity was stated to be similar, stimulated by fluoride, and unresponsive to catecholamines (Menon *et al.*, 1973).

The key to a reproducible stimulation of cyclases by catecholamines and serotonin in rat brain homogenates, observed in extensive studies by Von Hungen and Roberts, has apparently been the use of EGTA-inhibited preparations. Adenylate cyclase systems of brain tissue have been reviewed with an emphasis on amine responses in cell-free preparations in the presence of EGTA (Von Hungen and Roberts, 1974). In these studies (McCune *et al.*, 1971; Von Hungen and Roberts, 1973a,b, 1974; Von Hungen *et al.*, 1974, 1975a) norepinephrine and dopamine enhanced cyclic AMP formation in cell-free preparations from rat cerebral cortex, but the degree of activation was small, especially in the presence of optimal concentrations of calcium ions. EGTA was used to lower levels of calcium ions, and thereby enhanced the stimulatory effect of the amines. In many cell-free preparations, EGTA prevents hormonal activation of adenylate cyclases. However, in the studies by Von Hungen, Roberts and co-workers, EGTA was required for maximal expression of hormone responses. Indeed, calcium ions could activate the EGTA-inhibited cyclase to an extent similar to the activation by catecholamines. A small response to norepinephrine and dopamine was manifest in homogenates from rat cerebral cortex, subcortex, and cerebellum. The *d*-isomers of (nor)epinephrine were much less effective than the natural *l*-enantiomers. Addition of phosphatidyl serine to the incubations enhanced the response of the cyclase to the catecholamines. Relatively high concentrations of catecholamines (500 μM) were required for maximal activation of the membranal cyclases (McCune *et al.*, 1971). The effect of norepinephrine was blocked by β-antagonists. Activation of adenylate cyclase by norepinephrine and dopamine in homogenates from rat cerebral cortex and hippocampus was inhibited by lysergic acid diethylamide, 2-bromolysergic acid diethylamide, and methysergide (Von Hungen *et al.*, 1975a). Norepinephrine activated cyclases from the following subcortical brain regions from 6-day-old rats: striatum > hippocampus > midbrain > colliculus, hypothalamus (Von Hungen and Roberts, 1974). The development of basal, calcium-activated, fluoride-activated, and amine-activated adenylate cyclases in rat brain has been studied in detail with homogenate preparations (Von Hungen *et al.*, 1974, see Section 2.1.8).

The binding of $(\pm)[^3H]$propranolol to chick cerebral synaptosomes and the antagonism of this binding by β-adrenergic agonists and antagonists (Nahorski, 1976) closely reflected the potencies of such compounds in eliciting or blocking accumulation of cyclic AMP in slices from chick cerebrum (Nahorski *et al.*, 1975c). The binding of $[^3H]$dihydroalprenolol to sites in homogenates from different regions of rat brain has also been proposed to reflect levels of β-adrenergic receptors controlling adenylate cyclases (Alexander *et al.*, 1975; see, however, Skolnick and Daly, 1976c).

Dopamine*

The activation of dopamine-sensitive adenylate cyclases, particularly in cell-free preparations from striatum (caudate nucleus), has been the object of extensive research with dopaminergic agonists and antagonists. Responses of dopamine-sensitive cyclases from rat striatum and their blockage by dopaminergic antagonists has been studied with homogenates and synaptosomes from striatum, caudate nucleus, and caudate putamen (Kebabian *et al.*, 1972; Walker and Walker, 1973a,b; Carenzi *et al.*, 1975a,b; Clement-Cormier *et al.*, 1974, 1975; Clouet *et al.*, 1975; Horn *et al.*, 1974; Karobath, 1974, 1975; Karobath and Leitich, 1974; Lippmann *et al.*, 1975; Miller and Iversen, 1974a,b; Miller *et al.*, 1974a,b, 1975; Mishra *et al.*, 1974; Sheppard and Burghardt, 1974a,b; Von Hungen and Roberts, 1974; Walker, 1974; Burkard, 1975; Gessa and Tagliamonte, 1975; Govoni *et al.*, 1975; Van Inwegen *et al.*, 1975; Makman *et al.*, 1975a,b; Miller and Hiley, 1975, 1976; Puri *et al.*, 1975; Rotrosen *et al.*, 1975; Von Hungen *et al.*, 1975a; Iversen *et al.*, 1976; Laduron *et al.*, 1976). A number of recent reviews are available (Iversen, 1975; Iversen *et al.*, 1975a,b; Kebabian *et al.*, 1975b). In the pioneering studies by Greengard and co-workers dopamine (EC_{50}, 4 μM) and norepinephrine (EC_{50}, 28 μM) elicited a twofold increase in activity of adenylate cyclases in homogenates of rat caudate nucleus (Kebabian *et al.*, 1972). Isoproterenol had no effect, and apomorphine (EC_{50}, 2 μM) elicited a 1.5-fold increase. Combinations of dopamine and norepinephrine at maximal stimulatory concentrations did not have

---

*For structures of dopaminergic agonists and antagonists see Appendix.

additive effects. Chlorpromazine, haloperidol, and to a lesser extent phentolamine antagonized the dopamine and norepinephrine response. Promethazine and β-adrenergic antagonists did not block the responses. The results indicated the presence of a dopamine-sensitive cyclase in striatum which could also be activated by norepinephrine. Fluphenazine has been reported to inhibit the activation of striatal cyclases by both dopamine and norepinephrine (Rotrosen *et al.*, 1975). In another study the effects of dopamine were prevented by haloperidol and the very small effects of norepinephrine by β-antagonists (Walker and Walker, 1973a,b). Norepinephrine has been reported to inhibit cyclases from rat caudate (Walker, 1974). Others have reported that isoproterenol has no effect on cyclases from rat caudate (Mishra *et al.*, 1974; Tell *et al.*, 1975). Isoproterenol stimulated caudate adenylate cyclase from Cebus monkey to a lesser extent than dopamine (Makman *et al.*, 1975b). Propranolol, however, did not block the response to isoproterenol while the dopaminergic antagonist, pimozide, did block the response. Isoproterenol had little or no effect on caudate cyclases from rat, cat, rabbit, or rhesus monkey. Dopamine stimulated caudate cyclases from all these species (Makman *et al.*, 1975a,b). Dopamine (EC$_{50}$, 10 μM) elicited a twofold increase in adenylate cyclase activity in homogenates of mouse striatum (Von Voightlander *et al.*, 1973; Ginos *et al.*, 1975).

Dopamine-sensitive adenylate cyclases were present in mitochondrial fractions from rat striatum and appeared partially separated from lighter fractions containing dopamine and dopa decarboxylase (Laduron *et al.*, 1976). Synaptosomal fractions from rat caudate nucleus contained high levels of dopamine-sensitive adenylate cyclases (Clement-Cormier *et al.*, 1975). Stimulation of adenylate cyclases in homogenates of rat caudate nucleus by dopamine was maximal at 30°C, pH 7–8, and a magnesium-to-ATP ratio of greater than 4. In contrast, another group reported that the enhancement of basal adenylate cyclase activity in rat striatal preparations by dopamine was about twofold over a range of temperatures from 15 to 37°C (Miller, 1976). The Q_{10} for basal and dopamine-sensitive cyclase activity in rat striatal preparations was only about 1.5. Manganese ions greatly activated the cyclase from caudate, and further effects of dopamine were no longer observed (Clement-Cormier *et al.*, 1975). Dopamine did activate cyclases with cobalt present as the divalent cation. EGTA inhibited basal enzyme activity but had no effect on dopamine stimulation. In the presence of calcium ions dopamine had no effect. Thus, for dopamine in striatum, as for norepinephrine and serotonin in other brain regions, stimulation of cell-free brain adenylate cyclases was maximal in the presence of the inhibitory chelator. Activation of adenylate cyclase by dopamine and fluoride was reduced after phosphorylation-dependent release of calcium-dependent protein from striatal synaptosomes (Gnegy *et al.*, 1976c).

Structure–activity relationships of dopamine-agonists for activation of striatal cyclases have been extensively studied (Miller *et al.*, 1974b; Sheppard and Burghardt, 1974b; Burkard, 1975; Ginos *et al.*, 1975; Iversen, 1975; Iversen *et al.*, 1975a,b; Makman *et al.*, 1975b). *N*-Methyldopamine (epinine) was about as active as dopamine. Larger *N*-alkyl substituents or di-alkyl *N*-substitution reduced the activity of dopamines. At a concentration of 10 μM, dopamine, *N*-methyldopamine, and certain *N,N*-dialkyldopamines had nearly the same stimulatory effect on cyclases in homogenates of mouse caudate nucleus (Ginos et al., 1975). A catechol moiety was essential in phenethylamines. *dl*-α-Methyldopamine had very low activity. (*S*)α-Methyldopamine was inactive, while the *R*-isomer retained some activity. 2-Methyldopamine was active, but a 2-phenyl substituent or methyl substituents in other ring positions resulted in complete loss of activity.

The lack of activity of tetrahydroquinolines, such as salsolinol, and the high activity of apomorphine suggest that the active form of dopamine is the *trans* conformer. Certain of the tetrahydroquinolines were, however, rather good antagonists (Sheppard and Burghardt, 1974a). 2-Amino-6,7-dihydroxy-1,2,3,4-tetrahydronaphthalene, a bicyclic analog of dopamine with the nitrogen fixed in the *trans* conformation with respect to the phenyl ring, was an active agonist (Miller *et al.*, 1974b). A variety of apomorphine alkaloids were investigated as agonists and antagonists with dopamine-sensitive cyclases from rat striatum (Miller *et al.*, 1976b). Only apomorphine and *N*-propylnorapomorphine were active as agonists, while a number of alkaloids including apomorphine, bulbocapnine, and nuceferine had antagonist activity.

Piribedil (1-(3,4-methylenedioxybenzyl)-4-(2-pyrimidinyl)piperazine) yields a catecholic metabolite, S-584 (see Appendix), which has been shown to be a dopaminergic agonist towards adenylate cyclases in homogenates of rat striatum (Miller and Iversen, 1974a; Mishra *et al.*, 1974; Iversen *et al.*, 1975b; Makman *et al.*, 1975b). The metabolite is probably responsible for dopaminergic effects of piribedil *in vivo*. The *in vitro* effects of this metabolite on dopamine-responsive cyclases were blocked by chlorpromazine, spiroperidol, and other dopaminergic antagonists.

Responses of cyclases from rat striatum to dopamine and apomorphine have in many studies (see above) been shown to be blocked by dopaminergic antagonists. Many of these dopaminergic antagonists are effective antipsychotics, but correlations between their clinical efficacy and inhibition of cyclases have not in all cases been apparent. The very effective antipsychotics, fluphenazine and α-flupenthixol, were the most potent dopamine antagonists, causing at a 1 μM concentration a complete inhibition of the response to 100 μM dopamine (Karobath and Leitich, 1974; Miller *et al.*, 1974a; Miller and Iversen, 1974b). β-Flupenthixol was much more potent than the clinically inactive α-isomer in antagonizing the dopamine stimulation of cyclases. Chlorpromazine was less active than fluphenazine as were haloperidol, pimozide, spiroperidol, and droperidol. Promazine had very weak antagonist activity. There is, thus, little apparent correlation between the clinical efficacy of the butyrophenones and their rather low potency as antagonists of dopamine-sensitive cyclases in homogenates of caudate nucleus. Inhibition of dopamine-sensitive cyclase from rat striatum by a variety of butyrophenones has been studied (Iversen *et al.*, 1976). Bromperidol was sixfold more potent than haloperidol. Inhibition of dopamine-sensitive cyclases from rat striatum by various dibenzodiazepines, such as clothiapine > loxapine > clozapine, has been reported (Miller and Hiley, 1976). Thioridazine and clozapine, antipsychotic agents with little neuroleptic activity, were in many studies about as effective as chlorpromazine in inhibiting the dopamine-sensitive cyclases. Anticholinergic effects of these drugs are probably quite significant to their *in vivo* pharmacological profiles. Thus, agents such as thioridazine and clozapine which clinically rarely elicit extrapyramidal side effects have high potencies as antagonists at muscarinic receptors, while agents such as chlorpromazine, which clinically often elicit such side effects (muscular rigidity, tremor, and reduction in voluntary motion), are not potent muscarinic antagonists (cf. Iversen, 1975; Miller and Hiley, 1975, 1976). The inhibition of dopamine-sensitive striatal cyclases by pimozide, α-flupenthixol, α-chlorprothixene, and haloperidol was competitive with dopamine, rapid in onset, and rapidly reversed by addition of high concentrations of dopamine (Miller, 1976). Although differing somewhat in different investigations, the potency of various psychoactive agents as inhibitors of dopamine-elicited activation of striatal adenylate cyclases can be rank ordered, with approximate IC_{50} values given in parentheses: α-flupenthixol (1 nM) > fluphenazine (5 nM) > (+)butaclamol (10 nM) > trifluoperazine, chlorpromazine, α-chlorprothixene (50 nM) > spiroperidol, prochlorperazine, thioridazine (100 nM) > pimozide, clozapine, β-chlorprothixene, droperidol, chlorimipramine (200 nM) > promazine.

Various tricyclic antidepressants, of which amitriptyline, doxepine, chlorimpramine, and nortriptyline were most potent, inhibited dopamine-sensitive adenylate cyclases in homogenates of rat striatum (Karobath, 1974, 1975; Karobath and Leitich, 1974). The active antidepressants were less potent than antipsychotic phenothiazines but nearly equipotent with butyrophenones. The crystal conformations of dopamine agonists and of various tricyclic dopamine antagonists including α-flupenthixol, β-flupenthixol, chlorpromazine, trifluoperazine, and imipramine have been discussed in terms of interaction with the dopamine-binding site of dopamine-sensitive adenylate cyclases (Horn *et al.*, 1975; Post *et al.*, 1975; Snyder, 1976). Amphetamine, *p*-hydroxyamphetamine, and *p*-hydroxynorephedrine had no effect on basal or dopamine-stimulated cyclases from striatum (Carenzi *et al.*, 1975a). The "serotonin antagonists," 2-bromo- and 1-methyl-lysergic acid diethylamide and cyproheptadine, antagonized the activation of striatal adenylate cyclases by dopamine and lysergic acid diethylamide (Von Hungen *et al.*, 1975a, see below). At high concentrations serotonin, mescaline, bufotenine, psilocin, and *N,N*-dimethyltryptamine appeared to inhibit responses of striatal cyclases to dopamine (Von Hungen *et al.*, 1975a).

Effects of morphine on adenylate cyclases from striatum have not been consistent. In one study morphine had a stimulatory effect similar to that of dopamine on striatal cyclases (Puri *et al.*, 1975). The response appeared additive with dopamine only when both agents were used at submaximal concentrations. These preliminary results suggested that morphine might stimulate striatal dopamine receptors. In another study, no stimulation of cyclase by morphine was seen (Miller *et al.*, 1974a). Morphine did inhibit basal and dopamine-sensitive cyclases. In other studies, morphine and various narcotic analgesic agonists and antagonists did not inhibit either basal or dopamine-sensitive cyclases from rat striatum (Clouet *et al.*, 1975; Carenzi *et al.*, 1975b; Iwatsubo and Clouet, 1975; Tell *et al.*, 1975). Certain narcotic analgesics such as fentanyl (IC_{50}, 1 μM) > dextromoramide, etorphine > dextropropoxyphene > *dl*-methadone have been reported to inhibit dopamine-sensitive adenylate cyclases in homogenates of rat striatum (Gessa and Tagliamonte, 1975; Govoni *et al.*, 1975).

The stimulation of adenylate cyclases by dopamine and dopaminergic agonists and the efficacy of antipsychotics and other agents as antagonists have been studied in homogenates of the olfactory tubercle and nucleus accumbens of rat, guinea pig, hamster, and mouse (Kebabian *et al.*, 1972, 1975b; Clement-Cormier *et al.*, 1974; Horn *et al.*, 1974; Miller *et al.*, 1974a; Carenzi *et al.*, 1975a) in addition to the above mentioned studies on cyclases from striatum (caudate nucleus). Isoproterenol had no effect on adenylate cyclases in homogenates of rat olfactory tubercle, while norepinephrine (EC_{50}, 30 μM) at high concentrations caused a similar activation to that caused by dopamine (EC_{50} 7μM) or apomorphine. The stimulatory effects of the two catecholamines were not additive at maximal concentrations, suggestive of an interaction with the same receptor. The effect of dopamine was competitively inhibited by low concentrations of fluphenazine in homogenates of rat olfactory tubercle and rat or guinea pig nucleus accumbens. Chlorpromazine, haloperidol, and clozapine were less effective. Pimozide, promethazine, phentolamine, and imipramine were virtually ineffective. Propranolol had no effect. The antipsychotic (−)butaclamol inhibited dopamine-sensitive adenylate cyclase in homogenates from striatum and olfactory tubercle, while the pharmacologically ineffective (+)-isomer was inactive (Lippmann *et al.*, 1975; Miller *et al.*,

1975). It has been proposed (1) that the antipsychotic efficacy of various drugs correlates with their efficacy as antagonists of dopaminergic receptors in the mesolimbic system (olfactory tubercle, nucleus accumbens), (2) that the extrapyramidal side effects of neuroleptics are related to antagonism of dopaminergic receptors in the caudate nucleus, and (3) that their endocrinological side effects are related to antagonism of dopaminergic function in the median eminence of the hypothalamus. However, clozapine and thioridazine, clinically effective agents which have a low incidence of extrapyramidal side effects, were equally as effective as antagonists of dopamine-sensitive cyclases in homogenates of caudate nucleus as in those of olfactory tubercle.

Dopamine and apomorphine stimulated cyclases in homogenates of the anterior amygdala (Racagni and Carenzi, 1976). Haloperidol and clozapine antagonized the response to dopamine. Serotonin had no effect, and norepinephrine had only a minimal effect on cyclases from amygdala.

Adenylate cyclase in homogenates of monkey caudate nucleus was stimulated by dopamine and by isoproterenol, whereas only dopamine was effective in the rat caudate (Makman *et al.,* 1975a,b). Epinine, *N*-isopropyl-dopamine, apomorphine, the catecholic metabolite of piribedil, and norepinephrine stimulated cyclases from monkey caudate. Dopamine stimulated adenylate cyclases in homogenates of anterior limbic cortex, olfactory tubercle, and nucleus accumbens from rhesus monkey (Mishra *et al.,* 1975). With homogenates of anterior limbic cortex, dopamine, apomorphine, and the catecholic metabolite of piribedil elicited a similar twofold activation of cyclases, while norepinephrine and isoproterenol had only marginal effects. With olfactory tubercle of rhesus monkey and with anterior limbic cortex of Cebus monkey, dopamine, norepinephrine, and isoproterenol all activated cyclases twofold or more. Responses to dopamine were blocked in preparations of anterior limbic cortex and olfactory tubercle by fluphenazine but not by propranolol or phentolamine.

Dopamine-responsive cyclases have not been extensively studied in brain regions other than the limbic system. In rat brain homogenates or synaptosomes, dopamine had no effect (Izumi *et al.,* 1975a; Tell *et al.,* 1975). The stimulation of cyclase activity by dopamine in homogenates of caudate > cerebellum, hippocampus, cortex was not inhibited by lithium (Walker, 1974). Dopamine had no effect in brain stem. In earlier studies dopamine had virtually no effect in preparations from rat cortex, hippocampus, and cerebellum (Walker and Walker, 1973b) or in rat cerebellum (Kebabian *et al.,* 1972). Dopamine elicited a small response of cyclases in homogenates of rat cerebral cortex, hippocampus, striatum, subcortex, and cerebellum (McCune *et al.,* 1971; Von Hungen *et al.,* 1975a). The effect of dopamine was antagonized by haloperidol. Dopamine activated cyclases from striatum > hippocampus > midbrain > colliculi, hypothalamus of 6-

day-old rats to an extent similar to the activations by norepinephrine (Von Hungen and Roberts, 1974). Further pharmacological evaluation of dopamine-elicited activation of cyclases from brain areas other than the limbic system is clearly required.

Dopamine elicited small increases in cyclase activity in homogenates from rat cerebral cortex and in lysed neuronal fractions from rat cerebral cortex, midbrain, and striatum and in lysed glial fractions from cerebellum and striatum (Palmer, 1973a; Palmer et al., 1976b). In a subsequent study, dopamine activated cyclases in lysed neuron- and glia-enriched fractions from rat cerebral cortex and thalamus and in lysed neuron fractions from striatum (Palmer and Manian, 1976). Haloperidol and phenothiazines including various dihydroxy analogs of the latter compounds inhibited dopamine-sensitive cyclases in all preparations.

Lysergic acid diethylamide (EC_{50}, 1 μM) like dopamine increased adenylate cyclase activity in homogenates from rat striatum, nucleus accumbens, olfactory tubercle, and limbic cortex, but not in homogenates from cerebellum (Spano et al., 1975b). The 2-bromo derivative was inactive. The combined response to lysergic acid diethylamide and dopamine was less than that elicited by dopamine alone in striatal homogenates. Lysergic acid diethylamide mimicked the dopamine agonist, apomorphine, in eliciting contralateral circling in rats with unilateral lesions of the nigrostriatal system (Pieri et al., 1974) and activated adenylate cyclase in homogenates of rat striatum (W. P. Burkard, unpublished, cited in Pieri et al., 1974). A third group (Von Hungen et al., 1975a) reported that lysergic acid diethylamide antagonized the activation of adenylate cyclase by dopamine in homogenates from striatum, cerebral cortex, and hippocampus and in addition caused a small but significant activation of striatal cyclases. The stimulatory effects of dopamine and of lysergic acid diethylamide were antagonized in striatal cyclase preparations by trifluoperazine, thioridazine, chlorpromazine, haloperidol, 2- bromo, and 1-methyl-lysergic acid diethylamide and cyproheptadine. Lysergic acid diethylamide stimulated cyclases from rat colliculi.

Serotonin*

Significant stimulations of adenylate cyclases by serotonin in cell-free preparations from brain have been reported by Von Hungen, Roberts, and co-workers (McCune et al., 1971; Von Hungen and Roberts, 1974; Von Hungen et al., 1973, 1975a,b). EGTA was present to inhibit cyclase activity. Others have reported no effect of serotonin on cyclases in rat brain homogenates (Burkard and Gey, 1968; Duffy and Powell, 1975) or in

---

*For structures of serotonergic agonists and antagonists see Appendix.

synaptosomes from rat cerebral cortex (Izumi *et al.*, 1975a). In initial studies by Von Hungen, Roberts, and co-workers, serotonin had only small stimulatory effects on cyclase activity in homogenates from rat cerebral cortex, subcortex, and cerebellum. In subsequent more detailed studies, serotonin had only a small effect on cyclases from rat midbrain and hypothalamus and a somewhat larger effect on cyclases from colliculi and hippocampus. Serotonin, mescaline, bufotenine, psilocin, and N,N-dimethyltryptamine had little or no effect on striatal adenylate cyclase activity. In preparations from 1-day-old rats, serotonin stimulated cyclases from cortex, hippocampus, hypothalamus, cerebellum, and medulla-pons, but not striatum. These responses declined and virtually disappeared during development. The stimulatory effects of serotonin (EC_{50}, 1 μM) were relatively large, a 1.4- to 1.7-fold increase, with cyclases from the anterior and posterior colliculi of 1- to 3-day-old rats. Bufotenine, N-methylserotonin, 5-methoxytryptamine, and tryptamine also activated the cyclases in colliculi preparations. α-Methylserotonin, 6-hydroxytryptamine, psilocin, dopamine, and norepinephrine were less effective, while N,N-dimethyltryptamine and α-ethyltryptamine had no effect. Lysergic acid derivatives including lysergic acid diethylamide, 2-bromolysergic acid diethylamide, and methysergide, cyproheptadine, and chlorpromazine antagonized the response to serotonin, while haloperidol, propranolol, morphine, and phenoxybenzamine were ineffective. Lysergic acid diethylamide, cyproheptadine, and chlorpromazine had agonist activity toward cyclases from colliculi. The stimulatory effect of serotonin on cyclases from colliculi declined during maturation of rats.

Histamine*

Responses of cyclases in cell-free preparations from brain to histamine have now been established. In initial studies histamine had no effect on cyclases in rat cerebral homogenates or synaptosomes (Burkard and Gey, 1968; Izumi *et al.*, 1975b). Histamine had only a marginal effect on EGTA-inhibited cyclases in rat cerebral cortex (Von Hungen and Roberts, 1973a,b). Histamine had no effect on levels or release of cyclic AMP from rat cerebral cortical synaptosomes (De Belleroche *et al.*, 1974). Recently, however, effects of histamine on adenylate cyclases in homogenates from guinea pig brain have been reported (Hegstrand *et al.*, 1976). GTP was used to augment histamine responses. Histamine (EC_{50}, 20 μM) enhanced activity of adenylate cyclases from guinea pig hippocampus about twofold. Metiamide competitively inhibited the response to histamine. Pyrilamine (1 μM), propranolol, phentolamine, fluphenazine, and atropine had no effect

*For structures of histaminergic agonists and antagonists see Appendix.

on the response. Histamine markedly stimulated cyclases from neocortex, hippocampus, and striatum but had no effect in cerebellum, hypothalamus, thalamus, midbrain, pons, and medulla. Histamine had no effect on cyclases from rat neocortex, hippocampus, striatum, or cerebellum.

Histamine elicited small increases in cyclase activity in lysed neuronal fractions from rabbit cortex and hippocampus and in lysed glial fractions from rabbit hippocampus (Palmer, 1973a; Spiker et al., 1976). Thioridazine, chlorpromazine, and hydroxy analogs of chlorpromazine inhibited histamine-sensitive cyclases in lysed neuronal and glial enriched fractions from rabbit cerebral cortex. Haloperidol was effective only in the lysed glial fractions.

Histamine activated adenylate cyclases in homogenates of brain capillaries (Joo et al., 1975a). Both H_1- and H_2-antagonists inhibited the response.

Acetylcholine

Acetylcholine had no effect or inhibited rat brain cyclases (Von Hungen and Roberts, 1973a,b; Duffy and Powell, 1975) and inhibited cyclases in homogenates in rat striatum (Walker and Walker, 1973a).

Amino Acids and Peptides

Glutamate had no effect on cyclase activity in guinea pig brain homogenates (Shimizu et al., 1974). γ-Aminobutyrate had no effect on cyclase activity in rat cerebral cortical homogenates (Von Hungen and Roberts, 1973a,b). Various polypeptide hormones such as thyrotropin, adrenocorticotropin, luteinizing hormone, insulin, and glucagon had no effect on brain cyclases (Burkard and Gey, 1968; Williams et al., 1969; Von Hungen and Roberts, 1973a,b).

The polypeptide, substance P(EC_{50}, 0.2 μM), was reported to activate cyclases from rat brain (Duffy and Powell, 1975). No response to substance P was observed when the calcium-chelating agent, EGTA, was present. Substance P stimulated adenylate cyclases in homogenates from various human cortical regions, cerebellum, hypothalamus, substantia nigra, and pineal gland (Duffy et al., 1975). Stimulations were observed in both white and gray matter.

Prostaglandins*

Prostaglandin E_1 was first reported to stimulate cyclase in rat brain homogenates in 1972 (Abdulla and McFarlane, 1972). In a subsequent

---

*For structures of prostaglandins and antagonists including narcotic analgesics see Appendix.

detailed study prostaglandins E_1 and E_2 have been reported to enhance adenylate cyclase activity in rat brain homogenates (Collier and Roy, 1974a,b). The maximal stimulation was about twofold. Prostaglandin $F_{2\alpha}$ was ineffective. Morphine, heroin, levorphan, etorphine, and certain other analgesics were effective, apparently competitive, antagonists of the stimulation of adenylate cyclase by the prostaglandins, while dextrorphan was ineffective. The potency of these compounds correlated quite well with their *in vivo* analgesic potency and their affinity for opiate receptors in rat brain homogenates. The morphine antagonist, naloxone, prevented the inhibitory effect of morphine. Naloxone at 1 mM in combination with a phosphodiesterase inhibitor, isobutylmethylxanthine, stimulated cyclic AMP formation in rat brain homogenates (Collier *et al.*, 1975). Morphine had no effect on fluoride-stimulated cyclases from rat brain. The central analgesic effects of morphine have been proposed to be due to antagonism of the activation of central cyclase systems by prostaglandin and have been discussed (Collier and Roy, 1974a,b; Roy and Collier, 1975) in terms of *in vivo* interactions of morphine, prostaglandins, inhibitors of prostaglandin synthetase, cyclic AMP, and phosphodiesterase inhibitors. In the studies with homogenate preparations, very high concentrations of prostaglandins were employed and the concentration of radioactive ATP was very low (1.2 μM), especially for 30-min incubations in the absence of an ATP-regenerating system.

Another group (Duffy and Powell, 1975) has reported the activation of rat brain cyclases by prostaglandins E_1 and E_2. Prostaglandin $F_{2\alpha}$ had no effect. A third group reported that prostaglandin had only a marginal effect on activity of adenylate cyclases from rat cerebral cortex either in the absence or presence of GTP (Van Inwegen *et al.*, 1975). Morphine did not antagonize this response or responses to catecholamines or GTP. A fourth group (Tell *et al.*, 1975) was unable to demonstrate any effect of prostaglandin E_1 or E_2 or morphine on adenylate cyclase activity in rat brain homogenates either assayed under conditions described by Collier and Roy or with higher concentrations of ATP and addition of an ATP-regenerating system. Prostaglandins and morphine also had no effect on adenylate cyclase activity assayed in rat caudate homogenates in the presence or absence of dopamine and/or GTP. Effects of morphine on dopamine-sensitive cyclases from striatum have been inconsistent (see above). Chou *et al.* (1971a) reported the activation of adenylate cyclases in mouse cerebral cortical homogenates by morphine. Brain adenylate cyclase activity was stated to be inhibited by the prostaglandin antagonists, 17-oxa-13-prostynoic acid and polyphoretin phosphate (Hynie *et al.*, 1975).

Enkephalins, pentapeptides (Tyr-Gly-Gly-Phe-Met and Tyr-Gly-Gly-Phe-Leu) isolated from pig brains, have been shown to be natural agonists for opiate receptors (Hughes *et al.*, 1975). Enkephalins have been cited as antagonizing the activation of brain adenylate cyclase by prostaglandins (Goldstein, 1976).

Depolarizing Agents

Ouabain was reported to elicit a small increase in cyclase activity of cell-free preparations from rat cerebral cortex, but only with suboptimal concentrations of manganese and with calcium ions absent (Katz and Tenenhouse, 1973b). Electrical pulsation or high concentrations of potassium ions had no significant effect on levels or release of cyclic AMP from rat cerebral synaptosomes (De Belleroche *et al.*, 1974).

GTP

Hormone responses of various adenylate cyclases from peripheral organs are potentiated by GTP, which in addition often activates basal cyclase activity. GTP was reported to slightly stimulate adenylate cyclases from rat cerebral cortex (Van Inwegen *et al.*, 1975). GTP, GDP, GMP, and guanylylimidodiphosphate inhibited basal and to a lesser extent dopamine-stimulated adenylate cyclases in homogenates of rat caudate nucleus (Clement-Cormier *et al.*, 1975). In synaptosomal fractions from caudate, GTP no longer inhibited basal cyclase activity and potentiated the response to dopamine. GTP inhibited basal cyclase activity in rat caudate homogenates with maximal inhibition at 100 μM (Tell *et al.*, 1975). Adenylate cyclase activity assayed in the presence of 100 μM dopamine was not inhibited by GTP. GTP thus "potentiated" the dopamine responses. Isoproterenol had no effect on cyclase activity in caudate homogenates either in the absence or presence of GTP. At a 100 μM concentration GTP was stated to increase adenylate cyclase activity in hippocampal homogenates and to markedly potentiate the stimulation by histamine (Hegstrand *et al.*, 1976). GTP levels in mammalian tissues are about 100 μM, whereas potentiative effects of GTP on adenylate cyclase activities often pertain at 1 μM. A recent mechanism for GTP-regulation of adenylate cyclase might explain this apparent paradox (Blume and Foster, 1976b).

Vesicular Preparations from Brain

In view of the large, often complete, and certainly variable loss of receptor-mediated activation of adenylate cyclases which occurs during cellular disruption of nervous tissue, caution must be exercised in any extrapolation of *in vitro* results to the actual levels and responsiveness of the cyclases in a particular brain region. However, a method of brain homogenation in Krebs–Ringer buffer that affords vesicular preparations which retain receptor-modulated adenylate cyclases and which in other ways exhibit characteristics of intact brain cell systems has been reported (Chasin *et al.*, 1974). Thus, a resuspended Krebs–Ringer particulate preparation from guinea pig cerebral cortex, cerebellum, and hippocampus labeled with radioactive adenine (see Section 3.1) responded to various agents with large accumulations of intravesicular radioactive cyclic AMP. Epinephrine (EC_{50}, 1 μM) elicited 2-fold, 6- to 20-fold, and 1.3-fold increases in cyclic AMP levels in preparations from cortex, cerebellum, and hippocampus, respectively, while histamine (EC_{50}, 10 μM) caused elevations of 3- to 4-fold in cortical and 3- to 8-fold in hippocampal preparations and had no effect in cerebellar preparations. Both adenosine and exogenous cyclic AMP elicited a 2-fold increase in radioactive cyclic AMP in hippocampal preparations. In one experiment, epinephrine elevated endogenous levels of cyclic AMP in cerebellar preparations by 32-fold while elevating radioactive cyclic AMP by 17-fold. The effects of epinephrine in cerebellar preparations were antagonized by a β-antagonist, propranolol, while in cortical preparations an α-antagonist, dibenamine, was most effective. The stimulatory effects of adenosine (EC_{50}, 10 μM) and cyclic AMP were antagonized by theophylline. Histamine and epinephrine had additive effects in hippocampal preparations in contrast to the synergistic effect which pertains in brain slices. Fluoride did not stimulate cyclic AMP formation, nor did exogenous ATP serve as a substrate for the responsive adenylate cyclases. The responses apparently were occuring in vesicular entities with sedimentation properties similar to those reported for synaptosomes. Another group has reported that with such vesicular preparations from guinea pig cortex, norepinephrine, adenosine, histamine, veratridine, glutamate (EC_{50}, 20 μM), and an analog of glutamate, cysteine sulfinate, elicited increases in levels of radioactive cyclic AMP (Shimizu *et al.*, 1975a). Combinations of various agents had additive or somewhat less than additive effects on levels of cyclic AMP. As in sliced preparations (see Section 3.1), the stimulatory effect of glutamate was blocked by theophylline and the effect of the depolarizing agent, veratridine, by theophylline or tetrodotoxin. The results suggest that depolarization of neuronal entities by veratridine elicits the release of substances that stimulate cyclase in the homogenate preparation in a sequence perhaps similar to that which pertains in brain slices. Vesicular preparations of this type from rat limbic forebrain responded to (nor)epinephrine, isoproterenol, and α-methylnorepinephrine with a two-fold increase in accumulations of cyclic AMP (Horn and Phillipson, 1976). The response to catecholamines was stereospecific, with the *d*-isomers being relatively inactive. Dopamine, *d*-isoproterenol, octopamine, normetanephrine, salbutamol (*N-tert*-butyl-4-hydroxy-3-hydroxymethylphenethanolamine) and carbuterol (*N-tert*-butyl-4-hydroxy-3-ureidophenethanol amine) had no effect. The response to norepinephrine was blocked by a variety of β-antagonists in the following order of potency: $(-)$propranolol (IC_{50}, 0.7 μM) > $(-)$alprenolol (IC_{50}, 5 μM) > $(+)$alprenolol > $(+)$propranolol > practolol, dichlorisoproterenol, sotalol. The β-antagonists, nifenalol (IPNEA) and N-isopropyl-α-methyl-p-methylphenethanolamine (H35/25), were ineffective. At a 10 μM concentration promazine, $(+)$butaclamol, clozapine, β-chlorprothixene, thioridazine, chlorpromazine, α- and β-clopenthixol, α-chlorprothixene, pimozide, phentolamine, haloperidol, and trifluoperazine caused a 40 to 80% inhibition of the response to 50 μM norepinephrine, with promazine the most effective and trifluoperazine the least effective antagonists. The α- and β-isomers of flupenthixol were both relatively inactive, eliciting only about a 35% inhibition. $(-)$Butaclamol was even less active as an antagonist, and desipramine and 7-hydroxychlorpromazine were inactive. Large numbers of vesicular entities along with classical synaptosomes—some with attached postsynaptic vesicular entities—were present in these preparations (Horn and Phillipson, 1976).

In a study on synaptosomes prepared in the usual fashion in isotonic sucrose, accumulation of cyclic AMP from what appeared to be intrasynaptosomal ATP was measured (Harris, 1976). Synaptosomes were prepared from adenine-labeled rat cortical, hindbrain, and striatal slices. Isoproterenol, norepinephrine, and to a lesser degree dopamine elicited accumulations of radioactive cyclic AMP. β-Antagonists, but not a dopaminergic antagonist, trifluoperazine, inhibited the amine responses in striatal synaptosomes. The results suggest a specific labeling by adenine of compartments of intracellular nucleotides associated with β-adrenergically controlled cyclases. This prelabeled synaptosomal preparation would appear worthy of further study.

2.1.8 Developmental Changes in Adenylate Cyclases and Cyclic AMP in Brain

Endogenous levels of brain cyclic AMP and both basal and fluoride-activated cyclase in homogenates increased in rats after birth until about 9 to 20 days of age (Schmidt *et al.*, 1970, Hommes and Beere, 1971; Weiss, 1971; Kauffman *et al.*, 1972; Schmidt and Robinson, 1972; Kohrman, 1973; Perkins and Moore, 1973b; Singhal *et al.*, 1973a,b). The basal levels of cyclase were then usually found to decline markedly, while fluoride-activated levels declined less markedly. Thus, in neonatal rats there was virtually no fluoride activation of brain adenylate cyclases. Maximal levels of fluoride-stimulated adenylate cyclase activity were attained in rat cerebrum and brain stem at about Day 15, while in cerebellum maximal levels were not attained until about Day 30 (Weiss, 1971). Levels of cyclase in cerebrum and brain stem declined while cerebellar levels were maintained. Hommes and Beere (1971) reported that fluoride-stimulated cyclase increased markedly after 30 days of age in rats. Cyclic AMP levels in rat cerebrum and brain stem reached a maximum 10 to 15 days after birth and then declined, while levels in cerebellum did not reach a maximum until Day 30 and then did not decline with age (Weiss and Strada, 1973). In another study, levels of cyclic AMP in rat cerebrum were maximal at about 2 months of age and then declined to much lower levels which were maintained from 6 months to at least 2 years of age (Zimmerman and Berg, 1973; Zimmerman and Isaacs, 1975). Maximal serum levels of testosterone were attained at 3 months of age and then markedly declined. It was suggested that the two phenomena might be interrelated.

Levels of cyclic AMP increased during maturation of mice, with a large increase in forebrain and smaller increases in cerebellum and brain stem (Steiner *et al.*, 1972). In another study, cyclic AMP levels did not appear to increase in mouse brain during development (Orenberg *et al.*, 1976). In hamster cerebrum, adult levels of cyclase were threefold greater than in young animals (Weiss *et al.*, 1971). Adenylate cyclase activity in chick cerebrum increased fourfold during development (Nahorski *et al.*, 1975c). Cyclic AMP levels in chick cerebrum decreased fourfold during the first 4 weeks after birth, while the postdecapitation increase in cyclic AMP nearly doubled.

A detailed comparison of adenylate cyclase activity in homogenates of different brain regions from 2-month-old, adult, and 2-year-old "senescent" Sprague–Dawley rats has been reported (Walker and Walker, 1973b). Basal cyclase levels remained the same during aging in cortex and hippocampus and actually increased in caudate and cerebellum. Fluoride-stimulated levels of cyclase remained nearly the same during aging in caudate and hippocampus but had increased in cortex and cerebellum. Thus, there was an age-dependent increase in the degree of stimulation of adenylate cyclase by fluoride in cortex and an age-dependent decrease in caudate. In homogenates from adult hippocampus, both dopamine and norepinephrine caused a 20% activation of adenylate cyclases. The response to norepinephrine disappeared on aging. In adult cortex, neither catecholamine caused more than a 20% activation of cyclases, and no stimulatory effects were seen in senescent cortex. In homogenates from adult cerebellum both catecholamines activated cyclase by nearly 100%; the amines had no stimulatory effect in senescent cerebellum. According to other workers (Kebabian *et al.*, 1972), dopamine did not activate cyclases in homogenates of rat cerebellum. In homogenates of caudate from adult rats, dopamine caused an activation of cyclases, but this activation was nearly absent in homogenates from senescent rats. The results of Walker and Walker (1973b) suggest either that adenylate cyclases of brain became less responsive to catecholamines during senescence or that hormonal sensitivity was less well preserved in homogenates from senescent rats.

The development of basal, calcium-activated, fluoride-activated, and amine-activated adenylate cyclases in homogenates of rat brain has been studied in great detail (Von Hungen *et al.*, 1973, 1975b). In cerebral cortex and subcortex, the latter representing combined hippocampus, thalamus, midbrain, striatum, and hypothalamus, basal levels of cyclase increased from birth to Day 14, while in cerebellum and medulla-pons-brain stem, levels were nearly maximal at Day 1 after birth. Levels of fluoride-, calcium-, norepinephrine-, and dopamine-stimulated cyclase in cortical preparations increased to maxima during the first 2 weeks after birth followed by modest declines to adult levels. Responses of cyclases from cortex and subcortex to serotonin were greatest at Day 1 and subsequently declined to virtually undetectable levels by 42 days of age. Marginal responses of cyclases to norepinephrine and dopamine were detected at Day 1 in preparations from all brain regions, while responses to serotonin were detected at Day 1 in cortex, hippocampus, hypothalamus, cerebellum, and medulla-pons-brain stem, but not in striatum. Many of these amine responses were no longer significant in 42-day-old rats. Responses of cyclases to serotonin in preparations from anterior and posterior colliculi declined during maturation and were minimal by Day 14.

2.1.9 Ganglia and Peripheral Neurons

Ganglia

Cyclases in homogenates from bovine superior cervical ganglion were activated less than twofold by dopamine or norepinephrine (Kebabian and Greengard, 1971). Fluoride activated adenylate cyclases in homogenates of chick sensory ganglia (Hier *et al.*, 1973). Adenylate cyclase activity was detectable only in the presence of fluoride in homogenates of the abdominal ganglia of the mollusc *Aplysia californica* (Cedar and Schwartz, 1972). Possible activation of basal enzyme activity by serotonin could not, therefore, be studied. Octopamine, serotonin, and dopamine effectively stimulated adenylate cyclases in homogenates of cockroach thoracic ganglia (see Section 3.3.2).

Retina

Cyclases in homogenates of mammalian retina are activated by (nor)epinephrine, dopamine, and apomorphine but not by histamine, isoproterenol, or phenylephrine (Brown and Makman, 1972, 1973; Chader *et al.*, 1973; Bucher and Schorderet, 1975). The activation by dopamine was blocked most effectively by fluphenazine, haloperidol, and chlorpromazine and somewhat less effectively by α-antagonists, such as ergotamine and phentolamine. Other ergot alkaloids which are not α-antagonists also blocked the response to dopamine. The effect of epinephrine was inhibited by both α- and β-antagonists. The activation of adenylate cyclases from mammalian retina by dopamine has been studied in further detail (Makman *et al.*, 1975a,b). Dopamine and fluoride-sensitive cyclases were present in homogenates of retina from rat, mouse, rabbit, calf, cat, and monkey. The potency of various catecholamines towards rat retinal cyclases was as follows: dopamine > epinine, epinephrine >> isoproterenol. Isoproterenol stimulated cyclases from monkey retina, while having marginal effects on cyclases from calf retina. Apomorphine and the catechol metabolite of piribedil activated retinal cyclases. Pimozide and other dopaminergic antagonists effectively blocked responses to the dopaminergic agonists. The presence of EDTA or EGTA was stated to enhance both basal and dopamine-sensitive cyclase activity in retinal homogenates. Lysergic acid diethylamide was stated to activate cyclases in retinal homogenates from various species (Spano *et al.*, 1975b). Dopamine, but not either epinine, apomorphine, (nor)epinephrine, or octopamine, stimulated cyclases in homogenates of octopus retina (Makman *et al.*, 1975a).

Development of dopamine-sensitive cyclases in rat and rhesus monkey retina has been reported (Makman *et al.*, 1975a). In rat, maximal levels of dopamine-sensitive cyclases in retina were attained at Day 14 after birth. Levels of basal, dopamine- and fluoride-stimulated cyclase activity in homogenates of mouse retina increased significantly during development, reaching maximal levels in DBA mice by 10 to 15 days of age (Lolley *et al.*, 1974). Dopamine-stimulated cyclase then greatly decreased to adult levels. In contrast, in a strain of C3H mice in which photoreceptor cells degenerate, levels of retinal cyclase activities continued to increase to adulthood and reached maximal levels far greater than in DBA mice with normal visual input (Lolley *et al.*, 1974; Makman *et al.*, 1975a). Cyclic AMP levels were also higher in retina from the sightless mice. Similar results pertained in a mutant strain of C57B1/6J mouse whose photoreceptor cells have undergone degeneration. It would appear that concomitant with photoreceptor cell degeneration and hence cessation of visual input to the bipolar and ganglion cells of the inner retina, cyclic AMP-generating systems of the inner retinal cells become hyperresponsive to dopamine. Adenylate cyclase and cyclic AMP are associated to a significant extent with the bipolar and ganglion layer of normal retina. However, in one study, the dopamine-sensitive cyclases did not appear elevated in homogenates from retina of sightless C3H mice and were reduced in retina of sightless C57B1/6J mice

(Makman *et al.,* 1975a). In rats in which neonatal treatment with glutamate was used to destroy inner retinal layers, retinal cyclase activity was decreased by about 50%.

High levels of adenylate cyclase are present in membranes from the photosensitive portion of photoreceptor cells of vertebrate retina (Bitensky *et al.,* 1971, 1972). Early data suggested a light-induced inactivation of this cyclase, but subsequent studies demonstrated that the true phenomenon involved was a light-induced activation of an associated phosphodiesterase (see Section 2.3.10). Lolley *et al.,* (1974) observed little reduction in total retinal adenylate cyclase activity when dark-adapted preparations were exposed to light. This had appeared to indicate that adenylate cyclase of the rod outer segments represented only a minor portion of total retinal adenylate cyclase activity.

Peripheral Neurons

Adenylate cyclase and to a lesser extent phosphodiesterase activity increased proximal to a constriction of the sciatic nerve (Bray *et al.,* 1971). The cyclase was associated with particulate fractions. The results suggest a synthesis of adenylate cyclase in neuronal cell bodies, followed by axonal transport to distal cholinergic nerve terminals of the chicken.

2.1.10 Cultured Cells

In contrast to the marginal activations with homogenates of nervous tissue, cultured glioma cells yield homogenates whose adenylate cyclase activity assayed with exogenous ATP was increased four- to twelvefold by catecholamines via interaction with a β-receptor (Schimmer, 1971, 1973; Jard *et al.,* 1972; Opler and Makman, 1972; Schwartz *et al.,* 1973; Maguire *et al.,* 1976a,b). High concentrations of dopamine, phenylephrine, ephedrine, and octopamine were stimulatory, while histamine, serotonin, tyramine, tryptamine, prostaglandin, and acetylcholine had no effect and adenosine and theophylline at high concentrations were inhibitory. Cyclases in homogenates of human glioma cells were activated by prostaglandin and adenosine (Clark *et al.,* 1975; Perkins *et al.,* 1975). Lithium and sodium ions (10 mM) were reported to significantly enhance both basal activity of glioma cyclases and the stimulatory effects of epinephrine (Schimmer, 1971, 1973). Fluoride stimulated cyclases in glioma homogenates (Perkins *et al.,* 1971; Schimmer, 1971; Jard *et al.,* 1972; Opler and Makman, 1972). Astrocytes from newborn hamsters contained levels of adenylate cyclases twofold higher than those of virus-transformed astrocyte cells from newborn hamsters (Weiss *et al.,* 1971).

Binding of radioactive norepinephrine to particulate fractions of rat glioma cell lines showed no obvious correlations with activation of cyclic AMP-generating systems in these cells by norepinephrine or isoproterenol (Maguire *et al.*, 1974a). Hydroxybenzylpindolol and its iodo-derivative were potent competitive antagonists of isoproterenol-sensitive cyclases in particulate preparations from rat glioma cells (Maguire, 1976a,b). Dissociation of hydroxyiodopindolol occurred very slowly with a half-time of about 50 min. Pindolol, propranolol, dichlorisoproterenol, and practolol were less potent antagonists. Chlorpromazine and desipramine inhibited both basal and isoproterenol-sensitive cyclases. Binding of radioactive hydroxyiodopindolol to β-receptors correlated under a variety of conditions with its inhibitor effects on isoproterenol-sensitive adenylate cyclases in particulate preparations from the rat glioma cells. GTP and guanylylimidodiphosphate decreased the affinity of agonists for the adenylate cyclase but had no effect on the binding of the pindolol derivative. Based on the binding studies, each glioma cell was estimated to contain approximately 4000 β-receptor sites, each presumably coupled to one adenylate cyclase enzyme. A neuroblastoma cell line unresponsive to catecholamines did not contain a measurable number of binding sites for the radioactive pindolol derivative.

In homogenates from neuroblastoma cells, prostaglandins, adenosine, and, to a lesser extent, catecholamines have been reported to activate adenylate cyclases. Adenosine (K_m, 70 μM) and its 2-chloro (K_m, 7 μM), 2-hydroxy, and 8-dimethylamino derivatives activated cyclases in homogenates of mouse neuroblastoma cells (Blume and Foster, 1975, 1976a; Penit *et al.*, 1976). Inosine, guanosine, cytosine, 2'-, 3'-, and 5'-deoxyadenosine, adenine arabinofuranoside, xylopyranoside, and tubercidin (7-deazadenosine) had no effect. 5'-AMP was either ineffective (Blume and Foster, 1975) or inhibitory (Penit *et al.*, 1976). An inhibitory component to adenosine action was apparent at high concentrations of this nucleoside. Theophylline (K_i, 35 μM) competitively inhibited the response to 2-chloroadenosine, while having no effect on prostaglandin-sensitive cyclase activity. 2'- and 5'-deoxyadenosine inhibited basal, 2-chloroadenosine, and prostaglandin-sensitive cyclases. Prostaglandins E_1 and E_2 caused a very large activation of cyclases from neuroblastoma cells, while prostaglandin $F_{2\alpha}$ was nearly inactive. Combinations of prostaglandin and either adenosine or 2-chloroadenosine had less than additive effects and indeed adenosine in high concentrations slightly inhibited the response to prostaglandin. Norepinephrine and dopamine had marginal stimulatory effects on cyclase activity which were not potentiated by adenosine. Isoproterenol had no effect. The magnitude of the activation of cyclases by either prostaglandin or 2-chloroadenosine was greatest at low concentrations of magnesium ions. Calcium ions inhibited adenylate cyclases from neuroblastoma cells (Blume and Foster, 1976a).

Acetylcholine, prostaglandin E_1, dopamine, and GTP activated adenylate cyclases in homogenates of certain neuroblastoma cell lines (Prasad *et al.*, 1975c,d). GTP potentiated the response to prostaglandin E_1 in homogenates from cells induced to differentiate by treatment with a phosphodiesterase inhibitor but had no effect in homogenates from undifferentiated cells. Dopamine, apomorphine, norepinephrine, and isoproterenol enhanced adenylate cyclase activity in neuroblastoma homogenates (Prasad and Gilmer, 1974; Prasad *et al.*, 1974). Characterization of the catecholamine-sensitive adenylate cyclases was carried out with homogenates of neuroblastoma cells differentiated by culturing in the presence of prostaglandin E_1 or the phosphodiesterase inhibitor, RO 20-1724. Differentiation resulted in enhanced basal levels of cyclase and enhanced activity of prostaglandin and epinephrine-sensitive cyclases. Basal cyclase levels and responses to dopamine and norepinephrine were enhanced in cells differentiated by culture with butyrate, but not in cells differentiated by culture in serum-free medium. Cyclases in homogenates from differentiated neuroblastoma cells no longer responded to isoproterenol, while still exhibiting an enhanced sensitivity to norepinephrine. The response of the cyclases to norepinephrine was completely blocked by a 10 μM concentration of either phentolamine or propranolol, but it was only partially blocked by haloperidol. The response to dopamine was effectively blocked by phentolamine and haloperidol. Very high concentrations of propranolol were required to block the dopamine response. Combinations of norepinephrine and dopamine had additive effects on cyclase activity. Prostaglandin E_1 also activated cyclases in homogenates of differentiated neuroblastoma cells. The response to prostaglandin was blocked by phentolamine, was additive with the response to norepinephrine, but was not additive with the response to dopamine. In these "adrenergic" neuroblastoma cell lines, acetylcholine had no effect on adenylate cyclase activity. In homogenates from two other neuroblastoma cell lines, a "cholinergic" line and a line containing neither tyrosine hydroxylase nor choline acetyltransferase, acetylcholine and cholinergic agonists stimulated cyclase activity (Prasad *et al.*, 1974). In the latter cell line, dopamine, norepinephrine, and prostaglandin E_1 stimulated cyclase activity, while serotonin and histamine were ineffective. Combinations of acetylcholine and either dopamine or norepinephrine had additive effects on cyclase activity. The stimulatory effects of acetylcholine and/or dopamine were effectively blocked by the muscarinic antagonist, atropine. Atropine had only marginal inhibitory effects on the stimulation of cyclase by norepinephrine. Nicotinic "antagonists," such as hexamethonium and nicotine, also reduced the stimulatory effect of acetylcholine, while haloperidol, phentolamine, and propranolol had no antagonistic action. Catecholamines and acetylcholine have either no or only minimal effects on cyclic AMP-generating systems in intact neuroblastoma cells (see Section 3.5.2).

2.2 Guanylate Cyclases

The enzyme, guanylate cyclase, catalyzes the conversion of GTP to cyclic GMP and pyrophosphate. Manganese-GTP is an excellent substrate for guanylate cyclases and manganese thus often appears a requisite activator (cf. Chrisman *et al.*, 1975). Magnesium is much less effective. Soluble guanylate cyclases from most tissues are activated by calcium ions, while particulate cyclases are inhibited. Fluoride ions have no effect on activity of guanylate cyclases, nor has activation in cell-free preparations by hormones been reported.

2.2.1 Regional Distribution of Guanylate Cyclase and Cyclic GMP in Brain

Guanylate Cyclase

Levels of guanylate cyclase were in general lower than the levels of adenylate cyclase in brain tissue (Hardman and Sutherland, 1969; White and Aurbach, 1969; Boehme, 1970; Gorodis and Morgan, 1973; Kimura and Murad, 1975a,b; Nakazawa and Sano, 1974; Krishna and Krishnan, 1975; Spano *et al.*, 1975a; Krishnan and Krishna, 1976). Most data have been from rat (see Table 1) and mouse brain. Guanylate cyclase activity in rat brain was highest in telencephalon, diencephalon, midbrain, and cerebellum with lower activity in pons-medulla and lowest activity in spinal cord (Nakazawa and Spano, 1974; Nakazawa *et al.*, 1976). The levels of GTP, the substrate for guanylate cyclase, were much lower in brain tissue than levels of ATP (Mandel and Harth, 1961; Goldberg *et al.*, 1970, 1973; Steiner *et al.*, 1972). Levels of ATP in brain were about 14 to 40 nmol/mg protein or 1.4 to 4 mM, while GTP levels were about 1.5 to 2.5 nmol/mg protein or 0.15 to 0.25 mM. In neuroblastoma cells ATP levels were 15 to 30 nmol/mg protein, while GTP levels were only one-tenth as high (Wintzerith *et al.*, 1976). The K_m for GTP with rat cerebellar guanylate cyclase was about 150 μM (Nakazawa *et al.*, 1976). Guanylate cyclase activity was very low in a detergent-dispersed adenylate cyclase preparation from porcine brain, both before and after cellulose chromatography (Brostrom *et al.*, 1975).

Cyclic GMP

Levels of cyclic GMP were usually markedly lower than levels of cyclic AMP in various brain regions (Goldberg *et al.*, 1969, 1970, 1973; Ishikawa *et al.*, 1969; Ferrendelli *et al.*, 1970, 1972, 1973b; Steiner *et al.*, 1970, 1972; Kuo *et al.*, 1972; Mao *et al.*, 1974a,b,c; Spano *et al.*, 1975a;

Ohga and Daly, 1976a). Most data have been from rat (see Table 1) and mouse brain. Very high levels of cyclic GMP were found in cerebellum where levels of cyclic GMP approached or equaled levels of cyclic AMP. Changes in cyclic GMP levels in brain after decapitation were not as marked as those of cyclic AMP (Goldberg *et al.*, 1970; Steiner *et al.*, 1970, 1972; Kimura *et al.*, 1974). Postdecapitation increases in both nucleotides were greatest in cerebellum. An extremely sensitive assay permitted determination of cyclic GMP levels in hypothalamus, locus coeruleus, and raphe nuclei from individual rats (Cailla *et al.*, 1976). Cyclic AMP and cyclic GMP levels were cited as being codetermined in less than 1 mg of brain tissue.

2.2.2 Subcellular and Morphological Distribution of Guanylate Cyclase in Brain

In brain as in most other tissues, a major portion of guanylate cyclase activity appeared in soluble fractions of homogenates (Gorodis and Morgan, 1973; Bensinger *et al.*, 1974; Nakazawa and Sano, 1974; Kimura and Murad, 1974, 1975a,b; Nakazawa *et al.*, 1976). High levels were associated with synaptosomes. Guanylate cyclase was markedly activated upon solubilization. However, recent data indicated that membrane and soluble guanylate cyclases from brain represent distinct enzymes (Troyer and Ferrendelli, 1976). The distribution of guanylate cyclase in homogenate fractions from brain was similar to that of soluble neuronal marker enzymes such as glutamate decarboxylase and tyrosine hydroxylase; i.e., the highest specific activity of the enzyme was associated with the soluble fraction from lysed synaptosomes (Goridis and Morgan, 1973). The specific activity of guanylate cyclase associated with the synaptosomal membrane fragments was eightfold lower than the activity in the soluble synaptosomal fraction.

Cyclic GMP levels were greatly reduced in cerebella of "nervous" mutant mice in which Purkinje cells are virtually absent (Mao *et al.*, 1975b). The results indicate that high levels of cyclic GMP are normally present in Purkinje cells. Levels of guanylate cyclase and cyclic GMP phosphodiesterase were stated to be unaltered in the cerebellum of the "nervous" mutant mice. Cerebella of mutant mice were at least 30% smaller than normal mouse cerebella. Levels of cyclic GMP in mouse cerebellum were twofold higher in the molecular layer containing Purkinje dendrites than in the granular layer (Rubin and Ferrendelli, 1976).

Guanylate cyclase activity was higher in cultures of cells from neonatal rat cerebral cortex enriched in neurons than in cultures enriched in glial cells (cited in Goridis and Morgan, 1973). Guanylate cyclase activity was not detected in chick embryo brain cell cultures that contained only glial elements (Goridis *et al.,* 1974). Cultures from 8- to 12-day-old embryos which consisted of both glial and neuronal elements did contain guanylate cyclase.

2.2.3 Activation and Inhibition

Manganese and to a much smaller extent magnesium ions activated brain guanylate cyclases, while ATP and other nucleoside triphosphates were inhibitory (White and Aurbach, 1969; Boehme, 1970; Goridis and Morgan, 1973). Maximal activation by manganese or magnesium occurred at a concentration of about 10 mM. Calcium ions inhibited some of these guanylate cyclase preparations, presumably as in other tissues by inhibitory effects on particulate cyclases. A partially purified soluble guanylate cyclase from rat brain required manganese ions for activity (Nakazawa and Sano, 1974). Calcium stimulated enzyme activity, particularly in the presence of suboptimal concentrations of manganese. Another group also reported that soluble guanylate cyclase from rat brain was stimulated by calcium ions in the presence of suboptimal concentrations of manganese ions, but that calcium ions were inhibitory to the enzyme in the presence of magnesium ions (Olson *et al.,* 1976). The soluble guanylate cyclase was separated from four calcium-binding proteins including calcium-dependent activator protein (see Sections 2.1.6 and 2.3.5) by DEAE-cellulose and Sephadex chromatography (Figure 2). Readdition of the calcium-dependent activator protein to purified guanylate cyclase had no effect on enzyme activity in the presence of calcium ions at concentrations from 0.5 to 1 mM and of manganese ions at 0.1 mM.

Hormone or drug activation of particulate or soluble guanylate cyclases from brain has not been reported. Hormonal activation of cyclic GMP-generating systems in brain slices as in other tissues may, therefore, reflect only hormone-elicited increased access of calcium ions to intracellular guanylate cyclase. Recently, azide and hydroxylamine were reported to activate particulate, but not soluble guanylate cyclases from rat cerebral cortex (Kimura *et al.,* 1975). Halide and cyanide ions had no effect. The nature of activation of particulate guanylate cyclase by azide was not determined but was stated to involve neither preservation of GTP nor inhibition of phosphodiesterases. In the presence of a heat-labile macromolecule isolated from liver, azide markedly activated the soluble guanylate cyclase from rat cerebral cortex (Mittal *et al.,* 1975). At a concentration of

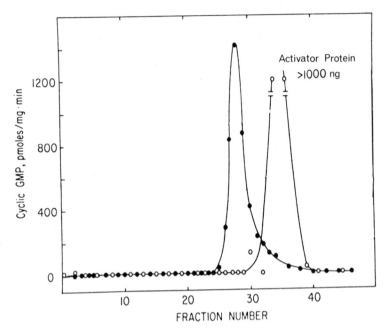

Figure 2. Guanylate cyclase from rat cerebrum. An ammonium sulfate fraction of soluble proteins was chromatographed on DEAE-cellulose and the fractions were assayed for guanylate cyclase (●——●). Boiled fractions were assayed for a calcium-dependent activator protein of adenylate cyclases and phosphodiesterases, and the results are expressed as nanograms of activator protein (○——○). (Modified from Olson *et al.*, 1976, *Life Sciences*, copyright Pergamon Press.)

500 μM, promethazine, chlorpromazine, imipramine, and diphenhydramine inhibited guinea pig cerebellar guanylate cyclases by about 30% (Ohga and Daly, 1976b). Fluphenazine had no effect.

2.2.4 Developmental Changes in Guanylate Cyclase and Cyclic GMP in Brain

Guanylate Cyclase

Levels of guanylate cyclase in rat cerebellum were unchanged during development, while levels decreased slightly in cerebral cortex (Kimura and Murad, 1975b). In another study, levels of guanylate cyclase in rat cerebellum appeared to decrease markedly from Day 8 to adulthood (Spano *et al.*, 1975a). Guanylate cyclase activity increased sixfold in chick embryo cerebrum between Day 12 and Day 16 after fertilization, followed by a threefold decrease during the subsequent few days including the first 24 hr after hatching (Goridis *et al.*, 1974).

Cyclic GMP

Cyclic GMP levels in rat cerebellum were low at birth and began a profound increase at the eighth day after birth (Steiner *et al.*, 1972). Increases in other brain regions were less marked. Indeed, in rat forebrain, levels of cyclic GMP appeared to decline between Days 3 and 7 after birth followed by a slight increase during the next 2 weeks. Another group (Spano *et al.*, 1975a) reported a 20-fold increase in cerebellar levels of cyclic GMP during development of rats from Day 8 to adulthood.

2.2.5 Ganglia

A major portion of guanylate cyclase in bovine retinal preparations was particulate (Bensinger *et al.*, 1974). High levels of guanylate cyclase and cyclic GMP have been found in rod outer segments of rabbit photoreceptor cells (Pannbacker, 1973; Krishnan and Krishna, 1976; Frandsen and Krishna, 1976). Indeed, about 90% of retinal guanylate cyclase appeared associated with membranes of the rod outer segments (Virmaux *et al.*, 1976). In retina of mice, cyclic GMP levels increased during development, reaching maximal levels at about Day 15 (Farber and Lolley, 1974). However, in the C3H strain of mice in which the high K_m phosphodiesterase of photoreceptor cells does not develop normally and in which the photoreceptor cells subsequently degenerate, cyclic GMP levels transiently attained very high levels during development at about Day 15. This transient accumulation occurred in the abnormal photoreceptor cells, prior to degeneration.

2.3 Phosphodiesterases

A variety of phosphodiesterases exist in nervous tissue as in other tissues. Certain enzymes, because of specificity or intracellular localization, are probably involved with cyclic AMP metabolism, some with cyclic GMP metabolism, and some with metabolism of both cyclic nucleotides. Phosphodiesterases occur as both soluble and particulate enzymes. Phosphodiesterases require magnesium ions or manganese ions for activity. Calcium ions play an important regulatory role for many phosphodiesterases, being required for activity, but are often inhibitory at high concentrations. Inhibition of phosphodiesterases by EGTA appears due to chelation of calcium. With certain phosphodiesterases activation by calcium requires a calcium-dependent protein activator. Both "low K_m" and "high K_m" cyclic AMP phosphodiesterase activities have been extensively studied, but it is usually unclear as to whether these activities represent different enzymes or one enzyme with two sites for cyclic AMP. Most studies on phosphodiesterases from nervous tissue have been with cyclic AMP as a substrate, and unless otherwise noted the following citations have been based on results with cyclic AMP. A comprehensive review on phosphodiesterases is available (Appleman et al., 1973).

2.3.1 Regional Distribution in Brain

Levels of cyclic AMP-phosphodiesterase varied considerably in different brain regions of various species. Levels of cyclic AMP-phosphodiesterases have been studied in brain regions of rabbit (Drummond and Perrott-Yee, 1961; Breckenridge and Johnston, 1969); rat (Weiss and Costa, 1968; Williams et al., 1971; Weiss and Strada, 1973); mouse (Schmidt and Lolley, 1973; Sattin, 1975); monkey (Williams et al., 1969, 1971); human (Williams et al., 1969, 1971); cat (Krishna et al., 1970; Dalton et al., 1974); dog (Butcher and Sutherland, 1972); steer (Cheung et al., 1975b); and trout (Yamamoto and Massey, 1969), while cyclic GMP-phosphodiesterases have been studied in brain regions of rat (Nakazawa and Sano, 1974) and cat (Dalton et al., 1974). Regional distribution of calcium-independent and calcium-dependent phosphodiesterase activity in bovine brain has been reported (Cheung et al., 1975b). Levels of high K_m cyclic AMP-phosphodiesterase were stated to be similar in brain homogenates from mouse, rat, rabbit, steer, sheep, and chicken (Breckenridge and Johnston, 1969). Levels of phosphodiesterase were in most species high in gray matter of cortex and in hypothalamus, lower in cerebellum, medulla, and pons, and very low in spinal cord. In rat brain a sixfold range of low K_m cyclic AMP-phosphodiesterase was observed with levels decreasing in the following order: neocortex, hippocampus > caudate nucleus, septum-fornix > olfactory tubercle, thalamus, hypothalamus > olfactory bulb > medulla-pons, cerebellum, spinal cord (Weiss and Costa, 1968). Highest levels of cyclic GMP-phosphodiesterase were detected in rat telencephalon and diencephalon, with low levels in midbrain, cerebellum, pons-medulla, and spinal cord (Nakazawa and Sano, 1974). Levels of phosphodiesterases in various regions of rat brain are summarized in Table 1. No correlations between levels of adenylate cyclase and cyclic AMP-phosphodiesterases in different brain regions have been apparent, although high levels of both enzymes were observed in the neocortex. In rabbit cortex levels of high K_m phosphodiesterase were sixfold greater than in cerebellum (Drummond and Perrott-Yee, 1961). Levels of cyclic AMP and cyclic GMP-phosphodiesterase activity in homogenates of mouse caudate nucleus were reported to be nearly equal (Prasad *et al.*, 1975a). The regional distribution of cyclic AMP and cyclic GMP phosphodiesterase activity using 5 μM cyclic nucleotide was quite similar in 15 areas of cat brain (Dalton *et al.*, 1974). In contrast to other species cerebellar levels of phosphodiesterase in cat were relatively high. Cyclic AMP and cyclic GMP-phosphodiesterase activities in human cerebrospinal fluid were similar as was the case in cerebral cortex but were present at very low levels, even when compared to those in blood plasma (Hidaka *et al.*, 1975).

2.3.2 Morphological Localization in Brain

A histochemical assay demonstrated that most of the cyclic AMP phosphodiesterase activity which survived glutaraldehyde fixation in rat cerebral cortical slices was localized at postsynaptic membranes on dendritic processes (Florendo *et al.*, 1971). The assay was based on the conversion of cyclic AMP to adenosine and inorganic phosphate by the action of tissue phosphodiesterases and exogenous 5'-nucleotidase. The phosphate was precipitated as the lead salt. Such assays requiring high concentrations of cyclic AMP probably detect only high K_m phosphodiesterases. The assay consisted of incubation of slices with cyclic AMP, lead ions, and a snake venom 5'-nucleotidase. The lead salt of phosphate formed from 5'-AMP precipitated at sites of phosphodiesterase activity. Theophylline apparently inhibited this high K_m phosphodiesterase activity. Theophylline and other methylxanthines have, however, been found to effectively inhibit 5'-nucleotidase (Tsuzuki and Newburgh, 1975). This lead-precipitate histochemical procedure was subsequently used (Adinolfi and Schmidt, 1974) to demonstrate the consistent presence of phosphodiesterase at emerging postsynaptic sites on dendritic processes in the molecular layer of the developing mouse brain (5 to 35 days of age). Similar results were obtained with tissue in which loss of phosphodiesterase activity was minimized by omission of the initial fixation with glutaraldehyde. It would appear likely that only a small portion of the postsynaptic sites containing phosphodiesterase could be undergoing innervation by rather scarce noradrenergic fibers of the cerebral cortex. In an earlier study by another group with a similar assay, glial cells were found to be stained heavily compared to neuronal cells in slices of rabbit cerebral cortex and cerebellum (Shanta *et al.*, 1966). Synaptic areas on neurons were, however, strongly stained. Intense staining was seen in the neuropile of the plexiform layer of cerebral cortex and the molecular layer of the cerebellum. Lead ions used in such histochemical assays have been shown to inhibit phosphodiesterase (cf. Breckenridge and Johnston, 1969), although Florendo *et al.* (1971) did not observe further inhibition by lead in glutaraldehyde-treated preparations. Phosphodiesterase activity assayed in homogenates from the gray matter of rabbit cerebral cortex or olfactory bulb did not appear uniquely associated with particular layers (Breckenridge and Johnston, 1969). Low levels appeared associated with myelinated nerve processes, such as in cerebral and cerebellar white matter, optic nerve, and dorsal column of spinal cord.

Cyclic AMP-phosphodiesterase activity in cerebral cortex was not decreased after lesion of the medial forebrain nerve bundle, nor did it decrease in the denervated superior cervical ganglion (Breckenridge and Johnston, 1969) or pineal gland (Weiss, 1971); all of which was consonant with a postsynaptic localization for a significant portion of this enzyme in such tissues. A soluble phosphodiesterase increased proximal to a constriction of the sciatic nerve, suggestive of synthesis in cell bodies and axonal transport to distal nerve terminals (Bray *et al.*, 1971).

2.3.3 Subcellular Distribution in Brain

Phosphodiesterase activity was found in both soluble and membrane fractions from brain homogenates and was associated with both soluble and membrane fractions from lysed synaptosomes (Cheung and Salganicoff, 1967; De Robertis *et al.*, 1967; Weiss and Costa, 1968; Yamamoto and Massey, 1969; Gaballah and Popoff, 1971a, Thompson and Appleman, 1971b; Campbell and Oliver, 1972; Miki and Yoshida, 1972; Weller *et al.*, 1972; Johnson *et al.*, 1973; Cheung *et al.*, 1975b). The high K_m cyclic AMP-phosphodiesterase activity of rat brain was nearly equally distributed between soluble and particulate fractions (Cheung and Salganicoff, 1967). About one-third of the high K_m phosphodiesterase activity from rat brain was found in soluble fraction (Gaballah and Popoff, 1971a). About one-half of the synaptosomal enzyme was found to be associated with membrane. Cyclic GMP-phosphodiesterase activity was also found in soluble and particulate fractions from rat brain (Nakazawa and Sano, 1974). In subcortical regions a relatively higher proportion of the cyclic GMP-phosphodiesterase activity was present in the soluble fractions. High and low K_m activities for both cyclic AMP and cyclic GMP have been compared in particulate and soluble fractions from rat brain (Beavo *et al.*, 1970). At high substrate concentrations rates of hydrolysis of both nucleotides were similar, although cyclic AMP was hydrolyzed slightly faster than cyclic GMP in the supernatant fraction. At low substrate concentrations cyclic GMP was hydrolyzed faster than cyclic AMP in both particulate and supernatant fractions.

2.3.4 Multiplicity of Brain Phosphodiesterases

A number of different phosphodiesterases were present even in the soluble fractions from homogenates of brain tissue (Brooker *et al.*, 1968; Beavo *et al.*, 1970; Cheung, 1970; Kakiuchi *et al.*, 1971, 1972; Monn and Christiansen, 1971; Thompson and Appleman, 1971a,b,c; Campbell and Oliver, 1972; Cehovic *et al.*, 1972; Russell *et al.*, 1972; Uzunov and Weiss, 1972a; Appleman *et al.*, 1973; Weiss and Strada, 1973; Lin *et al.*, 1975). A phosphodiesterase with a high affinity ($K_m \sim 2-4$ μM) for cyclic AMP and another with a low affinity ($K_m \sim 100$ μM) occurred in most brain regions. Usually only a single K_m of 20 μM or less was observed with cyclic GMP. High and low K_m cyclic AMP-phosphodiesterases were detected from rat cerebrum, cerebellum, caudate nucleus, and spinal cord (Weiss and Strada, 1973). Cyclic AMP-phosphodiesterase from cortex and hypothalamus of DBA and C3H mice appeared to have a single K_m of about 80 μM (Schmidt and Lolley, 1972). Roberts and Simonsen (1970) and Breckenridge and Johnston (1969) had reported a single K_m of about 300 μM and 120 μM, respectively, for mouse brain phosphodiesterase. Only a single K_m for human phosphodiesterases was apparent (Kodama *et al.*, 1971). In human fetal brain, however, both high and low K_m phosphodiesterases were detected (Weiss and Strada, 1973).

Starch gel electrophoretic patterns with an assay based on lead precipitation of phosphate and using 5'-nucleotidase and high concentrations of cyclic AMP indicated the presence of one major, one minor, and two trace bands of phosphodiesterase activity in homogenates of rat or rabbit brain (Monn and Christiansen, 1971). Only one cyclic AMP-phosphodiesterase was detected after starch gel electrophoresis of human brain supernatants (Pichard *et al.*, 1972).

The proportions of the various phosphodiesterases vary in different rat brain regions and their activation and inhibition profiles differ markedly. At least six different forms of phosphodiesterase have been isolated by polyacrylamide gel electrophoresis of sonicated soluble fractions from rat cerebral and cerebellar homogenates (Uzunov and Weiss, 1972a; Uzunov *et al.*, 1974; Weiss *et al.*, 1974; Weiss, 1975). Profiles of phosphodiesterase enzymes from rat cerebrum and cerebellum are shown in Figures 3 and 4. In addition, the calcium-dependent activator protein which is required for activation of certain phosphodiesterases was isolated. The phosphodiesterase isozymes of peaks I–IV all exhibited linear kinetics with cyclic AMP. Peak II had a K_m of 50 μM, peaks I, III, IV a K_m of 100 μM. The low K_m enzymes apparently present in the original rat cerebral homogenate were not detected after gel electrophoresis. Peaks III and IV were the least stable, peak I the most stable of the four isolated isozymes—only peak II was activated by calcium, while both peaks II and VI were activated by

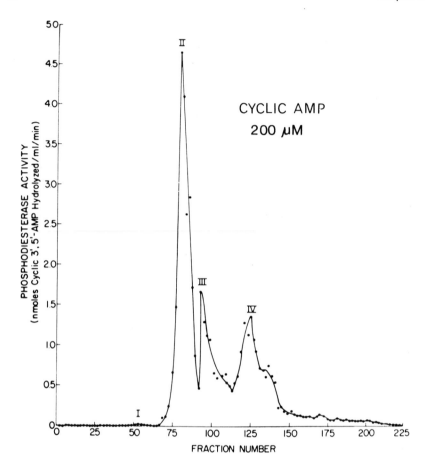

Figure 3. Phosphodiesterases from rat cerebrum. Homogenates were sonicated and soluble proteins were fractionated on a polyacrylamide gel column and assayed in the presence of calcium ion and the calcium-dependent activator protein. (Modified from Weiss *et al.,* 1974, *Molecular Pharmacology,* copyright Academic Press.)

calcium plus activator protein. The activator protein in the concentrations tested increased the V_{max} of peak II without affecting the K_m for cyclic AMP. In the absence of calcium and activator protein, peak III appeared to represent the major enzyme in rat cerebellum (Figure 4), but after addition of calcium and activator protein the activity of peak II was increased fivefold and then represented the major enzyme in cerebellum as had been the case in cerebrum. Only one major (peak III) and one minor peak of phosphodiesterase activity appeared to be present in homogenates of rat caudate nucleus (Fertel and Weiss, 1974, Figure 5).

Isoelectric focusing allowed isolation of at least six cyclic phosphodiesterase enzymes from rat cerebrum (Pledger *et al.*, 1975, Figure 6). Only four enzymes were detected if the cerebral homogenate was first dialyzed with EGTA (Figure 7). One of the isolated enzymes (peak C) was now dependent on calcium ion and activator protein with both cyclic AMP and cyclic GMP as substrate. This enzyme, a major isozyme in rat cerebrum,

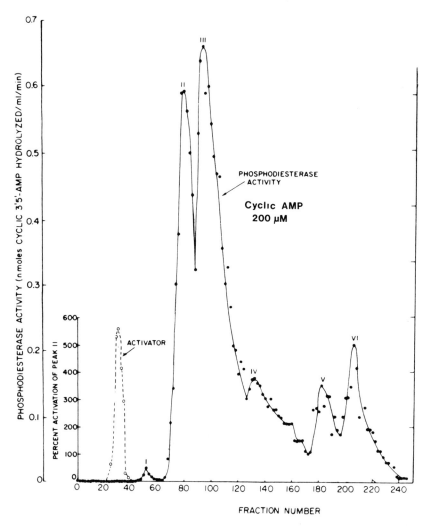

Figure 4. Phosphodiesterases from rat cerebellum. Homogenates were sonicated and soluble proteins were fractionated on a polyacrylamide gel column and assayed in the absence of calcium-dependent activator protein. The elution pattern of the calcium-dependent activator protein, assayed in boiled fractions, is plotted as percent activation of peak II. (Modified from Uzunov and Weiss, 1972, *Biochimica Biophysica Acta*, copyright Elsevier Publishing Co.)

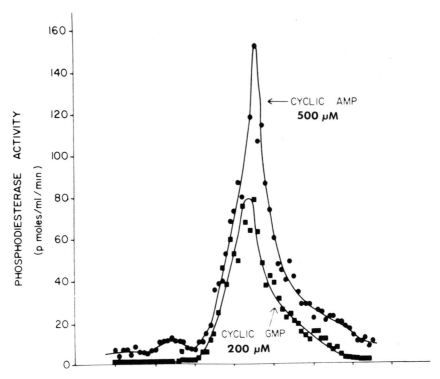

Figure 5. Phosphodiesterases from rat caudate nucleus. Homogenates were sonicated and soluble proteins were fractionated on a polyacrylamide gel column and assayed with cyclic AMP or cyclic GMP. (Modified from Fertel and Weiss, 1974, *Analytical Biochemistry,* copyright Academic Press.)

exhibited both a low and high K_m for cyclic AMP. The same six cyclic AMP-phosphodiesterases were apparently detected in rat cerebellum by isoelectric focusing (Pledger *et al.*, 1974, Figure 8). Three of these enzymes (B,C,D) exhibited activity towards cyclic GMP and cyclic AMP. All enzymes except that of peak E showed kinetics indicative of high and low K_m forms. The K_m for cyclic AMP with the peak E isozyme was 7 μM. This is in marked contrast to the results with phosphodiesterases isolated by gel electrophoresis where all peaks exhibited kinetics indicative of only high K_m forms (Uzunov *et al.*, 1974). When sonication of homogenates was omitted prior to centrifugation, only three phosphodiesterases (B,D, and E) were detected by isoelectric focusing. These three enzymes, therefore, appeared to be primarily soluble in rat cerebellum, while the remaining three (A,C, and F) appeared to be primarily membrane bound.

Phosphodiesterase activity in supernatant fractions from rat cortex was separated into three fractions by gel filtration (Thompson and Appleman, 1971a,b,c). A high molecular weight fraction exhibited a K_m of 100 μM for cyclic AMP and 13 μM for cyclic GMP, while a lower molecular weight fraction exhibited a K_m of 5 μM for cyclic AMP and 11 μM for cyclic GMP. The rate of hydrolysis of cyclic GMP with the lower molecular weight fraction was, however, barely measurable. It was suggested that the high K_m (high molecular weight) enzyme was cytoplasmic and physiologically concerned with cyclic GMP hydrolysis, while the low K_m (low molecular weight) enzyme was membranal and concerned with cyclic AMP hydrolysis.

Two major fractions of phosphodiesterase isolated from rat brain had the following properties: The lower molecular weight fraction exhibited a higher affinity for cyclic AMP than for cyclic GMP, while the higher

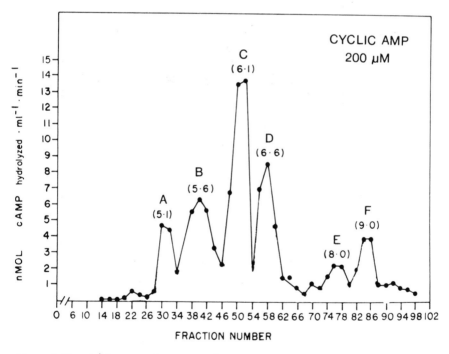

Figure 6. Phosphodiesterases from rat cerebrum. Homogenates were sonicated and soluble proteins were fractionated on an isoelectric focusing column. Numbers in parentheses refer to isoelectric points. Activator protein had little effect on enzyme activities which were, however, inhibited by EGTA. (Modified from Pledger *et al.,* 1975, *Biochimica Biophysica Acta,* copyright Elsevier Publishing Co.)

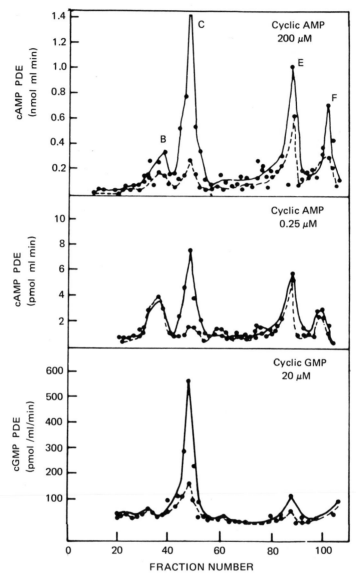

Figure 7. Dialyzed phosphodiesterases from rat cerebrum. Homogenates were sonicated and soluble proteins were fractionated on an isoelectric focusing column after dialysis versus EGTA. Assays were in the presence (●——●) or absence (●----●) of activator protein and calcium ion. (Modified from Pledger *et al.*, 1975, *Biochimica Biophysica Acta*, copyright Elsevier Publishing Co.)

molecular weight fraction had a higher affinity for cyclic GMP, and kinetic properties with cyclic AMP suggestive of the presence of low and high K_m enzymes (Russell *et al.*, 1972). Alternatively, the kinetics could be rationalized in terms of one enzyme with two sites for cyclic AMP and exhibiting negative cooperativity.

After separation by Sephadex chromatography, three apparent peaks of phosphodiesterase activity were isolated from rat cerebral cortex (Kakiuchi *et al.*, 1975, Figure 9). Similar results pertained with rat cerebellum where two or perhaps three peaks were detected. The lowest molecular weight isozyme was nearly completely dependent on calcium and activator protein. The activator protein was estimated to have a molecular weight of 30,000, while the calcium-dependent phosphodiesterase was estimated to have a molecular weight of 150,000. At high concentrations of cyclic nucleotide, hydrolysis of cyclic AMP was faster than cyclic GMP with this phosphodiesterase, while the reverse pertained with low concentrations. Cerebellum contained slightly more activator protein than cerebral cortex, but in both regions the activator protein was in great excess compared to the phosphodiesterase. During and after purification brain phosphodiesterases, particularly calcium-dependent phosphodiesterases, were found to be quite labile.

Three fractions containing phosphodiesterase activity were isolated by Sephadex chromatography of dog cerebral cortical homogenates (Sheppard *et al.*, 1972). Apparent molecular weights were about 50,000, 120,000, and 450,000. All three fractions exhibited a low K_m for cyclic AMP of 10 μM, but the two higher molecular weight fractions also showed a high K_m. The high molecular weight phosphodiesterase fractions were found to be activated by snake venom. Presumably, this activation is due to proteolytic enzymes (cf. Cheung, 1969). Phosphodiesterase activity towards cyclic GMP was also enhanced by the treatment of these fractions with snake venom.

Beef cerebrum appeared, like rat cerebrum, to contain by gel electrophoresis only four peaks of cyclic AMP-phosphodiesterase activity (Weiss, 1975).

A calcium-dependent phosphodiesterase has been described from pig brain (Brostrom *et al.*, 1975; Egrie and Giegel, 1975). Calcium-dependent phosphodiesterase activity represented greater than 60% of total cyclic AMP-phosphodiesterase activity and greater than 50% of total cyclic GMP-phosphodiesterase activity in homogenates of porcine brain (Brostrom and Wolff, 1976). The calcium-dependent phosphodiesterase, isolated by protamine-Sepharose and ECTEOLA-cellulose chromatography from porcine brain, hydrolyzed both cyclic AMP and cyclic GMP. Addition of calcium and calcium-dependent activator protein increased basal enzyme activity

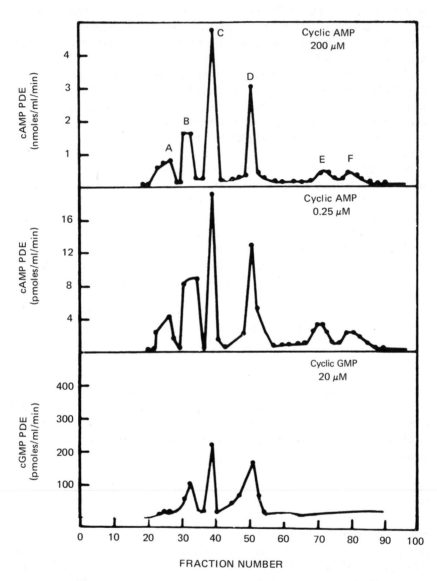

Figure 8. Phosphodiesterases from rat cerebellum. Homogenates were sonicated and soluble proteins were fractionated on an isoelectric focusing column and assayed with cyclic AMP or cyclic GMP. (Modified from Pledger *et al.*, 1974, *Biochimica Biophysica Acta,* copyright Elsevier Publishing Co.)

about sixfold. A variety of studies indicated that only one phosphodiesterase was present. These studies included isoelectric focusing, polyacrylamide gel electrophoresis, thermal stabilities, competitive inhibition between cyclic AMP and cyclic GMP and identical K_m values for cyclic AMP (180 μM) and cyclic GMP (8 μM) for basal enzyme activity and for enzyme fully activated by calcium and calcium-dependent activator protein.

Only one major phosphodiesterase peak was detected in human cortical homogenates after Sepharose chromatography, using either cyclic AMP or cyclic GMP as substrate (Hidaka *et al.*, 1975). This enzyme exhibited a high and low K_m with cyclic AMP, but only a low K_m with cyclic GMP. Both cyclic AMP and cyclic GMP-phosphodiesterase activities were stimulated by snake venom. Sepharose chromatography indicated the presence of more than one phosphodiesterase in human cerebrospinal fluid.

Affinity chromatography with a Sepharose gel coupled after cyanogen bromide activation to calcium-dependent activator protein was used to isolate calcium-dependent phosphodiesterases from rat cerebrum (Miyake *et al.*, 1976). Calcium-dependent phosphodiesterase appeared to be the major enzyme in both soluble and particulate fractions. The isolated enzyme was activated by calcium and activator protein only at low substrate concentrations of cyclic AMP and cyclic GMP. Chromatography on a succinylated aminopropyl agarose column coupled after *N*-hydroxysuccinimide activation to the activator protein was not satisfactory for affinity separation of calcium-dependent phosphodiesterases.

The presence of such a variety of phosphodiesterases in brain homogenates with differing affinities for cyclic nucleotides and influenced *in situ* to varying degrees by calcium ions, protein activators, and ATP makes difficult any extrapolation of results on phosphodiesterase activity in homogenates to phosphodiesterase-controlled degradation of cyclic nucleotides in morphological compartments of the intact functioning brain.

2.3.5 Activation

Brain phosphodiesterases require magnesium ions for maximal activity. Manganese ions can substitute for magnesium. Brain tissue also contains high levels of nucleoside 2',3'-cyclic phosphate phosphodiesterases (Drummond and Perrott-Yee, 1961) which is associated mainly with myelin (Kurihara and Tsukada, 1967). This enzyme which forms 2'-phosphates is not concerned in metabolism of cyclic AMP and cyclic GMP and does not require a metal ion for activity. Cyclic AMP-phosphodiesterases exhibited a relatively low effect of temperature on their activity: Q_{10} values of 1.2 to

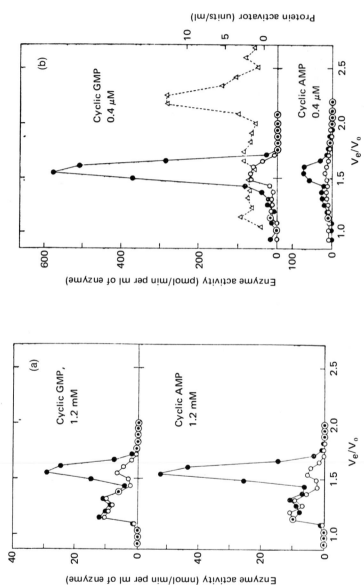

Figure 9. Phosphodiesterases and calcium-dependent activator protein from rat cerebral cortex. Homogenates were fractionated on a Sepharose G-200 column (V_o = void volume) and assayed with (a) high concentrations and (b) low concentrations of cyclic nucleotides. Activator protein and calcium ions were present in all assays and EGTA was either present ($\circ$——$\circ$) or absent ($\bullet$——$\bullet$). Activity of the stable calcium-dependent activator protein ($\triangle$----$\triangle$) was assayed with boiled fractions. (Modified from Kakiuchi *et al.*, 1975, *Biochemical Journal*, copyright Biochemical Society.)

1.5 have been reported for brain enzymes (Sheppard and Wiggan, 1971; Sheppard *et al.*, 1972). Certain brain phosphodiesterases could be activated by imidazole, dithiothreitol, proteolytic enzymes, endogenous protein factors, or calcium ions (Cheung, 1967b, 1969, 1970, 1971a,b; Kakiuchi and Yamazaki, 1970a,b,c; Beavo *et al.*, 1970; Williams *et al.*, 1971; Kakiuchi *et al.*, 1972, 1973; McNeill *et al.*, 1972; Miki and Yoshida, 1972; Uzunov and Weiss, 1972; Hidaka *et al.*, 1975). Imidazole stimulated the high K_m phosphodiesterase from bovine cerebrum: maximal stimulation was observed at 10 to 20 mM imidazole (Cheung, 1971a). Neither imidazole nor nicotinic acid (1 mM) had any effect on either low or high K_m cyclic AMP-phosphodiesterases isolated by gel filitration from rat cortical supernatants (Thompson and Appleman, 1971b). Imidazole stimulated cyclic GMP hydrolysis in a rat brain preparation (Williams *et al.*, 1971), while in another study imidazole was reported to noncompetitively inhibit rat brain cyclic GMP-phosphodiesterase and to have no effect on cyclic AMP hydrolysis (Goldberg *et al.*, 1970). Imidazole acetic acid has been reported to uncompetitively activate high K_m cyclic AMP-phosphodiesterase from mouse brain (Roberts and Simonsen, 1970). Cyclic AMP-phosphodiesterase activity from cockroach brain was activated by imidazole (Rojakovick and March, 1974). A phosphodiesterase purified from rat cerebral cortex was stimulated by imidazole, inhibited by EGTA, and stimulated by low concentrations of calcium ions (Miki and Yoshida, 1972). Trypsin treatment had no effect on the stimulation by imidazole, but EGTA no longer inhibited trypsin-treated brain phosphodiesterase. Miki and Yoshida (1972) proposed the presence of a trypsin-sensitive inhibitory factor, whose inhibition was overcome by calcium ions. The activity of a purified bovine brain phosphodiesterase could be greatly enhanced by treatment with trypsin (Cheung, 1971b). This activation was time dependent and the mechanism involved was unclear. The purified phosphodiesterase could also be activated by reconstitution with a very stable brain protein (mol wt 240,000). The relationship of this protein to the stable calcium-dependent activator protein (see below) is uncertain. The activity of "partially purified" phosphodiesterase from bovine brain was also greatly enhanced in a time-dependent process by protein factors present in snake venoms (Cheung, 1967b, 1969). A heat stable factor, present in rat adipocytes after stimulation of cyclic AMP formation, inhibited hydrolysis of cyclic AMP and cyclic GMP by rat brain phosphodiesterase (Ho *et al.*, 1975b). The factor copurified and appeared to be identical with a factor that inhibited cyclic AMP formation in rat adipocytes (Ho and Sutherland, 1971) and a factor that inhibited adenylate cyclase, activated protein kinase, and stimulated membrane phosphorylation in various preparations (Ho and Sutherland, 1975). The chemical nature of this factor is unknown. The hydrolysis of 1 mM cyclic GMP by bovine cerebral phosphodiesterase was stimulated by magnesium ion and low concentrations of calcium ion and inhibited by high concentrations of calcium ion (Cheung, 1971a). Cyclic GMP-phosphodiesterase activity (K_m, 10 μM) in rat cerebral homogenates was also inhibited by calcium ions (Fertel and Weiss, 1974). Strontium ions could replace calcium ions in reversing the inhibition of cyclase by EGTA (Bradham *et al.*, 1970). Bovine brain phosphodiesterase (mol wt 200,000) after column purification and dialysis still contained nearly one equivalent of calcium and zinc ions (Cheung, 1971a). Both of these cations at low concentrations were stimulatory to the enzyme. Presumably, the inhibition of phosphodiesterase by EGTA and other chelating agents was due to removal of these two cations. EGTA at 100 μM did not inhibit the enzyme completely. It appears likely that EGTA removed only the calcium ion effectively.

The stimulatory effects of calcium ions on brain phosphodiesterase activity have now been investigated in detail. Independently, a heat stable calcium-dependent protein activator for phosphodiesterases was detected in brain homogenates by two groups (Kakiuchi and Yamazaki, 1970a,b; Cheung, 1970). Calcium-dependent and -independent phosphodiesterases were then isolated from rat brain homogenates by gel filtration (Kakiuchi and Yamazaki, 1971; Kakiuchi *et al.*, 1972). Further studies confirmed that activation of the hydrolysis of cyclic AMP or cyclic GMP by the calcium-dependent phosphodiesterase required the presence of the activator protein (Kakiuchi *et al.*, 1973). Half maximal activation of hydrolysis of cyclic AMP and cyclic GMP in the presence of activator protein occurred at calcium concentrations of 8 and 4 μM, respectively, Calcium ions and activator protein decreased the high K_m for cyclic AMP hydrolysis from 90 to 50 μM, while not affecting the low K_m (4 μM). The K_m for cyclic GMP hydrolysis was decreased from 20 to 2 μM by calcium ions plus activator protein. It was proposed that the calcium-dependent phosphodiesterase might *in vivo* be concerned with calcium-dependent regulation of cyclic GMP-hydrolysis rather than with hydrolysis of cyclic AMP. The nature of the activation of phosphodiesterase by calcium ions plus activator protein has not yet been completely defined, but it probably involves an activated ternary complex of enzyme–activator protein–calcium ion. Activation of bovine cerebral cortical phosphodiesterase required both activator protein and calcium ions, and kinetic analysis was compatible with positive cooperativity between calcium and activator protein for binding to enzyme (Wickson *et al.*, 1975). Binding of calcium to the activator protein appeared to increase the affinity of this protein for the catalytic unit of calcium-dependent phosphodiesterase (Teshima and Kakiuchi, 1974). Brain phosphodiesterase can be activated by calcium-dependent activator protein from other tissues (Cheung, 1971b; Uzunov *et al.*, 1975). Similarly, calcium-dependent activator protein from brain has been demonstrated to activate phosphodiesterases from other tissues. Complex kinetics were observed with a purified calcium-dependent phosphodiesterase from porcine brain under conditions where the enzyme was only partially activated by addition of submaximal concentrations of activator protein (Brostrom and Wolff, 1976). Under such conditions the K_m's for cyclic AMP and for cyclic GMP were greatly *increased*. Less calcium-dependent activator protein was required for maximal activation of the enzyme at high substrate concentrations of both cyclic AMP and cyclic GMP. Addition of the activator appeared to greatly decrease the apparent K_m of the enzyme for magnesium ions. Less activator protein was required for activation at high concentrations of magnesium ions. Cyclic GMP was hydrolyzed faster than cyclic AMP at low substrate concentrations, while the converse was true at high substrate concentrations. The calcium-dependent phosphodiesterase from porcine brain was activated in a calcium-independent, rapid and reversible process by certain lipids such as lysophosphatidyl choline, phosphatidyl inositol, and fatty acids (Wolff and Brostrom, 1976). Lysophosphatidyl ethanolamine and serine were ineffective. Sodium dodecyl sulfate at low concentrations had a modest stimulatory activity, while other detergents had none. The maximal activation of the enzyme by the phospholipids and by calcium plus calcium-dependent activator protein were similar, and both types of activation resulted in stabilization of the enzyme. Activation of cyclic AMP hydrolysis required higher concentrations of phosphatidyl inositol than did activation of cyclic GMP hydrolysis. Activation of cyclic GMP hydrolysis by lysophosphatidyl choline exhibited a high degree of positive cooperativity. This was probably also true for phosphatidyl inositol. At maximal concentrations of phospholipids or calcium-dependent activator, no additivity of their stimulatory effects on phosphodiesterase were observed. In contrast to the lack of effect of calcium-dependent activator protein on the K_m of maximally activated phosphodiesterase for cyclic AMP or cyclic GMP, the phospholipids increased the K_m for both cyclic nucleotides from those observed with unactivated enzyme. The effect was most pronounced with lysophosphatidyl choline which increased the K_m for cyclic AMP from a basal value of 180 μM to about 1000 μM and the K_m for cyclic GMP from 8 μM to 30 μM. Phosphatidyl inositol had much smaller effects. The apparent K_m for magnesium of 3 μM was not influenced with varying concentrations of phospholipid. Fluphenazine competitively inhibited activation of the enzyme by both lysophosphatidyl choline or calcium-dependent activator protein. The physiological significance of activation of calcium-dependent phosphodiesterases by phospholipids in unclear. It should be noted that the calcium-activator protein is a negatively charged (phospho)protein (see below). Earlier studies had demonstrated that several naturally occurring lipids, of which lysolecithin and phosphatidyl inositol were most effective, stimulated the activity of high K_m cyclic AMP-phosphodiesterases in the soluble fraction of homogenates of rat brain (Bublitz, 1973). After separation of phosphodiesterases by Sephadex chromatography, lysolecithin had virtually no stimulatory effect on the highest molecular weight fraction but stimulated hydrolysis of high and low concentrations of cyclic AMP and of cyclic GMP by phosphodiesterases in the lower molecular weight fractions.

Calcium-dependent activator protein in bovine brain (Cheung *et al.*, 1975b) and rat brain (Gnegy *et al.*, 1976a) was nearly equally distributed between soluble and membranal fractions. The activator protein was released from membrane fractions of rat brain or striatum under phosphorylating conditions with cyclic AMP present (Gnegy *et al.*, 1976a,b).

The apparent molecular weight of the calcium-dependent activator protein has been reported in various studies to be from 15,000 to 30,000. The protein activator (mol wt 15,000) was purified to homogeniety from bovine brain (Lin *et al.*, 1974). Four binding sites for calcium appeared to be present. The activator stimulated cyclic AMP hydrolysis to a greater extent than cyclic GMP hydrolysis. In later studies it was reported that in the presence of EGTA to chelate calcium, the calcium-binding activator protein eluted at a volume corresponding to a molecular weight of 33,000 on a Sephadex column, completely separated from calcium-dependent phosphodiesterase activity which eluted as two peaks, one at the void volume and the other at a volume corresponding to a molecular weight of 170,000 (Lin *et al.*, 1975). In the presence of calcium ions, the activator remained virtually completely associated with the phosphodiesterases which emerged at the void volume and at a volume corresponding to a molecular weight of 230,000. EGTA was in another study reported to cause a reversible dissociation of activator with an apparent molecular weight of 30,000 from the catalytic (mol wt 150,000) subunit (Teshima and Kakiuchi, 1974). The molecular weight of purified activator protein based on amino acid analysis was about 19,000 (Cheung *et al.*, 1975b).

A calcium-binding phosphoprotein had been isolated from pig brain (Wolff and Siegel, 1972). It had a molecular weight of 11,500, contained ten phosphate groups and bound 1 mol of calcium/mol of protein with a K_a of about 25 μM. This protein was reported to have properties identical with those of the calcium-dependent phosphodiesterase activator protein (Wolff and Brostrom, 1974). Other calcium-binding proteins, such as S-100 protein and troponin, did not affect calcium-dependent phosphodiesterases. Activation of phosphodiesterases by the pig brain calcium-binding protein was readily reversible by EGTA. It has appeared that only the calcium-activator protein complex interacts well with the phosphodiesterase. Removal of calcium from the activator protein by EGTA resulted in a change in the protein's tertiary structure as evidenced by a decrease in α-helical content as measured by circular dichroism. A calcium-binding protein with similar molecular weight, electrophoretic mobility, and phosphorous content was recently isolated from electroplax of the electric eel (Childers and Siegel, 1975). Calcium-dependent activator proteins isolated from brain by others did not contain phosphate (Liu and Cheung, 1976; Watterson et al., 1976).

2.3.6 Inhibitors

Inhibition of brain phosphodiesterases has been reported for a variety of compounds including methylxanthines such as theophylline, caffeine, 3-isobutyl-1-methylxanthine, and 1,3,7- trisubstituted xanthines (Cheung, 1967a; Honda and Imamura, 1968; Vernikos-Danellis and Harris, 1968; Yamamoto and Massey, 1969; Goldberg et al., 1970; Lespagnol et al., 1970; Roberts and Simonsen, 1970; Mizon et al., 1971; Amer et al., 1972; Beer et al., 1972; Pichard et al., 1972; Sheppard et al., 1972; Weinryb et al., 1972; Harris et al., 1973; Nahorski et al., 1973; Dalton et al., 1974; MacDonald, 1974; Rojakovick and March, 1974; Shimizu et al., 1974; Stefanovich, 1974; Stefanovich et al., 1974; Teshima et al., 1974; Weiss et al., 1974; Du Moulin and Schultz, 1975; Tsuzuki and Newburgh, 1975; Hayashi et al., 1976; Levin and Weiss, 1976); 3,4-dialkoxybenzyl-2-imidazolidinones such as RO 20-1724 (Sheppard et al., 1972; Weinryb et al., 1972; Dalton et al., 1974; Du Moulin and Schultz, 1975; Francis et al., 1975; Schwabe et al., 1976a; a 3,4-dialkoxyphenyl-2-pyrrolidone ZK 62711 (Schwabe et al., 1976a); 1-H-pyrazolo[3,4b]pyridines such as SQ 20009 (Beer et al., 1972; Chasin et al., 1972; Dalton et al., 1974; Rojakovick and March, 1974; Du Moulin and Schultz, 1975; Hess et al., 1975; Kakiuchi et al., 1975a); benzodiazepines such as diazepam, medazepam, and chlordiazepoxide (Beer et al., 1972; Weinryb et al., 1972; Dalton et al., 1974; Du Moulin and Schultz, 1975; Levin and Weiss, 1976); phenothiazines such as fluphenazine, chlorpromazine, trifluoperazine, and promethazine (Honda and Imamura, 1968; Yamamoto and Massey, 1969; Roberts and Simonsen, 1970; Uzunov and Weiss, 1971; Williams et al., 1971; Beer et al., 1972; Weinryb et al., 1972; Berndt and Schwabe, 1973; Levin and Weiss, 1976); thioxanthenes such as chlorprothixene (Honda and Imamura, 1968; Berndt and Schwabe, 1973); tricyclic antidepressants such as nortriptyline, imipramine, and desipramine (Honda and Imamura, 1968; Abdulla and Hamadah, 1970; Roberts and Simonsen, 1970; Kodama et al., 1971; Beer et al., 1972; Pichard et al., 1972; Weinryb et al., 1972; Berndt and Schwabe, 1973; Somerville, 1973; Levin and Weiss, 1976; Palmer, 1976); papaverine and related alkaloids (Goldberg et al., 1970; Poech and Kukovetz, 1971; Amer *et al.*, 1972; Sheppard *et al.*, 1972; Weinryb *et al.*, 1972; Weller *et al.*, 1972; Furlanut *et al.*, 1973; Nahorski *et al.*, 1973; Dalton *et al.*, 1974; Shimizu *et al.*, 1974; Weiss *et al.*, 1974; Du Moulin and Schultz, 1975; Furatani *et al.*, 1975; Kakiuchi *et al.*, 1975; Levin and Weiss, 1976; Montecucchi, 1976); apomorphine (Nahorski *et al.*, 1973); reserpine and reserpine derivatives (Honda and Imamura, 1968; Yamamoto and Massey, 1969; Williams *et al.*, 1971; Beer *et al.*, 1972; Weinryb *et al.*, 1972; Rojakovick and March, 1974); ergot alkaloids such as dihydroergotamine (Iwangoff and Enz, 1971, 1972; Montecucchi, 1976); catechols and catecholamines (Sheppard *et al.*, 1972; Nahorski *et al.*, 1973); morphine (Weinryb *et al.*, 1972; Puri *et al.*, 1975); imidazopyrazines (Mandel, 1971); a benzopyrimidine, quazodine (Amer and Browder, 1971); tolbutamide (Goldfine *et al.*, 1971); dipyridamole (Pichard *et al.*, 1972; Weinryb *et al.*, 1972; Dalton *et al.*, 1974); phentolamine (McNeill *et al.*, 1972; Roberts and Simonsen, 1970); triazolopyrazines and triazolopyrimidines such as ICI 58301 and ICI 63197 (Somerville, 1973; Arbuthnott *et al.*, 1974); imidazole (Goldberg *et al.*, 1970); reticulol (Furatani *et al.*, 1975); 6-mercaptopurine (Pichard *et al.*, 1972; Weinryb *et al.*, 1972), puromycin (Goldberg *et al.*, 1970); adenosine, guanosine, and 2'-deoxy analogs (Roberts and Simonsen, 1970; Sattin and Rall, 1970; Shuman *et al.*, 1973); various steroids (Weinryb *et al.*, 1972); 1-[(*tert*-butylimino)methyl]-2-(3-indolyl)indoline (Amer *et al.*, 1972); protamine (Shimizu *et al.*, 1974); diphenylhydantoin, chloramphenicol, pyrvinium pamoate, bunamidine, amphotercin B, protoveratrine A, quinacrine, vinblastine, pentazocine, and indomethacin (Weinryb *et al.*, 1972). Inhibition of phosphodiesterases by analogs of cyclic AMP and cyclic GMP is discussed in Section 2.3.7. Table 2 presents a survey of the relative activity of some of the more active and widely used phosphodiesterase inhibitors. Structures are presented in Figure 10.* A survey of inhibitors and substrates of phosphodiesterases from a variety of mammalian and nonmammal tissues has been published (Amer and Kreighbaum, 1975).

A total of 158 compounds representing 49 classes of therapeutic agents, were screened as inhibitors of low K_m rat brain phosphodiesterase (Weinryb *et al.*, 1972). Correlations between potency as *in vitro* inhibitors of low K_m rat brain phosphodiesterase and efficacy in a conflict test for a number of compounds led to a proposal that antianxiety drugs may act via elevations of brain cyclic AMP (Beer *et al.*, 1972; Horovitz *et al.*, 1972; Hess *et al.*, 1975). The rank order of potency of the most active inhibitors of phosphodiesterase was SQ 20009 >> diazepam > fluphenazine > chlordiazepoxide, theophylline; while the rank order of effectiveness in a

---

*Structures of other compounds with inhibitory activity towards phosphodiesterases are to be found among various agonists and antagonists in the Appendix.

TABLE 2. Inhibitors of Brain Phosphodiesterases[a]

| | IC$_{50}$ values (μM) | | |
| | Cyclic AMP | | |
Inhibitor	Low K_m	High K_m	Cyclic GMP
Methylxanthines			
Theophylline	120–600[b]	300–800[b]	1200
Caffeine	300–900	—	—
Isobutylmethylxanthine	25–40	10–70	50
Imidazolidinones			
RO 20-1724	30–200	—	>200
RO 72956	140	—	—
Pyrrolidones			
ZK 62711	10–100	—	>200
Pyrazolopyridines			
SQ 20009	2[b]	30	25[b]
SQ 20006	50	—	—
SQ 66007	20–70	35–60	—
Benzodiazepines			
Medazepam	25		—
Diazepam	30–50	100	—
Chlordiazepoxide	100	100	—
Phenothiazines			
Fluphenazine	50	—	—
Chlorpromazine	120[c]	—	—
Alkaloids			
Papaverine	2[b]–40[c]	50–300[c]	2[b]–100
Apomorphine	15	—	—
1-Diethylamino-ethylreserpine	—	25	—
Other compounds			
Nortriptyline	200[b]	—	—
Dipyridamole	4–12	—	—
Reticulol	—	40	—
6-Mercaptopurine	30	—	—

[a] IC$_{50}$ values are based on values from the references cited in the text and are meant only to provide indices of the relative activities of the various inhibitors. Values reported by different investigators have varied considerably.
[b] Competitive inhibition.
[c] Noncompetitive inhibition.

conflict test was diazepam > chlordiazepoxide, SQ 20009 > theophylline, fluphenazine. Combinations of chlordiazepoxide and either theophylline or SQ 20009 had additive effects in the conflict test. Not all potent antianxiety agents were phosphodiesterase inhibitors, for example, meprobamate and pentobarbital. Very high concentrations of tricyclic antidepressants were required to inhibit high K_m phosphodiesterases in homogenates of neuronal

Methylxanthines

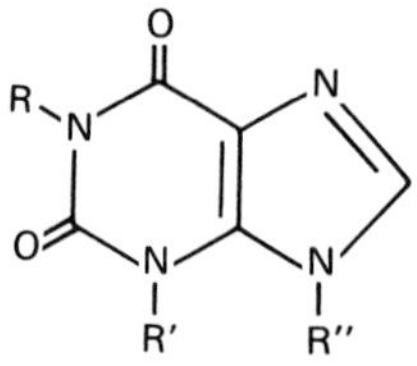

Theophylline
R,R'=CH₃,R''=H
Caffeine
R,R',R''=CH₃
3-Isobutyl-1-methylxanthine
R=CH₃,R'=CH CH₃C₂H₅

Imidazolidinones

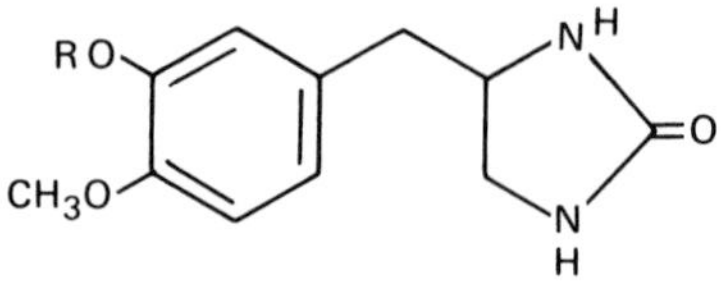

RO 20-1724
R = (CH₂)₃CH₃
RO 72956
R = CH₃

Pyrrolidones

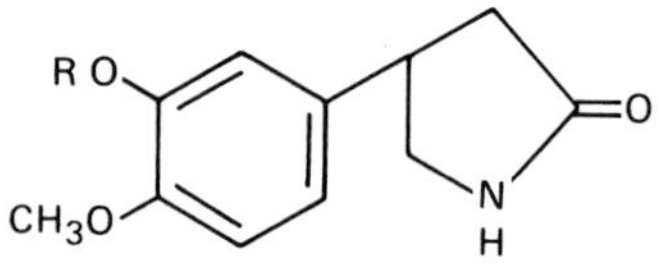

ZK 62711

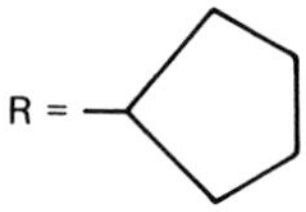

R = (cyclopentyl)

Pyrazolopyridines

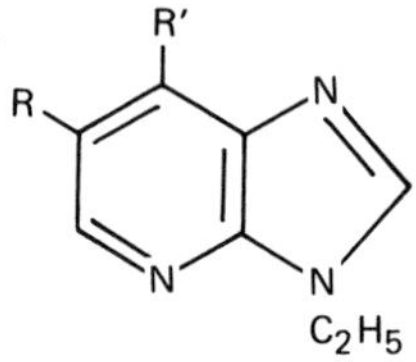

SQ 20009
R = CO₂C₂H₅,R'=NHN=C(CH₃)₂
SQ 20006
R = CO₂C₂H₅,R'=NHNH₂
SQ 66007
R = COCH₃,R'=SC₂H₅
SQ 65442
R = CO₂C₂H₅,R'=SC₂H₅

Benzodiazepines

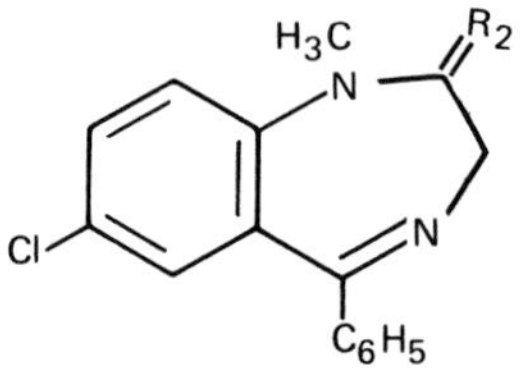

Medazepam
R₂ = H₂
Diazepam
R₂ = O

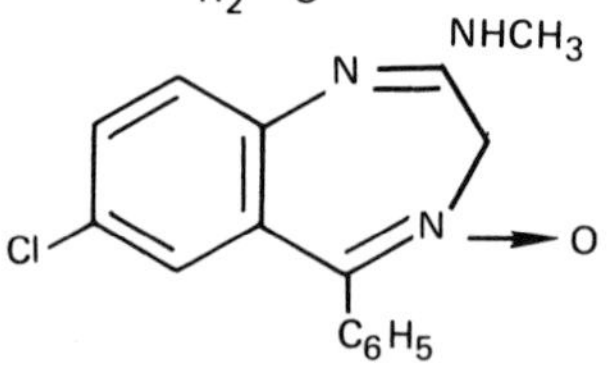

Chlordiazepoxide

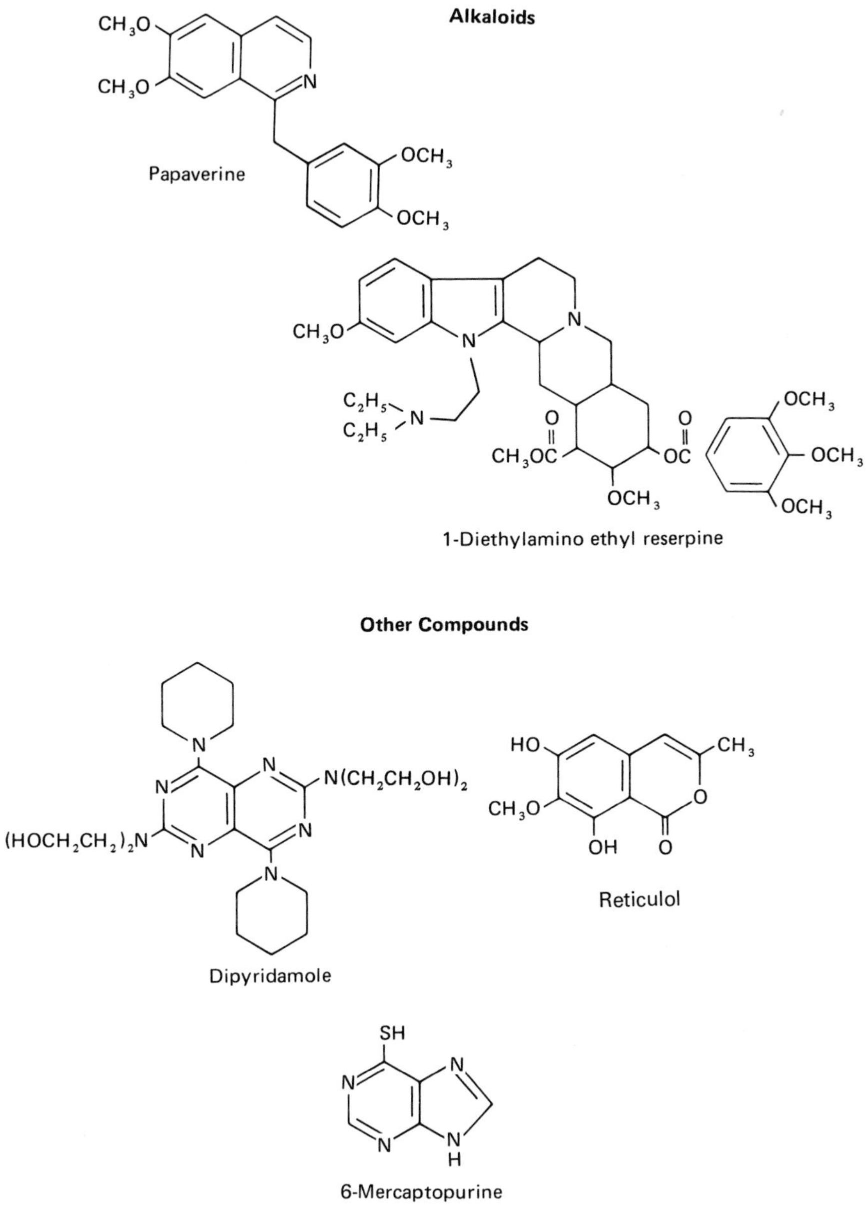

Figure 10. Structures of phosphodiesterase inhibitors. For structures of fluphenazine, chlorpromazine, apomorphine, and nortriptyline see Appendix.

or glial fractions from rat cerebral cortex (Palmer, 1976). The only excep-
tions were 2-hydroxydesipramine with an IC_{50} of about 100 μM for both
neuronal and glial phosphodiesterases and nortriptyline and iprindole with
IC_{50}'s of 100 μM for neuronal phosphodiesterases.

Imidazopyrazines have been reported to inhibit phosphodiesterases of
various sources (Mandel, 1971). Inhibition of phosphodiesterases was probably responsible for the enhanced accumulation of radioactive cyclic AMP
during incubation of bovine brain homogenates with 1 mM 5-chloro-6-
(ethylamino)-1,3-dihydro-2H- imidazo [4,5b] pyrazin-2-one and radioactive
ATP. Fluoride ion and theophylline were present in the incubation media.

Inhibition of phosphodiesterase by ATP and other nucleoside triphosphates (Cheung, 1966; Yamamoto and Massey, 1969) appeared only partially dependent on chelation of magnesium ions (Cheung, 1971a), while in
subsequent studies the inhibition of phosphodiesterase by ATP appeared to
be due exclusively to chelation of magnesium and calcium ions (Teshima *et
al.*, 1974).

Inhibition of rat brain high K_m phosphodiesterase by various sulfhydryl reagents, such as mersalyl, meralluride, ethacrynic acid, and phenyl-
mercuric acetate, has been reported (Gadd *et al.*, 1973).

Rat brain phosphodiesterases were inhibited by a heat stable protein
from rod outer segments of bovine retina (Dumler and Etingof, 1976).

Electrical pulsation or high concentrations of potassium ions had no
significant effect on high K_m phosphodiesterase activity of rat cerebral
cortical synaptosomes (De Belleroche *et al.*, 1974). Theophylline slightly
decreased synaptosomal levels of cyclic AMP.

Differential Effects of Inhibitors on Various Brain Phosphodiesterases

Trifluoperazine inhibited phosphodiesterases from rat cerebrum and
brain stem more effectively than phosphodiesterases from cerebellum
(Uzunov and Weiss, 1971, see below). No marked regional differences in
the efficacy of benzodiazepines (medazepam, chlordiazepoxide, diazepam) as phosphodiesterase inhibitors were noted in studies on cat brain
preparations (Dalton *et al.*, 1974). Benzodiazepines inhibited hydrolysis of
low concentrations (5 μM) of cyclic AMP and cyclic GMP equally effectively. Theophylline inhibited soluble phosphodiesterases from brains of
rats of various ages to a similar extent (Schmidt *et al.*, 1970). Morphine
was a weak inhibitor of high K_m phosphodiesterase, but not of low K_m
enzyme in homogenates of rat striatum (Puri *et al.*, 1975).

Certain phosphodiesterase inhibitors possessed quite different inhibitory activity toward the various isolated isozymes (Uzunov *et al.*, 1974;
Weiss *et al.*, 1974). A calcium-dependent phosphodiesterase from rat
cerebrum (peak II, Figure 3) was more strongly inhibited by trifluoperazine

than a calcium-independent phosphodiesterase (peak III), while theophylline and papaverine were more effective as inhibitors of the latter enzyme. Peak I was not significantly inhibited by 25 μM trifluoperazine (Weiss and Greenberg, 1975). Cyclic GMP inhibited both peak II and III enzymes, but was more effective against the calcium-activated peak II phosphodiesterase. Trifluoperazine was much less effective as an inhibitor of unactivated peak II enzyme, and its inhibition of the calcium-activated enzyme was overcome by increasing the concentration of the activator protein. Inhibitions of cyclic AMP hydrolysis by trifluoperazine were mixed in character, while inhibitions by theophylline, papaverine, and cyclic GMP were competitive. The results suggest that trifluoperazine inhibits brain phosphodiesterases in general, but much more effectively inhibits the calcium-dependent phosphodiesterase, through some type of interaction with binding of the activator protein.

The selective inhibition of brain calcium-dependent phosphodiesterases by phenothiazines, such as chlorpromazine and trifluoperazine, was competitive with calcium-activator protein and was not reversed by high concentrations of calcium ions (Levin and Weiss, 1976). Chlorpromazine was about threefold more potent in inhibiting activated hydrolysis of cyclic AMP (IC_{50}, 45 μM) than in inhibiting activated hydrolysis of cyclic GMP (IC_{50}, 140 μM). A variety of antipsychotics selectively and effectively inhibited the calcium-dependent phosphodiesterase: pimozide (IC_{50}, 7 μM), trifluoperazine > thioridazine, chlorprothixene > chlorpromazine, benperidol (dihydrodroperidol). Promethazine, benzodiazepines, such as medazepam and chlordiazepoxide, and tricyclic antidepressants, such as amitriptyline, protriptyline, and desipramine, also selectively inhibited the calcium-dependent enzyme but were much less potent with IC_{50} values from 100 to 300 μM. Theophylline (IC_{50}, 1500 μM) and papaverine (IC_{50}, 130 μM) inhibited both calcium-independent and calcium-activated hydrolysis of cyclic AMP. Fluphenazine competitively inhibited the activation of calcium-dependent cyclic GMP phosphodiesterase by a phospholipid, lysophosphatidyl choline (Wolff and Brostrom, 1976).

Papavarine had the following order of potency an an inhibitor of various cyclic AMP phosphodiesterases from rat cerebrum: peak IV > peak III > peak II (calcium-dependent) > peak I (Weiss, 1975). At low concentrations papaverine was a competitive inhibitor (see above), while at higher concentrations inhibition was noncompetitive. Papaverine and various analogs were somewhat more potent as inhibitors of the particulate high K_m cyclic AMP-phosphodiesterases than of the corresponding soluble enzymes from guinea pig brain (Furlanut et al., 1973). Only benzyl-isoquinolines were effective as inhibitors. The calcium-dependent phosphodiesterase activity with 0.4 μM cyclic GMP as substrate was inhibited most effectively by papaverine and SQ 20009 and least effectively by theophylline (Kakiuchi et al., 1975a,b). Inhibition of the calcium-dependent phosphodiesterase from bovine brain by caffeine was not affected by increasing the concentration of the activator (Lin *et al.*, 1974).

A series of 4-(3,4-dialkoxybenzyl)-2-imidazolidinones have been developed as potent phosphodiesterase inhibitors (Sheppard *et al.*, 1972). The 3-butoxy-4-methoxy-analog (RO 20-1724) has been used extensively. It was an extremely potent inhibitor of erythrocyte phosphodiesterase (IC_{50}, 0.1 μM), but was much less effective with brain phosphodiesterases. The IC_{50} values of RO 20-1724 versus 5 μM cyclic AMP with phosphodiesterases in three Sephadex fractions from dog cerebral cortical homogenates ranged from about 25 to 100 μM. The most effective inhibition was seen with the lowest molecular weight fraction. Interestingly, the inhibitor at 50 μM had little or no effect on the rate of hydrolysis of 5 μM cyclic GMP. Only the two high molecular weight fractions were studied with cyclic GMP. RO 20-1724 and a structurally related dialkoxyphenyl-2-pyrrolidone, ZK 62711, were compared as inhibitors of low K_m cyclic AMP-phosphodiesterase activity from rat cerebral cortex (Schwabe *et al.*, 1976a). At concentrations of 0.1 to 1 μM, ZK 62711 caused substantially more inhibition of soluble calcium-dependent cyclic AMP-phosphodiesterases than did RO 20-1724, but both compounds at 100 μM caused about 50% inhibition. The IC_{50} values for soluble calcium- independent cyclic AMP-phosphodiesterase were for both compounds less than 10 μM, while the IC_{50} values for particulate cyclic AMP-phosphodiesterase activity assayed in the presence of calcium ions and activator protein were about 100 μM. Neither compound was a potent inhibitor of cyclic GMP-phosphodiesterases.

The effects of various inhibitors on two phosphodiesterase preparations from rat cerebral cortex have been investigated with both low and high concentrations of cyclic AMP (Du Moulin and Schultz, 1975). One preparation consisted of the calcium-dependent phosphodiesterase (K_m, 2 μM) isolated by Sephadex chromatography, the other was a relatively crude preparation (K_m, 20 μM) obtained by ammonium sulfate precipitation from homogenates. Isobutylmethylxanthine was a significantly more active inhibitor with the calcium-dependent enzyme than with the crude phosphodiesterase preparation. Isobutylmethylxanthine, papaverine, SQ 66007, diazepam, and chlordiazepoxide were effective inhibitors of the enzymes with IC_{50} values of 100 μM or less, while theophylline, RO 20-1724, and clonazepam (a desmethyl 2'-chloro-7-nitro analog of diazepam) had no inhibitory effect when tested at a 80 μM concentration.

2.3.7 Analogs of Cyclic AMP and Cyclic GMP*

Certain phosphodiesterases of brain appear to hydrolyze both cyclic AMP and cyclic GMP, while other enzymes appear to be more or less

---

*For structures of dibutyryl analogs of cyclic AMP and cyclic GMP see Appendix.

specific for one of the cyclic nucleotides (Drummond and Perrott-Yee, 1961; Drummond *et al.*, 1964a; Cheung, 1967a, 1970, 1971a,b; Brooker *et al.*, 1968; Beavo *et al.*, 1970, 1971; Roberts and Simonsen, 1970; Kakiuchi *et al.*, 1971, 1973; Thompson and Appleman, 1971b,c; Williams *et al.*, 1971; Campbell and Oliver, 1972; Appleman *et al.*, 1973; Goldberg *et al.*, 1973; Dalton *et al.*, 1974). Hydrolysis of cyclic AMP by rat brain phosphodiesterases was either unaffected (Goldberg *et al.*, 1970) or slightly inhibited by cyclic GMP (Harris *et al.*, 1973). The hydrolysis of cyclic AMP by certain phosphodiesterases including particulate low K_m rat brain phosphodiesterase and ganglion phosphodiesterase was, however, stimulated by low concentrations of cyclic GMP (Beavo *et al.*, 1971; Boudreau and Drummond, 1975; Hidaka *et al.*, 1975). Conversely, the hydrolysis of cyclic GMP by rat brain phosphodiesterases was competitively inhibited by cyclic AMP (Goldberg, *et al.*, 1970; Williams, *et al.*, 1971). Hydrolysis of cyclic AMP by mouse brain phosphodiesterases was inhibited by cyclic GMP (Roberts and Simonsen, 1970). Cross inhibition of cyclic AMP and cyclic GMP hydrolysis occurred with human cerebral phosphodiesterases (Hidaka *et al.*, 1975). Cyclic GMP inhibited hydrolysis of cyclic AMP with peak II and peak III phosphodiesterases (see Figure 3) from rat brain (Weiss *et al.*, 1974). The K_i values were 10 and 25 μM, respectively. Cyclic IMP has relatively high activity as both a substrate and inhibitor of brain phosphodiesterases (Campbell and Oliver, 1972; Harris *et al.*, 1973). Cyclic UMP, cyclic CMP, and cyclic TMP have little or no activity as substrates or inhibitors of brain phosphodiesterase. 2′,3′-Cyclic nucleoside phosphates also have virtually no activity.

The activity of a variety of other cyclic nucleotides including the butyryl derivatives of cyclic AMP as substrates and/or inhibitors of brain phosphodiesterases has been reported (Drummond and Powell, 1970; Muneyama *et al.*, 1971; Cehovic, 1972; Meyer *et al.*, 1972; Harris *et al.*, 1973; Jastorff and Bar, 1973; Miller *et al.*, 1973a–c; Shuman *et al.*, 1973; Simon *et al.*, 1973; Sasaki *et al.*, 1976). Based on these studies and data with phosphodiesterases from other tissues, the various analogs can be grouped according to activity as substrates roughly as follows:

High activity (velocity 60 to 120% of that of cyclic AMP): cyclic GMP, cyclic IMP, tubercidin (7-deazaadenosine) cyclic phosphate, toyocomycin (7-cyano-7-deazaadenosine) cyclic phosphate, and 6-thiopurine riboside cyclic phosphate.

Moderate activity (velocity 30 to 60% of that of cyclic AMP): 8-amino, 2′-deoxy, 2′-O-methyl, and 1-alkyloxy cyclic AMPs, sangivamycin (7-deaza-7-carbamoyladenosine) cyclic phosphate, 6-methoxy, and 6-alkylthio purine riboside cyclic phosphates.

Low to no activity (velocity 0 to 30% of that of cyclic AMP): N^6-alkyl, N^6-dialkyl, N^6-alkoxy, 8-bromo, 8-halo, 8-alkylamino, 8-azido, 8-methoxy, 8-hydroxy, 8-thio, 8-alkylthio, 1-methyl, 2-methyl, 2′-O-butyryl, N^6-butyryl, 2′-O,N^6-dibutyryl, and 1,N^6-etheno cyclic AMPs, adenine arabinoside, and xylofuranoside cyclic phosphates, 8-substituted cyclic GMPs.

The various analogs as inhibitors of cyclic AMP-phosphodiesterases can be grouped according to activity roughly as follows:

Potent inhibitor (IC_{50} less than that of theophylline): 8-bromo, 2-methyl-8-alkylthio, and 2'-O-butyryl cyclic AMPs, 8-bromo, 8-alkylthio, and 8-alkylamino cyclic AMPs and IMPs, tubercidin, toyocomycin, and sangivamycin cyclic phosphates.

Moderate inhibitor (IC_{50} comparable to theophylline): 8-methylthio, 8-azido, N^6-alkyloxy, N^6-butyryl, 1-methyl, 1-alkyloxy, $1,N^6$-phenyletheno, 2'-deoxy, and 2'-O-methyl cyclic AMPs.

Weak or no activity: 8-amino, 8-thio, 8-methoxy, and $2'-O,N^6$-dibutyryl cyclic AMPs, adenine arabinoside, and xylofuranoside cyclic phosphates.

Structure–activity correlations for cyclic AMP and cyclic GMP analogs as substrates and inhibitors of mammalian phosphodiesterases have been reviewed (Cehovic *et al.*, 1972; Meyer and Miller, 1974; Amer and Kreighbaum, 1975). The relative activity of these analogs can vary considerably depending on the source of the phosphodiesterase.

2.3.8 Developmental Changes in Brain Phosphodiesterases

The phosphodiesterase activity in brain increased during maturation of rodents (Schmidt *et al.*, 1970; Gaballah and Popoff, 1971a; Weiss, 1971; Weiss *et al.*, 1971; Kauffman *et al.*, 1972; Schmidt and Robison, 1972; Schmidt and Lolley, 1973; Smoake *et al.*, 1973; Weiss and Strada, 1972, 1973; Dewar *et al.*, 1975), although in one study no postnatal change and a prenatal decrease was reported for rats (Hommes and Beere, 1971). Levels of phosphodiesterase were similar in brain of two strains of albino rats, Wistar and Campbell, and increased to similar extents during maturation (Dewar *et al.*, 1975). The latter strain has retinal dystrophy. Levels and development of cyclic AMP-phosphodiesterase were similar in DBA and C3H mice (Schmidt and Lolley, 1972). The latter strain has retinal dystrophy. Phosphodiesterase activity in chick cerebrum increased markedly during development (Nahorski *et al.*, 1976).

Activity of particulate and of soluble phosphodiesterases in rat brain homogenates increased from birth to Day 24 roughly in parallel (Schmidt *et al.*, 1970). High K_m rat brain phosphodiesterase activity in both homogenates and in particulate fractions (synaptosomes, mitochondria) increased at least twofold between 10 and 20 days of age, after which there was little further change (Gaballah and Popoff, 1971a). Differences in developmental patterns of low and high K_m brain phosphodiesterases have been noted in rat (Weiss, 1971; Weiss and Strada, 1972, 1973; Strada *et al.*, 1974). In cerebellum, levels of cyclic AMP-phosphodiesterase were maximal at Day 1 after birth and declined with age due to decreases in both low and high K_m enzymes. Levels in rat cerebrum and brain stem increased to maximal values by about Day 20 after birth with a much greater fold increase for the high K_m enzyme. The profile of phosphodiesterase activity after polyacrylamide gel electrophoresis of cerebral preparations from 1-day-old and adult rats differed markedly. The greatest increase, 20-fold, was in the calcium- dependent phosphodiesterase (peak II of Figure 3) with lesser 5-fold increases in peaks III and IV. Peak I was not detectable in preparations from 1-day-old rats. In rat cerebellum, increases in high and low K_m phosphodiesterases during development were not significant. The profile of phosphodiesterase activity after electrophoresis of cerebellar preparations from 1-day-old rats did not differ markedly from that of adult rats. Peak I was absent and peak II was relatively lower in the preparations from 1-day-old rats. The effect of the activator protein on the various phosphodiesterases from cerebellum was similar in newborn and adult rats; only peak II and to a lesser extent peak VI were activated. Levels of the activator protein appeared lower in cerebellum than in cerebrum or brain stem of newborn rats, while in adults levels had become similar in all three brain regions. Total levels of brain phosphodiesterases increased to a much greater extent than the levels of the calcium-dependent activator protein during development in rats (Smoake *et al.*, 1974). However, even in adult the activator protein appeared to be present in excess in brain homogenates.

2.3.9 Strain Differences in Brain Phosphodiesterases

Wistar and Campbell rats had similar levels of brain phosphodiesterases (Dewar *et al.*, 1975). Levels of cortical and hypothalamic phosphodiesterases were similar in DBA and C3H mice (Schmidt and Lolley, 1972). In both strains levels of the enzyme were significantly higher in cortex than in hypothalamus. Sattin (1974) reported that phosphodiesterase activity measured with either 1 mM cyclic AMP or cyclic GMP in the presence of EGTA was substantially higher in cortical homogenates from C57B1/6J as compared to DBA mice. Enzyme activity in DBA-C57 hybrids was similar to the C57 parent.

2.3.10 Ganglia and Peripheral Neurons

Sympathetic Ganglion

Soluble cyclic AMP and cyclic GMP-phosphodiesterases in homogenates of bovine or canine superior cervical ganglia were only slightly stimulated by calcium ions (Boudreau and Drummond, 1975). Three isozymes were isolated by DEAE-cellulose chromatography. The calcium-dependent activator protein, present in substantial amounts in the ganglia homogenates, remained on the column. The isolated isozymes were inhibited by calcium ions, and this inhibition was reversed by the activator protein. One isozyme was relatively specific for cyclic GMP, while the other two hydrolyzed both cyclic nucleotides; all displayed complex kinetics. Compound 48/80, an agent which causes release of histamine from mast cells, was reported to effectively inhibit cyclic AMP-phosphodiesterases from rat superior cervical ganglia (Lindl *et al.*, 1974).

Retina

Different forms of phosphodiesterases have been reported in mammalian retina, a preparation that includes both photoreceptor, bipolar, and ganglion cells (Pannbacker *et al.*, 1972; Farber and Lolley, 1973; Schmidt and Lolley, 1973). High levels of phosphodiesterase were present in the photosensitive rod outer segments of photoreceptor cells (Pannbacker *et al.*, 1972; Chader *et al.*, 1974). In these studies only a high K_m enzyme was detected. At low substrate concentrations cyclic GMP was hydrolyzed more rapidly than cyclic AMP, The hydrolysis of cyclic AMP and cyclic GMP was not stimulated by calcium ions and was inhibited by various compounds: papaverine > isobutylmethylxanthine > dibutyryl cyclic AMP, theophylline, caffeine, triiodothyronine, ATP. In contrast, others (Coquil *et al.*, 1975) have reported a single K_m for cyclic AMP and complex kinetics for cyclic GMP with phosphodiesterases from bovine rod outer segments. Gel electrophoresis gave evidence for only one enzyme. At low concentrations cyclic AMP stimulated cyclic GMP hydrolysis, but it was inhibitory at higher concentrations. In another study high and low K_m's for cyclic AMP and a high K_m for cyclic GMP were reported (Manthorpe and McConnell, 1975). Calcium-dependent activator protein from rat brain enhanced the activity of phosphodiesterase from bovine rod outer segments (Dumler and Etingof, 1976). A heat-stable inhibitor protein (mol wt 38,000) for phosphodiesterases has been isolated from bovine rod outer segments (Dumler and Etingof, 1976). The inhibitor protein inhibited phosphodiesterases from rod outer segments and rat brain. Inhibition of the phosphodiesterase from rod outer segments was immediate and more effective with cyclic AMP than with cyclic GMP as substrate, and with solubilized rather than membrane phosphodiesterases. There was no effect on the K_m for cyclic AMP. A calcium-dependent activator protein was also isolated from rod outer segments. The inhibitor protein inhibited activated phosphodiesterase more effectively than unactivated enzyme. A light- and ATP-dependent formation of a phosphodiesterase activator in rod outer segments has been described (see Section 4.3.2). Thus, illumination of rod outer segment membranes of *Rana pipiens* resulted in a marked decrease in formation of cyclic AMP due to an activation of phosphodiesterase (Miki et al., 1973). Activation of phosphodiesterase appeared to occur in two steps: (1) light-dependent formation of a trypsin-resistant, heat-labile, nondialyzible macromolecule activator; (2) ATP-dependent activation of phosphodiesterase by this macromolecule. The activator had no effect on phosphodiesterase activity in homogenates from brain or other tissues. It increased the V_{max} but had no effect on the K_m for hydrolysis of cyclic AMP and cyclic GMP by photoreceptor phosphodiesterases. Cyclic GMP was hydrolyzed 33-fold faster than cyclic AMP at 0.1 μM concentrations by the activated phosphodiesterase. Phosphodiesterase inhibitors such as theophylline, iso-butylmethylxanthine, dipyridamole, SQ 20009, and papaverine had similar inhibitory effects on basal and light-activated phosphodiesterases. The phosphodiesterase from frog rod outer segment disc membranes has been solubilized and purified (Miki et al., 1975). The solubilized enzyme (mol wt 240,000) was no longer activated in the presence of ATP by light but was activated by protamine and polylysine. Protamine and heparin activated cyclic GMP-dependent phosphodiesterase from disc membranes, and a model stressing a possible relationship of activation of phosphodiesterase by such polyanions and activation by ATP plus light in rod outer segments was developed (Bitensky et al., 1975). Other nucleotide triphosphates could replace ATP, but α,β-methylene ATP, γ-methylene ATP, and adenylyl imidodiphosphate were ineffective, suggesting that a phosphorylation reaction is involved in ATP-dependent light activation of phosphodiesterase.

Cyclic GMP and high K_m cyclic AMP phosphodiesterase activities developed in retina during maturation of DBA mice, but not in C3H mice, the latter a strain whose photoreceptor cells undergo degeneration (Farber and Lolley, 1973). In DBA mice, the high K_m phosphodiesterase was detected only 6 days after birth and then increased markedly, concommitant with differentiation of the photoreceptor outer segments. In C3H mice, the high K_m phosphodiesterase did not develop and was apparently absent in the retina of adult mice. Levels of phosphodiesterase were nearly fivefold lower in C3H mice. The levels of low K_m cyclic AMP phosphodiesterase were similar in retina of DBA and C3H mice. Gel electrophoresis, followed by histochemical staining for phosphodiesterase with high concentrations of cyclic AMP as substrate demonstrated that retinal homogenates from adult C3H mice contained only one band of enzyme activity, while homogenates from adult DBA mice contained two additional bands. Lack of development of the high K_m phosphodiesterase, which is primarily localized in the photoreceptor cell layer, preceded degeneration of the photoreceptor cells in the C3H strain of mouse. The low K_m phosphodiesterase was present primarily in the inner layers of the retina consisting of bipolar and ganglion cells. Lack of development of the high K_m phosphodiesterase apparently resulted in very high levels of cyclic GMP in the photoreceptor layer of the C3H mouse (Farber and Lolley, 1974). Subsequently, the high levels of cyclic GMP fell precipitously in retina of C3H mice to values below those of DBA mice. This decrease appeared linked to the degeneration and loss of photoreceptor cells in the former strain. Similar data have been obtained with Campbell and Hunter rat strains. In normal retina of adult Wistar (albino) and PVG (pigmented) rats, both low and high K_m phosphodiesterases were present, while in the dystrophic retina of adult Campbell (albino) and Hunter (pigmented) rats only the low K_m enzyme was detected (Dewar *et al,,* 1975). Postnatal increases in retinal phosphodiesterases in retina of Wistar and PVG rats appeared due mainly to increases in the high K_m enzyme. The postnatal increases in retinal phosphodiesterases were greatly decreased in the dystrophic albino strain even before histological evidence for retina degeneration was detectable. In the dystrophic pigmented strain, phosphodiesterase levels did increase markedly during the first 4 weeks after birth and then declined markedly during degeneration of the photoreceptor cell layer. However, in the rats of a Royal College of Surgeons strain, levels of the highest K_m cyclic AMP-phosphodiesterase in the dystrophic retina exceeded those of normal Fischer and Sprague–Dawley rats during degeneration of rod outer segments and then declined below normal levels as photoreceptor cells disappeared (Lolley and Farber, 1975). It was proposed that the debris from rod outer segments containing the high K_m enzyme retained the capacity to hydrolyze cyclic AMP. Two K_m values for cyclic GMP-phosphodiesterase were observed in control and dystrophic retina for the first 2 weeks after birth. During retinal degeneration only a high K_m enzyme was observable. In control retina the high K_m enzyme for cyclic GMP appeared associated with particulate fractions from whole retina and in photoreceptor cells of dissected retina. The low K_m enzyme was soluble and associated with the bipolar and ganglion layer. In dystrophic retina both particulate and soluble enzyme exhibited a high K_m, but after dissection of retina a high K_m enzyme in photoreceptor cells and low K_m enzyme in inner layers were observed. Further data indicated that a heat-labile macromolecular factor from dystrophic retina increased the K_m of the low K_m cyclic GMP phosphodiesterase. It would appear that in the Royal College of Surgeons rat, dystrophy of the retina precedes rather than follows marked changes in levels of phosphodiesterases. In other dystrophic strains the lack of degradation of cyclic nucleotides might be involved in the initiation of degeneration.

In rats in which neonatal treatment with glutamate was used to selectively destroy inner retinal layers, phosphodiesterase activity of the retina was only decreased by 30% (Makman *el at.,* 1975a).

Peripheral Neurons

Soluble phosphodiesterase activity increased above a constriction in the sciatic nerve (Bray et al., 1971). Low K_m cyclic AMP-phosphodiesterases from bovine splenic nerve were inhibited by papaverine, isobutyl-methylxanthine, and cyclic AMP analogs (Cubeddu et al., 1975).

2.3.11 Cultured Cells

Phosphodiesterases were present in homogenates from cultured glioma and neuroblastoma cells (Perkins et al., 1971; Benda et al., 1972; Jard et al., 1972; Schwartz et al., 1973; Uzunov et al., 1973). Both particulate and soluble forms were present in human glioma cells: the soluble enzyme(s) had an apparent K_m of 15 μM (Perkins et al., 1971). A very large proportion of phosphodiesterase activity was associated with the particulate fraction. At least two forms (high and low K_m) were present in rat glioma cells and apparently corresponded to peaks I and IV of rat brain (Uzunov and Weiss, 1973, see Figure 3). Subsequent studies with another rat glioma cell line revealed three phosphodiesterase fractions which corresponded to peaks I, II, and III of rat cerebrum (Uzunov et al., 1974). A soluble calcium-dependent phosphodiesterase has been investigated in homogenates of rat glioma cells (Brostrom and Wolff, 1974). The calcium-binding activator protein had properties identical to those of the activator protein from porcine brain. The degree of activation of cyclic AMP and cyclic GMP-phosphodiesterases with the calcium-binding activator protein did not differ markedly. Mouse neuroblastoma cells appeared to have only one phosphodiesterase which apparently corresponded to peak III of rat brain (Uzunov and Weiss, 1973, 1974, see Figure 3). Another group reported that cyclic AMP and cyclic GMP-phosphodiesterase activities were present in both soluble and particulate fractions from mouse neuroblastoma cells and that the kinetics were compatible with the presence of high and low K_m forms (Kumar et al., 1975; Prasad et al., 1975a). The specific activity of phosphodiesterases, in particular that of cyclic GMP-phosphodiesterases, decreased with increasing protein concentration in the assay of neuroblastoma homogenates.

Low K_m phosphodiesterase activity, but not high K_m activity increased greatly during the culture of rat glioma cells, followed by a marked decrease in both activities when the cells reached confluence (Benda et al., 1972). In glioma–fibroblast hybrid cells both high and low K_m phosphodiesterase activities increased rapidly during culture. Another group reported that phosphodiesterase activity remained fairly constant during culturing of glioma cells (Schwartz *et al.*, 1973). The activity of phosphodiesterases markedly increased during cyclic AMP-dependent differentiation of both glioma and neuroblastoma cells (see Section 4.1.4.). Levels of phosphodiesterase activity in astrocytes and virus-transformed astrocyte cells from newborn hamsters were similar (Weiss *et al.*, 1971).

Theophylline was a weak inhibitor of cyclic AMP phosphodiesterase from a human glioma cell line, while isobutylmethylxanthine and papaverine were potent inhibitors (Clark *et al.*, 1974). Adenosine had little effect on activity of phosphodiesterases from glioma cells (cited in Perkins *et al.*, 1975). Cyclic AMP-phosphodiesterases from mouse neuroblastoma cells were inhibited by dipyridamole > RO 20-1724 > papaverine > medazapam (Dalton *et al.*, 1974). Theophylline was a very weak inhibitor. Imidazole, surprisingly, inhibited the neuroblastoma phosphodiesterase (Kumar *et al.*, 1975). RO 20-1724 inhibited hydrolysis of cyclic AMP, but not cyclic GMP in homogenates of neuroblastoma cells (Prasad *et al.*, 1975a). Papaverine and very high concentrations of theophylline inhibited hydrolysis of both cyclic AMP and cyclic GMP.

2.4 Protein Kinases

Cyclic AMP- and cyclic GMP-dependent protein kinases appear to consist of an inactive complex of regulatory and catalytic units. Binding of cyclic AMP to its regulatory unit dissociates the complex to yield a fully active catalytic unit. A similar mechanism *probably* pertains for cyclic GMP. Activation of cyclic AMP-dependent kinases by cyclic GMP and activation of cyclic GMP-kinases by cyclic AMP can occur, but only at very high concentrations of the "incorrect" cyclic nucleotide. Such cross-activations probably have no physiological significance although activation of cyclic GMP-dependent kinases by cyclic AMP would appear possible. Cyclic nucleotide-dependent protein kinases require magnesium ion for activity and are inhibited by calcium ions. Both soluble and particulate kinases exist, the latter associated in nervous tissue with synaptosomes, microtubules, and nuclei. Substrate profiles, particularly for cyclic AMP-dependent kinases, have been extensively studied. Serine residues and to a lesser extent threonine residues are phosphorylated. Histones are excellent substrates for both cyclic AMP- and cyclic GMP-dependent kinases and have therefore usually been used as substrates for studies with these enzymes. Modulatory proteins exist which appear to inhibit cyclic AMP-dependent kinases and to activate cyclic GMP-dependent kinases. These changes in activity in the presence of modulator proteins reflect changes in substrate profiles for the kinases. Determination of the endogenous substrate or substrates of protein kinases in any particular tissue or cell type remains a difficult task. In many tissues, the cyclic AMP-dependent kinase appears to phosphorylate its own regulatory unit. Studies on intrinsic or autophosphorylation of proteins in membranal preparations by the cyclic AMP-dependent kinases present within such preparations represent one approach to the question of endogenous substrates, but this approach cannot, of course, be used for soluble protein kinases. *In vitro* studies can, however, provide insights into the possible nature of the various endogenous protein substrates whose state of phosphorylation is regulated by cyclic nucleotides in the nervous system. Investigations in intact cells or tissue slices are complicated by high rates of turnover of protein phosphate (see Section 4.5). The field of protein kinases and protein phosphorylation has been recently reviewed (Rubin and Rosen, 1975).

2.4.1 Cyclic AMP-Dependent Kinases

Regional Distribution in Brain

Levels of cyclic AMP-dependent protein kinases in different brain regions have not been studied extensively. Cyclic AMP-dependent kinases presumably occur in most brain regions including cerebral cortex, cerebellum, and hypothalamus (Sold and Hofman, 1974; McKelvy, 1975). Other protein kinases were present in brain which were not activated by cyclic AMP (Walinder, 1972, 1973; Inoue *et al.*, 1973): Both phosvitin and protamine kinases have been described. Phosvitin was an ineffective substrate for cyclic AMP-dependent enzymes.

Subcellular Distribution and Multiplicity of Cyclic AMP-Dependent Protein Kinases

Cyclic AMP-dependent protein kinases were found to be associated in brain homogenates with both soluble protein fractions and particulate fractions (Maeno *et al.*, 1971; Gaballah and Popoff, 1971b; Gaballah *et al.*, 1971, Uno *et al.*, 1976b). High activity was associated with synaptosome fractions, and the major portion of this activity was membrane bound rather than soluble. Only small amounts of the protein kinase activity were associated with nuclei. Protein kinase activity in rat brain particulate fractions could be solubilized and enhanced by treatment with a detergent. Others reported low levels of histone kinase activity in synaptosomal membrane preparations from ox brain and that little kinase activity could be removed from the synaptosomal membranes with detergents (Weller and Rodnight, 1973a). Autophosphorylation of synaptosomal membranes was, however, markedly increased by cyclic AMP (see below). Cyclic

AMP-dependent kinases have been found associated with myelin derived from obligodendroglial cells (Miyamoto and Kakiuchi, 1973; Miyamoto, 1975), with a membranal preparation presumably representing plasma membranes and containing high levels of Na$^+$,K$^+$-ATPase (Dowd and Schwartz, 1975), and with microtubules (Goodman *et al.*, 1970, see below). Protein kinases from nuclei of liver cells catalyzed the phosphorylation of histones and nonhistone chromatin protein (Kish and Kleinsmith, 1974). Phosphorylation of histones was inhibited by cyclic AMP, while phosphorylation of the nonhistones was stimulated by cyclic AMP. Such results are clearly relevant to the mechanism of control of RNA formation by cyclic AMP. Such nuclear protein kinases do not appear to have been investigated in brain tissue.

At least two soluble forms of cyclic AMP-dependent protein kinase, perhaps a monomer and a dimer, appeared to be present in homogenates from rat, guinea pig, and bovine brain (Miyamoto *et al.*, 1971; Inoue *et al.*, 1973; Kuo, 1974). Three to four protein kinases were detected after DEAE-cellulose chromatography of homogenates from rat brain using histone or casein as substrate (Takahashi *et al.*, 1975). Only one of these, the last to emerge, was stimulated by cyclic AMP (Figure 11). Cyclic AMP- and cyclic GMP-dependent protein kinases have been isolated from bovine cerebellum (Takai *et al.*, 1975, Figure 12). A readily dissociated cyclic AMP kinase was the major type in rat brain (Corbin *et al.*, 1975).

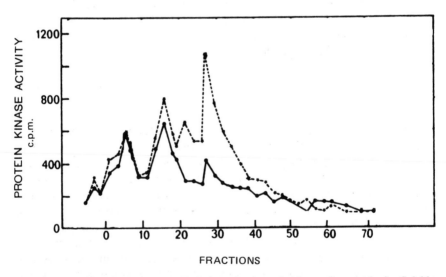

Figure 11. Cyclic AMP-dependent and -independent protein kinases from rat brain. Soluble proteins were fractionated on a DEAE-cellulose column and assayed with 0.2 mM [^{32}P]ATP and histone as cosubstrates in the absence (●———●) and presence of 5 μM cyclic AMP (*-----*). Modified from Takahashi *et al.*, 1975, *Journal of Neurochemistry*, copyright Pergamon Press.)

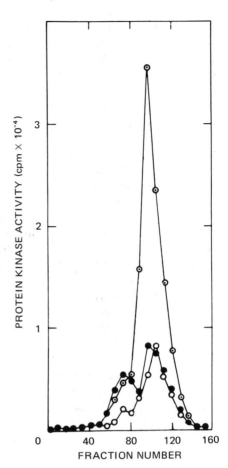

Figure 12. Cyclic AMP- and cyclic GMP-dependent protein kinases from bovine cerebellum. Soluble proteins were fractionated on a DEAE-cellulose column and assayed with [^{32}P]ATP and histone as cosubstrates in the absence of cyclic nucleotide (O——O), the presence of 0.1 μM cyclic AMP (⊙——⊙), or the presence of 0.1 μM cyclic GMP (●——●). (Modified from Takai *et al.*, 1975, *Journal of Biological Chemists,* copyright American Society of Biological Chemists.)

Substrates

Brain protein kinases activated by cyclic AMP have been reported to catalyze the phosphorylation of a variety of protein substrates including histones, protamine, casein, albumin, phosphorylase-b kinase, glycogen synthetase I, acetylcholinesterase, ribosomes, synaptosomes, synaptic vesicles, myelin basic protein, microtubules, and rod outer segments from retina (Drummond *et al.*, 1964b; Goldberg and O'Toole, 1969; Kuo and Greengard, 1969a,b, 1970a,b; Miyamoto *et al.*, 1969a,b, 1971; Goldberg *et al.*, 1970; Gaballah and Popoff, 1971b; Johnson *et al.*, 1971; Maeno *et al.*, 1971; Murray and Froscio, 1971; Schmidt and Robison, 1972; Inoue *et al.*, 1973; Miyamoto and Kakiuchi, 1975; Schmidt and Sokoloff, 1973; Weller and Rodnight, 1973a; Daile *et al.*, 1975; Miyamoto, 1975). Histones represent one of the best substrates for the brain enzymes and have been used in most studies on brain protein kinases. Protamine was a relatively good substrate, while casein was a relatively poor substrate. Phosphorylation of myelin fractions by brain protein kinases was not stimulated by cyclic AMP in contrast to marked stimulation of protein kinase-catalyzed phosphorylation of purified myelin basic protein (Miyamoto and Kakiuchi, 1973). The subcellular distribution of protein kinase substrates in rat cerebral homogenates has been studied (Johnson *et al.*, 1971). Synaptosomal membrane fractions were excellent substrates. The protein kinase substrates were not readily solubilized from these membrane preparations by detergents. A membranal preparation from bovine brain containing high levels of Na^+K^+-ATPase was a substrate for cyclic AMP-dependent protein kinases (Dowd and Schwartz, 1975). Phosphorylase-b kinase was present in rabbit and mouse brain and in dog cerebellum, medulla, spinal cord, diencephalon, cerebral cortex, and pons (Drummond *et al.*, 1964c; Drummond and Bellward, 1970). Levels of this substrate for a cyclic AMP-dependent kinase were at least tenfold lower in brain than levels in skeletal muscle. Levels of phosphorylase b followed a somewhat similar pattern to those of phosphorylase b kinase. Conversion of the glucose-6-phosphate-independent form (I) of glycogen synthetase to the glucose-6-phosphate-dependent form (D) was readily demonstrated with rat brain preparations in the presence of ATP, cyclic AMP, and a phosphodiesterase inhibitor, indicating the presence of a cyclic AMP-dependent glycogen synthetase–I kinase activity in brain (Goldberg *et al.*, 1970).

A purified cyclic AMP-dependent protein kinase from pig brain was highly specific for histones, having virtually no activity with bovine serum albumin, casein, phosphorylase b (kinase) and an RNA polymerase and only low activity with protamine (Nesterova *et al.*, 1975). A cyclic AMP-dependent protein kinase has been isolated from hypothalamus (McKelvy, 1975). Histone was an excellent substrate. Neurosecretory granules from the bovine stalk median eminence of the hypothalamus served as a substrate; they were phosphorylated on four different proteins which did not include the major proteins, neurophysin I and II, of the granules. A thyrotropin-releasing-hormone deamidase from the hypothalamus was a substrate for the enzyme while S-100 protein, nuclei, mitochondria, and synaptosomes were not.

Substrate specificity of soluble and membranal protein kinases from bovine brain and other tissues differed markedly with histone, the more active substrate for soluble enzymes, and protamine, the more active substrate for the particulate enzymes (Uno *et al.*, 1976b).

Protein kinase solubilized from myelin has been studied in detail (Miyamoto, 1975). Phosphorylation of histone by the kinase from myelin was strongly dependent on cyclic AMP, while the phosphorylation of protamine and myelin basic protein was only modestly enhanced by cyclic

AMP. The solubilized protein kinase from myelin differed, therefore, from the major soluble protein kinase of bovine brain in the magnitude of the stimulatory effect of cyclic AMP on phosphorylation of protamine. Cyclic AMP had markedly stimulated protamine phosphorylation with the bovine brain enzyme. Cyclic AMP-dependent phosphorylation of histone by the solubilized myelin protein kinase was markedly inhibited by protein kinase modulator protein.

A protein kinase associated with tubulin from microtubules has been extensively studied (Soifer *et al.*, 1972, 1975; Leterrier *et al.*, 1974a,b; Soifer, 1975; Lagnado *et al.*, 1975). This kinase catalyzed in the absence of cyclic AMP phosphorylation of casein, phosvitin > lysine-rich histones, protamine, and glycogen synthetase I, but did not phosphorylate actin, myosin, troponin, tropomysin, arginine-rich histone, bovine serum albumin, and synaptic vesicle membranes. Cyclic AMP stimulated phosphorylation of histone but not casein or phosvitin. Indeed, the presence of casein prevented cyclic AMP-dependent phosphorylation of histone. 5'-AMP effectively inhibited basal kinase activity towards histone, but not cyclic AMP-dependent phosphorylation. In contrast to soluble brain protein kinases the kinase associated with tubulin was not inhibited by calcium ions. The kinase associated with tubulin was inhibited by a protein factor from muscle. Protamine phosphorylation by the kinase associated with tubulin was reported to be either significantly (Soifer, 1975) or only slightly stimulated by cyclic AMP (Leterrier *et al.*, 1974a,b.) After lyophilization, the phosphorylation of histones by tubulin preparations was no longer stimulated by cyclic AMP. A protein kinase acitivity separated from tubulin preparations by DEAE-Sephadex chromatography showed a somewhat similar profile of substrate activity with phosvitin phosphorylation greatly reduced and cyclic AMP-dependent phosphorylation of protamine greatly increased (Leterrier *et al.*, 1974a). Purification of tubulin by vinblastine precipitation reduced basal and cyclic AMP-dependent kinase to very low levels. An inhibitory effect of magnesium was proposed to represent inactivation of kinase rather than separation of kinase from tubulin. The nature and significance of autophosphorylation of tubulin preparations by this intrinsic protein kinase has been a subject of intense investigation (see below). Phosphorylation of rat brain microtubular protein with brain protein kinase in the presence of cyclic AMP yielded a phosphorylated microtubular protein (Murray and Froscio, 1971). In the presence of heat- and trypsin-sensitive protein(s) contained in brain homogenates, the phosphorylated microtubular protein no longer adsorbed quantitatively to DEAE-Sephadex, indicating that phosphorylation had altered the interaction of microtubular proteins with certain other brain proteins.

Cyclic AMP-dependent protein kinase activity from nerve cords of tobacco hornworms *(Manduca sexta)* has been studied in detail (Albin and

Newburgh, 1975a). In most respects, the characteristics of the enzyme activity were similar to those of enzymes from mammalian brain. However, protamine was a better substrate than histone. The enzyme was inhibited by a sulfhydryl reagent, p-hydroxymercuribenzoate. Cyclic AMP was much more potent than cyclic GMP as an activator of histone phosphorylation with preparations from the insect nerve cords. At least two kinases were present.

The serine residues phosphorylated in lysine-rich histones by cyclic AMP-dependent protein kinase from porcine brain always occurred at a sequence X-Y-Ser, where X is a lysine or arginine residue and Y is either an acidic or neutral residue (Shylapnikov *et al.*, 1975). A synthetic peptide, Gly-Arg-Gly-Leu-Ser-Leu-Ser-Arg, contained as the first six residues a sequence whose serine in myelin basic protein had been phosphorylated (Daile *et al.*, 1975). The peptide proved to be a substrate for bovine brain protein kinase and was phosphorylated on the expected serine residue. Williams (1976) has reviewed the nature of the amino acid residues proximate to phosphorylated serines and threonines in substrates for cyclic AMP-dependent protein kinases. The serine residues phosphorylated in histone by cyclic AMP-dependent protein kinase from bovine cerebellum were not the same residues phosphorylated by a cyclic GMP-dependent protein kinase from the same source as demonstrated by autoradiographic analysis of tryptic digests of the phosphorylated histones (Takai *et al.*, 1975).

A cyclic AMP-dependent disphosphoinositide kinase consisting of a catalytic unit and an inhibitory regulatory unit which binds cyclic AMP has been described (Torda, 1972a,b). The enzyme catalyzes the formation of triphosphoinositide.

Activation and Inhibition

Cyclic AMP-dependent kinases from brain and from other tissues consisted of regulatory units which bind cyclic AMP and the functional catalytic units (Kuo *et al.*, 1970; Miyamoto *et al.*, 1971; Inoue *et al.*, 1973). The relatively inactive complex made up of regulatory and catalytic units was dissociated and thereby activated upon binding of cyclic AMP. The apparent K_m for cyclic AMP was in the order of 0.1 μM or less. Dissociation of the complex by cyclic AMP decreased the K_m of the kinase for ATP by more than tenfold but did not affect the K_m for a protein substrate, histone, or for magnesium ion. The K_m for ATP with the activated kinase was then about 10 μM and the V_{max} of the enzyme was more than doubled upon activation by cyclic AMP. Cyclic AMP dependency could be restored to the catalytic component of brain protein kinase upon addition of regulatory unit isolated from liver. Histones and to a lesser extent other basic proteins appeared to be able to cause dissociation of regulatory and catalytic units of brain protein kinases (Miyamoto *et al.*, 1971; Miyamoto and Kakiuchi, 1973). Such dissociation presumably occurs to some extent during purification of cyclic AMP-dependent protein kinases. Dissociation of certain protein kinase regulatory units required the presence of both cyclic AMP and histone (cf. Rappaport *et al.*, 1976; see p. 72).

Synaptic membrane fractions bound cyclic AMP at 0°C to at least two sites (Weller and Rodnight, 1975a). Low affinity sites were present in great excess. Acetylcholine, norepinephrine, dopamine, adenosine, ATP, AMP, and phosphodiesterase inhibitors had virtually no effect on binding, while high concentrations of cyclic AMP, cyclic IMP, and dibutyryl cyclic AMP inhibited binding at the high affinity site. Presumably, the high affinity binding represented at least in part sites on the regulatory unit of protein kinases.

A cyclic AMP-dependent protein kinase was isolated from pig brain and resolved into regulatory and catalytic subunits with apparent molecular weights of 40,000 and 90,000, respectively (Nesterova *et al.*, 1975). Another group had reported an apparent molecular weight for the regulatory unit of about 49,000 (Maeno *et al.*, 1974). A cyclic AMP-dependent protein kinase from bovine cerebellum had an apparent molecular weight of 180,000 (Takai *et al.*, 1975). A polyacrylamide gel coupled to cyclic AMP was used to separate bovine brain protein kinase regulatory and catalytic units (Rieke *et al.*, 1975). The regulatory unit could be partially recovered from the gel during incubation with 1 mM cyclic AMP,

Bovine brain cyclic AMP-dependent protein kinase was relatively insensitive to ethoxyformic anhydride inactivation in the absence of cyclic AMP (Witt and Roskoski, 1975). Dissociation of the regulatory unit by cyclic AMP rendered the enzyme sensitive to the anhydride. Magnesium ATP protected the enzyme. The results suggested that the catalytic site of the enzyme was protected when combined with the regulatory unit.

Cyclic AMP-dependent protein kinases from brain required magnesium or manganese ions and were inhibited by calcium ions, ADP, AMP, GDP, adenosine, and 2'-deoxyadenosine (Kuo and Greengard, 1969a; Miyamoto *et al.*, 1969b; Kuo *et al.*, 1970). Cobalt ions activated the enzyme. Concentrations of magnesium ions of 5 to 10 mM were required for maximal activity. In the presence of 2.5 mM calcium ions cyclic AMP inhibited the kinase. No effective inhibitors of the enzyme have been developed, but of course a chelating agent such as EDTA could completely block enzyme activity by removing the essential divalent cation. Adenosine and AMP at 50 μM were relatively ineffective as inhibitors of cyclic AMP activation of bovine brain protein kinase; ADP was somewhat more effective, and FMN even more effective. Indeed, cyclic AMP (5 μM) inhibited brain protein kinase in the presence of 50 μM FMN. The efficacy of the inhibitors versus cyclic AMP activation of kinases was dependent upon the tissue source of the kinase. At high concentrations cyclic AMP inhibited protein kinases apparently due to competition with ATP at the catalytic site (Miyamoto 1969; Donnelly *et al.*, 1973a). Sulfhydryl reagents were relatively ineffective inhibitors, but inhibition of a purified cyclic AMP-dependent enzyme from bovine cerebellum by sulfhydryl reagents has been described (Takai *et al.*, 1975). A cyclic AMP-dependent protein kinase isolated from hypothalamus was partially inhibited by 100 μM serotonin, dopamine, and norepinephrine (McKelvy, 1975). Hypothalamic releasing hormones and pituitary hormones had no effect on the kinase.

The cyclic AMP-dependent protein kinase from bovine brain has been shown to catalyze the phosphorylation of its own regulatory subunit (mol wt 48,000) (Maeno *et al.*, 1974). Cyclic AMP strongly inhibited the phosphorylation of the regulatory unit in the presence of zinc, calcium, nickel, or ferrous ions. In the presence of only magnesium or cobalt ions, cyclic AMP had no effect on phosphorylation of the subunit. The phosphorylated regulatory subunit had electrophoretic properties identical to a protein (see below) phosphorylated in synaptic membrane fractions in the presence of cyclic AMP. Phosphorylation of the regulatory unit of protein kinase from heart muscle facilitated cyclic AMP-dependent dissociation of regulatory and catalytic units (Ehrlichman *et al.*, 1974).

Adenylate cyclase-catalyzed formation of cyclic AMP in liver and other tissues was apparently accompanied by the formation of a compound which noncompetitively inhibited kinase-catalyzed activation of phosphorylase b by cyclic AMP (Murad *et al.*, 1969). The inhibitor was very similar in chromatographic properties to cyclic AMP and was inactivated by incubation with phosphodiesterase. Agents which increased cyclase-catalyzed formation of cyclic AMP also increased the formation of the inhibitor. High levels of the inhibitor appeared to be present in acid extracts of rat brain. The cyclic AMP antagonist isolated from liver inhibited cyclic AMP-dependent protein kinase from brain, and this inhibition could be overcome by cyclic AMP (Wasner, 1975).

Further activation of phosphorylase-b kinase did not occur in brain homogenates in the presence of cyclic AMP (Rall and Gilman, 1970), suggesting that this substrate of a cyclic AMP-dependent kinase was already phosphorylated. Further activation of phosphorylase-b kinase did occur with calcium (Drummond and Bellward, 1970). The activation by calcium was increased in the presence of activating factor isolated from skeletal muscle and was blocked by an inhibitory factor isolated from bovine heart. The activating factor has been isolated from brain and shown to be a calcium-activated proteinase which activates phosphorylase-b kinase by a proteolytic process (Drummond and Duncan, 1968). The inhibitory factor inhibited the proteinase activity of the activating factor. The physiological significance of this type of calcium-dependent activation of an enzyme important to metabolism in brain is not certain. Relatively low concentrations of calcium (EC_{50} 10 μM) were subsequently reported to activate brain phosphorylase-b kinase (Ozawa, 1973). The data are indicative of a possible independent control of physiological processes by cyclic AMP and calcium ions (cf. Rasmussen, 1970; Rasmussen and Goodman, 1975; Berridge, 1975).

A stable protein factor isolated from muscle inhibited cyclic AMP-dependent protein kinases (Walsh *et al.*, 1971). The protein inhibitor (mol wt 26,000) did not appear to bind cyclic AMP. The inhibitor was detected in highest amounts in brain and muscle and has been isolated from rat brain (Rappaport *et al.*, 1976). The mechanism of action of this inhibitor was not resolved. Inhibition was noncompetitive with ATP, protein substrate, or cyclic AMP and was accompanied by an apparent increase in the affinity of cyclic AMP for the regulatory unit of the kinase. This inhibitor would appear identical with inhibitory protein kinase modulators. In 1973, protein kinase modulator proteins from brain were found to inhibit cyclic AMP-dependent protein kinases and to activate cyclic GMP-dependent kinases (Donnelly *et al.*, 1973a,b). Similar modulator proteins have been isolated from a variety of sources. The kinase modulator protein from lobster tail muscle inhibited the phosphorylation of histone, catalyzed by the catalytic subunit of cyclic AMP-dependent protein kinase from bovine brain, but stimulated phosphorylation of protamine. Similarly, the modulator protein could either inhibit or stimulate cyclic GMP-dependent protein kinases, depending on the substrate. The effects of the modulator would thus appear to be due to interaction with the catalytic subunit of protein kinases, thereby changing the kinase activity with respect to various protein substrates (Kuo, 1975b). The affinity of ATP for the catalytic unit of cyclic AMP-dependent brain protein kinase was not altered by the modulator, while the apparent increase in binding of cyclic AMP to the corresponding holoenzyme in the presence of modulator was proposed to be due to modulator binding to the catalytic unit and thereby promoting dissociation of the regulatory unit. The protein kinase modulator from mammalian tissues including brain was separated by Sephadex chromatography into a "stimulatory" and an "inhibitory" modulator (Kuo *et al.*, 1976a,b). This is in contrast to the modulator from lobster tail muscle in which stimulatory and inhibitory activity appeared to reside in one protein. The mammalian "stimulatory" modulator stimulated cyclic GMP-dependent kinases and had no effect on cyclic AMP-dependent kinases. The "inhibitory" modulator inhibited cyclic AMP-dependent kinases, while having no effect on cyclic GMP-dependent kinases. Both "inhibitory" and "stimulatory" modulators appeared to be present in nearly equivalent amounts in brain.

Activation by Analogs of Cyclic AMP

The activation of brain cyclic AMP-dependent protein kinases by various analogs of cyclic AMP has been extensively studied (Miyamoto *et al.*, 1969b; Kuo and Greengard, 1970a; Kuo *et al.*, 1970; Bauer *et al.*, 1971; Muneyama *et al.*, 1971; Meyer *et al.*, 1972, 1973, 1975a,b; Jones *et al.*, 1973b; Miller *et al.*, 1973a,b,c, 1976a; Shuman *et al.*, 1973; Simon *et al.*, 1973; Kuo *et al.*, 1974; Miyamoto, 1974; Christensen *et al.*, 1975; Khwaja *et al.*, 1975; Panitz *et al.*, 1975; Severin *et al.*, 1975; Uno *et al.*, 1976a). Structure-activity correlations for activation of cyclic AMP (brain)- and cyclic GMP (lobster tail)-dependent protein kinases have been reviewed (Simon *et al.*, 1973; Meyer and Miller, 1974). Cyclic GMP activated the cyclic AMP-dependent kinases, but only at very high concentrations. Cyclic IMP was somewhat more potent than cyclic GMP, while other "natural" cyclic nucleotides were virtually inactive (Kuo *et al.*, 1970). Analogs of cyclic GMP and cyclic IMP were also relatively inactive with cyclic AMP-dependent kinases. The various analogs of cyclic AMP as activators of cyclic AMP-dependent protein kinases from brain can be grouped according to activity roughly as follows:

Potent activators (potency 2- to 18-fold greater than cyclic AMP): 8-(*p*-chlorophenylthio) > > 8-thio, 8-hydroxy > 8-benzylthio, 8-bromo, 2-methyl-8-bromo, 8-chloro, 8-methylthio, 8-amino, 2-methyl-8-(*p*-chlorophenylthio), 1,N^6-phenyletheno cyclic AMPs.

Moderate activators (potency from 0.5- to 1.5-fold that of cyclic AMP): 2-*n*-octyl, 2-styryl cyclic AMPs, 6-alkylthio purine riboside cyclic phosphate, tubercidin cyclic phosphate > cyclic AMP, 2-methyl-8-benzylthio > 8-alkylamino, 8-dialkylamino, 8-azido, 2-methyl-8-azido, 8-iodo, N^6-butyryl, N^6-hydroxy, N^6-alkoxy, N^6-alkyl, 1,N^6-etheno cyclic AMPs, 6-methoxy purine riboside cyclic phosphate, toyocomycin cyclic phosphate, 2-trifluoromethyl, 2-benzylthio cyclic AMPs, 8-(*p*-chlorophenyl)inosine cyclic phosphate.

Low activators (potency less than about one half that of cyclic AMP): cyclic IMP, various 2-substituted analogs, such as 2-chloro, 2-thio, 2-hydroxy, 2-methylthio, 2-alkyl cyclic AMPs, sangivamycin cyclic phosphate, 1-alkoxy, 1-alkyl cyclic AMPs, and the 5'-thio analog of cyclic AMP.

A 2'-hydroxy group in the ribose configuration was required for activation of bovine brain protein kinase (Miller *et al.*, 1973c, Khwaja *et al.*, 1975). Thus, dibutyryl cyclic AMP is inactive. Isosteres of cyclic AMP in which the 3'- or 5'-oxygen was replaced by NH or by CH_2 had very low activity towards brain protein kinase (Panitz *et al.*, 1975). Relative activities of analogs as activators of brain protein kinases have varied somewhat in different studies. In one study with bovine brain protein kinase the activities of various cyclic AMP derivatives were as follows: 8-hydroxy > 8-amino, 8-thio, 8-methylthio > cyclic AMP > 8-benzylamino > cyclic IMP (Kuo *et al.*, 1974). In the presence of the kinase modulator protein the stimulation by the cyclic AMP derivatives was inhibited. The potency of various compounds in activating the kinase paralleled their ability to dissociate the regulatory and catalytic subunits. The inability of the potent 8-substituted analogs to effectively compete against binding of radioactive cyclic AMP to bovine brain kinase was suggestive of multiple binding sites, one with a high affinity for cyclic AMP and another with high affinity for 8-subsituted analogs. Indeed, 8-thio and 8-methylthio cyclic AMP actually potentiated rather than decreased the binding of radioactive cyclic AMP to bovine brain cyclic AMP-dependent protein kinase. The regulatory subunit of bovine brain cyclic AMP-dependent protein kinase was selectively labeled upon irradiation with [^{32}P]-8-azido cyclic AMP (Pomerantz *et al.*, 1975). An excess of cyclic AMP virtually completely prevented the photoaffinity labeling.

Autophosphorylation of Membrane Proteins

A cyclic AMP-elicited increase in rates of autophosphorylation of membrane proteins by ATP occurred with synaptosomes, microtubule fractions, and certain microsomal preparations from brain, but not with synaptic vesicles or myelin fractions from brain or with membranes from peripheral crab nerves (Goodman *et al.*, 1970; Weller and Rodnight 1970, 1973a,b; Johnson *et al.*, 1971; Schmidt and Robison, 1972; Miyamoto and Kakiuchi, 1973; Schmidt and Sokoloff, 1973; Miyamoto, 1976). Cyclic AMP or various analogs did not potentiate intrinsic phosphorylation of rat brain myelin fractions but fluoride did, perhaps by inhibition of phosphatases (Miyamoto and Kakiuchi, 1973; Miyamoto, 1975). Autophosphorylation occurred exclusively on myelin basic protein. Cyclic AMP did activate phosphorylation of histone by protein kinases of myelin. A solubilized membranal preparation from bovine brain containing high levels of Na$^+$,K$^+$-ATPase was autophosphorylated by an intrinsic cyclic AMP-dependent protein kinase (Dowd and Schwartz, 1975). ATPase activity was less stable in this preparation than the protein kinase activity.

Cyclic AMP-dependent autophosphorylation of synaptosomal preparations has been studied extensively. Phosphorylation of two minor protein components of a rat cerebral synaptic membrane preparation was greatly increased by cyclic AMP (Johnson *et al.*, 1973; Ueda *et al.*, 1973; Maeno *et al.*, 1975; Malkinson *et al.*, 1975). These proteins had apparent molecular weights of 86,000 (protein I) and 49,000 (protein II) on gel electrophoresis (Figure 13). Protein I appeared unique to synaptic membranes, while protein II has been proposed to be identical with the regulatory subunit of cyclic AMP-dependent protein kinases. Maximal labeling of both proteins occurred very rapidly (<10 sec), both in the presence and absence of cyclic AMP. Radioactivity associated with protein I then remained elevated, while radioactivity associated with protein II returned within 2 min in the presence of cyclic AMP nearly to the levels seen in the absence of cyclic AMP. Rapid turnover of membrane phosphoproteins including protein I was clearly indicated by a rapid disappearance of all labeled protein bands

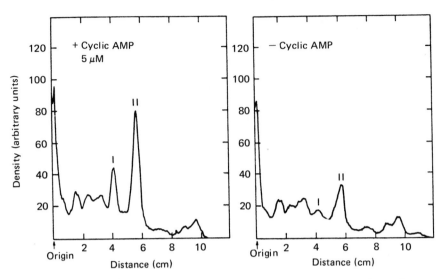

Figure 13. Cyclic AMP-dependent autophosphorylation of rat cerebral synaptic membranes. After a preincubation for 1 min, a membranal fraction was phosphorylated for 15 sec with 5 μM [^{32}P]ATP at pH 6. After treatment with sodium dodecylsulfate proteins were separated by polyacrylamide gel electrophoresis. Autoradiograms were scanned with a densitometer. (Modified from Ueda *et al.*, 1973, *Journal of Biological Chemistry*, copyright American Society of Biological Chemists.)

if the radioactive ATP was diluted with an excess of nonradioactive ATP after a 1-min incubation. High concentrations of cyclic IMP enhanced phosphorylation of both proteins, while high concentrations of cyclic GMP elicited a slight stimulation of phosphorylation of protein I. Magnesium ions were present in all incubations but could be replaced by manganese or cobalt. Replacement with zinc led to a stimulation of phosphorylation of proteins I and II in the absence of cyclic AMP. Cyclic AMP in the presence of zinc had no effect on phosphorylation of protein I and inhibited the phosphorylation of protein II. Calcium ion also prevented the stimulatory effect of cyclic AMP. Both zinc and calcium inhibit cyclic AMP-dependent protein kinases. Zinc ions also inhibit protein phosphatases (see Section 2.5). Adenosine, an inhibitor of cyclic AMP-dependent protein kinase, inhibited phosphorylation of proteins I and II as did adenine and AMP. ADP, an effective inhibitor of cyclic AMP-dependent protein kinase, was relatively ineffective in inhibiting phosphorylation of the two membrane components. The chelating agent, EDTA, blocked cyclic AMP-dependent phosphorylation. Cyclic AMP stimulated both phosphorylation and dephosphorylation of protein II. Addition of the regulatory unit of protein kinase to the synaptosomal membrane system did not inhibit phosphorylation of proteins I and II. Fluoride potentiated phosphorylation of both proteins probably due to the inhibition of ATPases and protein phosphatases by fluoride in the membrane preparation. The results are clearly consonant with a cyclic AMP-dependent activation of phosphorylation of two neuronal membrane proteins. Synaptosomal membrane fractions from rat, bovine, and turkey cerebrum, and from rat, bovine, human, and pig cerebral cortex gave similar results. With synaptosomal membrane fraction from rat cerebellum, the phosphorylation of protein I, but not that of protein II, was stimulated by cyclic AMP. With synaptosomal membrane fractions from rat caudate nucleus, incorporation of phosphate was much lower: phosphorylation of protein I was enhanced by cyclic AMP, while phosphorylation of protein II was inhibited by cyclic AMP. In a subsequent study with preparations from rat caudate nucleus cyclic AMP stimulated phosphorylation of three proteins with apparent molecular weights of 85,000, 80,000, and 49,000 (Krueger *et al.,* 1975). The two higher molecular weight proteins were present only in the subcellular fractions from caudate nucleus that contained synaptic membranes, i.e., the same fractions that contained dopamine-sensitive adenylate cyclases. Cyclic AMP-dependent phosphorylation of the lower molecular weight protein, presumably protein II, was observed in all subcellular fractions from caudate nucleus. Nonsynaptosomal membrane fractions from brain, membrane fractions from lingual nerves, and membrane fractions from liver, lung, kidney, and spleen showed minimal autophosphorylation (Johnson *et al.,* 1973; Malkinson *et al.,* 1975). Membranes from heart, kidney, and vas deferens and other tissues did exhibit a cyclic AMP-dependent phosphorylation of a protein corresponding to protein II, presumably the regulatory unit of cyclic AMP-dependent protein kinases.

Endogenous phosphorylation of brain soluble fraction led to one major phosphorylated protein with an apparent molecular weight of 49,000, presumably protein II (Malkinson, 1975). In the presence of magnesium ions, cyclic AMP stimulated phosphorylation of this protein. In the presence of calcium ions, cyclic AMP (10 μM) inhibited and cyclic GMP stimulated phosphorylation of this protein. At lower concentrations cyclic AMP stimulated phosphorylation even in the presence of calcium ions. In the presence of zinc, even 0.5 μM cyclic AMP was inhibitory. With detergent-solubilized preparations from synaptic membranes, cyclic AMP-dependent phosphorylation of protein II was detected along with minor phosphorylation of certain other proteins (Ueda *et al.,* 1975). Zinc ions stimulated phosphorylation of protein II, and cyclic AMP was inhibitory in the presence of zinc. With ammonium chloride-solubilized preparations, cyclic AMP inhibited phosphorylation of protein II both in the presence and absence of zinc ions. Cyclic AMP stimulated phosphorylation of protein I in ammonium chloride preparations. The dephosphorylation of protein II in solubilized preparations was stimulated by cyclic AMP. Analysis of kinetic data led to the proposal that a protein kinase, a protein phosphatase, and protein II exist as a complex in solubilized preparations from synaptic membranes. These three constituents were separable by ion-exchange chromatography (cited in Ueda *et al.*, 1975). It was suggested that protein II represents the regulatory component of cyclic AMP-dependent protein kinase. The nature and function of protein I, which appears to be an entity unique to synaptosomal membranes remains as yet undefined. Protein I has been solubilized and purified from bovine brain (cited in Greengard, 1976). Levels of protein I were very low in cerebrum of neonatal rats and increased "sharply" at 2–3 weeks of age, a time at which synapses increase markedly.

Another group using a different gel system detected three synaptosome membrane proteins whose phosphorylation was stimulated by cyclic AMP (Ehrlich and Routtenberg, 1974). In the absence of cyclic AMP, incorporation of radioactive phosphate from ATP was quite high and reached a maximum within 20 sec, falling to relatively low levels within 15 min. In the presence of cyclic AMP the time course was similar for all three proteins, and stimulation of net phosphorylation by cyclic AMP reached a maximum within 2 min. Net phosphorylation of protein I and II was still enhanced by cyclic AMP after 30 min of incubation. Further studies detected a total of four proteins in a synaptic membrane fraction from rat cerebral cortex whose phosphorylation was stimulated by cyclic AMP (Routtenberg and Ehrlich, 1975, Figure 14). Protein D (mol wt 83,000) appeared to correspond to protein I, and protein E (mol wt 53,000) to protein II. Autophosphorylation of protein F (mol wt 47,000) and protein G (mol wt 34,000) was also clearly stimulated by cyclic AMP. Protein H (mol wt 10,000–18,000) was prominent in myelin fractions, while proteins D to G were more prominent in synaptic membrane fractions. Rates of phosphorylation and dephosphorylation of proteins D,E, F, and G were influenced by cyclic AMP, zinc ions, and concentrations of magnesium and ATP. Cyclic GMP inhibited phosphorylation of protein E.

A third group has reported cyclic AMP-dependent autophosphorylation of three proteins in synaptosomal membranes (Weller and Morgan, 1976). A phosphorylated protein corresponding to protein I (mol wt 83,000) and a somewhat higher molecular weight phosphorylated protein appeared concentrated in the fractions from synaptosomes which were enriched in membranes of synaptic junctions, while a phosphorylated protein corresponding to protein II appeared concentrated in residual membrane fractions derived from synaptosomes.

Stimulation of autophosphorylation of microsomal and synaptosomal membrane fractions by cyclic AMP was greatest during short incubations (Weller and Rodnight, 1973b), suggesting that cyclic AMP-dependent autophosphorylation occurred rapidly at a limited number of serine residues,

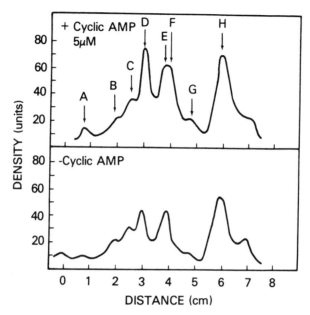

Figure 14. Cyclic AMP-dependent autophosphorylation of rat cerebral cortical synaptic membranes. After a preincubation for 2 min a membranal fraction was phosphorylated for 2 min with 7.5 μM [^{32}P]ATP at pH 6.5. After treatment with sodium dodecylsulfate, proteins were separated by polyacrylamide gel electrophoresis. Autoradiograms were scanned with a densitometer. (Modified from Routtenberg and Ehrlich, 1975, *Brain Research*, copyright Elsevier Publishing Co.)

while cyclic AMP-independent phosphorylation occurred more slowly, but at a much greater number of sites. Partial dephosphorylation of membranes enhanced the stimulatory effect of cyclic AMP but had no stimulatory effect on basal rates of phosphorylation. Turnover rates of phosphoserine residues were obviously influenced by both cyclic AMP-dependent and -independent kinases and by phosphatases. Certain membrane preparations contained cyclic AMP and/or adenylate cyclases capable of generating cyclic AMP under the conditions of assay (Weller and Rodnight, 1971, 1974; Weller *et al.*, 1972). The contribution of endogenous cyclic AMP to basal rates of autophosphorylation was, however, not clear. In microsomal and synaptosomal preparations, agents which might have increased intrinsic rates of cyclic AMP formation, such as biogenic amines, adenosine, prostaglandins, fluoride ions, theophylline, and papaverine, did not increase basal rates of autophosphorylation. Theophylline was actually inhibitory. Fluoride was stimulatory, but only in the presence of theophylline. Theophylline, adenosine, calcium ions, and certain other agents significantly inhibited autophosphorylation of synaptosomal membranes measured in the presence of cyclic AMP. Radioactive phosphate was incorporated into a tubulin-like component of pig cerebellar synaptic membranes (Lagnado et al., 1975). Cyclic AMP increased total incorporation of phosphate into proteins of synaptic membranes twofold but had no effect on phosphorylation of the tubulin-like component.

Cyclic AMP-elicited increases in autophosphorylation of synaptic membranes were stated to be markedly decreased in preparations from electrically shocked animals (Appel and Locher, 1973). Passive avoidance training of rats was stated to result in increased rates of incorporation of phosphate into protein F (Figure 14) of synaptosomal membrane preparations from temporal cortex and caudate nucleus, but not in preparations from cerebral cortex (Routtenberg et al., 1975).

Exogenous cyclic AMP-dependent protein kinase, cyclic AMP, and ATP were required for release of calcium-dependent phosphodiesterase activator protein from membrane fractions of rat brain (Gnegy et al., 1976a). The activator protein was not a substrate for the kinase, nor could in vivo incorporation of radioactive phosphate of intraventricular ATP into activator protein be demonstrated. It appeared probable that cyclic AMP-dependent phosphorylation of a membrane protein results in release of the activator protein from synaptosomal membranes. Cyclic AMP-dependent autophosphorylation of synaptosomal membrane fractions from rat striatum resulted in release of the calcium-dependent activator protein for phosphodiesterases into the cytoplasm (Gnegy et al., 1976b).

The autophosphorylation of microtubule protein by an associated protein kinase has been extensively studied (Goodman et al., 1970; Rappaport et al., 1972; 1975; Soifer et al., 1972, 1975; Eipper, 1974a,b; Leterrier et al., 1974a,b; Lagnado et al., 1975; Sloboda et al., 1975; Soifer, 1975; Rappaport et al., 1976). The objectives have been to determine (1) whether the kinase can be separated from tubulin, the major microtubular protein, (2) the nature of the proteins phosphorylated in tubulin preparations, and (3) the dependency of the phosphorylation on cyclic AMP.

Some workers have reported that a variety of different purification procedures did not remove the intrinsic protein kinase activity from tubulin (Sloboda et al., 1975; Soifer, 1975; Soifer et al,, 1975). However, a separation of tubulin and the associated kinase appeared to pertain on DEAE-cellulose chromatography (Leterrier et al., 1974; Rappaport et al., 1975) or on Sepharose chromatography (Shigekawa and Olsen, 1975). The kinase appeared to have a molecular weight based on Sepharose chromatography of about 280,000. A partial separation was also reported after sucrose gradient centrifugation (Leterrier et al., 1974a). Eipper (1974a,b) reported that the kinase could not be completely separated from rat brain tubulin aggregates, but that tubulin dimer could be isolated without an associated kinase. Recently, separation of cyclic AMP-dependent protein kinase from tubulin has been confirmed with chromatographic and ultra-centrifuge techniques (Rappaport *et al.* 1976). Both cyclic AMP and histone were required for dissociation of the regulatory and catalytic units of the separated kinase.

Cyclic AMP stimulated the autophosphorylation of purified brain tubulin, and a major portion of ^{32}P-radioactivity was associated with the tubulin band after disc gel electrophoresis (Rappaport *et al.*, 1972). However, the ^{32}P-labeled protein clearly separated from colchicine tubulin after ultracentrifugation. The results suggested that autophosphorylation of tubulin had not occurred, but that instead minor protein constituents had been phosphorylated. Microtubules from mouse brain contained a cyclic AMP-dependent protein kinase (Shigekawa and Olsen, 1975). Tubulin dimers and aggregates served as substrate for this cyclic AMP-dependent protein kinase, but the extent of phosphorylation was very low at about 0.1 mol of phosphate/mol of tubulin. Autophosphorylation of tubulin appeared to occur with nearly equal labeling of the two chains, α and β, of the protein (Leterrier *et al.*, 1974a,b; Lagnado *et al.*, 1975), but most of the phosphorylated protein appeared to remain aggregated on sucrose gradient centrifugation and separated from less highly labeled tubulin subunits and their associated protein kinase. Under the phosphorylation conditions only 8% of the tubulin molecules had incorporated one phosphate moiety. Similar results were reported by Eipper (1974a,b) with a rat brain tubulin preparation whose intrinsic kinase activity was independent of cyclic AMP. Another group (Sloboda *et al.*, 1975) presented evidence with chick brain microtubules that one of two high molecular weight proteins which copurify as minor constituents with tubulin during assembly–disassembly of microtubules was the preferred substrate for the cyclic AMP-dependent protein kinase associated with microtubules. Cyclic AMP-dependent autophosphorylation of tubulin was also detected, but this occurred at only a minute fraction of the rate of phosphorylation of the microtubule-associated protein. It would certainly appear that minor constituents of purified tubulin preparations undergo phosphorylation and can continue to copolymerize with tubulin. The significance of this phosphorylation is unknown, but phosphorylation did appear to alter interactions of microtubular proteins with certain other brain proteins (see above, Murray and Froscio, 1971). The effect of cyclic AMP-dependent phosphorylation of rat brain microtubular protein on the chromatographic properties of an associated phospholipase has been studied (Quinn, 1973). Recent data have confirmed that tubulin was not autophosphorylated, but that cyclic AMP did stimulate the phosphorylation of minor high molecular components of tubulin preparations (Rappaport *et al.*, 1976). These phosphorylated components copolymerize with tubulin. However, neither the rate nor extent of polymerization was influenced by the presence of ATP–cyclic-AMP or by the presence of a thermostable inhibitor of protein kinases (cf. Walsh *et al.*, 1971) which nearly completely inhibited basal and cyclic AMP-stimulated autophosphorylation of tubulin preparations.

The autophosphorylation of tubulin preparations has been reported by the various groups to be either independent of cyclic AMP or to be stimulated by cyclic AMP (see above). Manganese ions inhibited the kinase, while calcium ions had no effect. Vinblastine and vincristine which can cause polyaggregation of tubulin *in vitro* enhanced cyclic AMP-activated autophosphorylation of tubulin preparations (Lagnado *et al.*, 1975). Colchicine had no effect. AMP inhibited autophosphorylation.

Developmental Aspects

Levels of cyclic AMP-dependent protein kinases in rat brain appeared to decrease slightly during postnatal development (Gaballah *et al.*, 1971; Schmidt and Robison, 1972; Schmidt and Sokoloff, 1973; Takahashi *et al.*, 1975). With histone as a substrate, activity of protein kinases in both the presence and absence of cyclic AMP was found to double in rat brain during the first 21 days after birth (Gaballah *et al.*, 1971). However, the degree of activation of kinases by cyclic AMP (cyclic AMP-dependent activity) did not increase significantly for total, particulate, or soluble fractions. Indeed, especially with the soluble fraction, there appeared to be a decrease during maturation in the percent activation of kinase by cyclic AMP. Others (Schmidt and Sokoloff, 1973; Schmidt and Robison, 1972) found no significant changes in histone kinase activity, either in the presence or absence of cyclic AMP, when comparing microsomal preparations from newborn and 30-day-old rats. The percent activation of histone phosphorylation by cyclic AMP decreased during maturation. The decrease in the degree of activation of kinases by cyclic AMP during the development of rats might be a reflection of greater basal activation due to higher endogenous levels of cyclic AMP in older rats. Development of protein kinase activity with histone and casein as substrates was studied in rats from 5 to 30 days of age (Takahashi *et al.*, 1975). Basal levels of "histone kinase" activity increased with age, while cyclic AMP-dependent activity decreased. "Casein kinase" activity remained unaltered during development. Binding of radioactive cyclic AMP to homogenates, presumably at least in part to kinase regulatory protein, decreased with age. Thus, in contrast to other components of the cyclic AMP system, marked developmental changes in overall kinase activity did not appear to occur in brain. The ability of rat brain ribosomes to serve as substrates for a partially purified adult rat brain protein kinase did not change during postnatal development (Schmidt and Sokoloff, 1973). Cyclic AMP-dependent autophosphorylation of a partially purified protein kinase preparation from rat brain did increase during maturation (Schmidt and Robison, 1972).

Ganglia and Peripheral Neurons

Modest levels of phosphorylase-b kinase were present in superior cervical and stellate ganglia, while very low levels were detected in ganglia lacking synapses, the nodose ganglion, and in spinal and peripheral nerves (Drummond and Bellward, 1970). Levels of phosphorylase b followed a similar pattern. Cyclic nucleotide-dependent kinases have been reported in homogenates of bovine retina (Brown and Makman, 1972). Rod outer segments contained protein kinases which catalyzed phosphorylation of histones (Kuhn *et al.*, 1973; Pannbacker and Schoch, 1973; Frank and Bensinger, 1974). The data were contradictory as to whether histone phosphorylation by these kinases was stimulated by cyclic AMP. Phosphorylation of rhodopsin and protamine did not appear to be stimulated by cyclic AMP. Both GTP and ATP phosphorylated rhodopsin in rod outer segments, and both kinase-catalyzed reactions were stimulated by light (Chader *et al.*, 1976). Cyclic AMP, adenosine, AMP, and ATP had marked inhibitory effects on phosphorylation by GTP.

Cultured Cells

Cyclic AMP-activated protein kinases have been reported from glioma cells (Perkins *et al.*, 1971; Benda *et al.*, 1972; Jard *et al.*, 1972; Opler and Makman, 1972) and neuroblastoma cells (Greengard and Kuo, 1970c; Casola *et al.*, 1974). Cyclic AMP-dependent protein kinase activity increased markedly during culture of rat glioma cells. In homogenates of glioma cells less than 40% of the kinase activity was associated with the soluble fraction. Norepinephrine-elicited accumulation of cyclic AMP in a rat glioma cell line was accompanied by a translocation of protein kinase from cell cytoplasm to nuclear fractions (Salem and De Vellis, 1976). Autophosphorylation of a nuclear protein (mol wt 100,000) was enhanced with nuclear fractions from norepinephrine-treated cells. Cyclic AMP-dependent protein kinase activity was detected only in the soluble fraction from neuroblastoma cells while cyclic AMP binding was detected in both soluble and particulate fractions (Prasad *et al.*, 1975e, 1976). No cyclic AMP-dependent autophosphorylation of proteins was detected in neuroblastoma homogenates (Casola *et al.*, 1974). Histone and phosvitin present in the media of cultured glioma and glial cells underwent phosphorylation (Agren and Ronquist, 1974). The phosphorylation of histone, but not phosvitin, was enhanced by cyclic AMP. Thus, at least part of both cyclic AMP-dependent and -independent membrane protein kinases in these cells would appear to be exoenzymes. The "exohistone kinase" of glioma cells was activated by exogenous cyclic AMP and apparently by cyclic AMP released from cells during stimulation with norepinephrine (Schlaeger and Kohler, 1976).

2.4.2 Cyclic GMP-Dependent Kinases

Cyclic GMP-dependent kinases occur along with cyclic AMP-dependent kinases in brain, but they appear less stable. Little is known of their endogenous substrates and hence function.

Regional and Subcellular Distribution in Brain

Levels of cyclic GMP-dependent protein kinases appeared to be higher in cerebellum than in cortex (Sold and Hofmann, 1974). The enzyme was mainly present in soluble fractions. The binding of cyclic AMP and cyclic GMP to proteins, presumably at least in part representing regulatory units of protein kinases, was studied in these brain regions. In soluble fractions from rat cerebellum the ratio of cyclic AMP to cyclic GMP bound was about 3, while in cerebrum it was about 7. At least two different sites, one relatively specific for cyclic AMP and one relatively specific for cyclic GMP, were present. In an ammonium sulfate fraction from guinea pig brain cyclic AMP binding exceeded cyclic GMP binding 13-fold (Gill and Kanstein, 1975). The major binding sites for cyclic GMP in rat cerebellar homogenates were associated with cyclic GMP protein kinases (Lincoln *et al.*, 1976).

Properties

Cyclic GMP-dependent protein kinases (EC_{50} for cyclic GMP, 0.05 μM) catalyzing the phosphorylation of histones were present in soluble fractions from brain homogenates, required magnesium ions for activity, and were inhibited by calcium ions (Greengard and Kuo, 1970; Hofmann and Sold, 1972; Kuo, 1974). Manganese and cobalt ions could replace the magnesium. Cyclic GMP-dependent kinases appeared to be best assayed with phosphate buffer, with an arginine-rich histone as substrate, and with a protein kinase modulator present which inhibits cyclic AMP-dependent kinase activity and potentiates cyclic GMP-dependent kinase activity (Donnelly *et al.*, 1973a,b; Kuo, 1974, 1975b). The relatively unstable mammalian cyclic GMP-dependent kinase could be partially purified from brain and other tissue by column chromatography or ammonium sulfate fractionation (Kuo, 1974; Sold and Hofmann, 1974; Takai *et al.*, 1975). These procedures separated the cyclic GMP-dependent enzyme from one or two cyclic AMP-dependent kinases (cf. Figure 12). Binding of cyclic GMP was found to be specifically associated with two cyclic GMP-dependent kinases, one major, one minor, during DEAE-cellulose column purification of bovine cerebellar homogenates, while binding of cyclic AMP was specifically associated with a cyclic AMP-dependent protein kinase (Takai *et al.*, 1975). The purified cyclic GMP-dependent kinase (mol wt 140,000) required

100 mM magnesium for maximal activity and was inhibitied by sulfhydryl reagents. The serine residues phosphorylated in histone by this cyclic GMP-dependent kinase were different than those phosphorylated by the cerebellar cyclic AMP-dependent kinase. The K_m of ATP was about 7 μM, a value similar to the K_m of ATP for cyclic AMP-dependent kinases. Cyclic GMP-dependent kinase did not activate phosphorylase-b kinase. The minor cyclic GMP-dependent kinase in bovine cerebellum had an apparent molecular weight of about 90,000. The physiological substrates for cyclic GMP-dependent kinases in brain are unknown. Cyclic GMP-dependent phosphorylation of two membranal proteins has been reported for smooth muscle preparations (Casnellie and Greengard, 1974). These two phosphorylated proteins have not been detected in preparations from tissues other than smooth muscle (cited in Greengard, 1976).

The substrate profiles for cyclic GMP-dependent kinases like the profiles for cyclic AMP-dependent kinases can be altered by modulator proteins. In mammalian tissues, two kinase modulator proteins have been isolated (Kuo et al., 1976a,b). One was specific to cyclic AMP-dependent kinases and was referred to as the "inhibitory" modulator, while the other was specific to cyclic GMP-dependent kinases and was referred to as the "stimulatory" modulator. Both occurred in nearly equal amounts in brain. The modulator from lobster tail muscle stimulated the activity of the catalytic subunit of lobster tail cyclic GMP-dependent protein kinase with protamine or an arginine-rich histone as substrates and inhibited the enzyme with a histone mixture as substrate (Donnelly et al., 1973b). The same modulator protein from lobster tail was usually inhibitory to cyclic AMP-dependent protein kinases but could be stimulatory with protamine as substrate.

Activation by Analogs of Cyclic GMP

Most studies on analogs of cyclic GMP as activators of cyclic GMP-dependent protein kinases have been with the kinase isolated from lobster tail (Kuo and Greengard, 1970d). 8-Bromo cyclic GMP has been reported to be a potent activator of lung cyclic GMP-dependent kinase and cyclic AMP to be only one-twentieth as potent as cyclic GMP in activating the enzyme (Kuo, 1974). Reviews on the potency of cyclic GMP analogs as activators of the lobster tail muscle protein kinase are available (Simon et al., 1973; Meyer and Miller, 1973). In a recent study with the cyclic GMP-dependent protein kinase from lobster tail muscle, the potencies of various analogs were measured in the presence or absence of the lobster tail modulator protein (Kuo et al., 1974). The potencies of some of the most active compounds were as follows (compounds in italic activated the kinase to a greater extent in the presence of the modulator protein): *8-bromo cyclic*

GMP > *cyclic GMP* > *8-benzylamino cyclic AMP* > 8-bromo cyclic AMP > *8-thio cyclic AMP* > 8-methylthio cyclic AMP > *8-benzylamino cyclic GMP,* cyclic AMP, *8-bromo cyclic IMP, N⁶-benzyl cyclic AMP,* 2-hydroxy cyclic AMP, and 8-amino cyclic AMP. The dibutyryl analog of cyclic GMP was 10,000-fold less potent than cyclic GMP. Analogs other than 8-bromo cyclic GMP that were more potent than cyclic GMP include the 8-(*p*-chlorophenyl) thio, 8-benzylthio, 8-methylthio, 8-hydroxy, 8-carbamyl, and 8-(1-hydroxyethyl) cyclic GMPs (Miller *et al.,* 1973a; Christensen *et al.,* 1975). Cyclic AMP at very high concentrations inhibited the kinase from lobster tail by competition with ATP (Donnelly *et al.,* 1973a).

Developmental Aspects

Levels of cyclic AMP-dependent protein kinase were sixfold greater than cyclic GMP-dependent protein kinase in brain of adult guinea pig (Kuo, 1975a). In brains from fetal and neonatal guinea pigs levels of cyclic AMP-dependent kinases were respectively 20- and 10-fold greater than cyclic GMP-dependent kinases. It would appear that levels of the cyclic GMP-kinases increased considerably during development in contrast to levels of cyclic AMP-kinases which at least in rats (see above) had not appeared to undergo marked developmental changes.

2.5 Phosphoprotein Phosphatases

Dephosphorylation of specific proteins phosphorylated by the action of cyclic AMP- and cyclic GMP-dependent protein kinases presumably terminates the physiological effects of cyclic nucleotides in intact cells. The phosphoprotein phosphatases responsible for this dephosphorylation have not been extensively studied. Such enzymes are both membrane-bound and soluble, have differing substrate profiles, and do not appear to require a divalent cation. Cyclic AMP may in certain cases stimulate phosphoprotein phosphatase activity. The enzyme activity is inhibited by fluoride ion and zinc ion at least in cell-free preparations.

2.5.1 Regional and Subcellular Distribution in Brain

Phosphoprotein phosphatases in brain were present both in soluble and membrane fractions (Weller and Rodnight, 1971; Maeno and Greengard, 1972; Maeno *et al.,* 1975; Miyamoto and Kakiuchi, 1975). Levels of protein phosphatase in cerebral cortex were nearly threefold higher than in cerebellum or pons and sevenfold higher than in caudate nucleus. In rat cerebral cortical homogenates, at least three soluble phosphoprotein phosphatases were present (Figure 15), but a major portion of total activity was associated with synaptic membranes. The subcellular distribution of phosphoprotein phosphatases in homogenates of rat and guinea pig cerebral cortex, cerebellum, caudate nucleus, and medulla was similar, with about 50% of the enzyme associated with particulate fractions. Soluble phosphatases obtained by lysis of synaptosomes represented nearly one-half of the activity associated with this particulate fraction. The soluble phosphatases from synaptosomes apparently consisted of the same three phosphatases seen in cytoplasm-soluble fractions, but in somewhat different proportions. Histochemically the phosphatases were cited as being associated with postsynaptic dendrites in rat cortex (Greengard *et al.*, 1972).

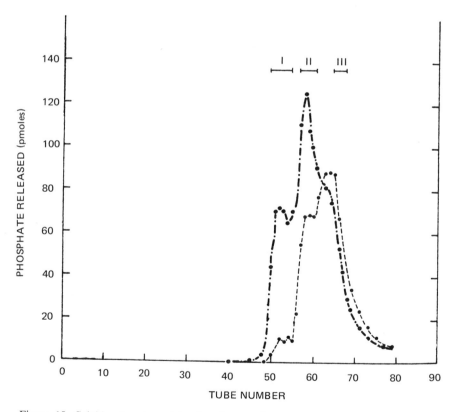

Figure 15. Soluble phosphoprotein phosphatases from rat cerebrum. Soluble proteins from cerebral homogenates were fractionated on a DEAE-cellulose column and assayed with phosphorylated protamine (●--●) or histone (●---●). The roman numerals refer to the three apparent isozymes. (Modified from Maeno and Greengard, 1972, *Journal of Biological Chemistry*, copyright American Society of Biological Chemists.)

A phosphatase which converted phosphorylase a to the b form was present in brain (Drummon et al., 1964b). A rat brain glycogen synthetase-D phosphatase activity has been reported (Goldberg and O'Toole, 1969). Phosphoprotein phosphatase activity for myelin basic protein was found in both soluble and myelin fractions from brain (Miyamoto and Kakiuchi, 1975). The myelin phosphoprotein phosphatase was solubilized with Triton X-100. At least two such phosphatases were present as soluble proteins in brain.

Phosphoprotein phosphatase activity from nerve cords of tobacco hornworms (Manduca sexta) has been studied in detail with a phosphoprotamine as substrate (Albin and Newburgh, 1975b). The properties of the enzymes were similar to those of enzymes from brain tissue. ATP, GTP, and fluoride and the sulfhydryl reagent, p-hydroxymercuribenzoate, inhibited enzyme activity.

2.5.2 Activation, Inhibition, and Substrates

Magnesium and calcium ions had little effect on basal activity of brain phosphoprotein phosphatases, while manganese ions increased enzyme activity of the three soluble enzymes from rat cerebral cortex (Maeno and Greengard, 1972). Zinc ions and fluoride were strongly inhibitory. The different enzymes differed in their substrate profiles. One of the soluble enzymes (I, Figure 15) had a V_{max} with protamine ninefold higher than with histone. Another soluble enzyme (III) had a nearly twofold higher V_{max} with the histone than with protamine. The third soluble phosphatase (II) and the particulate enzyme had an approximate 1.4- to 1.8-fold higher V_{max} with protamine than with histone. Solubilization of the particulate enzymes from synaptic membrane fragments with a detergent, Triton X-100, yielded enzymes which retained their original high affinities for protamine and exhibited a V_{max} with protamine about 1.8-fold higher than with the histone. Radioactive phosphorylated substrates for these studies were prepared with brain protein kinase, cyclic AMP, and [^{32}P]ATP. Two soluble phosphoprotein phosphatases and one associated with myelin fractions from brain showed highest activity towards phosphorylated myelin-basic protein and lower activity towards phosphorylated histone and protamine (Miyamoto and Kakiuchi, 1975). Preparation of the phosphorylated substrates was with bovine brain cyclic AMP-dependent protein kinase.

The apparent loss of inhibitory regulatory subunits of muscle phosphorylase phosphatase during purification yielded an active enzyme with an apparent molecular weight of 30,000 (Brandt et al., 1974). Whether inhibitory subunits occur with other phosphatases is unknown,

A compound with chromatographic properties similar to those of cyclic AMP, whose levels increase in liver and other tissues during formation of cyclic AMP, inhibited cyclic AMP-dependent protein kinases (Murad *et al.*, 1969; Wasner, 1975). The same factor stimulated a beef muscle phosphoprotein phosphatase (Wasner, 1975). Cyclic AMP inhibited the phosphatase. Cyclic AMP, has, however, in other systems appeared capable of stimulating phosphoprotein phosphatases (see below).

2.5.3 Dephosphorylation of Membranal Phosphoproteins

Dephosphorylation of synaptic membranes autophosphorylated by ATP in the presence of cyclic AMP was studied after addition of EDTA and excess ATP to block further incorporation of radioactivity by intrinsic protein kinases (Maeno and Greengard, 1972). Rapid dephosphorylation presumably due to the membranal phosphoprotein phosphatases was observed. The rate of autodephosphorylation was much greater than rates of dephosphorylation of exogenous phosphorylated substrates. The overall rate of dephosphorylation of membranal preparations by these intrinsic enzymes was not accelerated by cyclic AMP. Zinc ions were strongly inhibitory, as were fluoride ions. Subsequent studies revealed that cyclic AMP greatly accelerated the dephosphorylation of a specific protein in synaptic membrane fractions (Maeno *et al.*, 1975). Phosphorylated synaptic membranes were prepared in the presence of zinc ions, thereby completely inhibiting phosphoprotein phosphatases. Addition of EDTA removed the zinc ion, thereby preventing further action of the protein kinases in the absence of a divalent cation. Dephosphorylation of protein II, probably the regulatory subunit of cyclic AMP-dependent protein kinase (see Section 2.4.1) occurred only in the presence of cyclic AMP (EC$_{50}$, 0.7 μM) and was essentially complete within 2 min. Other cyclic nucleotides had no effect. Adenosine did not inhibit the dephosphorylation. The mechanism involved in stimulation of dephosphorylation of protein II by cyclic AMP is not yet resolved. However, since it occurred under conditions where endogenous protein kinase was inhibited by EGTA, it would appear to have been a direct effect, not related to activation of protein kinases.

3

Accumulation of Cyclic Nucleotides

The complexity of the interrelationships of the cyclases, phosphodiesterases, protein kinases, and phosphoprotein phosphatases with macromolecular factors, magnesium, manganese, and calcium ions, and levels of ATP and GTP and, in addition, the existence of multiple enzyme forms with differing properties even within one cell make it difficult or impossible to extrapolate results obtained with homogenates to the functional operation of cyclic nucleotide systems in intact cells. Studies on the accumulation of cyclic nucleotides in brain slices, ganglia, and cultured cells under various conditions can, however, provide pertinent information. The extent of accumulation of cyclic AMP in intact cells will be influenced by a number of factors: (1) the basal levels of adenylate cyclases and the availability of ATP as a substrate; (2) the degree of activation of this enzyme by biogenic amines, adenosine, and other compounds: (3) the levels and properties of cyclic nucleotide phosphodiesterases; and (4) the levels of cyclic AMP-dependent protein kinases with binding sites that presumably sequester cyclic AMP. The subcellular distribution and availability of ions such as calcium and magnesium with their abilities to inhibit or activate these systems will be important in determining the extent of accumulation of cyclic AMP. Similar factors would be involved in the function of cyclic GMP-generating systems of intact cells. Two methods have been extensively used to study the factors regulating accumulations of cyclic AMP in such preparations. Either endogenous levels of cyclic AMP are measured, or the extent of formation of radioactive cyclic AMP from intracellular radioactive adenine nucleotides labeled during a prior incubation of the preparation with radioactive adenine or adenosine is ascertained. Combination of the two methods can provide information relevant to compartmentalization of adenine nucleotides either within a cell or in different cells of a complex tissue such as that represented by a brain slice. The adenine or adenosine used in the prelabeling technique is incorporated into intracellular nucleotides by the action of adenine phosphoribosyltransferase or adenosine kinase, respectively (Shimizu and Daly, 1972a; Shimizu *et al.*, 1972). In the case of adenosine, a prior uptake process may be rate limiting at low concentrations (Huang and Daly, 1974a).

3.1 Cyclic AMP in Brain Slices

Accumulation of cyclic AMP and to a lesser extent cyclic GMP has been investigated in brain slices from different brain regions and a variety of species. The results indicate that in spite of its heterogeneity the brain slice provides a valuable tool for the study of the factors involved in the regulation of cyclic nucleotides in the central nervous system. After sacrifice, cyclic AMP levels rose rapidly in brain tissue (see Section 4.4.1). Fortunately, cyclic AMP in brain slices returned to low stable levels after incubation for 30 to 90 min in aerated medium. During this period, ATP levels were reestablished in levels (20 nmol/mg protein) approximately one-half those which pertained *in vivo*. Levels of ADP and AMP fell to relatively low values, 3 and 1 nmol/mg protein, respectively, in guinea pig cortical slices (Huang and Daly, 1974b). Investigation of cyclic AMP-generating systems in brain slices have been carried out after such prior "stabilizing" incubations. Basal levels of cyclic AMP in brain slices after the preincubations are relatively low, in most instances between 5 and 40 pmol/mg protein (Table 3). Long preincubations, especially at high ratios of media to tissue, adequate aeration, and avoidance of transfers of tissue immediately prior to addition of test agents resulted in the lowest basal levels of cyclic AMP in brain slices. Endogenous adenosine appeared to be primarily responsible for high basal levels of cyclic AMP. The cyclic AMP-generating systems in slices appear to remain functional for at least 2 hr.

Brain slices from rabbit, guinea pig, rat, and mouse have been extensively studied. In most investigations, chopped tissue of 200–300 μm has been used. In certain studies cross-chopped tissue has been used, and in some investigations on electrical stimulation tangential slices of cortex have been used. Slabs of tissue, particularly intact hypothalami, have also been investigated. Profound differences in the extent of accumulation of cyclic AMP elicited by stimulatory agents were observed in the various species and/or brain regions. Presumably, such differences in responses of brain slices to biogenic amines, adenosine, depolarization and drugs reflect similar differences in the intact brain. However, differential losses or alterations

TABLE 3. Levels of Cyclic AMP and Cyclic GMP in
Incubated Brain Slices[a]

Brain region	Cyclic AMP	Cyclic GMP
Rabbit		
Cerebral cortex	3–6	1–2
Cerebellum	5–10	1–2
Guinea pig		
Cerebral cortex	5–20	2–4
Cerebellum	6–30	10–30
Rat		
Cerebral cortex	10–50	0.3–3
Cerebellum	30–400	20–70
Hippocampus	10–25	2–5
Striatum	3–15	0.2–3
Hypothalamus	15–30	3–9
Brain stem	20–40	2–5
Mouse		
Cerebral cortex	10–50	0.7–1.0
Cerebellum	10–17	4–18

[a]Values are from the literature cited in the text and are meant to provide indices of
levels of cyclic nucleotides in incubated brain slices in picomoles per milligram of
protein. Values from different laboratories have varied considerably, but levels
with particular experimental paradigms have been quite reproducible.

in responses during preparation of brain slices cannot be excluded. Time
courses for the accumulation of cyclic AMP in response to biogenic
amines, adenosine, and depolarizing conditions have been reported for
slices from different species and different brain regions. Under most conditions, maximal accumulations were reached within 3 to 10 min. With
ouabain nearly 15 min was required, while with glutamate maximal accumulations were not reached even after 20 min. The maximal accumulation
of cyclic AMP was either maintained or decreased usually slowly during a
subsequent 10 to 20 min of incubation in the continued presence of the
stimulatory agent. Rates of disappearence of cyclic AMP from stimulated
slices after washing and subsequent incubation have also been investigated.
The results of such kinetic measurements in brain slices are, of course,
strongly influenced by the time required for a small molecule to permeate or
be removed from a 200–300 μm thick tissue; i.e., with a half-time of 2 to 3
min (Schultz and Daly, 1973a). It should be stressed that accumulations of
cyclic AMP have been frequently measured and compared at a single time
point between 4 and 20 min and at a single high concentration of the
stimulatory agent. The biogenic amines, histamine, norepinephrine, and
serotonin, had in most brain slice preparations an EC_{50} for accumulation of

cyclic AMP between 1 and 20 μM, while adenosine had an EC_{50} of about 30 μM. The true EC_{50} values for norepinephrine and adenosine were significantly lower because of active uptake processes within the brain slice. The increases in endogenous levels of cyclic AMP in brain slices were in most instances reflected in similar increases in levels of radioactive cyclic AMP derived from intracellular adenine nucleotides labeled during a prior incubation with radioactive adenine or adenosine. The following sections will discuss the effects of biogenic amines, adenosine, depolarization, and other factors on the accumulation of cyclic AMP in brain slices from the various species of animals.

The effects of various agonists and antagonists on levels of cyclic AMP differed remarkably in different brain regions and in the same region from different strains or species of animals. Some of these are summarized in Table 4 and illustrate not only the quantitative differences in accumulations of cyclic AMP, but also differences in the nature of the receptors that control cyclic AMP formation. However, even for slices from the same brain region of the same species the magnitude of accumulations of cyclic AMP reported in the literature often differed markedly. Such differences would appear to be due to many factors, among which the following appear to be relevant: (1) experimental variables involving methods for removal of brain tissue and slice preparation, length of preincubation periods, transfers of tissue, aeration of slices in the medium, measurement of either radioactive cyclic AMP in prelabeled slices or of endogenous cyclic AMP, method of determination of protein concentration, and, finally, subtle factors related to each individual investigator's experimental techniques; (2) biological variability of individual animals and of groups of animals dependent on source, strain, history, and season; (3) inadequate experimentation; i.e., insufficient to compensate for the biological and technical variables. Differences in endogenous levels of adenosine and/or calcium ions in tissue slices would appear to be of prime importance to the function and responses of cyclic AMP-generating systems. With low basal levels of cyclic AMP, the accumulation of cyclic AMP in picomoles per milligram of protein elicited by various agents, particularly biogenic amines, are usually much lower than in experiments where high basal levels of cyclic AMP pertained. Protein determinations with brain tissue can give quite different results, depending on the assay used. Thus, Biuret protein values are about 2.7-fold higher than Lowry values for cerebral cortical tissue using bovine serum albumin as the protein standard (Skolnick et al., 1975). Cyclic AMP values based on Biuret protein must be multiplied by 2.7 to make them comparable to values based on Lowry protein. Methodologies for use of brain slices in the study of accumulation of endogenous and radioactive AMP has been discussed in other reviews (Daly, 1972; Shimizu and Daly, 1972a; Skolnick and Daly, 1976b).

TABLE 4. Effect of Various Agents on Levels of Cyclic AMP in Incubated Brain Slices[a]

Brain region	Putative neuromodulators					
	Catecholamines (100 μM)	Serotonin (100 μM)	Histamine (100 μM)	Adenosine (100 μM)	Prostaglandin E_1 (85 μM)	Glutamate (2–10 mM)
Rabbit						
Cerebral cortex	±	±	+++	+	±	+
Cerebellum	++(β)	±	++		±	±
Guinea pig						
Cerebral cortex	±(α)	±	++($H_1>H_2$)	+++	±	
Cerebellum	++(β)	±	±	+++	±	+++
Hippocampus	±(α)	±	++(H_1,H_2)	+++		
Rat						
Cerebral cortex	++(α,β)	±	±(H_2)	+++	+	++
Cerebellum	+(β)	±	±	++	±	
Hippocampus	+	±	±		+	
Striatum	+(β,DA)	±	±	+	++	
Hypothalamus	++(αβ)	±	±			
Mouse						
Cerebral cortex	++(β)	±	±	+		
Cerebellum	++(α,β)	±	±	++		++

[a] A marginal or no accumulation of cyclic AMP (0 to 2-fold increase) is designated by ±; a small accumulation (2- to 4-fold increase) by +, an intermediate accumulation (4- to 15-fold increase) by ++, and a large accumulation (more than 15-fold increase) by +++. Types of receptors are designated in parentheses as α- and β-adrenergic, dopaminergic (DA), or H_1- or H_2-histaminergic based on agonist–antagonist data. References pertinent to these data are cited in the text.

3.1.1 Rabbit

Norepinephrine

In cerebral cortical slices, norepinephrine (EC_{50}, 4 μM) had no effect or elicited a less than 3-fold increase in the level of cyclic AMP, while in cerebellar slices a 3- to 15-fold increase in cyclic AMP occurred (Rall and Kakiuchi, 1966; Kakiuchi and Rall, 1968a,b; Shimizu *et al.*, 1969, 1970a; Forn and Krishna, 1971; Krishna *et al.*, 1970; Schmidt and Robison, 1971; Berti *et al.*, 1972; Kuo *et al.*, 1972). The effect of norepinephrine in cerebellar slices was completely blocked by a β-antagonist, dichlorisoproterenol, was unaffected by an α-antagonist, phenoxybenzamine, and was partially antagonized by relatively high concentrations of chlorpromazine or diphenhydramine (Kakiuchi and Rall, 1968b). Isoproterenol elicited an accumulation similar to that elicited by norepinephrine. The maximal accumulations elicited by norepinephrine declined more rapidly in cerebellar than in cortical slices (Kakiuchi and Rall, 1968a,b). Cyclic AMP-systems in cerebellar slices became refractory to restimulation by norepinephrine, but were at this time still responsive to histamine. Norepinephrine had either no effect or elicited only a 2-fold increase in cyclic AMP levels in slices from hypothalamus, hippocampus, caudate nucleus, and brain stem (Kakiuchi and Rall, 1968a; Krishna *et al.*, 1970; Schmidt and Robison, 1971). With adenine-labeled slices from caudate nucleus, a much larger stimulation by norepinephrine was reported (Shimizu *et al.*, 1969). The latter study was done in the presence of caffeine, a weak phosphodiesterase inhibitor. α-Methylnorepinephrine was nearly as active as norepinephrine in cerebellar slices (Shimizu *et al.*, 1970d). Norepinephrine elicited a 3-fold increase in cyclic AMP levels in slices from brachium-pontis-fornix-optic tract (Kakiuchi and Rall, 1968a). Norepinephrine elicited accumulations of cyclic AMP in slices from frontal cortex, hypothalamus, and hippocampus of newborn rabbits (Schmidt and Robison, 1971). The response reached a maximum 9 to 14 days after birth and then declined to finally disappear in slices from adults. The stimulatory effects of norepinephrine were nearly constant in cerebellar slices throughout maturation to adulthood. Schmidt and Robison (1971) discuss the fact that a much higher dose of chlorpromazine was required to block the alerting response of 9- to 14-day-old rabbits as compared to adults. Thus, the peak of *in vivo* subsensitivity to this phenothiazine coincided with the peak of responsiveness of norepinephrine-sensitive cyclic AMP-generating systems in rabbit cortical, hippocampal, and hypothalamic slices.

Histamine

Histamine (EC_{50}, 10 μM) elicited accumulations of cyclic AMP in cortical (5- to 30-fold increase), hypothalamic (20- to 30-fold), brain stem (35-fold), and cerebellar (3- to 10-fold) slices (Rall and Kakiuchi, 1966; Kakiuchi and Rall, 1968a,b; Shimizu *et al.*, 1969, 1970a,c; Forn and Krishna, 1971; Krishna *et al.*, 1970; Berti *et al.*, 1972; Kuo *et al.*, 1972; Palmer *et al.*, 1972b; Spiker *et al.*, 1976). Histamine elicited only a 3-fold increase in slices from brachium-pontis-fornix-optic tract (Kakiuchi and Rall, 1968). Cyclic AMP-systems in cerebellar slices became refractory to restimulation by histamine, while remaining responsive to norepinephrine. Histamine was antagonized by phenoxybenzamine, chlorpromazine, clozapine, thioridazine, haloperidol, diphenhydramine, tripellenamine (Kakiuchi and Rall, 1968a,b; Palmer *et al.*, 1972b; Spiker *et al.*, 1976), and lithium ions (Forn and Valdecasas, 1971). Histamine analogs and homologs such as 3-(2-aminoethyl)-pyrazole (betazole), 3-(2-aminoethyl)-1,2,4-triazole, ω-N-methylhistamine, and ω-N,N-dimethylhistamine elicited accumulations of cyclic AMP in cortical slices, while 1-methylhistamine was inactive (Shimizu *et al.*, 1970c). Histamine elevated levels of cyclic AMP by 6- to 8-fold in slices of caudate nucleus or hypothalamus. The accumulations of cyclic AMP elicited in cortical slices by histamine increased during the first 8 days postpartum and then declined to adult levels (Palmer *et al.*, 1972b). Histamine and norepinephrine had less than additive effects in cortical slices (Kakiuchi and Rall, 1968a).

Serotonin, Other Amines, Amino Acids

Serotonin had either no or only a small stimulatory effect on cyclic AMP levels in cerebellar or cortical slices (Kakiuchi and Rall, 1968a,b; Forn and Krishna, 1971; Shimizu *et al.*, 1970d). In cerebellar slices serotonin consistently elicited a two- to three-fold increase in cyclic AMP levels (Kakiuchi and Rall 1968b). β-Phenylethylamine and N-methyltryptamine had marginal activity in cerebellar slices (Shimizu *et al.*, 1970c,d). Dopamine, tyramines, octopamines, amphetamine, spermine, and other polyamines, glycine, γ-aminobutyrate, glutamate (4 mM), acetylcholine, and prostaglandin had virtually no effect on cyclic AMP levels in cortical and/or cerebellar slices (Kakiuchi and Rall, 1968a,b; Forn and Krishna, 1971; Shimizu *et al.*, 1970c,d; Berti *et al.*, 1972; Kuo *et al.*, 1972; Lee *et al.*, 1972). Indeed, some of these agents such as acetylcholine in cerebellar slices (Kuo *et al.*, 1972) caused a slight decrease in basal levels of cyclic AMP. Acetylcholine did not prevent the response of cyclic AMP-generating systems to norepinephrine or histamine in cerebellar slices (Kakiuchi and Rall, 1968b).

Adenosine

In adenine-labeled rabbit cortical slices adenosine elicited a 3.5-fold increase in radioactive cyclic AMP (Berti *et al.*, 1972).

Depolarizing Agents

Various depolarizing agents, which in brain slices from other rodents appear to elicit accumulations of cyclic AMP by mechanisms involving at least in part the formation and intermediacy of adenosine, elicited large accumulations of cyclic AMP in rabbit cerebral cortical slices (Rall and Sattin, 1970; Shimizu et al., 1970a,d; Shimizu and Daly, 1972b). Veratridine, batrachotoxin, and ouabain elicited 30-, 40-, and 100-fold increases, respectively, in cyclic AMP levels. Potassium ions (40 mM), in contrast, had much smaller effects. Potassium ions (100 mM) increased endogenous levels of cyclic AMP in rabbit cortical slices by only 50% (Kakiuchi and Rall, 1968), but this experiment was done in the presence of the adenosine antagonist, theophylline, which in guinea pig cortical slices is known to antagonize the response to potassium ions. Combinations of veratridine with either norepinephrine or histamine had greater than additive effects in rabbit cortical slices.

Phosphodiesterase Inhibitors

The effects of theophylline, a relatively weak inhibitor of brain phosphodiesterases and also an antagonist of adenosine, on accumulations of cyclic AMP in brain slices were first studied in cortical and cerebellar preparations from rabbit, where in slices prepared at 4° it potentiated the accumulation of cyclic AMP elicited by norepinephrine and histamine (Kakiuchi and Rall, 1968a,b). Potentiation of the response to histamine by theophylline was confirmed in adenine-labeled cortical slices prepared in the cold (Shimizu et al., 1970b). In later studies by Rall and Sattin (1970) using rabbit cortical slices prepared at room temperature, theophylline did not potentiate the response to histamine. It was suggested that theophylline potentiated amines only in slices prepared in the cold. However, others using adenine-labeled rabbit cortical slices reported no potentiation of histamine responses by theophylline, regardless of the temperature at which the slices were prepared (Forn and Krishna, 1971). Other quite active phosphodiesterase inhibitors have now proven more useful than theophylline in studies on the role of phosphodiesterase in brain slices (see below). However, theophylline is still useful in such preparations as an adenosine antagonist.

3.1.2 Guinea Pig

Norepinephrine

The catecholamines, norepinephrine and epinephrine, elicited only a small (Kakiuchi et al., 1969; Shimizu et al., 1969, 1970a, 1973; Sattin and

Rall, 1970; Chasin *et al.*, 1971, 1973; Huang *et al.*, 1971; Kodama *et al.*, 1971; Huang and Daly, 1972; Shimizu and Daly, 1972b; Zanella and Rall, 1973; Sattin *et al.*, 1975; Ohga and Daly, 1976a) or insignificant (Forn and Krishna, 1971; Schultz and Daly, 1973a; Huang and Daly, 1974a; Schultz, 1975) accumulation of cyclic AMP in cerebral cortical slices. The response was fully manifest at birth (Schmidt *et al.*, 1970). It has been proposed (Sattin *et al.*, 1975) that adenosine is necessary in order for norepinephrine to elicit an accumulation of cyclic AMP in guinea pig cortical slices. However, norepinephrine did elicit an accumulation of cyclic AMP in neocortical slices in the presence of isobutylmethylxanthine, a potent adenosine-antagonist and phosphodiesterase inhibitor (Dismukes *et al.*, 1976a). The stimulatory effects of epinephrine in cortical slices were blocked by α-antagonists, while being only slightly antagonized by antihistamines and unaffected by β-antagonists. Thus in guinea pig cortical slices, epinephrine apparently activated adenylate cyclases by interaction with a classical α-receptor. The marginal stimulatory activity of a pure β-agonist, isoproterenol (Chasin *et al.*, 1973; Sattin *et al.*, 1975), was compatible with this interpretation.

In cerebellar slices, norepinephrine (EC_{50}, 5 μM) elicited an 8- to 20-fold increase in levels of cyclic AMP (Chasin *et al.*, 1971, 1973; Zanella and Rall, 1973; Sattin *et al.* 1975; Ohga and Daly, 1976a,b). Isoproterenol elicited a larger accumulation of cyclic AMP than did norepinephrine in cerebellar slices. An α-agonist, phenylephrine, had virtually no effect. β-Antagonists blocked the stimulatory effect of the catecholamines in cerebellar slices, while α-antagonists were ineffective and antihistamines caused only a marginal inhibition. Prostaglandin E_1 did not antagonize the response to norepinephrine. Epinephrine elicited a small accumulation of cyclic AMP in slices from hippocampus and amygdala, but not from diencephalon and brain stem. The effects of epinephrine were blocked in hippocampus and amygdala by α-antagonists and partially blocked by chlorpheniramine. The β-antagonist, propranolol, partially antagonized the effect of epinephrine in slices from amygdala (Chasin *et al.*, 1973). Chlorpromazine and less effectively imipramine blocked the effect of epinephrine in hippocampal slices (Free *et al.*, 1974).

Histamine

Histamine (EC_{50}, 7 to 20 μM) elicited a 3- to 20-fold increase in levels of cyclic AMP in cortical slices (Kakiuchi *et al.*, 1969; Shimizu *et al.*, 1969, 1970a,c, 1973; Forn and Krishna, 1971; Krishna *et al.*, 1970; Rall and Sattin, 1970; Sattin and Rall, 1970; Shimizu and Daly, 1970, 1972b; Chasin *et al.*, 1971, 1973; Huang *et al.*, 1971; Kodama *et al.*, 1971; Huang and Daly, 1972, 1974b; Schultz and Daly, 1973a,b,c,d; Shimizu and Okayama, 1973; Zanella and Rall, 1973; Schultz, 1974a,b; Baudry *et al.*, 1975;

Schultz, 1975a,b; Rogers *et al.*, 1975; Dismukes *et al.*, 1976a,b). The effect of histamine was blocked by classical H_1-antihistamines, while α- and β-antagonists had marginal or no inhibitory action (Chasin *et al.*, 1971, 1973; Shimizu and Daly, 1972b; Schultz and Daly, 1973b; Zanella and Rall, 1973; Rogers *et al.*, 1975). ω-N-Methylhistamine, ω-N,N-dimethylhistamine, 3-(2-aminoethyl)-1,2,4-triazole, and 3-(2-aminoethyl)pyrazole (betazole) stimulated cyclic AMP formation in guinea pig cortical slices, while 1-methylhistamine was inactive (Shimizu *et al.*, 1970c). The accumulation of cyclic AMP elicited by histamine and histamine analogs has been studied in detail in cortical slices (Rogers *et al.*, 1975; Dismukes *et al.*, 1976b). The response to histamine in cortical slices was effectively blocked by H_1-antagonists such as *d*-brompheniramine, promethazine, chlorpheniramine, phenindamine, and pyrilamine, while H_2-antagonists were much less effective. *l*-Brompheniramine was much less effective than the *d*-isomer. Combinations of H_1- and H_2-antagonists completely blocked the response to histamine, while the H_1-antagonist alone blocked the response by 70 to 80%. The results were consonant with the presence of both H_1- and H_2-receptors in guinea pig cortex, with H_1-receptors predominant. In guinea pig cortical slices at 100 μM concentrations both 4-methylhistamine, a specific H_2-agonist, and 2-methylhistamine, a specific H_1-agonist, elicited accumulations of cyclic AMP (Dismukes *et al.*, 1976b). Other H_1-agonists such as 2-aminoethylthiazole, 2-aminoethylpyridine, and 2-phenyl, 2-amino, 2-fluoro, and 2-benzylhistamine were virtually inactive at this concentration. 2-Aminoethylthiazole and 2-fluorohistamine at a 1 mM concentration did elicit accumulations of cyclic AMP. Another group reported that the stimulation of cyclic AMP accumulation in guinea pig cortical slices by histamine could not be completely blocked by either H_1 (pyrilamine) or H_2 (metiamide) antagonists, but that a combination of the two antagonists completely blocked the histamine response (Baudry *et al.*, 1975). Maximal inhibition of the response to histamine by either agent was about 60% and was attained at 1 μM pyrilamine and at 100 μM metiamide. 4-Methylhistamine elicited a significant accumulation of cyclic AMP. The response was completely blocked by the H_2-antagonist and was unaffected by the H_1-antagonist.

In cerebellar slices, histamine had either marginal (Zanella and Rall, 1973; Ohga and Daly, 1976a) or no (Chasin *et al.*, 1971; Rogers *et al.*, 1975) effect on cyclic AMP levels. Histamine had no effect in slices from hypothalamus, medulla-pons, diencephalon, or brain stem and only a small effect in amygdala, while eliciting a greater than eightfold increase in cyclic AMP in hippocampal slices (Chasin *et al.*, 1973; Rogers *et al.*, 1975). Histamine elicited a fivefold accumulation of cyclic AMP in thalamic slices and a twofold accumulation in striatal slices. The response in hippocampus was not blocked by α- and β-antagonists and was only partially blocked by classical H_1-antihistamines such as chlorpheniramine and pyrilamine. The accumulation of cyclic AMP elicited by histamine in hippocampal slices was partially blocked by chlorpromazine and imipramine (Free et al., 1974). In hippocampal slices both the H_1-antagonist, d-brompheniramine, and the H_2-antagonist, metiamide, effectively inhibited the response to histamine by about 50% (Rogers et al., 1975; Dismukes et al., 1976b). Combinations of the two antagonists resulted in a greater inhibition of the response. The results were consonant with a nearly equal contribution of both H_1- and H_2-receptors to histamine responses in hippocampal slices. In hippocampal slices, histamine (EC_{50}, 12 μM), 2-aminoethylthiazole (EC_{50}, 250 μM), and 4-methylhistamine (EC_{50}, 100 μM) elicited accumulations of cyclic AMP (Dismukes et al., 1976b). Histamine elicited the largest maximal accumulation, 4-methylhistamine the smallest. The response to histamine was completely blocked by a combination of H_1- and H_2-antagonists, while the response to 4-methylhistamine was unaffected by an H_1-antagonist and was completely blocked by an H_2-antagonist. The response to the H_1-agonist, 2-aminoethylthiazole, was completely blocked by either d-brompheniramine, an H_1-antagonist or by metiamide, an H_2-antagonist. It was proposed that because of the low affinity of 2-aminoethylthiazole for H_1-receptors, its response could be blocked even by the H_2-antagonist.

In contrast to results with rabbit and rat cortical slices, histamine and (nor)epinephrine had much greater than additive effects on levels of cyclic AMP in guinea pig cerebral cortical slices (Huang et al., 1971, 1973; Chasin et al., 1973; Schultz and Daly, 1973a; Schultz, 1975b). The synergism occurred only with the physiologically active levorotatory catecholamine. A local anesthetic, cocaine, did not prevent the synergism, which was, however, completely blocked by α-antagonists and partially blocked by the H_1-antihistamine, diphenhydramine. Thus the synergism appeared to involve interaction of the catecholamine with α-receptors and histamine with H_1-receptors. Consonant with this interpretation, isoproterenol did not potentiate the accumulation of cyclic AMP elicited by histamine. The partial blockade of the effect of combinations of histamine and norepinephrine by theophylline (Huang et al., 1973; Schultz and Daly, 1973b; Huang and Daly, 1974a) suggested that adenosine is involved to some extent in this synergistic interaction. Histamine did increase somewhat the efflux of radioactive adenosine from adenine-labeled cortical slices (Pull and McIlwain, 1975). The magnitude of the synergistic interaction of histamine and norepinephrine steadily declined in guinea pig cortical slices preincubated with histamine prior to addition of norepinephrine (Schultz, 1975b). Preincubation with norepinephrine had, however, no effect on the magnitude of the accumulation of cyclic AMP elicited by histamine–norepinephrine. Similar synergisms between histamine and epinephrine were seen in slices of guinea pig hippocampus (Chasin et al., 1973). The threshold for responses of cyclic AMP-generating systems to histamine in hippocampal slices was greatly decreased by the presence of epinephrine. Slightly greater than additive effects may occur in cortical slices with combinations of histamine and serotonin (Huang *et al.*, 1971).

Serotonin, Other Amines, Amino Acids, Prostaglandins

Serotonin had either marginal (Shimizu *et al.*, 1970d; Chasin *et al.*, 1971) or no (Huang *et al.*, 1971; Huang and Daly, 1972; Schultz and Kleefeld, 1975) effect on cyclic AMP levels in cerebral cortical slices and had no effect in cerebellar slices (Chasin *et al.*, 1971). Marginal effects of serotonin have been reported with slices from hippocampus, amygdala, diencephalon, and brain stem (Chasin *et al.*, 1973). Even in the presence of a phosphodiesterase inhibitor, isobutylmethylxanthine, the response to serotonin was not significant in guinea pig cerebral cortical slices (Dismukes *et al.*, 1976a).

A variety of other agents including dopamine, phenethylamine, prostaglandin, polypeptide hormones, acetylcholine, glycine, γ-aminobutyrate, glutamate, and N,O-dibutyryl cyclic AMP had no significant effect on cyclic AMP levels in cerebral cortical slices (Shimizu *et al.*, 1970c,d; Chasin *et al.*, 1971, 1973; Zanella and Rall, 1973; Schultz and Kleefeld, 1975), nor did dopamine or acetylcholine have significant effects in slices from hippocampus, amygdala, diencephalon, and brain stem. Glutamate at very high concentrations did elicit significant accumulations of cyclic AMP in cortical slices (see p. 123).

Prostaglandins had no effect on basal or adenosine-elicited levels of cyclic AMP in guinea pig cortical or cerebellar slices, nor did a preincubation of slices with indomethacin, to inhibit synthesis of prostaglandins, alter subsequent responses to norepinephrine, adenosine, or potassium ions (Zanella and Rall, 1973). Prostaglandin E_1 at 85 μM did elicit a small accumulation of cyclic AMP in cerebellar slices (Ohga and Daly, 1976a). Prostaglandins had no effect on cyclic AMP levels in cortical slices from a variety of mammals (Robison *et al.*, 1970b; Shimizu *et al.*, 1970c,d; Berti *et al.*, 1972). However, in three independent investigations prostaglandins E_1 and E_2 elicited accumulations of cyclic AMP in cortical slices from Sprague–Dawley rats (Berti *et al.*, 1972; Kuehl *et al.*, 1972; Dismukes and Daly, 1975b) (see Section 3.1.3).

Adenosine

Adenosine (EC_{50}, 30 μM) and adenine nucleotides elicited a 15- to 50-fold increase in levels of endogenous cyclic AMP in cortical slices (Sattin and Rall, 1970; Somerville and Smith, 1972; Schultz and Daly, 1973a,b,c,d;

Zanella and Rall, 1973; Huang and Daly, 1974a,b; Schultz, 1974, 1975a,b; Ohga and Daly, 1976a). Theophylline competitively blocked the stimulatory effect of adenosine (Sattin and Rall, 1970). In early studies with adenine-labeled slices, a relatively low 7- to 10-fold increase in radioactive cyclic AMP levels was elicited by adenosine (Shimizu *et al.*, 1969, 1970a,d; Shimizu and Daly, 1970, 1972b; Huang *et al.*, 1971, 1972), but in later experiments from the same laboratory (Shimizu *et al.*, 1973; Schultz and Daly, 1973a,b,c; Huang and Daly, 1974a,b) and by Somerville and Smith (1972) 20- to 30-fold increases were consistently observed with adenine-labeled slices. The reason for the differences was not apparent. Adenosine, AMP, ADP, and ATP elicited 3- to 4.4-fold accumulations of cyclic AMP in slices of guinea pig olfactory cortex (Kuroda and Kobayashi, 1975). Theophylline blocked the response. Adenosine elicited a 12- to 60-fold increase in cyclic AMP in cerebellar slices (Zanella and Rall, 1973; Ohga and Daly, 1976a). The response was blocked by theophylline and unaffected by sotalol or phentolamine. Adenosine elicited an 11-fold increase in levels of cyclic AMP in hippocampal slices (Dismukes *et al.*, 1976b).

Adenosine, in addition to stimulating formation of cyclic AMP from intracellular radioactive adenine nucleotides, was incorporated by phosphorylation into nucleotides which then serve as precursors of cyclic AMP (Sattin and Rall, 1970; Shimizu and Daly, 1970; Schultz and Daly, 1973a). In guinea pig cortical slices incorporation of exogenous 0.1 mM adenosine into cyclic AMP represented less than 20% of the total accumulation of cyclic AMP after 10 min of incubation (Schultz and Daly, 1973a), while in mouse cortical slices it represented about 40% (Skolnick and Daly, 1974c). Theophylline, which blocked the stimulatory effect of adenosine in cortical slices, did not significantly inhibit the incorporation of adenosine into intrecellular nucleotides which served as precursors of cyclic AMP (Shimizu *et al.*, 1969; Sattin and Rall, 1970; Huang and Daly, 1974a). Furthermore, agents such as dipyridamole, papaverine, hexobendine, and 6-(*p*-nitrobenzylthio)guanosine, which effectively inhibited active uptake of adenosine into cortical slices concomitantly potentiated the accumulation of cyclic AMP elicited by low concentrations of adenosine (Huang and Daly, 1974a). These and other observations have provided strong evidence for an extracellular adenosine receptor which serves to activate a cyclic AMP-generating system(s) in brain slices. Attempts to demonstrate such an extracellular site for adenosine action using a nonpermeating quaternary analog of the blocking agent, theophylline, were not successful (Schultz and Daly, 1973b), apparently because the polar quaternary analog, 7-(2'-diethylmethylammoniumethyl)theophylline iodide, was no longer an effective antagonist at the extracellular adenosine receptor. In fat cells, the inhibitory effects of adenosine on the cyclic AMP-generating system occur at very low concentrations of adenosine and are blocked by theophylline

TABLE 5. *Structure–Activity Relationships for Adenosine Analogs and Methylxanthines as Agonists or Antagonists of Adenosine-Sensitive Cyclic AMP-Generating Systems in Guinea Pig Cerebral Cortical Slices*[a]

Compound	Agonist activity	Antagonist activity
Adenosine	+++	
Purine analogs		
1-Chloro	++++	
2-Hydroxy	++	
2-Amino (isoguanosine)	++	
2-Fluoro	++	
6-Methylamino	++	
6-Dimethylamino	−	
6-Phenylamino	++++	
6-Benzylamino	+++	
6-Phenylisopropylamino	+++	
1-Methyl	−	−
1,N^6-Etheno	−	−
8-Bromo	−	−
7-Deaza (tubercidin)	−	−
7-Deaza-8-aza (formycin)	−	−
8-Aza	−	−
Inosine	−	−
Guanosine	−	−
Ribose analogs		
L-Ribofuranosyl	−	+
Arabinofuranosyl	−	++
Xylofuranosyl	−	+++
2′-Deoxy	−	++
3′-Deoxy	−	++
2′,5′-Dideoxy	+	++
5′-Deoxy	++	++
2′-*O*-Methyl	−	−
3′-*O*-Methyl	−	
3′-Deoxy-3′-methyl	−	
2′,3′-Isopropylidene	−	
5′-Deoxy-5′-amino	−	
5′-Deoxy-5′-azido	−	
5′-*O*-Acetate	−	
5′-*O*-Nicotinate	−	
5′-Carboxylic acid	−	−
5′-Ethyl-5′-carboxylate	−	−
Carbocyclic analog	−	−
Phosphorylated derivatives		
ATP	+++	
α,β-Methylene ATP	−	−
β,γ-Methylene ATP	−	−
ADP	++	
5′-AMP	+++	

TABLE 5. (continued)

Compound	Agonist activity	Antagonist activity
Phosphorylated derivatives (continued)		
2'-AMP	++	
3'-AMP	++	
3',5'-Cyclic AMP	+++	
N^6-Benzylcyclic AMP	+	
2'-Deoxycyclic AMP	−	+
N^6-Butyryl cyclic AMP	−	−
8-Bromocyclic AMP	−	−
8-Benzylthiocyclic AMP	−	−
1,N^6-Ethenocyclic AMP	−	−
Methylxanthines		
Theophylline	−	+++
Caffeine	−	++
Isobutylmethylxanthine	−	+++

[a] Agonist activity was measured at 0.1 mM concentrations and is expressed on a scale of −(no activity) to ++++ relative to the activity of adenosine. Antagonist activity versus 0.1 mM adenosine was measured using 0.2 to 0.3 mM concentrations of analog or methylxanthine. The most effective inhibitors (+++) inhibit by >75%, the least effective (+) by <40%, while inactive compounds are designated by −.

and potentiated by uptake inhibitors (Ebert and Schwabe, 1973; Fain, 1973). Whether adenosine has similar inhibitory effects on certain cyclic AMP systems in brain slices is unknown and would probably be masked by its marked stimulatory effects on overall levels of cyclic AMP.

A large number of compounds structurally related to adenosine have been screened for agonist or antagonist activity in guinea pig cortical slices (Sattin and Rall, 1970; Shimizu *et al.*, 1970d; Huang *et al.*, 1972; Huang and Daly, 1974a; Sturgill *et al.*, 1975; Mah and Daly, 1976). A summary is presented in Table 5. Alterations in the purine portion of adenosine, as in 1-methyladenosine, 8-bromoadenosine, tubercidin, formycin, and 8-azadenosine, resulted in virtual loss of both agonist and antagonist activity. Among natural nucleosides only adenosine exhibited agonist activity. Certain purine-modified adenosine analogs such as the 2-chloro, 2-hydroxy, 2-amino, N^6-methyl, or 8-methylamino derivitives did retain agonist activity. Indeed, 2-chloroadenosine and adenosines with a bulky N^6-substituent were as potent or more potent than adenosine. N^6-Dimethyladenosine was inactive. Alterations in the ribose moiety of adenosine as in 3'-*O*-methyl-derivative, 5'-esters other than phosphates, and 2'-deoxy, 3'-deoxy, arabinoside, xylofuranoside, and carbocyclic analogs resulted in a nearly complete loss of stimulatory activity. 5'-Deoxyadenosine, however, retained approximately one-third the agonist activity of adenosine. 5'-Deoxyadenosine, 2-chloroadenosine, and N^6-phenyladenosine, like adenosine, interacted synergistically with amines, had their effects blocked by theophylline, and were potentiated by an adenosine-uptake inhibitor, hexobendine (Huang and Daly, 1974a). Most of the ribose-modified analogs, including 5'-deoxy-adenosine, were adenosine antagonists. In certain instances, as with the xylofuranoside, these adenosine analogs may have general inhibitory effects on responses of cyclic AMP-generating systems in brain slices (Mah and Daly, 1976). ATP, ADP, and AMP were active in stimulating cyclic AMP formation, but their activity appeared to be dependent on a prior hydrolysis to adenosine. Certainly, significant hydrolysis of exogenous adenine nucleotides to adenosine occurred during incubation with slices (Sattin and Rall, 1970). The presence of adenosine deaminase has been used as a method of assessing to what extent adenosine was involved in stimulations of cyclic AMP-generating systems by various agents (Huang et al., 1973a; Mah and Daly, 1976; Schwabe et al., 1976a,b). Responses to adenosine, ATP, cyclic AMP, and an adenosine-histamine combination were antagonized by the deaminase, suggesting that ATP and cyclic AMP must be hydrolyzed to adenosine prior to activating cyclic AMP-generating systems. ATP and cyclic AMP are not substrates for this enzyme, which converts adenosine to an inactive metabolite, inosine. N^6-Phenylisopropyl-adenosine is not a substrate for the deaminase, and the response of cyclic AMP-generating systems to this agent were not antagonized by adenosine deaminase in guinea pig cortical slices. Only the analogs of cyclic AMP which could be hydrolyzed to an active adenosine analog stimulated accumulations of radioactive cyclic AMP in adenine-labeled guinea pig cerebral cortical slices. Various methylxanthines inhibited adenosine-elicited accumulations of cyclic AMP. Theophylline and isobutylmethylxanthine were more effective antagonists than caffeine. Antagonism of adenosine responses by theophylline appeared competitive, being overcome by high concentrations of adenosine.

In guinea pig cortical slices, a variety of adenosine "antagonists" such as theophylline, isobutylmethylxanthine, 2'-deoxyadenosine, and adenine xylofuranoside antagonized the response of cyclic AMP-generating systems to adenosine, ATP, cyclic AMP, and adenosine–amine combinations (Shimizu et al., 1975; Mah and Daly, 1976). The inhibitory effects of adenine xylofuranoside, however, appeared to be nonspecific, since this adenosine analog also greatly inhibited the response to histamine and to histamine–norepinephrine. Adenosine antagonists and adenosine deaminase have been used to investigate the role of adenosine "release" in the accumulations of cyclic AMP elicited by depolarizing agents, psychotropic agents, metabolic inhibitors, and glutamate in guinea pig cerebral cortical slices (see below).

The effects of adenosine in cortical slices were not antagonized by α- or β-antagonists or by antihistamines (Somerville and Smith, 1972; Schultz and Daly, 1973d). In fact, compounds of this type which have local anesthetic activity such as phentolamine, propranolol, and pheniramine and local anesthetics such as procaine and cocaine slightly potentiated the effects of adenosine. Such stimulatory effects might be related to the enhanced responses to adenosine observed in the absence of calcium ions (see below). Sattin *et al.* (1975) reported little potentiation of the response to adenosine by phentolamine or diphenhydramine in cortical slices but did mention a potentiation by phenoxybenzamine. In another study cocaine had no apparent effect on adenosine-elicited accumulation of radioactive cyclic AMP in adenine-labeled cortical slices (Shimizu *et al.*, 1973). Cocaine did potentiate the effects of low but not high concentrations of biogenic amines in cortical slices (Huang *et al.*, 1971; Shimizu *et al.*, 1973). A β-antagonist, sotalol, which has little local anesthetic activity, was stated to partially block the effect of adenosine in guinea pig cerebellar slices (Zanella and Rall, 1973).

Adenosine–Amine Combinations

In cerebral cortical slices, combinations of adenosine with (nor)epinephrine, histamine, or serotonin had much greater than additive effects on accumulations of cyclic AMP (Sattin and Rall, 1970; Shimizu *et al.*, 1970a; Huang *et al.*, 1971; Schultz and Daly, 1973a,b,c,d; Zanella and Rall, 1973; Huang and Daly, 1974a,b; Sattin *et al.*, 1975; Schultz, 1975a,b; Mah and Daly, 1976; Dismukes *et al.*, 1976a). Combinations of cyclic AMP or ATP with histamine had greater than additive effects on cyclic AMP levels in guinea pig cerebral cortical slices. Combinations of adenosine with norepinephrine or histamine had additive or greater than additive effects in cerebellar slices (Zanella and Rall, 1973; Ohga and Daly, 1976a). The effects of adenosine with either norepinephrine or isoproterenol in cerebellar slices were stated to be no greater than additive (Sattin *et al.*, 1975). Dopamine had no effect on cyclic AMP levels in the presence of low concentrations of adenosine in cortical slices, but under these conditions dopamine did appear to increase the response to 10 μM norepinephrine (Sattin *et al.*, 1975), perhaps due to inhibition of uptake or metabolism of norepinephrine by the tenfold higher concentrations of dopamine. Representative results for amine- and/or adenosine-elicited accumulations of cyclic AMP are shown in Table 6. Clearly, the magnitude of amine-elicited accumulations would be strongly influenced by the level of endogenous adenosine within the slice. Indeed, the magnitudes of amine responses were greatly increased by the presence of compounds that would inhibit reuptake of adenosine, and this increase was antagonized by theophylline (Huang and Daly, 1974a). Synergistic effects of amine–adenosine combinations were blocked by an adenosine antagonist, theophylline (Sattin *et al.*, 1975;

TABLE 6. Representative Effects of Various Agents on the
Accumulation of Cyclic AMP in Guinea Pig Cerebral Cortical or
Cerebellar Slices[a]

| | Cyclic AMP (pmol/mg protein) | | |
| | Cerebral cortex | | Cerebellum |
Agent	(A)	(B)	(C)
None	11	14	6
Histamine	80	75	8
Norepinephrine	18	13	140
Serotonin	—	14	—
Adenosine	300	220	350
Adenosine + histamine	800	900	470
Adenosine + norepinephrine	600	900	560
Adenosine + serotonin	—	600	—

[a]Data from (A) Sattin and Rall (1970), (B) Schultz and Daly (1973a), (C) Zanella and Rall
(1973). All agents were 0.1 mM. Data in (B) based on Biuret protein (see p. 100).

Mah and Daly, 1976). At low concentrations of adenosine, the synergistic
effects of amine–adenosine combinations were greatly potentiated by compounds that blocked uptake of the adenosine (Huang and Daly, 1974a).
Stimulatory effects of adenosine on accumulation of cyclic AMP were
detected at lower concentrations of the riboside when histamine was
present in the incubation medium (Huang et al., 1971). The EC_{50} for
adenosine for potentiative interaction with a histamine–norepinephrine
combination was about 16 μM (Schultz, 1975a).

The synergistic interactions between adenosine and catecholamines
appeared to be mediated in guinea pig cortical slices by receptors in many
respects similar to those mediating the effect of adenosine or amines alone.
l-Norepinephrine was much more effective than the d-isomer. Isoproterenol, a pure β-agonist, had virtually no effect on cyclic AMP-generating
systems in guinea pig cortical slices and did not synergistically interact with
adenosine (Schultz and Daly, 1973d). A synergistic interaction of isoproterenol and adenosine in guinea pig cortical slices has been reported (Sattin et
al., 1975), but it occurred only at a very high concentration of the catecholamine and might have been due to the weak α-activity of isoproterenol. A
marginal response pertained with isoproterenol alone. The synergistic
effects of adenosine–(nor)epinephrine combinations in cortical slices were
blocked by α-antagonists, partially blocked by chlorpromazine and dromoran, either partially blocked or unaffected by H_1-antihistamines and unaffected by β-antagonists (Huang and Daly, 1972; Schultz and Daly, 1973d;
Sattin et al., 1975).

The synergistic effect of the adenosine-histamine combination in cortical slices was antagonized by dromoran, chlorpromazine, and H_1-antihistamines, either partially blocked or unaffected by α-antagonists, and unaffected by a β-antagonist (Huang and Daly, 1972; Schultz and Daly, 1973d). In the presence of adenosine, 2-aminoethylthiazole, 2-methylhistamine, and 2-fluorohistamine at 100 μM concentrations elicited accumulations of cyclic AMP in guinea pig cerebral cortical slices nearly as great as those elicited by histamine, while 2-phenyl, 2-benzyl, and 2-aminohistamine and the H_2-agonist, 4-methylhistamine, elicited much smaller accumulations (Dismukes *et al.*, 1976b). The H_1-agonists had virtually no effect at this concentration in the absence of adenosine (see above). The results suggest that adenosine increases the affinity of H_1-agonists for histamine receptors and that the synergism between adenosine and histaminergic agonists in guinea pig cerebral cortex involves mainly H_1-receptors. In hippocampal slices, adenosine potentiated the responses of cyclic AMP-generating systems to histamine, 2-aminoethylthiazole, and 4-methylhistamine (Dismukes *et al.*, 1976b). The response to histamine in hippocampal slices had been inhibited by about 50% with either H_1- or H_2-antagonists in the absence of adenosine, while in the presence of adenosine, the H_1-antagonist, d-brompheniramine, inhibited the response by about 70% and the H_2-antagonist, metiamide, by only about 20%. The EC_{50} of 2-aminoethylthiazole was decreased tenfold to 24 μM in the presence of adenosine. The response to this H_1-agonist was blocked in the presence of adenosine by an H_1-antagonist, but not by an H_2-antagonist, metiamide. Dose–response curves for 4-methylhistamine exhibited in the presence of adenosine two maxima corresponding to EC_{50} values of 10 and 100 μM. Data on antagonists indicated that the high affinity interaction was with H_1-receptors, whose properties must have been altered in the presence of adenosine so as to permit activation by 4-methylhistamine. Thus, in hippocampus as in cortex, synergistic interactions of adenosine and histamine appeared to involve primarily H_1 receptors, which in the presence of adenosine exhibited enhanced affinity for the H_1-agonist, 2-aminoethylthiazole, and even interacted with the H_2-agonist, 4-methylhistamine. Burimamide was a much less effective H_2-antagonist than metiamide in these experiments and had no effect on responses to any of the adenosine–amine combinations.

The synergistic effect of adenosine–serotonin combinations in cortical slices was blocked by methysergide, was either unaffected or partially blocked by phenoxybenzamine, and was unaffected by β-antagonists, chlorpromazine and dromoran (Huang and Daly, 1972; Schultz and Daly, 1973d). Serotonin appeared to enhance the accumulation of cyclic AMP elicited by an adenosine–norepinephrine combination (Huang *et al.*, 1971). Surprisingly, Sattin *et al.* (1975), using a low concentration of adenosine, were unable to confirm extensive studies on the adenosine-serotonin interactions in guinea pig cortical slices.

Adenosine elicited repetitive accumulations of cyclic AMP in guinea pig cortical slices (Sattin and Rall, 1970; Schultz and Daly, 1973c; Schultz, 1975a). However, biogenic amines elicited only one accumulation, after which the slices were unresponsive to amines unless adenosine was present (Schultz and Daly, 1973c; Schultz, 1975a,b). Thus, it appeared that the presence of adenosine maintained amine-receptor mechanisms in a responsive state. An intermediate incubation with adenosine did not restore amine responsiveness to slices previously incubated with amines, although these slices would respond normally to an adenosine–amine combination. A prior incubation of guinea pig cortical slices with histamine–norepinephrine rendered the cyclic AMP-generating systems refractory to restimulation for at least 1.5 hr (Schultz, 1975a). An adenosine–histamine–norepinephrine combination, however, elicited a full response in these slices at that time. Responses to histamine–norepinephrine in unstimulated slices did not decline during this prolonged incubation. The coaddition of a phosphodiesterase inhibitor such as diazepam, isobutylmethylxanthine, or SQ 66007 with histamine–norepinephrine partially restored the response. The partial restoration of amine-responsiveness in amine-stimulated slices by phosphodiesterase inhibitors and the lack of effect of many phosphodiesterase inhibitors on adenosine-mediated accumulations of cyclic AMP led to the proposal that loss of amine-responsiveness was due to an amine or cyclic AMP-mediated increase in phosphodiesterase activity and that adenosine prevented or negated this increased activity of phosphodiesterase (Schultz and Daly, 1973b,c; Schultz, 1975a,b). Recently, however, certain phosphodiesterase inhibitors (RO 20-1724, benzodiazepines, ZK 62711) have been shown to be effective in potentiating adenosine-mediated accumulation of cyclic AMP (Schultz, 1974a,; Schwabe et al., 1976a). In addition, adenosine in cell-free brain preparations did not significantly inhibit phosphodiesterases (Clark et al., 1974).

Depolarizing Agents

Depolarizing agents, such as batrachotoxin, veratridine, ouabain, and high concentrations (30 to 140 mM) of potassium ions elevated cyclic AMP levels by 10- to 40-fold in guinea pig cortical slices (Rall and Sattin, 1970; Shimizu et al., 1970a,b,d, 1973; Shimizu and Daly, 1970, 1972a,b; Huang et al., 1972, 1973a; Huang and Daly, 1972, 1974b; Schultz and Daly, 1973a,b,c; Zanella and Rall, 1973; Shimizu et al., 1974b). Electrical pulsation (Kakiuchi et al., 1969; Somerville and Smith, 1972; Huang et al., 1973a; Kuroda and McIlwain, 1973; Reddington et al., 1973; Zanella and Rall, 1973) elevated concentrations of cholinium and ammonium ions or replacement of sodium ions with sucrose (Rall and Sattin, 1970; Shimizu and Daly, 1972b) also increased cyclic AMP levels. Depolarization was apparently requisite to the resultant accumulation of cyclic AMP since compounds with local anesthetic activity such as procaine, cocaine, chlorpromazine, dromoran, diphenhydramine, dichlorisoproterenol, and propranolol antagonized the effects of the depolarizing agents and of electrical pulsation (Kakiuchi *et al.*, 1969; Shimizu *et al.*, 1970d, 1973; Huang *et al.*, 1972; Shimizu and Daly, 1972b; Somerville and Smith, 1972; Zanella and Rall, 1973; Shimizu *et al.*, 1974b). The order of inhibitory potency of a series of local anesthetics versus veratridine-elicited accumulations of cyclic AMP was dibucaine > tetracaine > cocaine > lidocaine > procaine. Dibucaine alone at high concentrations (0.5 mM) elicited a small accumulation of cyclic AMP in cerebral cortical slices. The β_1-adrenergic antagonist, practolol, a compound without significant local anesthetic activity, did not block the response to electrical pulsation. Veratridine elicited accumulations of cyclic AMP in slices from brain stem and basal ganglia and cocaine antagonized these accumulations (cited in Shimizu *et al.*, 1973). The stimulatory effects of veratridine, batrachotoxin, electrical stimulation, and to a lesser extent ouabain, were antagonized in cerebral cortical slices by agents such as tetrodotoxin and saxitoxin which specifically block sodium channels in neurons (Shimizu *et al.*, 1970d; Huang *et al.*, 1972; Shimizu and Daly, 1972b; Reddington *et al.*, 1973). These agents had little effect on the accumulation elected by elevated concentrations of potassium ions or histamine. Replacement of sodium with lithium ions antagonized the effects of batrachotoxin and ouabain, while the stimulatory effect of histamine was unchanged (Shimizu and Daly, 1972b). Lithium ions have been reported to antagonize the accumulation of cyclic AMP elicited by histamine in rabbit cortical slices and by norepinephrine in rat cortical and hypothalamic slices, but not by norepinephrine in rat brain stem (Forn and Valdecasas, 1971; Palmer *et al.*, 1972a). The effects of a variety of analogs of ouabain, veratridine, and batrachotoxin and in addition certain other types of depolarizing agents on cyclic AMP accumulation in adenine-labeled cortical slices have been reported (Huang *et al.*, 1972). Effects of various compounds with local anesthetic activity on the accumulations of cyclic AMP elicited by ouabain, veratridine, and high potassium ions were also reported.

Membrane depolarization might itself have activated adenylate cyclases, but it would appear more likely that depolarization-evoked formation or release of specific activators was involved. Depolarization in brain slices by batrachotoxin, veratridine, ouabain, potassium ions, or electrical pulsation reduced ATP levels and resulted in increased levels of adenosine within the slice and enhanced efflux of adenosine from the slice (Pull and McIlwain, 1972a,b, 1973; Shimizu *et al.*, 1970a, 1972a; Heller and McIlwain, 1973; Huang *et al.*, 1973a; Kuroda and McIlwain, 1973; Schultz and Daly, 1973a; Huang and Daly, 1974b). Tetrodotoxin only blocked by 70 to

80% the increase in release of adenosine elicited by electrical pulsation (Pull and McIlwain, 1973) while virtually completely blocking the accumulation of cyclic AMP elicited by electrical pulsation (Reddington et al., 1973). The magnitude of release of adenosine during electrical pulsation (Pull and McIlwain, 1972a) or incubation with depolarizing agents (Schultz and Daly, 1973a) was sufficient to account for the observed accumulations of cyclic AMP in guinea pig brain slices. The release of adenosine elicited by electrical pulsation was markedly enhanced by the presence of papaverine or 2'-deoxyadenosine presumably by inhibition of adenosine reuptake (McIlwain, 1972). Exogenous adenosine increased both the basal rate and the rate of electrically stimulated efflux of radioactive adenosine from adenine-labeled guinea pig cortical slices, presumably again by competition with reuptake and incorporation mechanisms (Pull and McIlwain, 1973). If "released" adenosine was responsible for the enhanced accumulation of cyclic AMP elicited by depolarizing agents and electrical pulsation, then the responses to such agents should have been blocked by theophylline and other adenosine antagonists. The responses to batrachotoxin, veratridine, and electrical pulsation in cortical slices were, indeed, blocked by greater than 70% by theophylline or isobutylmethylxanthine (Kakiuchi et al., 1969; Shimizu et al., 1970b; Shimizu and Daly, 1972b; Somerville and Smith, 1972; Huang et al., 1973a; Zanella and Rall, 1973; Mah and Daly, 1976). Theophylline had no effect on efflux of adenosine from electrically pulsed cortical slices (Pull and McIlwain, 1976). 2'-Deoxyadenosine was less effective than theophylline in antagonizing veratridine-elicited accumulation of cyclic AMP. The accumulation elicited by ouabain or potassium ions was blocked by only 40 to 50% by theophylline, isobutylmethylxanthine, or 3'-deoxyadenosine, indicating that with certain depolarizing agents, factors other than adenosine were involved in the activation of cyclic AMP-generating systems. Adenine xylofuranoside inhibited responses to veratridine and ouabain probably because of nonspecific effects on cyclases (Mah and Daly, 1976). Adenosine deaminase in the medium reduced by 70 to 90% the accumulation of cyclic AMP elicited by veratridine, 100 mM potassium ions, or electrical pulsation in cortical slices, while having little effect on accumulations of cyclic AMP elicited by ouabain or a histamine–norepinephrine combination (Huang et al., 1973a; Mah and Daly, 1976). Such results provided evidence for the release of adenosine into extracellular space as a requisite to the accumulation of cyclic AMP elicited by certain depolarizing agents.

The accumulations of cyclic AMP elicited in cortical slices by adenosine and by electrical pulsation were similar in magnitude, while the maximal accumulations elicited by veratridine, batrachotoxin, ouabain, and potassium ions were much greater, but again for all depolarizing agents of a similar magnitude (Shimizu et al., 1970b; Shimizu and Daly, 1972b;

Somerville and Smith, 1972; Huang *et al.*, 1973a; Zanella and Rall, 1973). Combinations of 40 mM potassium ions with adenosine or in one case with 5'-AMP had much greater than additive effects on cyclic AMP levels in cortical slices (Rall and Sattin, 1970; Huang *et al.*, 1971; Shimizu and Daly, 1972b; Zanella and Rall, 1973). Combinations of submaximal stimulatory concentrations of the other depolarizing agents either with each other or with 40 mM potassium ions or with adenosine had nearly additive effects, while at supramaximal concentrations their effects were not additive (Shimizu *et al.*, 1970b; Shimizu and Daly, 1972b). Combinations of adenosine and electrical pulsation had either less than additive (Zanella and Rall, 1973) or at least additive (Somerville and Smith, 1972) effects. Availability of ATP and differential effects of exogenous adenosine or adenosine "released" during depolarization at both receptor and catalytic sites of adenylate cyclases could be involved in some of the observed differences in extent of accumulation of cyclic AMP with the various depolarizing agents. Although adenosine did not appear to inhibit adenylate cyclases in cell-free brain preparations from guinea pig (Sattin and Rall, 1970), it has been reported to inhibit cyclases in another brain preparation (McKenzie and Bar, 1973) and in preparations from other tissues (cf. references in Huang and Daly, 1974a). As a substrate for adenosine and adenylate kinases, incorporated adenosine might compete effectively with cyclase for ATP in a small membrane-associated pool and thereby inhibit formation of cyclic AMP. Blockade of the uptake of adenosine by *p*-nitrobenzylthioguanosine did prevent the apparent inhibitory effects of high concentrations of adenosine on cyclic AMP accumulation in blood platelets (Haslam and Rosson, 1975). Thus, these inhibitory effects of adenosine on cyclic AMP accumulation appeared to occur at an intracellular site, whereas the stimulatory effects in platelets as in brain slices appear to be at an extracellular site. Inhibitory effects of low concentrations of adenosine on cyclic AMP-generating systems in fat cells occurred at an extracellular site (Ebert and Schwabe, 1973; Fain 1973).

Combinations of a depolarizing agent such as batrachotoxin, veratridine, ouabain, potassium and cholinium ions, or electrical pulsation with a biogenic amine such as norepinephrine, histamine, or serotonin had greater than additive effects on levels of cyclic AMP in guinea pig cortical slices (Kakiuchi *et al.*, 1969; Rall and Sattin, 1970; Shimizu *et al.*, 1970a,d; Huang *et al.*, 1971; Huang and Daly, 1972, 1974b; Shimizu and Daly, 1972a,b; Schultz and Daly, 1973a,c; Zanella and Rall, 1973).

The effects of a variety of catecholamines, phenolic amines, serotonin analogs, histamines, and various antagonists have been studied in the presence of 40 mM potassium ions (Shimizu *et al.*, 1970; Huang *et al.*, 1971; Huang and Daly, 1972). The results were similar to those discussed above for amine agonists and antagonists except that the effects of the amines were much more pronounced and blocking agents with local anesthetic activity were more active as antagonists against amine–potassium ion combinations than against the amine itself. (Nor)epinephrine, isoproterenol, N-methylepinephrine, and α-methylnorepinephrine exhibited activity. Dopamine, adrenalone, 6-hydroxydopamine, 5-hydroxydopamine, and 2-methyl, 5-methyl, or 6-methyl-norepinephrine had no activity. Only two phenolic amines, N-methyl-m-octopamine and 4-hydroxy-3-methanesulfonamidophenethanolamine exhibited activity. Tyramines, octopamines, (nor)metanephrine, and other monophenolic amines had no activity. Serotonin, N-methylserotonin, α-methylserotonin and 4-hydroxytryptamine exhibited activity, while bufotenine, 6-hydroxy-, or 2-hydroxytryptamine and 5,6-dihydroxytryptamine had no activity. Histamine, ω-N-methylhistamines were active, while α-methylhistamine was inactive. The synergism between histamine and potassium ions, unlike that between histamine and adenosine, was only partially blocked by theophylline (Rall and Sattin, 1970).

Initially, the observations that the accumulation of cyclic AMP elicited by depolarizing agents in cortical slices was antagonized in calcium-free medium and by magnesium ions were interpreted to be indicative of a presynaptic excitation–secretion step requiring calcium ion prior to postsynaptic activation of adenylate cyclase by a released neurotransmitter. In the mammalian central nervous system magnesium ions have, however, pronounced postsynaptic effects (Kato and Somjen, 1969). In addition, more recent studies with brain slices have revealed effects of calcium-free conditions on basal levels of cyclic AMP and on accumulations of cyclic AMP elicited directly by amines and adenosine (see below). Partial dependency of accumulations of cyclic AMP on extracellular calcium ions occurred with 40 mM and 100 mM potassium ions and with ouabain, batrachotoxin, and veratridine (Shimizu et al., 1970b; Shimizu and Daly, 1972b; Zanella and Rall, 1973; Shimizu et al., 1974b). In another study, the accumulation of cyclic AMP elicited by ouabain or 125 nM potassium ions in guinea pig cerebral cortical slices was completely blocked with calcium-free EGTA-containing media, while the response to veratridine was only marginally reduced (Schultz, 1975b; Schultz and Kleefeld, 1975). Calcium ions were apparently not required for the stimulatory effect of electrical pulsation (Zanella and Rall, 1973). The response to electrical pulsation was only slightly decreased in calcium-free EGTA-containing medium. High concentrations of magnesium ion, a calcium antagonist probably at both pre- and postsynaptic sites, blocked the increase in cyclic AMP elicited by 40 mM potassium ions and ouabain, had little effect on the increase elicited by veratridine and batrachotoxin, and potentiated the response to electrical pulsation (Rall and Sattin, 1970; Shimizu and Daly, 1972b; Zanella and Rall, 1973). Magnesium ions appeared to either decrease (Shimizu and Daly,

1972b) or increase (Rall and Sattin, 1970) the accumulation of cyclic AMP elicited by 100 mM potassium ions. The absence of calcium ions greatly increased the basal "release" of adenosine from cortical slices, while partially or completely antagonizing further increases in efflux of adenosine elicited, respectively, by veratridine (H. Shimizu, unpublished results) or electrical pulsation (McIlwain, 1972; Pull and McIlwain, 1973).

Clearly, the nature of the effects of depolarizing agents on cyclic AMP levels and the involvement of adenosine formation, calcium ions, and other factors in this enhanced accumulation of cyclic AMP have not been fully resolved even in guinea pig cerebral slices where the phenomena have been extensively studied. Further differences appeared with slices from other brain regions. In cerebellar slices, electrical pulsation elicited a 6- to 14-fold increase in cyclic AMP levels which was antagonized by the adenosine antagonist, theophylline (Zanella and Rall, 1973). The response of cyclic AMP-generating systems to electrical pulsation in cerebellar slices was additive with the response to adenosine, in contrast to cortical slices where no additivity was observed. An attempt to delineate whether or not substances released by electrical pulsation might be interacting with responses of cyclic AMP-generating systems to exogenous adenosine in cerebellar slices has been made (Zanella and Rall, 1973). A partial blockade of response to the combination of adenosine and electrical pulsation by the β-antagonist, sotalol, suggested that release of norepinephrine might be involved. An alternative approach, namely depletion of endogenous norepinephrine by prior treatment of animals with reserpine or 6-hydroxydopamine, led to ambiguous results because of the greatly enhanced responses to electrical pulsation in cerebellar slices from drug-treated animals (see Section 3.1.13). Responses to adenosine also appeared to be enhanced after drug treatments, as was the response to a combination of adenosine and electrical pulsation. Ouabain and veratridine elicited, respectively, fourfold and eightfold increases in cyclic AMP levels in cerebellar slices. Potassium ions (40 mM) had no effect on levels of cyclic AMP in cerebellar slices and partially antagonized the increase in levels of cyclic AMP elicited by adenosine. It would appear that in cortical slices high concentrations of potassium ions increase "release" of unknown substances which potentiate adenosine responses, while in guinea pig cerebellar slices potassium ions increase "release" of substances which inhibit adenosine responses. In both cortical and cerebellar slices, combinations of potassium ions and amines or of adenosine and amines had greater than additive effects on cyclic AMP levels. The response to electrical pulsation in cerebellar slices was only slightly decreased in calcium-free EGTA-containing medium or by the presence of 14 mM magnesium ion. In a more recent study veratridine elicited a three- to fourfold accumulation of cyclic AMP in guinea pig cerebellar slices (Ohga and Daly, 1976a,b). The response to veratridine was dependent on calcium ions and was blocked by theophylline. High concentrations of magnesium ion had little effect on the response to veratridine. The response was not antagonized by atropine, strychnine, diethyl glutamate, picrotoxin, or sotalol, but was reduced by phentolamine, chlorpromazine, and promethazine, probably because of local anesthetic effects of the latter drugs.

Studies with depolarizing agents and metabolic inhibitors (see below) have not provided clear insights into the morphological compartments associated with cyclic AMP accumulation in brain slices. The enhanced release of adenosine with neuronal depolarizing agents such as veratridine and the blockage by tetrodotoxin suggested that adenosine formation and release were occurring primarily from neuronal compartments. Potassium ions would conversely be expected to depolarize both neuronal and glial cells. A reduction of ATP in compartments associated with adenylate cyclases of the slice would be expected to result in decreased responses of cyclic AMP-generating systems, while reductions of ATP in other morphological compartments could result in adenosine "release" and resultant increased levels of cyclic AMP in another compartment. Unfortunately, depolarizing agents or metabolic inhibitors with specific effects on presynaptic or postsynaptic entities of neurons or on glia have not been defined. At present, with respect to the role and regulation of cyclic AMP in the central nervous system *in vitro,* investigations of the various depolarizing agents and metabolic inhibitors have posed more questions than they have answered. Furthermore, the relevance of such artificial depolarizations to regulatory mechanisms in the intact brain has not been established. A study of the formation of cyclic AMP in the isolated piriform cortex or superior colliculus on stimulation of their respective innervating tracts might provide exciting results. Stimulation of the tracts does result in enhanced "release" of adenosine into the medium from the isolated preparations (Heller and McIlwain, 1973). Adenosine stimulated cyclic AMP accumulation and inhibited transsynaptic potentials elicited in olfactory cortex after stimulation of the innervating tract, but it had no inhibitory effects on potentials in similar experiments with the superior colliculus (Kuroda and Kobayshi, 1975; Okada and Kuroda, 1975; Kuroda *et al.,* 1976, see Section 4.3.1).

Metabolic Inhibitors

Certain psychotropic drugs in high concentrations have been reported to elicit accumulation of cyclic AMP in guinea pig cerebral cortical slices. These included prenylamine, phenothiazines such as chlorpromazine, and tricyclic antidepressants such as desipramine and chlorimipramine (Huang and Daly, 1972, 1974b). In another report, only tricyclic antidepressants appeared to increase cyclic AMP levels (Kodama *et al.,* 1971). Many of these compounds have been reported to be inhibitors of phosphodiesterases and adenylate cyclases (see Sections 2.1.6 and 2.3.6), but their effects on levels of cyclic AMP appeared due primarily to their ability to cause depletion of ATP and resultant formation and efflux of adenosine (Huang and Daly, 1974b; Pull and McIlwain, 1976). Low concentrations of chlorpromazine and desipramine inhibited efflux of radioactive adenosine from control and electrically stimulated adenine-labeled guinea pig cerebral cortical slices, while high concentrations greatly increased release of adenosine. The maximal accumulation of cyclic AMP elicited by these agents occurred only after 7 to 15 min and was blocked by theophylline, but not a local anesthetic, cocaine, or by adrenergic antagonists. Attempts to demonstrate the expected synergistic interactions between "released" adenosine and biogenic amines were presumably thwarted in the case of chlorpromazine and chlorimipramine by antagonism of amine receptors by such tricyclic compounds. It was proposed that these various compounds reduced ATP levels by a nonspecific interference with oxidative phosphorylation and that the resultant "release" of adenosine elicited accumulations of cyclic AMP from intracellular ATP associated with cyclic AMP-generating systems. Chlorpromazine and promethazine caused increases in cyclic AMP levels in guinea pig cerebellar slices during 15-min but not during 45-min incubations (Ohga and Daly, 1976b). Other psychoactive drugs such as amphetamine, methylphenidate, monoamine oxidase inhibitors, reserpine, tetrabenazine, and droperidol had no or only marginal effects on cyclic AMP levels in cortical slices (Huang and Daly, 1972).

Certain metabolic inhibitors such as 2,4-dinitrophenol, cyanide, and azide elicited small accumulations of cyclic AMP, while others such as 2-deoxyglucose, malonate, and oligomycin had no effect or in the case of quinones (2-bromo-1,4-benzoquinone, 1,2-naphthoquinone-8-sulfonate) prevented accumulations of cyclic AMP in cerebral cortical slices. 2,4-Dinitrophenol and cyanide partially antagonized accumulations of cyclic AMP elicited by other agents (Shimizu and Daly, 1972b; Huang and Daly, 1974b). The accumulation of cyclic AMP elicited by 2,4-dinitrophenol was blocked by theophylline. It would appear that certain inhibitors reduce ATP in cyclic AMP-generating compartments, while others such as 2,4-dinitrophenol, in addition, elicit release of adenosine from other compartments. Lack of oxygen or glucose during incubations of guinea pig cortical slices has been cited as having little effect on levels of cyclic AMP (Kakiuchi and Rall, 1968a).

Glutamate

The putative excitatory neurotransmitters, glutamate and aspartate, elicited a 40- to 80-fold increase in levels of cyclic AMP in guinea pig cerebral cortical slices (Shimizu *et al.*, 1974). The rate of accumulation of cyclic AMP was linear for at least 30 min and the EC_{50} for these amino acids was about 1.5 mM, with maximal responses at 10 mM. The responses to amino acids were not decreased under calcium-free (EGTA) conditions or by the presence of local anesthetics such as tetrodotoxin or cocaine, but were effectively blocked by the adenosine antagonist, theophylline. The response to the amino acids was synergistic with that evoked by biogenic amines. Alanine at a prodigous concentration of 20 mM elicited a small accumulation of cyclic AMP. Restimulation of cyclic AMP formation by glutamate was possible after washing of glutamate-stimulated slices. The results suggest that the lowering of ATP levels within the slice due to consumption of ATP during uptake of the amino acids (cf. Banay-Schwartz *et al.*, 1974) had led to an increase in efflux of adenosine and a resultant activation of adenosine-sensitive cyclases. Glutamate did potentiate the rate of efflux of radioactivity, primarily adenosine, from adenine-labeled guinea pig cortical slices (Pull and McIlwain, 1975). However, the responses to adenosine and either glutamate or aspartate were greater than additive (Shimizu *et al.*, 1974, 1975b), a result difficult to rationalize in terms of adenosine as an intermediate in glutamate- or aspartate-elicited accumulation of cyclic AMP. The structure–activity dependency of the glutamate–aspartate response in guinea pig cortical slices has been extensively examined (Shimizu *et al.*, 1974, 1975b). The D-isomers were somewhat less active than the natural L-amino acids. Cysteine sulfinic acid appeared to be somewhat more efficacious than cysteate, glutamate, or aspartate, and the maximal accumulation elicited by this analog was two- to threefold greater than those elicited by the natural amino acids. Antagonists of glutamate-elicited excitation of central neurons such as diethyl glutamate, taurine, glycine, or γ-aminobutyrate had no effect on glutamate-elicited accumulations of cyclic AMP. Agonist activity for accumulation of cyclic AMP and excitation of central neurons by glutamate analogs, in contrast, showed a relatively good correlation. The accumulation of cyclic AMP elicited by glutamate in guinea pig cerebral cortical slices was effectively inhibited by 2,3-diaminopropionate, 2,4-diaminobutyrate, and ornithine (Shimizu *et al.*, 1975c). The diaminopropionate and diaminobutyrate had no effect on accumulations of cyclic AMP elicited by adenosine, histamine, or a histamine–norepinephrine combination, but did inhibit the response to aspartate. The accumulations of cyclic AMP elicited by kainic and ibotenic acid were not antagonized by 2,3-diaminopropionate, nor could the response to glutamate be completely inhibited by the diamino acid. The diamino acids would appear to represent useful specific antagonists for the study of glutamate-elicited accumulations of cyclic AMP in brain slices. Such compounds could be used to study the involvement of released glutamate and aspartate in the response of cyclic AMP-generating systems to depolarizing agents and metabolic inhibitors in brain slices.

The interrelationship of adenosine- and glutamate-elicited accumulations of cyclic AMP in guinea pig cortical slices requires further study. The inhibition of glutamate responses by theophylline, isobutylmethylxanthine, and adenosine deaminase (Mah and Daly, 1976) was clearly consonant with the intermediacy of adenosine. However, 2'-deoxyadenosine, another adenosine antagonist, had no effect on glutamate responses. 2'-Deoxyadenosine inhibited the accumulation of cyclic AMP elicited by adenosine, ATP, and adenosine–amine combinations in guinea pig cortical slices, but had little or no effect on responses to histamine, norepinephrine, glutamate, or kainic acid (Shimizu *et al.*, 1975c). Theophylline and isobutylmethylxanthine inhibited responses to adenosine, glutamate, asparate, and cysteine sulfinate, while having no effect on the response to histamine. At least three explanations of these anomalous results can be advanced: (1) Glutamate at high concentrations causes release of adenosine at cyclic AMP sites within the slice that are not reached because of metabolic or uptake barriers by exogenous adenosine or 2'-deoxyadenosine; (2) in the presence of glutamate, adenosine and 2'-deoxyadenosine activate receptors normally activated only by adenosine; (3) glutamate activates cyclic AMP systems independent of adenosine by mechanisms that are inhibited by methylxanthines or adenosine deaminase. The latter explanation has the corollary that methylxanthines and adenosine deaminase should no longer be considered as specific adenosine antagonists.

Calcium Ions

Early studies indicated that the accumulations of cyclic AMP elicited by histamine or adenosine in guinea pig cerebral cortical slices were little affected by the absence of calcium ions in the medium (Shimizu *et al.*, 1970b,d). High concentrations of magnesium, a pre- and postsynaptic calcium antagonist in brain tissue, however, potentiated accumulations of cyclic AMP elicited by histamine, norepinephrine, adenosine, or an adenosine–norepinephrine combination (Rall and Sattin, 1970; Shimizu and Daly, 1972b; Zanella and Rall, 1973; Sattin *et al.*, 1975). Basal levels of cyclic AMP were somewhat increased by the presence of high concentrations of magnesium ion, perhaps due to enhanced release of adenosine under these conditions.

The effects of the absence of calcium ions on the responses of cyclic AMP-generating systems in guinea pig cortical slices to amines and adenosine have now been investigated in some detail. In slices preincubated for 10 min in calcium-free medium plus 1 mM EGTA, the absence of calcium resulted in enhanced responses to histamine, norepinephrine, histamine–norepinephrine, and adenosine (Schultz, 1975b; Schultz and Kleefeld, 1975). During the initial 5 to 10 min of stimulation with the biogenic amines, cyclic AMP levels were similar under normal and "calcium-free" conditions, but cyclic AMP levels then declined in normal slices while continuing to rise under calcium-free conditions. Restimulation of cyclic AMP formation by histamine or histamine–norepinephrine was possible under calcium-free conditions, while restimulation was marginal under normal conditions. Similarly, the decline in the magnitude of the response to histamine–norepinephrine due to prior incubation of guinea pig cortical slices with histamine under normal conditions did not occur under calcium-free conditions. Norepinephrine had no effect on cyclic AMP levels in guinea pig cortical slices in the presence of calcium but elicited a twofold accumulation through interaction with an α-adrenergic receptor in calcium-free (EGTA) medium (Schultz and Kleefeld, 1975). Dopamine, serotonin, and prostaglandin E_1 (3–30μM) had no effect on cyclic AMP levels either in the presence or absence of calcium ions. In calcium-free (EGTA) medium cyproheptadine, normally considered a serotonin and histamine antagonist, elicited a threefold accumulation of cyclic AMP. Basal levels of cyclic AMP in guinea pig cortical slices increased after incubation in calcium-free (EGTA) medium for a total of 25 min. The results were interpreted in terms of activation of calcium-dependent phosphodiesterases under normal conditions due to an amine or adenosine-elicited influx of calcium. However, subsequent studies indicated that during prolonged incubation of slices with EGTA or calcium-free medium adenosine efflux had increased and that the enhanced responses to amines were primarily due to the presence of higher levels of extracellular adenosine (Ohga and Daly, 1976a; Schwabe et al., 1976b). Thus, prolonged incubation in calcium-free media greatly elevated basal levels of cyclic AMP in cortical slices and potentiated the response to norepinephrine. Theophylline reduced basal levels under both control and calcium-free conditions. Even during short incubations with EGTA, basal levels of cyclic AMP and responses to norepinephrine, adenosine, and N^6-phenylisopropyladenosine increased in guinea pig cerebral cortical slices, while responses to histamine remained virtually unaffected (Schwabe et al., 1976b). If both adenosine deaminase and EGTA were present, a response to norepinephrine and histamine was no longer detectable, while the response to N^6-phenylisopropyladenosine was virtually unchanged. Thus, in guinea pig as in rat (see Section 3.3.1), responses of cyclic AMP-generating systems to biogenic amines in cerebral cortical slices appeared to require the presence of either extracellular calcium or adenosine. In the absence of extracellular calcium ions formation of adenosine is enhanced. Perhaps the adenosine them in some way mobilizes calcium ions from membranal or intracellular compartments to provide for maintenance of adenylate cyclases in a responsive state. Elevated concentrations of extracellular calcium antagonized adenosine-elicited accumulations of cyclic AMP in olfactory cortical slices (Kuroda et al., 1976).

Verapamil, a putative calcium antagonist, increased levels of cyclic

AMP in slices from guinea pig cerebral cortex and cerebellum, but the mechanism involved was not investigated (Ohga and Daly, 1976b). An analog of verapamil, prenylamine, enhanced cyclic AMP levels in guinea pig cortical slices apparently via adenosine release (Huang and Daly, 1974b).

Levels of cyclic AMP were increased threefold in guinea pig cerebellar slices after incubation in calcium-free (EGTA) medium (Zanella and Rall, 1973), but were little affected by prolonged incubation in calcium-free medium without EGTA (Ohga and Daly, 1976a). Responses to norepinephrine, isoproterenol, and histamine were virtually unaffected by the prior prolonged incubation in calcium-free medium. The calcium ionophore, A-23187, had little effect on levels of cyclic AMP in cerebellar slices, while another calcium ionophore, X-537A, markedly reduced cyclic AMP levels (Ohga and Daly, 1976b).

Phosphodiesterase Inhibitors

Definitive studies on the role of phosphodiesterases in the responses on cyclic AMP-generating systems in brain slices have now begun. In the early studies, theophylline or caffeine were often routinely added to incubation media, but the effects were variable. Theophylline was subsequently found to be relatively ineffective in brain slices as a phosphodiesterase inhibitor and, in addition, to be an adenosine antagonist. Caffeine was less active as an adenosine antagonist (Shimizu *et al.*, 1969; Sattin and Rall, 1970; Huang *et al.*, 1972), but was also less active as a phosphodiesterase inhibitor. Theophylline had little or no effect on norepinephrine-elicited accumulation of cyclic AMP in guinea pig cortical slices (Shimizu and Daly, 1972b; Sattin *et al.*, 1975). Rall and Gilman (1970) stated that theophylline increased the accumulation of cyclic AMP elicited by low concentrations of norepinephrine in guinea pig cerebellar slices. Theophylline had little or no effect on histamine responses in guinea pig cortical slices prepared either at room temperature or in the cold (Kakiuchi *et al.*, 1969; Rall and Sattin, 1970; Shimizu *et al.*, 1970a; Shimizu and Daly, 1972b; Schultz and Daly, 1973b; Huang and Daly, 1974a). Caffeine, was, however, reported to potentiate histamine responses in guinea pig cortical slices (Shimizu *et al.*, 1969).

More potent and effective phosphodiesterase inhibitors have now been studied extensively in brain slices. Those include papaverine, RO 20-1724, and benzodiazepines such as diazepam. The pyrazolopyrimidine, SQ 20009, has been found to be relatively ineffective as a phosphodiesterase inhibitor in brain slices, in contrast to its high potency as an inhibitor of phosphodiesterases in brain homogenates. Isobutylmethylxanthine is a potent phosphodiesterase inhibitor, but its utility for studies on phosphodiesterases in brain slices is negated because of its high potency as an adenosine antagonist (Huang *et al.*, 1972; Schultz and Daly, 1973b; Mah and Daly, 1976). Many of the phosphodiesterase inhibitors appear to increase basal levels of cyclic AMP and potentiate amine responses in part because of inhibition of adenosine uptake. Thus, low concentrations of the phosphodiesterase inhibitors, papaverine, dipyridamole, and hexobendine, were found to potentiate amine responses primarily by inhibition of adenosine-reuptake processes, resulting in synergistic amine-endogenous adenosine interactions (Huang and Daly, 1974a). Such potentiations of amine responses were antagonized by theophylline. Papaverine increased the net efflux of adenosine from perfused brain preparations (McIlwain, 1972; Heller and McIlwain, 1973). A variety of phosphodiesterase inhibitors such as dipyridamole > papaverine, diazepam, chlordiazepoxide, SQ 20009 > RO 20-1724, inhibited uptake of radioactive adenosine by guinea pig cerebral cortical slices, indicating that in part stimulatory effects of such inhibitors on cyclic AMP levels in brain slices could be due to increases of extracellular adenosine levels within the slice (Mah and Daly, 1976). Even with RO 20-1724, adenosine mechanisms appeared of primary importance to its effects on accumulation of cyclic AMP in rat cortical slices (Schwabe *et al.*, 1976a,b, see Section 3.3.1). In rat cortical slices a related compound, ZK 62711, appeared the agent of choice for the specific inhibition of phosphodiesterases.

The phosphodiesterase inhibitors, isobutylmethylxanthine, papaverine, and dibutyryl cyclic AMP, significantly potentiated amine-elicited accumulations of cyclic AMP in guinea pig cerebral cortical slices (Schultz and Daly, 1973b,d; Mah and Daly, 1976). None of these inhibitors potentiated responses to maximal concentrations of adenosine, nor did isobutylmethylxanthine or papaverine significantly retard the disappearance of cyclic AMP in slices previously stimulated with a combination of adenosine–histamine–norepinephrine–phosphodiesterase inhibitor. Papaverine partially inhibited the accumulation of radioactive cyclic AMP elicited by cyclic AMP, perhaps by interfering with its conversion to adenosine. Papaverine had no effect on the accumulation of cyclic AMP elicited by glutamate.

Potent phosphodiesterase inhibitors such as diazepam and RO 20-1724 have now been found to potentiate adenosine, amine, and glutamate-elicited accumulations of cyclic AMP in guinea pig cortical slices (Schultz, 1974a,b; Mah and Daly, 1976). The EC_{50} for RO 20-1724 in potentiating the responses to histamine, adenosine, or a histamine–norepinephrine combination in cerebral cortical slices was about 20 μM. RO 20-2926 (4-(3-ethoxyethoxy-4-methoxybenzyl)-2-imidazolidinone), a somewhat more water soluble analog of RO 20-1724, was less effective than RO 20-1724, but did potentiate both amine- and adenosine-elicited accumulations of cyclic AMP.

A variety of benzodiazepines have been studied with respect to accumulations of cyclic AMP elicited by histamine, histamine–norepinephrine, and adenosine in guinea pig cortical slices (Schultz, 1974a,b; Mah and Daly, 1976). Diazepam was the most effective in potentiating accumulations of cyclic AMP. Indeed, chlordiazepoxide had little effect on adenosine responses. Diazepam appeared somewhat less potent (EC_{50}, 40 μM) in potentiating the response to histamine than in potentiating the response to a combination of histamine and norepinephrine (EC_{50}, 16 μM). Adenosine mechanisms are involved to a greater extent in the latter response and diazepam inhibits reuptake of adenosine. The presence of 0.5 mM diazepam significantly retarded, but did not block the disappearance of cyclic AMP in cortical slices previously stimulated by norepinephrine–histamine–diazepam. Basal levels of cyclic AMP in guinea pig cortical slices were elevated by RO 20-1724 and diazepam, presumably in part due to blockage of reuptake of endogenous adenosine. In another study, chlordiazepoxide and diazepam elevated basal levels of cyclic AMP in cortical slices and potentiated amine responses (Hess *et al.*, 1975).

SQ 20009 was surprisingly ineffective in guinea pig cortical slices and only slightly potentiated the response to histamine, while having no significant effect on responses to histamine–norepinephrine and slightly inhibiting responses to adenosine and glutamate (Schultz, 1974a,b; Mah and Daly, 1976). Another group reported that SQ 20009 potentiated amine responses (Hess *et al.*, 1975). SQ 66007, an analog of SQ 20009, was stated to potentiate amine responses (Schultz, 1975).

None of the inhibitors potentiated responses to veratridine in cortical slices (Huang *et al.*, 1972; Mah and Daly, 1976). Indeed, papaverine, diazepam, and SQ 20009 inhibited the response to veratridine, while RO 20-1724 had no effect. Papaverine inhibited the response to high concentrations of potassium ions in cortical slices. Isobutylmethylxanthine inhibited the response to veratridine in cerebellar slices (Ohga and Daly, 1976b).

Protamine, a phosphodiesterase inhibitor in brain homogenates, caused accumulations of cyclic AMP in guinea pig cortical slices which were antagonized effectively by theophylline (Shimizu *et al.*, 1974). Since it was unlikely that this protein penetrates to intracellular phosphodiesterases, the elevation in cyclic AMP levels in brain slices in the presence of protamine would appear more likely to have been due to enhanced efflux of adenosine under these conditions.

RO 20-1724 and diazepam increased basal levels of cyclic AMP in guinea pig cerebellar slices, while isobutylmethylxanthine, papaverine, and SQ 20009 had no effect and theophylline reduced levels (Ohga and Daly, 1976b). Isobutylmethylxanthine potentiated the response to norepinephrine in cerebellar slices. Papaverine slightly increased basal levels of cyclic AMP in cerebellar slices and slightly potentiated the response to norepinephrine (Hess *et al.*, 1975). Imidazole acetic acid, a compound which like other imidazoles can activate phosphodiesterases (see Section 2.3.5) had no effect on levels of cyclic AMP in guinea pig cortical slices (Hess *et al.*, 1975).

3.1.3 Rat

Catecholamines

Norepinephrine (EC_{50}, 5 μM) elicited a 2- to 20-fold increase in cyclic AMP levels in cortical slices from Sprague–Dawley, Holtzman, Wistar, Fisher, Buffalo, and several other strains of rats (Forn and Krishna, 1971; Krishna *et al.*, 1970; Rall and Sattin, 1970; Schmidt *et al.*, 1970; Shimizu *et al.*, 1970a; Forn and Valdecasas, 1971; Uzunov and Weiss, 1971, 1972b; Palmer, 1972, 1973b; Schmidt and Robison, 1972; Weiss and Strada, 1972; French and Palmer, 1973; Huang *et al.*, 1973b; Kalisker *et al.*, 1973; Palmer *et al.*, 1973; Perkins and Moore, 1973a,b; Schultz and Daly, 1973e; Walker and Walker, 1973a; De Belleroche *et al.*, 1974; Munday *et al.*, 1974; Frazer *et al.*, 1974; Skolnick and Daly, 1974a, 1975b,c, 1976; Palmer and Scott, 1974; Schultz, 1974c; Dismukes *et al.*, 1975; French *et al.*, 1975a,b; Markstein and Wagner, 1975; Skolnick *et al.*, 1975; Perkins *et al.*, 1975; Montecucchi, 1976; Schwabe and Daly, 1976; Schwabe *et al.*, 1976a,b; Harris, 1976; Lewin *et al.*, 1976).

Isoproterenol (EC_{50}, 0.5 μM) elicited an accumulation of cyclic AMP in cerebral cortical slices that was only about one-half the magnitude of that elicited by norepinephrine (Huang *et al.*, 1973b; Perkins and Moore, 1973a, b; Schultz and Daly, 1973e; Schultz, 1974c; Markstein and Wagner, 1975; Palmer *et al.*, 1976b; Schwabe and Daly, 1976). Epinephrine elicited a maximal accumulation of cyclic AMP intermediate to those evoked by isoproterenol and norepinephrine. The response to isoproterenol in cortical slices was blocked by β-antagonists and was unaffected by α-antagonists. The response to (nor)epinephrine was only partially blocked by either α- or β-antagonists, but was completely blocked by combinations of the two types of adrenergic antagonists (see above references and reviews by Daly, 1976; Skolnick and Daly, 1976b). The response to norepinephrine in the presence of an α-antagonist was virtually identical in magnitude to the maximal response to isoproterenol. In most studies, β-antagonists have proven more effective than α-antagonists in inhibiting norepinephrine-elicited accumulations of cyclic AMP in rat cerebral cortical slices. In one study pindolol at 0.1 μM completely blocked the response to 5 μM norepinephrine or 0.5 μM isoproterenol, while phentolamine and dihydroergotamine blocked the response to norepinephrine by about 50 to 60% and had no effect on the response to isoproterenol (Markstein and Wagner, 1975; see also Schultz and Daly, 1973e; Skolnick and Daly, 1975b). High concentrations of ergot alkaloids such as dihydroergotamine, dihydroergotoxin, and nicergoline elicited accumulations of cyclic AMP in cortical slices and did not antagonize the response to norepinephrine (Montecucchi, 1976). In one study either propranolol or phentolamine completely blocked the response to norepinephrine in rat cerebral cortical slices (Palmer *et al.*, 1976b). Only propranolol antagonized the isoproterenol response. A twofold increase in cyclic AMP levels elicited by norepinephrine in thick cortical slices from Wistar rats was reported to be completely blocked by propranolol and to be unaffected by phenoxybenzamine (French and Palmer, 1973). In a recent detailed study, the accumulation of cyclic AMP elicited in rat cerebral cortical slices by (nor)epinephrine was partially blocked by α-antagonists such as phentolamine, phenoxybenzamine, and clonidine (see below) and by β-antagonists such as (+)alprenolol, (−)propranolol, and sotalol (Skolnick and Daly, 1976c). (−)Alprenolol, however, at a concentration of only 10 μM completely blocked the response to the catecholamines. (−)Alprenolol also blocked the accumulation of cyclic AMP elicited by the α-agonist, methoxamine. The results are consonant with interaction of (−)alprenolol with both α- and β-receptors controlling cyclic AMP-generation in brain tissue. An apparent slower time course for the accumulation of cyclic AMP elicited by norepinephrine and by a norepinephrine–propranolol combination as compared to the time course with isoproterenol led to the proposal that the α-adrenergic component of the norepinephrine response might be indirect (Perkins and Moore, 1973a). The rapid accumulation of cyclic AMP elicited by the α-adrenergic agonist, methoxamine, in rat cortical slices (Skolnick and Daly, 1975b) was not consonant with this proposal. Recent studies have shown that the α-component of the response of cyclic AMP-generating systems to norepinephrine in brain slices was dependent on extracellular calcium (Schwabe and Daly, 1976, see below). Variations in calcium levels in slices, depending on many factors, might thus profoundly affect the apparent proportion of α- and β- adrenergic components of the response to norepinephrine.

Clonidine and oxymetazoline, agents normally considered α-agonists, effectively inhibited the α-component of norepinephrine-elicited accumulations of cyclic AMP in rat cerebral cortical slices (Skolnick and Daly, 1975c, 1976a,c; Schwabe and Daly, 1976). Clonidine had no agonist activity towards cyclic AMP-generation in cerebral cortical slices. Combinations of clonidine and propranolol completely blocked the norepinephrine response, while combinations of clonidine and phenoxybenzamine had no greater inhibitory effect than phenoxybenzamine alone. Clonidine completely blocked responses to the α-agonist, methoxamine, and had no effect on responses to high concentrations of isoproterenol. Clonidine, however, potentiated the response to submaximal concentrations of isoproterenol apparently by increasing the affinity of the α-receptor for the catecholamine. The potentiative interaction of clonidine and isoproterenol was blocked by phenoxybenzamine. Phentolamine also appeared to potentiate accumulations of cyclic AMP elicited by low concentrations of isoproterenol in rat cerebral cortical slices (Perkins and Moore, 1973a). Both the inhibitory effects of clonidine on norepinephrine-elicited accumulations of cyclic AMP and the potentiative effects on isoproterenol-elicited accumulations of cyclic AMP appeared to occur at postsynaptic sites since both effects were present to the same extent in cortical slices from 6-hydroxydopamine-treated rats (Skolnick and Daly, 1976a). Phenoxybenzamine at high concentrations elicited a small accumulation of cyclic AMP in cortical slices from control rats but not in slices from 6-hydroxydopamine-treated rats. The presence of either clonidine or sotalol blocked the accumulation of cyclic AMP elicited by phenoxybenzamine. It was proposed that blockade by phenoxybenzamine of presynaptic α-adrenergic receptors which modulate release enhanced the efflux of norepinephrine, which then activated postsynaptic β-receptors. Clonidine is known to decrease release of norepinephrine by interaction with presynaptic α-receptors.

The α-adrenergic agonist, methoxamine, has been reported to elicit a twofold accumulation of cyclic AMP in cerebral slices of the F-344 rat strain (Skolnick and Daly, 1975b,c; Skolnick *et al.*, 1975; Skolnick and Daly, 1976c). Methoxamine elicited only minimal responses in three other rat strains (ACI, BUF, and Sprague–Dawley). The response to methoxamine was very rapid and was not altered by a membrane stabilizer, tetracaine, suggesting a direct effect on cyclic AMP-generating systems. Maximal accumulations were elicited by 100 μM methoxamine and were inhibited by α-adrenergic antagonists, but not by a β-antagonist, propranolol. ($-$)Alprenolol, however, blocked the response to methoxamine (see above). Combinations of methoxamine and isoproterenol had additive effects on accumulation of cyclic AMP, consonant with the activation of α-receptors by the former amine and of β-receptors by the latter. However, combinations of methoxamine and norepinephrine also had additive effects, suggesting that in the absence of adenosine the two amines do not activate the same sets of α-adrenergic receptors (see below). Phenylephrine had virtually no α-agonist or antagonist activity in rat cerebral cortical slices (Skolnick and Daly, 1975c). In another study with longer preincubations both methoxamine and phenylephrine elicited significant accumulations of cyclic AMP in cortical slices of Sprague–Dawley rats, and even dopamine elicited a 1.4-fold accumulation (Schwabe and Daly, 1976; Schwabe *et al.*, 1976a). In the presence of the phosphodiesterase inhibitor, RO 20-1724, dopamine but not apomorphine elicited a small accumulation of cyclic AMP in rat cortical slices (Dismukes and Daly, 1974; Harris, 1976). Dopamine (100 μM) alone elicited a twofold increase in cyclic AMP levels in rat cortical slices (Munday *et al.*, 1974). In the presence of 1 mM caffeine, 500 μM norepinephrine, but not 500 μM dopamine, elicited a significant accumulation of radioactive cyclic AMP in adenine-labeled cortical slices (Walker and Walker, 1973a). No characterization of the small responses to dopamine in rat cerebral cortical slices has been reported, and it is possible that such responses are due to partial agonist activity of dopamine at noradrenergic receptors.

Both isoproterenol and metaproterenol at 100 μM concentrations elicited fivefold accumulations of cyclic AMP in rat cerebral cortical slices, while two β_1-agonists, salbutamol and terbutaline, were much less effective (Schwabe and Daly, 1976).

No response to norepinephrine or isoproterenol was seen in cortical slices of newborn rats (Schmidt *et al.*, 1970; Schmidt and Robison, 1972; Perkins, 1973; Perkins and Moore, 1973b). The responses to both amines developed in parallel between 6 and 13 days after birth and then declined to adult levels.

Norepinephrine elicited two- to eightfold increases in cyclic AMP levels in slices from cerebellum (Krishna *et al.*, 1970, Rall and Sattin, 1970; Forn and Krishna, 1971; Uzunov and Weiss, 1971, 1972; Palmer *et al.*, 1973; Hoffer *et al.*, 1976; Skolnick *et al.*, 1976; Schwabe and Daly, 1976; Schwabe *et al.* 1976b). Isoproterenol was more potent than norepinephrine in cerebellar slices, but it elicited a lower maximal accumulation of cyclic AMP. β-Adrenergic antagonists completely blocked catecholamine responses in cerebellar slices. However, at submaximal concentrations of norepinephrine, phentolamine significantly reduced the response to norepinephrine in rat cerebellar slices (Schwabe and Daly, 1976). No potentiative interaction of clonidine and isoproterenol occurred in cerebellar slices (Skolnick and Daly, 1975a), nor did clonidine inhibit norepinephrine responses in cerebellum (Skolnick *et al.*, 1976). Dopamine had no effect on cyclic AMP levels in rat cerebellar slices (Skolnick *et al.*, 1976).

Basal levels of cyclic AMP in rat cerebellar slices in some reports (Palmer, 1972; Palmer *et al.*, 1973; Ohga and Daly, 1976a; Skolnick *et al.*, 1976) were as high as 200 to 400 pmol/mg protein and were reduced by 50% or more on incubation with theophylline. Basal levels of cyclic AMP in rat cerebellar slices have also been reported as low as 60 pmol/mg protein (Rall and Sattin, 1970). Cerebellar levels of cyclic AMP were in all reports about tenfold higher than cortical levels. Even in the presence of theophylline levels of cyclic AMP remained quite high (70 pmol/mg protein) in cerebellar slices from Sprague–Dawley rats, but were much lower (10 pmol/mg protein) in slices from Wistar CFN rats (Hoffer *et al.*, 1975). Prolonged preincubation of cerebellar slices from Sprague–Dawley rats resulted in a reduction of basal levels of cyclic AMP to a value of only 30 pmol/mg protein (Schwabe and Daly, 1976; Schwabe *et al.*, 1976b). It would appear

that in rat cerebellar slices, high adenosine efflux and low phosphodiesterase activity contribute to maintenance of elevated levels of cyclic AMP.
Cyclic AMP levels were similar in cerebellar slices from control and X-
irradiated rats (Hoffer *et al.*, 1976). Thus, elimination of the neurons which
normally comprise the granular layer had little effect on basal levels of
cyclic AMP in cerebellar tissue.

Fluphenazine at 100 μM concentrations inhibited norepinephrine- and
isoproterenol-elicited accumulations of cyclic AMP in Sprague–Dawley rat
cerebellum by only 30% (Skolnick *et al.*, 1976). At fivefold higher concentrations fluphenazine completely inhibited cyclic AMP accumulation, but
from dose–response relationships this appeared to be a nonspecific effect.
α-Flupenthixol inhibited the norepinephrine response by 30% while β-
flupenthixol and promethazine were ineffective. Fluphenazine, α-flupen-
thixol, and β-blockers, but not β-flupenthixol and promethazine, antagonized the inhibitory effects of norepinephrine on firing of cerebellar Purkinje cells. Thus, although both β-blockers and fluphenazine antagonized a
β-adrenergic electrophysiological effect mediated by cyclic AMP, only
the β-blocker completely inhibited norepinephrine-elicted accumulations of
cyclic AMP in rat cerebellar slices with fluphenazine inhibiting the norepinephrine responses by only 30%. In order to rationalize these results it was
proposed that at least two populations of β-controlled cyclases exist in
cerebellum and that fluphenazine inhibits only one population which
includes the cyclases of Purkinje cells. To test this hypothesis, CFN-strain
Wistar rats were X-irradiated neonatally to destroy the late maturing
granule, basket, and stellate cells, while sparing the early maturing Purkinje
cells. In control CFN rats, fluphenazine inhibited the accumulation of
cyclic AMP elicited by norepinephrine in cerebellar slices by about 50%
while in cerebellar slices from X-irradiated rats in which Purkinje cells were
the predominant neuron, fluphenazine now completely inhibited the norepinephrine response (Hoffer *et al.*, 1976). The magnitude of the accumulation
of cyclic AMP elicited by norepinephrine was reduced in X-irradiated
cerebellum. The results were consonant with the proposal of a β-adrenergic
controlled cyclic AMP system in Purkinje cells which is inhibited by
antipsychotics and which mediates β-elicited inhibition of firing rates of the
Purkinje cells. The other β-controlled cyclase system which was not inhibited by fluphenazine would appear to have been associated with the granule, basket, and/or stellate neurons of the granular layer of cerebellum.
Theophylline was present in all experiments with cerebellar slices to reduce
basal levels of cyclic AMP.

Norepinephrine elicited a two- to eightfold accumulation of cyclic
AMP in slices from rat hypothalamus (Forn and Krishna, 1971; Palmer and
Burks, 1971; Palmer *et al.*, 1971, 1972a, 1973; Palmer, 1972, 1973b).
Isoproterenol elicited an accumulation of cyclic AMP lower than that

elicited by norepinephrine (Palmer *et al.*, 1973). Epinephrine and α-methyl-norepinephrine elicited accumulations of cyclic AMP intermediate in magnitude to those elicited by norepinephrine and isoproterenol. Responses to norepinephrine in hypothalamus were blocked nearly completely by either α-antagonists or β-antagonist. It was stated that responses to isoproterenol were also antagonized by either phentolamine or propranolol. In whole hypothalami from young female Holtzman rats norepinephrine, epinephrine, and dopamine slightly increased levels of cyclic AMP (Gunaga and Menon, 1973; Weissman *et al.*, 1975) as did norepinephrine in whole hypothalami from adult Sprague–Dawley rats (Schwabe *et al.*, 1976b).

Norepinephrine elicited a two- to fourfold accumulation of cyclic AMP in slices of striatum (caudate nucleus) (Forn and Krishna, 1971; Palmer *et al.*, 1973; Walker and Walker, 1973a; Schwabe *et al.*, 1976b). Evidence for the presence of both dopaminergic and β-adrenergic receptors in slices of caudate nucleus have been obtained (Forn *et al.*, 1974; Krueger *et al.*, 1976). Thus, in the presence of the phosphodiesterase inhibitor, isobutyl-methylxanthine, norepinephrine (EC_{50}, 30 μM), and isoproterenol (EC_{50}, 0.3 μM) elicited three- to fivefold increases in levels of cyclic AMP, while dopamine (EC_{50}, 60 μM) elicited nearly a twofold increase. The presence of cocaine, an inhibitor of uptake of catecholamines into nerve terminals, decreased the EC_{50} for norepinephrine to 4 μM, but surprisingly, neither cocaine nor an inhibitor of dopamine uptake, benztropine, affected the EC_{50} for dopamine. Inhibition of enzymes concerned with dopamine metabolism also had no effect on the dose–response curve for dopamine. Catechol-*O*-methyltransferase was inhibited by tropolone; monoamine oxidase by pargyline. The reason for the low efficacy of dopamine in slice preparations as compared to its high efficacy in homogenates (EC_{50}, 7 μM) thus remained undefined. Basal levels of cyclic AMP in these studies with caudate slices were extremely low at less than 3 pmol/mg protein and were increased three- to fourfold by the phosphodiesterase inhibitor. Similar elevations of basal levels and similar responses to dopamine were cited to occur in caudate slices in the presence of either of two other phosphodiesterase inhibitors, RO 20-1724 or SQ 20009. The response to dopamine in slices of caudate nucleus was readily blocked by fluphenazine, and less readily by chlorpromazine and haloperidol. Propranolol had no effect on the dopamine response. The response to norepinephrine was partially blocked by fluphenazine and nearly completely blocked by propranolol. The response to isoproterenol was unaffected by fluphenazine and was completely blocked by propranolol. In toto, the results indicated that dopamine activated cyclases controlled by dopaminergic receptors in caudate slices, while norepinephrine activated both dopaminergic and β-adrenergic controlled cyclic AMP-generating systems. Isoproterenol activated only the β-adrenergic systems. After prolonged preincubation of rat caudate slices, dopamine (EC_{50}, 1 μM) elicited a twofold accumulation of cyclic AMP (Wilkening and Makman, 1975). Isoproterenol (EC_{50}, 3 μM) elicited a similar accumulation of cyclic AMP. It was stated that isobutylmethylxanthine potentiated the response to isoproterenol much more than the response to dopamine. Another group reported that in the presence of 1 mM caffeine and 500 μM amine, both norepinephrine and dopamine elicited a significant accumulation of radioactive cyclic AMP in caudate slices (Walker and Walker, 1973a). In contrast, dopamine and 2-amino-6,7-dihydroxy-1,2,3,4-tetrahydronaphthalene, but not norepinephrine, were reported to elicit accumulations of cyclic AMP in slices of rat striatum (Munday et al., 1974).

With adenine-labeled slices of rat striatum, the potency of catecholamines in eliciting accumulations of cyclic AMP was l-isoproterenol > l-epinephrine, l-norepinephrine > > N-isopropyldopamine > d-norepinephrine, dopamine > apomorphine (Harris, 1976). Responses to combinations of dopamine and norepinephrine were not additive and were antagonized by β-antagonists. Responses to dopamine were unaffected by phentolamine, chlorpromazine, or trifluoperazine. The phosphodiesterase inhibitor, RO 20-1724, was present in all incubations. These results contrast with other reports in which dopamine elicited accumulations of cyclic AMP in slices of caudate by interaction with dopaminergic receptors (Forn et al., 1974). It would appear possible that radioactive adenine did not significantly label adenine nucleotides in compartments associated with dopamine-sensitive cyclases in striatal slices.

In spite of the fact that piribedil had no effect on cyclases in homogenates from rat caudate, the drug did increase levels of cyclic AMP in caudate slices (Makman et al., 1975b). Whether this effect in slices was due to metabolic conversion by demethylation to a dopaminergic agonist or to some indirect mechanism was not determined.

Norepinephrine, but not dopamine, elicited accumulations of cyclic AMP in slices of the limbic forebrain (amygdala, olfactory tubercle, preoptic area, nucleus accumbens, nucleus interstitialis, stria terminalis) (Blumberg et al., 1975; Vetulani and Sulser, 1975). The response to norepinephrine was blocked by the antipsychotics, pimozide and clozapine.

Norepinephrine elicited increases in levels of cyclic AMP in slices of hippocampus (threefold) (Palmer et al., 1973), midbrain (fourfold) (Palmer et al., 1973) combined midbrain–striatum (two- to sixfold) (Skolnick and Daly, 1974a), and brain stem (two- to fivefold) Palmer and Burks, 1971; Uzunov and Weiss, 1971, 1972b; Palmer, 1972; Palmer et al., 1973).

A variety of agents have been reported to inhibit responses to norepinephrine in slices from different brain regions. These include lysergic diethylamide and 2-bromolysergic acid diethylamide in hypothalamus and brain stem (Palmer and Burks, 1971), chlorpromazine and other psychoactive phenothiazines, but not promethazine, in cerebrum, brain stem, cerebellum, and hypothalamus (Palmer et al., 1971, 1972a; Uzunov and Weiss, 1971, 1972b), chlorprothixene and impramine in hypothalamus and brain stem (Palmer et al., 1972a; Uzunov and Weiss, 1972b), protriptyline in cortex and hypothalamus (Palmer, 1973), haloperidol in brain stem (Palmer et al., 1971), and lithium ions in cerebral cortex and hypothalamus, but not in brain stem (Forn and Valdecasas, 1971; Palmer et al., 1972a). The effects of a variety of antagonists on the accumulations of cyclic AMP elicited by norepinephrine in slices of cerebral cortex and of lateral and medial hypothalamus have been reported (Palmer and Manian, 1974a,b). In all three regions both an α-adrenergic blocker, phentolamine, and a β-blocker, propranolol, partially antagonized the response to norepinephrine. Various phenothiazines including chlorpromazine, fluphenazine, promethazine, promazine and mono- and di-phenolic phenothiazines partially blocked responses to norepinephrine. Haloperidol was relatively ineffective and blocked responses to norepinephrine significantly only in slices from cerebral cortex and medial hypothalamus. Thiothixene was an effective noradrenergic antagonist. Imipramine, a compound known to have α-antagonist activity, partially blocked the responses to norepinephrine in cortical slices, but had no effect on the response to isoproterenol (Frazer et al., 1974). Tricyclic antidepressants such as desipramine, iprindole, amitriptyline, nortriptyline, protriptyline, (chlor)imipramine, and opipramol inhibited norepinephrine-elicited accumulations of cyclic AMP in rat cerebral cortical slices (Palmer, 1976). The following compounds have been reported not to affect responses to norepinephrine: amphetamine and prostaglandin in slices from various brain regions, protriptyline in hypothalamus and brain stem, haloperidol in hypothalamus, imipramine in brain stem, and cocaine and pargyline in cerebral cortex, hypothalamus, and brain stem (Palmer and Burks, 1971; Palmer et al., 1971, 1972a, 1973; Palmer, 1973b). Amphetamine did antagonize the response to norepinephrine in hypothalamic slices.

Histamine

In rat cerebral cortical slices histamine had either marginal (Krishna et al., 1970; Rall and Sattin, 1970; Shimizu et al., 1970a; Berti et al., 1972; French et al., 1975a; Dismukes and Daly, 1976a) or no significant (Forn and Krishna, 1971; Palmer et al., 1973; Schultz and Daly, 1973e; De Belleroche et al., 1974) effect on cyclic AMP levels. Histamine did elicit significant accumulations of cyclic AMP in the presence of a phosphodiesterase inhibitor (Schultz and Daly, 1973e; Dismukes and Daly, 1974; Dismukes et al., 1975). In rat neocortical slices, the response to a histamine–isobutylmethylxanthine combination was blocked by the H_2-antagonist, metiamide, and only marginally reduced by the H_1-antagonist, d-brompheniramine (Dismukes *et al.*, 1975). Theophylline, propranolol, and phentolamine had no effect on the histamine response. Earlier studies (Schultz and Daly, 1973e) reported blockade of histamine responses in rat cortical slices with high concentrations of H_1-antagonists.

Histamine had no significant effect in slices from cerebellum, hypothalamus, midbrain, or hippocampus, but did elicit a small increase in slices from caudate nucleus (Forn and Krishna, 1971; Krishna *et al.*, 1970; Palmer *et al.*, 1973). Histamine was, in another study, reported to elicit a small accumulation of cyclic AMP in hippocampal slices (Dismukes *et al.*, 1975).

Combinations of histamine and norepinephrine had effects no greater (Schultz and Daly, 1973e) or only marginally greater (Huang *et al.*, 1971; Palmer *et al.*, 1973; French *et al.*, 1975a) than those elicited by norepinephrine alone in rat cerebral cortical slices.

The histamine releasing agent, compound 48/80, increased cyclic AMP levels in slices of rat cerebral cortex, brain stem, and hypothalamus (Lindl *et al.*, 1976). The increase elicited by compound 48/80 was blocked by propranolol in slices of cortex, brain stem, and cerebellum and by diphenhydramine in hypothalamus.

Serotonin, Other Amines, Amino Acids

Effects of serotonin, dopamine (see above), amphetamine, carbamylcholine, glutamate, and ACTH on accumulations of cyclic AMP were not detected in studies on slices from various brain regions (Forn and Krishna, 1971; Krishna *et al.*, 1970; Huang *et al.*, 1973b; Palmer *et al.*, 1973; Palmer, 1973b; Schultz and Daly, 1973e). A variety of amines including dopamine, phenylephrine, metaraminol, octopamine, norephedrine, and p-hydroxynorephedrine had no effect or lowered levels of cyclic AMP in hypothalamic slices (Palmer *et al.*, 1973). Serotonin had no or only marginal stimulatory effects on levels of cyclic AMP in rat cerebral cortical slices even in the presence of either isobutylmethylxanthine or RO 20-1724 (Dismukes and Daly, 1974; Dismukes *et al.*, 1975; French *et al.*, 1975a). Serotonin had no effect on levels of cyclic AMP in slices of limbic forebrain (Blumberg *et al.*, 1975) or in whole hypothalami from young female rats (Gunaga and Menon, 1973). Serotonin has been reported to inhibit the response to norepinephrine in slices from hypothalamus and midbrain but not cerebrum (Palmer *et al.*, 1973). Bufotenine, N,N-dialkyltryptamines, lysergic acid diethylamide, mescaline, psilocybin, and ibotenic acid were reported to elicit a twofold increase in cyclic AMP in slices of brain stem (Uzonov and Weiss, 1971, 1972b). These increases were blocked by trifluoperazine, regardless of whether the phenothiazine was added to the brain slice incubation or administered to the animal prior to sacrifice and preparation of slices. The monoamine oxidase inhibitor, pargyline, increased levels of cyclic AMP in slices from cerebral cortex, hypothalamus, and brain stem (Palmer, 1973b; Palmer *et al.*, 1973).

Glutamate and aspartate elicited sixfold increases in radioactive cyclic AMP in adenine-labeled rat cortical slices, while a more potent amino acid analog, cysteine sulfinic acid, elicited a twelvefold increase (Shimizu *et al.*, 1974). γ-Aminobutyrate had no stimulatory effects, but did inhibit responses to norepinephrine in rat cortical slices (French *et al.*, 1975a).

Prostaglandins

Prostaglandins E_1 and E_2 at 100 μM were reported to elicit a four- to fivefold increase in levels of radioactive cyclic AMP in adenine-labeled cortical slices from Sprague–Dawley rats (Berti *et al.*, 1972; Kuehl *et al.*, 1972). Theophylline potentiated the effect of the prostaglandin. Prostaglandin $F_{2\alpha}$ had no effect, nor did the E series prostaglandins stimulate formation of cyclic AMP in cerebral cortical slices from rabbit, guinea pig, or man. The lack of effects of E series prostaglandins on cyclic AMP levels in rat brain slices reported by other workers (see p. 108) presumably was due to the use of low concentrations of the prostaglandin. Such concentrations in most preparations are sufficient for maximal stimulation of prostaglandin-sensitive cyclic AMP-generating systems, but in brain slices very high concentrations are required. Preliminary data with brain slices (M. Mensah- Dwumah and J. W. Daly, unpublished results) suggested the presence and formation of endogenous prostaglandin antagonists. Prostaglandins E_1 (EC_{50}, 30 μM), and E_2 and 15(S)-15-methylprostaglandin E_2 methyl ester elicited a twofold accumulation of cyclic AMP in rat cerebral slices, while prostaglandins A_1 and B_1 had marginal effects and $F_{1\alpha}$ was inactive (Dismukes and Daly, 1975a). Prostaglandin E_1 elicited accumulations of cyclic AMP in slices from neocortex, striatum, hippocampus, and midbrain–thalamus–hypothalamus and medulla-pons, while having marginal effects in cerebellum. In cerebral slices, the response to prostaglandin was unaffected by theophylline and potentiated by RO 20-1724. Various antagonists including 7-oxa-13-prostynoic acid and the dibenzooxazepine hydrazide, SC 19220, α- and β-antagonists, and a local anesthetic had no effect on prostaglandin responses. Morphine slightly potentiated the prostaglandin response, while naloxone had no effect. The response of cyclic AMP-generating systems to combinations of prostaglandin E_1 with isoproterenol, norepinephrine, adenosine, or veratridine was not significantly greater than the response to one agent alone. Responses to a combination of prostaglandin with a norepinephrine–sotalol combination were additive. Isoproterenol had no significant effect on levels of cyclic AMP in the presence of 17

μM prostaglandin E_1 until the concentration of the catecholamine was 5 μM or greater. In the absence of prostaglandin, isoproterenol had stimulatory effects at 0.1 μM. It was proposed that prostaglandin inhibited isoproterenol responses.

Adenosine

Adenosine increased cyclic AMP levels 2- to 25-fold in rat cortical slices (Rall and Sattin, 1970; Murray and Froscio, 1971; Berti *et al.*, 1972; Huang *et al.*, 1973b; Perkins and Moore, 1973b; Schultz and Daly, 1973a; Dismukes and Daly, 1974; Schultz, 1974a,b; Skolnick and Daly, 1974a; Lewin *et al.*, 1976; Montecucchi, 1976; Schwabe *et al.*, 1976b), 3-fold in cerebellar slices (Rall and Sattin, 1970), and 5- to 6-fold in midbrain–striatal slices (Skolnick and Daly, 1974a). N^6-Phenylisopropyladenosine and 2-chloroadenosine increased the levels of cyclic AMP in cerebral cortical slices (Lewin *et al.*, 1976; Schwabe *et al.*, 1976b). Responses to adenosine were absent in cortical slices from newborn rats and developed slowly between days 6 and 14 after birth followed by a decline in adult responsiveness (Perkins, 1973; Perkins and Moore, 1973b). 2-Chloroadenosine (EC$_{50}$, 100 μM) elicited at least a threefold accumulation of cyclic AMP in rat caudate slices (Wilkening and Makman, 1975). The response to 2-chloroadenosine was antagonized by 3'-deoxyadenosine, theophylline, isobutylmethylxanthine, and SQ 20009. Propranolol and phentolamine did not potentiate the response to adenosine in rat cerebral cortical slices (Schultz and Daly, 1973e). The absence of extracellular calcium also did not significantly increase the response to adenosine (Schwabe *et al.*, 1976b). These results contrast with the data with guinea pig where potentiation of adenosine responses by local anesthetics and by absence of calcium were clearly evident (see Section 3.3.2). Adenosine deaminase with rat cerebral cortical slices greatly reduced the responses to norepinephrine and/or N^6-phenylisopropyladenosine in contrast to results with guinea pig cortical slices where only amine responses were reduced by the deaminase (Schwabe *et al.*, 1976b).

Adenosine–Amine Combinations

Adenosine and norepinephrine had greater than additive effects on cyclic AMP levels in cortical, cerebellar, and midbrain–striatal slices (Rall and Sattin, 1970; Huang *et al.*, 1973b; Perkins and Moore, 1973b; Schultz and Daly, 1973e; Skolnick and Daly, 1973a; Schwabe and Daly, 1976; Schwabe *et al.*, 1976b). A combination of N^6-phenylisopropyladenosine and norepinephrine had greater than additive effects in cerebral cortical slices as did combinations of adenosine and isoproterenol. Perkins *et al.*

(1975) stated that for potentiative interactions with adenosine in rat cerebral cortex the following order pertained: phenylephrine > norepinephrine > isoproterenol. Phentolamine antagonized the potentiative interaction of norepinephrine with adenosine to a greater extent than did propranolol, while in the absence of adenosine propranolol was a more effective antagonist than phentolamine. The data were clearly consonant with a primary involvement of α-receptors in the potentiative interaction of norepinephrine and adenosine in rat cerebral cortex. The α-agonist, methoxamine, in combination with adenosine, however, had only additive effects on levels of cyclic AMP in rat cortical slices (Skolnick and Daly, 1975b). In the absence of adenosine, methoxamine, and norepinephrine had additive effects on levels of cyclic AMP, while in the presence of adenosine, no additivity of the amine effects were observed. It was proposed that methoxamine activated a set of α-adrenergic receptors, which were not normally activated by norepinephrine, but that in the presence of adenosine these α-receptors were now capable of activation by norepinephrine. Responses to adenosine–norepinephrine combinations steadily increased in cortical slices during Days 5 to 14 after birth (Perkins and Moore, 1973b). Responses to the combination of amine and adenosine were seen at least 5 days before norepinephrine alone elicited an accumulation of cyclic AMP. Responses to 2-chloroadenosine and isoproterenol were greater than additive in slices of rat caudate (Wilkening and Makman, 1975).

Adenosine and histamine combinations have been reported to have effects marginally (Rall and Sattin, 1970) or significantly (Huang *et al.*, 1973b; Schultz and Daly, 1973e) greater than those of adenosine alone in cortical slices. Adenosine–serotonin combinations had effects no greater than adenosine alone. The effects of histamine and catecholamines in the presence of adenosine were generally antagonized by the same agents that antagonized responses to the amine alone in cortical slices (Perkins and Moore, 1973b; Schultz and Daly, 1973e).

In an initial experiment, the response to norepinephrine in cortical slices could be elicited only once (Schultz and Daly, 1973a), but the preparation remained responsive to norepinephrine in combination with adenosine. In a subsequent study norepinephrine and an α-agonist, methoxamine, were found to be fully able to restimulate accumulation of cyclic AMP in the absence of exogenous adenosine in cerebral cortical slices from both Sprague–Dawley and F-344 rat strains (Skolnick *et al.*, 1975).

Depolarizing Agents

The depolarizing agents, veratridine, batrachotoxin, ouabain, and potassium ions increased cyclic AMP levels 3- to 20-fold in rat cortical slices (Shimizu *et al.*, 1970; Huang *et al.*, 1973b; Skolnick and Daly, 1974a;

Montecucchi, 1976). Combinations of potassium ions and an ergot alkaloid had stimulatory effects no greater than either agent alone. Combinations of veratridine with either histamine or norepinephrine or potassium ions with norepinephrine had greater than additive effects. Another group reported that 80 mM potassium ions had no effect on cyclic AMP levels in rat cortical slices (Kimura *et al.*, 1975). Electrical stimulation of rat cortex *in vivo* increased adenosine levels nearly 2-fold, but cyclic AMP levels were not ascertained (Rubio *et al.*, 1975). Electrical stimulation of adenine-labeled rat hypothalamic slices led to enhanced efflux of radioactive hypoxanthine > inosine > adenosine (Sun *et al.*, 1976). Tetrodotoxin blocked the stimulated efflux.

The convulsant, pentylenetetrazole, at a 100 mM concentration elevated cyclic AMP levels in rat cortical slices (Lewin *et al.*, 1976). The response was inhibited by theophylline, while the responses to combinations of pentylenetetrazole with (2-chloro)adenosine or norepinephrine were additive or greater than additive. Anticonvulsants such as diphenylhydantoin, phenobarbital, and ethosuximide did not antagonize the response to pentylenetetrazole.

Estrogens and Other Hormones

Catecholamines, including dopamine, and estrogens increased levels of cyclic AMP in whole hypothalami from young female rats (Gunaga and Menon, 1973). The twofold increase in cyclic AMP elicited by estradiol occurred only after 40 min of incubation. This delayed effect was prevented by either phentolamine or propranolol. It was reported that diethylstilbestrol and 17-β-estradiol, but not less active estrogens such as 17-α-estradiol, estratriol, or estrone elicited twofold accumulations of cyclic AMP in incubated hypothalami from immature female rats (Weissman *et al.*, 1975; Weissman and Skolnick, 1975). The accumulation of cyclic AMP elicited by diethylstilbestrol followed a delayed time course and did not commence until after 50 min, reaching a maximum by 70 min. Clomiphene added together with the estrogen blocked the accumulation of cyclic AMP, but clomiphene added 40 min after the estrogen had no effect. Clomiphene had no effect on responses to norepinephrine. Phenoxybenzamine, propranolol, and haloperidol antagonized the accumulation of cyclic AMP elicited by diesthylstilbestrol, regardless of whether added at the beginning of or after 40 min of incubation. Combinations of estrogens and norepinephrine had less than additive effects on cyclic AMP levels in incubated hypothalami. The results were interpreted as follows: Estrogens interact with receptors on hypothalamic catecholamine cell bodies which in a time-dependent process leads to enhanced release of catecholamines at distal terminals and catecholamine-elicited accumulations of cyclic AMP at postsynaptic sites (Figure 16). Consonant with this proposal, estrogens had no effects in

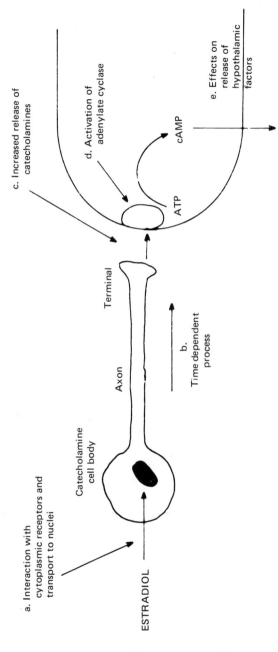

Figure 16. Estrogen and catecholamine-elicited accumulation of cyclic AMP in the hypothalamus. (From Weissman *et al.*, 1975, *Endocrinology*, copyright J. B. Lippincott Co.)

chopped hypothalami. The response of estrogens appeared specific to hypothalami, since no response was observed in incubated slabs of rat cerebral cortex.

Diethylstilbestrol, in addition to enhancing cyclic AMP accumulations in incubated hypothalami from immature female rats via a catecholamine-dependent mechanism, appeared to have a second stimulatory effect on cyclic AMP levels which was manifest only at high concentrations of the estrogen (Weissman et al., 1975). The second component of the response to diethylstilbestrol was blocked by theophylline and thus appeared to involve the intermediacy of adenosine.

The stimulation of cyclic AMP-generating systems in anterior pituitary gland by hypothalamic releasing factors from the hypothalamus and by catecholamines and prostaglandins (Zor et al., 1969; Sato et al., 1974; Borgeat et al., 1974 and references therein) is beyond the scope of the present review, but it is certainly relevant to certain central vegetative responses elicited by cyclic AMP-dependent mechanisms (see Section 4.5.2).

Calcium Ions

In rat cortical slices the response of cyclic AMP-generating systems to (nor)epinephrine was markedly reduced under calcium-free (EGTA) conditions, while the response to adenosine and N^6-phenylisopropyladenosine was marginally increased (Schwabe and Daly, 1976; Schwabe et al., 1976b). The inhibitory effect of EGTA on responses to norepinephrine was readily reversed by addition of excess calcium ions. Synergistic effects of the adenosines and either norepinephrine or isoproterenol on accumulations of cyclic AMP in rat cortical slices were no longer manifest in the presence of EGTA. Responses to norepinephrine and adenosine were increased in rat cortical slices after a prolonged prior incubation in calcium-free media in the absence of EGTA. Prolonged incubations with calcium-free media either in the presence or absence of EGTA led to increased basal levels of cyclic AMP which were reduced by theophylline, isobutyl-methylxanthine, or adenosine deaminase. Thus, enhanced release of adenosine from brain slices under calcium-free conditions and its stimulatory effects on cyclic AMP- generating systems tended to obscure direct effects of the absence of extracellular calcium on amine-sensitive cyclases, especially during prolonged incubations. EGTA decreased the response to norepinephrine in slices from cerebral cortex, cerebellum and striatum, but not in whole hypothalami. In both cortical and cerebellar slices, phentolamine and other α-antagonists no longer inhibited responses of cyclic AMP-generating systems to norepinephrine when EGTA was present. Propranolol, which in many studies had only partially blocked the response to norepinephrine in cortical slices, caused a complete blockade in the presence of EGTA. The responses to isoproterenol and another β-agonist, metaproterenol, were only slightly reduced by EGTA. The response to methoxamine was virtually abolished by EGTA. The results were consonant with a complete dependence of α-adrenergic elicited accumulations of cyclic AMP in brain slices on extracellular calcium ions. However, the presence of both EGTA and adenosine deaminase completely blocked the response to norepinephrine, while greatly reducing the response to N^6-phenylisopropyladenosine, an adenosine analog which is not a substrate for the deaminase. The latter results are more difficult to interpret, but would appear to indicate that in the absence of extracellular calcium ions and endogenous adenosine, responses of cyclic AMP-generating systems in rat cortical slices are greatly reduced and responses of catecholamine-sensitive cyclases are not detected. Possible effects of adenosine on mobilization of intracellular calcium should be considered.

Phosphodiesterase Inhibitors

The various inhibitors of phosphodiesterases have not been studied in detail in rat brain slices, but the available data are consonant with results from guinea pig. Norepinephrine-elicited accumulations were not potentiated in rat cerebral slices by theophylline (Forn and Krishna, 1971; Montecucchi, 1976). The effects of norepinephrine, isoproterenol, and histamine in cortical slices were potentiated by the phosphodiesterase inhibitors, papaverine and isobutylmethylxanthine (Schultz and Daly, 1973e). In later studies, isobutylmethylxanthine was found to antagonize norepinephrine-elicited accumulations of cyclic AMP in rat cerebral cortical slices due probably to its activity as as adenosine antagonist (Schwabe *et al.*, 1976a). Papaverine has been reported to elevate basal levels of cyclic AMP in cortical slices, but to have little effect on the response to norepinephrine (Montecucchi, 1976). Isobutylmethylxanthine inhibited the response to 2-chloroadenosine in caudate slices (Wilkening and Makman, 1975). RO 20-1724 enhanced responses to norepinephrine, isoproterenol, and histamine and marginally increased adenosine and dopamine responses in rat cerebral cortical slices (Dismukes and Daly, 1975; Schwabe *et al.*, 1976a,b). The potentiative effect of RO 20-1724 on the response to amines appeared, however, to be due mainly to enhanced adenosine-dependent activation of cyclic AMP-generating systems, which could be antagonized by theophylline or adenosine deaminase. Diazepam and chlordiazepoxide potentiated the response to norepinephrine, isoproterenol, and adenosine in cortical slices with diazepam slightly more effective (Schultz, 1975c). Both compounds increased basal levels of cyclic AMP. In another study chlordiazepoxide, but not diazepam or the inhibitor SQ 20009 (etazolate), was reported to enhance basal levels of cyclic AMP in cortical slices (Hess *et al.*, 1975). SQ 20009 inhibited the response to 2-chloroadenosine in slices of rat caudate and was stated to potentiate the response to dopamine (Wilkening and Makman, 1975).

A dialkoxyphenyl-2-pyrrolidone, ZK 62711, was extremely potent (EC_{50}, 1 μM) in enhancing norepinephrine-elicited accumulations of cyclic AMP in rat cerebral cortical slices (Schwabe *et al.*, 1976a). Indeed, it was nearly 100-fold more potent than the structurally related phosphodiesterase inhibitor, RO 20-1724. The pyrrolidone was, in addition, much more effective than RO 20-1724 in inhibiting calcium-dependent cyclic AMP-phosphodiesterases in homogenates from rat cerebral cortex. ZK 62711 effectively enhanced the accumulations of cyclic AMP elicited in rat cortical slices by isoproterenol and histamine. ZK 62711 was somewhat less potent (EC_{50}, 10 μM) with respect to enhancement of adenosine responses and had no effect on dopamine responses. Basal levels of cyclic AMP were elevated by ZK 62711 in cortical and cerebellar slices, but in contrast to RO 20-1724 (Schwabe *et al.*, 1976b) adenosine deaminase or theophylline did not prevent the ZK 62711-elicited increase in basal levels of cyclic AMP or the enhanced response to norepinephrine. ZK 62711, but not RO 20-1724, significantly enhanced the accumulation of cyclic AMP elicited by veratridine in rat cerebellar slices. In view of the potency of ZK 62711 in potentiating the accumulation of cyclic AMP elicited in brain slices by biogenic amines and adenosine and in view of the apparent lack of significant involvement of release of adenosine in its potentiative effects, ZK 62711 would appear to be the agent of choice for investigating the involvement of phosphodiesterases in cyclic AMP-phenomena in nervous tissue.

Strain Differences

The effects of norepinephrine, isoproterenol, adenosine, an adenosine–norepinephrine combination, and veratridine on cyclic AMP levels in cortical and midbrain–striatal slices have been compared in four strains of rats (Skolnick and Daly, 1974a). The responses of the norepinephrine-sensitive cyclic AMP-generating systems in midbrain–striatal slices were inversely correlated in Sprague–Dawley and three inbred rat strains (F-344, BUF, and ACI) with the responses of the corresponding systems in cerebral cortical slices. The magnitude of the norepinephrine responses in midbrain–striatal slices (BUF > Sprague–Dawley > ACI >> F344) was inversely correlated with the levels of tyrosine hydroxylase in this tissue. Such correlations were not observed with isoproterenol or other agents. The magnitude of responses to norepinephrine and to the α-agonist, methoxamine, in brain slices showed correlations with spontaneous behavioral activity in the four rat strains (Skolnick and Daly, 1974a, 1975; see Section 4.4.4, Figure 23).

3.1.4 Mouse

Catecholamines

Norepinephrine elicited a two- to twelvefold increase in cyclic AMP levels in cerebral cortical slices from various strains of mice (Krishna *et al.*, 1970; Rall and Sattin, 1970; Forn and Krishna, 1971; Israel *et al.*, 1972; Shimizu and Daly, 1972a; Wong and Henderson, 1972; Schultz and Daly, 1973e; Martres *et al.*, 1975; Skolnick and Daly, 1974b, 1975a; Sattin, 1975). Epinephrine elicited a response similar to that of norepinephrine, while isoproterenol elicited a significantly lower accumulation of cyclic AMP (Schultz and Daly, 1973e). Propranolol effectively antagonized all three catecholamines, while phentolamine had only marginal inhibitory effects. Dopamine was reported to elicit a small accumulation of cyclic AMP in cerebral cortical slices from Swiss albino mice (Martres *et al.*, 1975). Neither norepinephrine or isoproterenol elicited a significant accumulation of cyclic AMP in fetal mouse brain slices (Seeds and Gilman, 1971).

Norepinephrine elicited a 15- to 40-fold increase in cyclic AMP levels in cerebellar slices from Swiss Webster mice (Ferrendelli *et al.*, 1975). The norepinephrine response was nearly completely blocked by either α- or β-antagonists. Epinephrine elicited a response similar to that of norepinephrine, while isoproterenol and phenylephrine elicited much smaller responses. The response to a combination of isoproterenol and phenylephrine was additive. Dopamine at 1 mM had marginal effects on cyclic AMP levels in cerebellar slices. The response to norepinephrine was reduced in low sodium medium. Theophylline slightly reduced basal and norepinephrine-stimulated levels of cyclic AMP in mouse cerebellar slices.

Histamine

Histamine elicited a small accumulation of cyclic AMP in cortical slices from NIH general purpose mice (Krishna *et al.*, 1970; Forn and Krishna, 1971; Shimizu and Daly, 1972a; Schultz and Daly, 1973e) and had only a marginal effect in slices from C57B1/6J mice (Skolnick and Daly, 1974b, 1975a). Histamine elicited a marginal accumulation of cyclic AMP in slices of mouse forebrain (Rall and Sattin, 1970). Histamine at 1 mM concentration had marginal effects in cerebellar slices (Ferrendelli *et al.*, 1975).

Serotonin

In cerebral slices from Swiss albino mice, serotonin was reported to elicit a small accumulation of cyclic AMP (Martres *et al.*, 1975). In cerebellar slices from Swiss-Webster mice, serotonin at a 1 mM concentration had marginal effects (Ferrendelli *et al.*, 1975).

Adenosine

Adenosine elicited a 4- to 20-fold increase in cyclic AMP levels in cortical slices from mice of various strains (Rall and Sattin, 1970; Schultz and Daly, 1973e; Skolnick and Daly, 1974b, 1975a; Martres *et al.*, 1975; Sattin, 1975) and a 30-fold increase in cerebellar slices from Swiss-Webster mice (Ferrendelli *et al.*, 1973b, 1975). Combinations of adenosine and norepinephrine have additive or greater than additive effects on cyclic AMP in cortical slices, while the effects of combinations of adenosine and either histamine or serotonin were equal to or only marginally greater than those of adenosine alone. Combinations of adenosine and norepinephrine in cerebellar slices had much greater than additive effects.

Depolarizing Agents

Veratridine elicited a 4- to 18-fold increase in cyclic AMP levels in cortical slices from two mouse strains (Shimizu and Daly, 1972a; Skolnick and Daly, 1974b, 1975a). In cortical slices from three different mouse strains (C57B1/6J, NIH general purpose white, and Swiss-Webster), 40 to 64 mM potassium ions elicited, respectively, a marginal increase (Skolnick and Daly, 1974b), a 3-fold increase (Shimizu and Daly, 1972a), and a 60-fold increase (Ferrendelli *et al.*, 1973b) in levels of cyclic AMP. Combined effects of potassium ions and either norepinephrine or histamine appeared less than additive in cortical slices from NIH general purpose mice. In cerebellar slices from Swiss-Webster mice (Ferrendelli *et al.*, 1973b, 1975, 1976), 64 mM potassium ions elicited a transient 13-fold increase in cyclic AMP levels which returned to only a 3-fold above basal levels by 5 min. Higher concentrations of potassium ions elicited a 150-fold transient increase in cyclic AMP levels in Swiss Webster cerebellar slices. The effects of potassium ions were blocked by theophylline. Veratridine elicited a 20- to 25-fold increase in cyclic AMP levels in Swiss-Webster cerebellar slices. The response required sodium ions. Combinations of high potassium ions with norepinephrine had greater than additive effects on cyclic AMP levels.

Glutamate and Other Amino Acids

Glutamate (3 to 30 mM) elicited a significant increase in cyclic AMP levels in cerebellar slices from Swiss-Webster mice (Ferrendelli *et al.*, 1974, 1975). About a ninefold accumulation was elicited by 10 mM glutamate. This response was blocked by theophylline, suggesting that a "release" of adenosine in involved. Glycine (1 mM) elicited a transient small increase and γ-aminobutyrate (0.5 mM) a small decrease in cyclic AMP levels of cerebellar slices. The different amino acids did not appear to interact with respect to stimulation of cyclic AMP-generating systems. A combination of maximal stimulatory concentrations of potassium ions and glutamate elicited an accumulation of cyclic AMP smaller than that elicited by potassium alone. This result is reminiscent of the inhibitory effect of potassium ions on responses to adenosine in guinea pig cerebellar slices (see Section 3.1.2). A combination of glutamate and norepinephrine had greater than additive effects on cyclic AMP levels of cerebellar slices. γ-Aminobutyrate partially antagonized the norepinephrine response, while glycine had no effect.

Calcium Ions

Basal levels of cyclic AMP increased in mouse cerebellar slices under calcium-free conditions, and responses of cyclic AMP-generating systems to potassium ions and glutamate were markedly reduced while the response to norepinephrine was unaffected (Ferrendelli et al., 1974, 1975, 1976). The γ-aminobutyrate-elicited decrease in levels of cyclic AMP was still manifest under calcium-free conditions. Strontium or manganese ions could restore the response to potassium ions in calcium-free medium, while magnesium, barium or cobalt could partially restore the response. The calcium ionophore, A-23187, had no effect on cyclic AMP levels in mouse cerebellar slices.

Strain Differences

The responses of cortical cyclic AMP-generating systems to norepinephrine, adenosine, and an adenosine–norepinephrine combination have been compared in three inbred strains of mice, C57B1/6J, DBA/2J, and SEC/ReJ, and in C57-DBA and C57-SEC hybrid mice (Sattin, 1975). Basal levels in slices from C57B1/6J mice were markedly lower than those reported by Skolnick and Daly (1974b, 1975a). Differences in methods of protein determination (cf. Skolnick et al., 1975) and technical aspects of preparation and incubation of slices undoubtably account for lack of correspondence of basal levels between these two laboratories. In the C57, SEC, and DBA strains, norepinephrine elicited a 1.6-, 2.0-, and 4.6-fold increase in levels of cyclic AMP in cortical slices, respectively; adenosine a 6.0-, 12.2-, and 13.8-fold increase; and adenosine–norepinephrine a 24-, 35-, and 53-fold increase (Sattin, 1975). Thus, the C57 strain could be characterized as exhibiting relatively low accumulations, the DBA strain as exhibiting relatively high accumulations, and the SEC strain as exhibiting intermediate accumulations of cyclic AMP. Interestingly, responses in the C57-DBA hybrid resembled the "low accumulation" C57 parent, while responses in the C57-SEC hybrid resembled closely the "high accumulation" SEC parent. The DBA strain which exhibited high accumulations of cyclic AMP had significantly lower levels of cortical phosphodiesterase activity than the "low accumulation" C57 strain. In the C57-DBA hybrid mice which had shown low accumulations of cyclic AMP, the phosphodiesterase levels were as high as in the "low accumulation" parent. Strain differences in phosphodiesterase activity were more pronounced when cyclic GMP was used as substrate. The C57 mouse exhibits a low rate of active avoidance learning, while both the SEC and DBA strains exhibit high rates of learning. The magnitude of accumulation of cyclic AMP elicited by adenosine in the three strains and the hybrids appeared to be inversely correlated with the rates of acquisition of active avoidance learning (see Section 4.4.4, Figure 25). When extended to eight inbred strains of mice no correlations of the magnitude of norepinephrine- or adenosine-elicited accumulations of cyclic AMP in cerebral slices with active avoidance learning pertained (Stalvey *et al.*, 1976). Adenosine-elicited accumulations of cyclic AMP in five strains were inversely correlated with spontaneous activity. In individual mice of a randomly bred strain adenosine-responses and active avoidance learning showed an inverse correlation.

The responses of cyclic AMP-generating systems to amines, adenosine, and veratridine have been compared in cortical slices from C57B1/6J mice, "quaking" mutants of this strain, and heterozygous mice which do not exhibit the tremor and hypomyelination of the quaking mouse (Skolnick and Daly, 1974b). Adenosine-elicited accumulations of cyclic AMP were lower in the quaking and heterozygous mice, probably due primarily to decreased incorporation of adenosine into the cyclic AMP compartment (see Section 3.1.11).

3.1.5 Primates

Rhesus Monkey

In rhesus monkey, norepinephrine and histamine had either a marginal effect (Shimizu and Daly, 1972a) or no effect (Forn and Krishna, 1971) on accumulations of radioactive cyclic AMP in adenine-labeled cortical slices. Norepinephrine elicited a twofold increase in levels of cyclic AMP in cerebellar slices and a fivefold increase in hypothalamic slices, but had no effect in slices from caudate nucleus (Forn and Krishna, 1971). Histamine did not have significant effects in slices from cerebellum, caudate nucleus, or hypothalamus. Serotonin, dopamine, and carbamylcholine had no significant effects in any region. Depolarizing agents such as 40 mM potassium ions, batrachotoxin, and veratridine elicited three- to fivefold increases in cyclic AMP levels (Shimizu and Daly, 1972a). Ouabain elicited a tenfold increase. A combination of veratridine and histamine appeared to have greater than additive effects.

Squirrel monkey

In squirrel monkey, the effects of various agents and combinations of agents on the levels of radioactive cyclic AMP in adenine-labeled slices from functional neocortical areas (polysensory, auditory, and visual) and from limbic cortex have been investigated (Skolnick *et al.*, 1973). Norepinephrine elicited a four- to fivefold increase in all regions. Histamine had no significant effects in the neocortical slices. Serotonin elicited a twofold increase in slices from polysensory cortex and had smaller effects in other regions. Combinations of adenosine and norepinephrine had greater than additive effects, while the effects of combinations of adenosine and serotonin were not significantly greater than the effects of adenosine alone.

Human

Two different groups, one in Italy (Fumagalli *et al.*, 1971; Berti *et al.*, 1972) and one in Japan (Shimizu *et al.*, 1971; Kodama *et al.*, 1973) have studied the formation of cyclic AMP in slices from human brain tissue. Tissue was obtained as surgical samples during operations for aneurysm, glioma, glioblastoma, meningioma, medulloblastoma, and acoustic neurinoma. Most of the results were obtained with adenine-labeled slices. In cortical slices, norepinephrine elicited either 3- to 4-fold increases (Fumagalli *et al.*, 1971; Berti *et al.*, 1972) or 12- to 40-fold increases in levels of cyclic AMP (Shimizu *et al.*, 1971; Kodama *et al.*, 1973). Norepinephrine was shown to increase endogenous levels of cyclic AMP 15-fold (Kodama *et al.*, 1973). Epinephrine and isoproterenol elicited greater increases in levels of radioactive cyclic AMP than did norepinephrine (Shimizu *et al.*, 1971; Kodama *et al.*, 1973). β-Antagonists (propranolol) prevented the response to norepinephrine, while α-antagonists (phentolamine, dibenamine) were much less effective. Theophylline caused a slight inhibition of the response to norepinephrine. Norepinephrine elicited a 2- to 5-fold increase in radioactive cyclic AMP in cerebellar slices (Fumagalli *et al.*, 1971). Histamine either had no effect (Fumagalli *et al.*, 1971) or elicited a 2- to 6-fold increase (Shimizu *et al.*, 1971; Kodama *et al.*, 1973) in levels of radioactive cyclic AMP in cortical slices. Histamine had marginal effects in cerebellar slices (Fumagalli *et al.*, 1971). Serotonin had no effect in cortical or cerebellar slices (Fumagalli *et al.*, 1971) or elicited a marginal accumulation of radioactive cyclic AMP in cortical slices (Shimizu *et al.*, 1971; Kodama *et al.*, 1973). Adenosine elicited either a 2-fold (Berti *et al.*, 1972) or a 5- to 6-fold increase in cyclic AMP (Kodama *et al.*, 1973) in cortical slices. Veratridine elicited 20- to 40-fold increases in cortical slices (Shimizu *et al.*, 1971; Kodama *et al.*, 1973), but had no effect in slices of white matter. A combination of veratridine and norepinephrine elicited a 50-fold increase in levels of radioactive cyclic AMP, which then repre-sented a remarkable 70% of the total radioactive nucleotides in the cortical slice. Prostaglandins had no effects in cortical slices (Berti *et al.*, 1972). Desipramine at high concentrations was stated to enhance cyclic AMP levels in human cerebral slices (Kodama *et al.*, 1971).

3.1.6 Pig

In pig cerebral cortical slices epinephrine and dopamine elicited small accumulations of cyclic AMP, while norepinephrine, serotonin, isoproter-enol, histamine, prostaglandin E_2, and acetylcholine had virtually no effect (Sato *et al.*, 1974). In medial hypothalamic slices, norepinephrine, dopa-mine, and serotonin elicited small increases in cyclic AMP levels and histamine a threefold increase, while the other agents had no significant effect. All incubations were in the presence of theophylline.

3.1.7 Cat

In cat brain slices labeled with adenine, norepinephrine elicited signifi-cant increases in levels of radioactive cyclic AMP in tissue from cortex (fivefold), cerebellum (fivefold), and hypothalamus (less than threefold) and had no significant effect in slices from caudate nucleus (Forn and Krishna, 1971). Histamine elicited significant increases only in cerebellar (twofold) and hypothalamic (twofold) slices. Serotonin, dopamine, and carbamylcho-line had no significant effects in cat brain slices. Electrical stimulation of cat sensorimotor cortex resulted in a marked increase in "release" of radioac-tive adenosine and 5'-AMP (Sulakhe and Phillis, 1975).

3.1.8 Chicken

Catecholamines

Epinephrine and isoproterenol elicited a 3- to 4-fold increase in cyclic AMP levels in chick cerebral slices, while norepinephrine was quite ineffec-tive and required a concentration of 100 μM to elicit a 3-fold increase (Edwards *et al.*, 1974; Nahorski *et al.*, 1974). In subsequent studies in slices from chick cerebrum, epinephrine (EC_{50}, 2 μM) and isoproterenol

(EC$_{50}$, 0.3 μM) elicited 15- to 30-fold accumulations of cyclic AMP, while norepinephrine (EC$_{50}$, 20 μM) and the β-agonist, salbutamol, elicited a 10-fold accumulation (Nahorski *et al.*, 1975b). Dopamine and clonidine had little or no effect. The maximal response to isoproterenol was antagonized by norepinephrine and by propranolol, but not by phentolamine. The response to epinephrine was also selectively blocked by the β-antagonist. Responses to catecholamines were not blocked by H$_2$-antagonists. It was stated that isoproterenol elicited large accumulations of cyclic AMP in slices from cerebellum and smaller responses in slices from medulla, diencephalon, and optic lobes. Isoproterenol responses were maximal in cerebral slices from 3-day-old chicks and declined during further development (Nahorski et al., 1976).

Histamine

Histamine elicited a 3- to 20-fold increase in levels of cyclic AMP in slices of chick cerebrum (Edwards *et al.*, 1974; Nahorski *et al.*, 1974). The response to histamine was effectively blocked by the H$_2$-antagonists, metiamide, and burimamide, while an H$_1$-antagonist, pyrilamine, was ineffective except at very high concentrations. Histamine responses like those of isoproterenol were maximal at 3 days of age and then declined (Nahorski *et al.*, 1976).

Adenosine

In chick cerebral slices, adenosine was virtually ineffective, eliciting only a 1.3-fold increase in cyclic AMP levels at 10 μM and none at 100 μM (Edwards *et al.*, 1974). Adenosine responses, however, increased with age and became maximal at 19 days of age (Nahorski *et al.*, 1976).

3.1.9 Amphibians

In adenine-labeled brain slices from the frog *Rana pipiens*, (nor)epinephrine, histamine, serotonin, and carbamylcholine had no significant effect on levels of radioactive cyclic AMP (Forn and Krishna, 1971).

3.1.10 Conversion of Adenine and Adenosine-Labeled Nucleotides to Cyclic AMP

Guinea Pig

After incubation of guinea pig cortical slices with low concentrations of radioactive adenine virtually all of the radioactivity was converted to adenine nucleotides (Shimizu *et al.,* 1969; Shimizu and Daly, 1972a; Pull and McIlwain, 1972a). The initial accumulation of adenine into nucleotides in the slice showed a K_m of about 20 μM, which is remarkably similar to that of adenine phosphoribosyltransferase from the same tissue (Shimizu and Daly, 1972a). A large fraction (30 to 40%) of the adenine-labeled nucleotides in guinea pig cortical slices could be subsequently converted to cyclic AMP with certain stimulatory agents. Unfortunately, attempts to define the morphological distribution of radioactivity in these labeled slices have not been successful. Results of autoradiographic studies on guinea pig cortical slices labeled by incubation with radioactive adenine at first suggested that a major fraction of the radioactivity in the slice was associated with synaptic structures (F. Bloom, M. Huang, and J. W. Daly, unpublished results). However, subsequent studies indicated that from 50 to 60% of the total radioactivity had been lost from the slice during fixation. Attempts to minimize these losses were not particularly successful, but did afford autoradiographs in which significant radioactivity was detected in nonsynaptic structures. Greater than 60% of the total radioactivity in homogenates from control and electrically stimulated adenine-labeled guinea pig cortical slices was found in soluble fraction, while only much smaller percentages were found to be associated with mitochondrial and synaptosomal fractions (Kuroda and McIlwain, 1973). Metabolism and probably translocation of nucleotides during separation of subcellular fractions on ficoll gradients clearly rendered any assessment of the association of radioactive cyclic AMP, adenosine, inosine, etc. with a particular fraction difficult. However, adenosine-labeled nucleotides were associated to a significantly greater extent with synaptosomal fractions than were the adenine-labeled nucleotides. This result is perhaps relevant to the observations that adenosine-labeled nucleotides were less effective than adenine-labeled nucleotides as precursors of cyclic AMP in guinea pig cortical slices (Shimizu *et al.,* 1969; Shimizu and Daly, 1970). Radioactive adenine and adenosine were incorporated into adenine nucleotides of synaptosome preparations from guinea pig cerebral cortex (Kuroda and McIlwain, 1974). The rate of incorporation of adenosine was fourfold higher than that of adenine in contrast to results with guinea pig cortical slices where incorporation rates of the two precursors were similar. This provides further evidence suggestive of preferential uptake of adenosine into presynaptic sites. Incorporation of radioactive adenine into guinea pig cortical slices was not inhibited by the copresence of a neuronal depolarizing agent, veratridine, during short incubations (H. Shimizu, unpublished results). Incorporation of low concentrations of adenine was partially blocked by the following adenine analogs: N^6-methyladenine, hypoxanthine, 6-hydrazino-purine, and 8-bromoadenine (Mah and Daly, 1975). 1,N^6-Ethenoadenine, 2-chloroadenine, 8-azaadenine, 8-mercaptoadenine, 2-aminoadenine, and an adenine phosphoribosyltransferase inhibitor, 4-amino-pyrazolo [4,5d]-

pyrimidine had no or only marginal effects on uptake of adenine. Prior incubations of guinea pig cortical slices with high concentrations of adenine did not reduce the subsequent incorporation of 4 μM radioactive adenine (Schultz and Daly, 1973a), indicating that the levels of phosphoribosyl pyrophosphate, the cosubstrate of the transferase enzyme, were not depleted during the prior incubation. Furthermore, the rates of incorporation of radioactive adenine into steady-state levels of cyclic AMP elicited by histamine, adenosine, a combination of histamine and norepinephrine, or a combination of adenosine, histamine, and norepinephrine were in all instances proportional to the steady-state levels of cyclic AMP, suggesting that even when adenine was incorporated into cyclic AMP at rates of greater than 10 pmol/mg protein/min the steps from adenine to ATP prior to the adenylate cyclase reaction were not rate limiting (Schultz and Daly, 1973a). The subsequent percent conversion of adenine-labeled nucleotides to cyclic AMP elicited by veratridine was unaffected by a twofold change in the concentration (7 to 13 μM) of the radioactive adenine used to label guinea pig cortical slices (Shimizu and Daly, 1970). The percent conversion elicited by histamine was relatively independent of the duration of the adenine-labeling period (Shimizu et al., 1969) except when short labeling periods of less than 10 to 15 min were employed (Shimizu and Okayama, 1973). After short labeling periods, the subsequent percent conversion of labeled nucleotides to cyclic AMP appeared much greater, suggestive of an initial incorporation of adenine into a small compartment of nucleotides intimately associated with adenylate cyclases, followed by equilibration with a somewhat larger compartment. However, in another study the percent conversion of radioactive adenine nucleotides formed from [³H]adenine *during* stimulation with histamine either alone or in combination with norepinephrine, adenosine, or veratridine was not markedly greater than the percent conversion of the nucleotides labeled in the same guinea pig cortical slices during a prior 40-min incubation with [¹⁴C]adenine (Schultz and Daly, 1973a). The compartments of nucleotides which serve as precursors for cyclic AMP and which were labeled during a prior 40-min incubation with radioactive adenine did not undergo further equilibration with other compartments, as reflected in the constancy of the 35 to 40% conversion of labeled nucleotides elicited by a veratridine–histamine combination at various time intervals of up to 50 min after the prior labeling of the slice (Shimizu et al., 1970c).

Incorporation of adenosine into intracellular nucleotides in guinea pig cortical slices appeared to be dependent on both an active uptake process and on the action of adenosine kinase. Virtually all of the intracellular radioactivity was present as adenine nucleotides after incubation with low concentrations of radioactive adenosine (Shimizu et al., 1972). The apparent K_m for the uptake and incorporation of radioactive adenosine was about 20 μM in guinea pig cortical slices, a value which was similar to that of adenosine kinase from the same source. Analogs of adenosine such as N^6-benzyladenosine, N^6-phenyladenosine, 8-azaadenosine, 2-fluoroadenosine, formycin, 8-bromoadenosine, 3'-deoxyadenosine, 5'-deoxyadenosine adenine arabinofuranoside, and a carbocyclic analog of adenosine effectively inhibited incorporation of adenosine (McIlwain, 1972; Shimizu et al., 1972; Huang and Daly, 1974a; Mah and Daly, 1975). Many of these analogs inhibit adenosine kinase. 2'-Deoxyadenosine, 2-chloroadenosine, tubercidin, adenine xylofuranoside, and $1,N^6$-ethenoadenosine were less effective or ineffective in inhibiting uptake of adenosine. Other compounds such as dipyridamole and hexobendine that have been reported to be weak inhibitors of adenosine kinases were potent inhibitors of incorporation of low concentrations of radioactive adenosine, presumably at uptake sites. Various phosphodiesterase inhibitors, such as papaverine, diazepam, RO 20-1724, and SQ 20009 inhibited uptake of adenosine. In toto, the results suggest that an uptake process is rate limiting for incorporation of low concentrations of adenosine into intracellular nucleotides of brain slices. The copresence of a neuronal depolarizing agent, veratridine, inhibited incorporation of adenosine (Shimizu and Daly, 1970), while another depolarizing agent, ouabain, had virtually no effect (Shimizu et al., 1972). Cleavage of adenosine to adenine followed by incorporation of the adenine did not appear to be a significant pathway with guinea pig cortical slices (Shimizu et al., 1972).

Analogs of adenine and adenosine have been investigated as precursors of abnormal cyclic nucleotides in guinea pig cortical slices (Mah and Daly, 1975). Radioactive $1,N^6$-ethenoadenine or $1,N^6$-ethenoadenosine were not incorporated into intracellular nucleotides. 2-Chloroadenine was incorporated at a low rate and no evidence for formation of 2-chloro cyclic AMP was obtained. N^6-Benzyladenosine was converted only to N^6-benzyl 5'-AMP. 2'-Deoxyadenosine was converted to both 2'-deoxyadenine nucleotides and adenine nucleotides. It was possible to then demonstrate formation of 2'-deoxy cyclic AMP upon incubation of 2'-deoxyadenosine-labeled slices with veratridine, histamine-norepinephrine, or adenosine–histamine–norepinephrine.

The percent conversion of [^{3}H]adenine-labeled nucleotides to cyclic AMP elicited by histamine, adenosine, veratridine, or 125 mM potassium ions in guinea pig cerebral cortical slices was in each case approximately 1.8 times greater than the percent conversions of [^{14}C]adenosine-labeled nucleotides (Shimizu et al., 1969; Shimizu and Daly, 1970). Such results clearly indicated a more specific incorporation of adenine into compartments of nucleotides serving as precursors of cyclic AMP, but gave no evidence for the existence of functional compartments labeled to differing extents and stimulatable by different agents. Levels of radioactive cyclic AMP in adenine-labeled slices after stimulation with biogenic amines, adenosine, veratridine, and combinations of these agents represented in each instance approximately 10% of the total endogenous cyclic AMP measured in guinea pig cortical slices in parallel experiments under the same conditions (Schultz and Daly, 1973a). The increase elicited by these agents in levels of radioactive cyclic AMP and in levels of endogenous cyclic AMP occurred over similar time courses and to similar extents in parallel experiments. The disappearance of radioactive and endogenous cyclic AMP after removal of the stimulatory agent(s) by washing also followed similar time courses (Schultz and Daly, 1973b). Basal levels of cyclic AMP were reached with a half-time of less than 10 min after a prior stimulation with histamine, histamine–norepinephrine, adenosine, and amine-adenosine combinations. Disappearance of cyclic AMP was slower after a prior stimulation with veratridine. During histamine stimulations, both radioactive and endogenous cyclic AMP were measured simultaneously (Schultz and Daly, 1973a, b). Endogenous levels of cyclic AMP reached a maximum 2 min after histamine, followed by a rapid decrease to a level only one-half of the maximal level. Radioactive cyclic AMP increased to maximal levels within 4 to 6 min and was then maintained at elevated levels for an extended period. The results were consonant with two compartments of adenine nucleotides responding to histamine, one of which responded with a transient accumulation of cyclic AMP from a less highly labeled compartment of nucleotides, superimposed on a more sustained accumulation of cyclic AMP from a more highly labeled compartment. Papaverine potentiated the histamine-elicited accumulation of both radioactive and endogenous cyclic AMP 2-fold. Isobutylmethylxanthine was a more effective inhibitor with respect to the endogenous cyclic AMP. The time course for the disappearance of cyclic AMP after histamine stimulation in the presence of isobutylmethylxanthine, followed by washing and further incubation in the presence of the phosphodiesterase inhibitor, was also suggestive of a two-compartment system, with one compartment containing phosphodiesterases which are inhibited less effectively by isobutylmethylxanthine. During repetitive restimulations of cyclic AMP accumulations in guinea pig cortical slices by adenosine or an adenosine–histamine–norepinephrine combination, the specific activity of cyclic AMP decreased slightly, presumably due to the continued incorporation of the nonradioactive stimulant, adenosine, into the cyclic AMP (Schultz and Daly, 1973c). The percent conversion of radioactive adenine nucleotides to cyclic AMP with amines, adenosine, veratridine, and combinations of these agents was approximately 3-fold higher than the percent conversion of total adenine nucleotides to cyclic AMP under the same conditions in parallel experiments (Schultz and Daly, 1973a). The results suggest that the specific activities of the cyclic AMP that accumulated after stimulation with each of the various agents were similar and were approximately 3-fold higher than the specific activity of total adenine nucleotides. The specific activities of cyclic AMP in adenine-labeled cortical slices stimulated by histamine, adenosine, or veratridine, or by combinations of either veratridine–histamine or of adenosine–histamine–norepinephrine were found to be quite similar (Shimizu and Okayama, 1973). However, the specific activity of the cyclic AMP in the stimulated slices appeared to be about 40% higher than in control slices. The specific activity of cyclic AMP in slices incubated with histamine was approximately 5-fold higher than that of ATP. In these experiments, no change in the specific activity of cyclic AMP was noted during the time course of stimulation with histamine. In experiments from another laboratory, the specific activities of cyclic AMP after stimulation of adenine-labeled guinea pig cortical slices with norepinephrine or histamine were similar, but in each case they appeared *lower* than the specific activity of cyclic AMP in control slices (Chasin *et al.,* 1973). In guinea pig hippocampal slices, specific activities of cyclic AMP in control and histamine-stimulated preparations were similar, while the specific activity in norepinephrine-stimulated slices appeared to be lower. The specific activities of cyclic AMP and ATP have also been compared in guinea pig cortical slices that have been pulse-labeled with radioactive adenine for 5 min under control conditions and in slices in which steady-state levels of cyclic AMP were already elevated 1.5- or 8-fold by the presence of norepinephrine or histamine, respectively (Rall and Sattin, 1970). The specific activity of cyclic AMP in control and norepinephrine-stimulated slices was 2.3 to 2.6 times that of ATP, while the specific activity of cyclic AMP in histamine-stimulated slices was 7 times that of ATP. Comparison of the specific activity of ATP–ADP to that of the cyclic AMP which accumulated in guinea pig cortical slices incubated with radioactive 0.1 mM adenosine revealed that the specific activity of cyclic AMP was about 3 times greater than that of ATP–ADP (Sattin and Rall, 1970). Adenosine was in other studies (Shimizu and Daly, 1970) shown to be incorporated less specifically than adenine into the compartments of nucleotides serving as precursors of cyclic AMP.

A close association of adenine phosphoribosyltransferase and to a lesser extent adenosine kinase with cyclic AMP-generating systems has thus been firmly established in guinea pig cerebral cortical slices. However, whether this association is fortuitous or of functional significance has not been established. It would appear that some evidence for distinct functional compartments in guinea pig cortical slices labeled to differing extents with adenine or adenosine and stimulatable to various degrees with different agents has been obtained, but the results from various laboratories have been contradictory and have as yet provided little in the way of insights into the morphological entities with which adenine or adenosine-labeled nucleotides are associated in guinea pig cortical slices. Studies of the effects of depolarizing conditions, which might affect neurons and glia differentially, on the levels of radioactive ATP and on the efflux of radioactive adenosine from adenine-labeled guinea pig cortical slices have also not provided unambiguous answers.

Radioactive adenosine was released under control conditions from adenine or adenosine-labeled guinea pig cortical slices, and this efflux was increased under a variety of depolarizing conditions (Shimizu *et al.,* 1970a, 1972; McIlwain, 1972; Pull and McIlwain, 1972a, b; Heller and McIlwain, 1973; Huang *et al.,* 1973b; Kuroda and McIlwain, 1973; Schultz and Daly, 1973a; Huang and Daly, 1974b; Pull and McIlwain, 1975). Both radioactive and endogenous ATP were decreased in the slices under these conditions (Huang *et al.,* 1973a; Huang and Daly, 1974b). Interestingly, the specific activity of the adenosine released by electrical stimulation was 1.4 to 2.7 times greater than the specific activity of the total adenine nucleotides in the adenine-labeled slice (Kuroda and McIlwain, 1973). Chlorpromazine, desipramine, amobarbital, and diphenylhydantoin inhibited efflux of radioactive adenosine from control and electrically-stimulated adenine-labeled guinea pig cortical slices (Pull and McIlwain, 1976). A possible ATP antagonist, 2,2′-pyridylisatogen, at low concentrations inhibited adenosine efflux, while increasing efflux at higher concentrations. Glutamate at high concentrations of 1 to 5 mM markedly increased efflux of radioactive adenosine from adenine-labeled guinea pig cortical slices (Pull and McIlwain, 1975). Histamine had only a small stimulatory effect on release of adenosine, while norepinephrine, γ-aminobutyrate, and acetylcholine plus carbamylcholine had no effect. Only a very small percentage of the total radioactivity (0.6%) in adenine-labeled slices was originally present as adenosine (Pull and McIlwain, 1972). Electrical pulsation caused a rapid increase in tissue levels of adenosine along with an efflux of adenosine and its metabolites, inosine and hypoxanthine, into the media. It is noteworthy that the specific activities of adenosine, inosine, and hypoxanthine released from adenine-labeled guinea pig cerebral cortical slices were not equal with the specific activity of adenosine > inosine > hypoxanthine. This result suggests that the "release" of adenosine occurred from different compartments with the adenosine released from compartments of lower specific activity undergoing more extensive metabolism to deaminated products. Detailed studies have not been carried out on the radioactive material released from adenine-labeled cortical slices during incubation with depolarizing agents. Adenosine did appear to represent a larger proportion of the released radioactivity with depolarizing agents than it did after electrical pulsation (compare Shimizu *et al.,* 1970; Huang and Daly, 1974b; and Pull and McIlwain, 1972). Increasing the rate of electrical stimulation caused an increase in the proportion of adenosine present in the released radioactivity. High adenylate deaminase is present in brain and the pathway, AMP → IMP → inosine → hypoxanthine, probably accounted for part of the apparent "release" of inosine and hypoxanthine during electrical pulsation (Pull and McIlwain, 1972b). Adenosine deaminase, the enzyme responsible for the conversion of adenosine to inosine, was detected as a soluble and particulate enzyme in rat cerebral cortex and in cultured glial, glioma, and neuroblastoma cells (Pull and McIlwain, 1974b; Trams and Lauter, 1975). In cortical homogenates some enzyme appeared to be associated with synaptosomes. Levels of adenosine deaminase were high in rat hypothalamus, intermediate in medulla, hippocampus, midbrain, and cerebellum, and low in neocortex and striatum (Sun *et al.*, 1976). The pathway, adenosine → inosine → hypoxanthine, is also undoubtedly involved in increased "release" of inosine and hypoxanthine during electrical pulsation of slices. Adenosine had been shown to be more readily incorporated into guinea pig cortical synaptosomes than adenine (Kuroda and McIlwain, 1974). Depolarization by electrical pulsation or high potassium ions increased the efflux of adenosine from adenosine-labeled synaptosomes. The potassium-elicited increase was prevented in calcium-free media, while the increase due to electrical pulsation was partially reduced by tetrodotoxin.

The mechanism involved in the "release" of adenosine from brain slices and synaptosomes remains unknown. Two possibilities can be formulated: (1) A quantal release of adenosine or an adenine nucleotide as a result of membrane depolarization. This release could occur independently or in association with release of biogenic amines or other neurotransmitters. The latter phenomenon, concomittant release of ATP and catecholamines, has been well established for sympathetic neurons. ATP and acetylcholine release occurs from motor neurons. (2) Passive diffusion of adenosine out of the cytoplasm of cells whose levels of adenosine have increased as a result of depolarization-evoked reduction of ATP levels and elevation of AMP levels (Huang and Daly, 1974b). The significance of the *in vitro* "release" of adenosine in brain preparations to physiological functions for adenosine has not been established. In toto, the results with adenine- and adenosine-labeled guinea pig cerebral cortical slices would appear most consonant with labeling of neuronal compartments by adenine and adenosine. Adenosine would appear to preferentially label presynaptic terminals, while cyclic AMP formation appears to be associated to a greater extent with adenine-labeled nucleotides probably in postsynaptic structures.

Rat

Radioactive adenine was incorporated into adenine nucleotides of rat neocortical and hypothalamic slices (Sun *et al.*, 1976). Rates of incorporation were higher in hypothalamus. In rat brain slices, prolonged incubation in the presence of a veratrum alkaloid, protoveratrine, reduced incorporation of radioactive adenine (Glick and Quastel, 1972). High concentrations of potassium ions had no effect on incorporation of adenine during prolonged incubations. Radioactive adenosine injected into the carotid artery of rat was effectively incorporated into intracellular adenine nucleotide pools (Shimizu *et al.*, 1972). No studies on the conversion of such labeled nucleotides to cyclic AMP have been reported.

Compartmentalization and disposition of labeled adenine nucleotides has not been studied extensively in rat brain slices. With adenine-labeled slices from rat cerebral cortex, a preliminary report indicated that during incubation with norepinephrine the specific activity of cyclic AMP increased markedly during the first minutes followed by a decrease to original values (Krishna *et al.*, 1970), suggestive of an initial utilization of more highly labeled adenine nucleotides. Another group reported that the specific activity of cyclic AMP was similar in control and isoproterenol- and norepinephrine-stimulated slices from rat cortex (Perkins, 1973; Perkins and Moore, 1973a,b). Certain of the latter data were, however, suggestive of an increase in specific activity of cyclic AMP with norepinephrine. The specific activity of cyclic AMP in adenine-labeled striatal slices during incubations with norepinephrine was fairly constant (Harris, 1976).

Mouse

The incorporation of radioactive adenine, hypoxanthine, and adenosine into intracellular nucleotides has been studied in detail in mouse brain slices (Wong and Henderson, 1972). Adenine and hypoxanthine were incorporated into adenine ribonucleotides, and norepinephrine was reported to increase the rate of incorporation of adenine. A stimulatory effect of norepinephrine on adenine incorporation was not observed in studies with guinea pig cortical slices (Schultz and Daly, 1973a).

The formation of cyclic AMP from endogenous nucleotides and from adenine- and adenosine-labeled nucleotides has been thoroughly studied in cortical slices from C57Bl/6J mice (Skolnick and Daly, 1975). In contrast to results with guinea pig cortical slices, the ratio of the percent conversion to cyclic AMP of [^{14}C]adenine-labeled nucleotides to that of [^{3}H]adenosine-labeled nucleotides was clearly dependent on the stimulatory agent; with veratridine the ratio was 1.4, with norepinephrine, 2.2, with adenosine–norepinephrine, 2.0, and with adenosine and adenosine–histamine, 3.0. The specific activity of cyclic AMP in both adenine- and adenosine-labeled slices after incubation with norepinephrine, adenosine, adenosine–amine combinations, and veratridine was dependent on the stimulatory agent. For example, in adenosine-labeled cortical slices the specific activity of cyclic AMP was about 50% lower in the norepinephrine-stimulated preparation compared to the veratridine-stimulated preparation. The specific activity of cyclic AMP was lowest when adenosine or adenosine–norepinephrine were used as the stimulatory agent, but, at least in part, this was due to a marked incorporation of the exogenous adenosine into the accumulating cyclic AMP. Thus, exogenous adenosine contributed approximately 40% of the adenine nucleotide precursor for cyclic AMP during 9- to 15-min incubation of mouse cortical slices with 0.1 mM radioactive adenosine. Cyclic AMP formation was also investigated in the quaking mouse, a mutant derived from the C57B1/6J strain (Skolnick and Daly, 1974b). Biochemical alterations in nucleotide metabolism were manifest in cortical slices from the quaking mouse and from heterozygous mice, which contain one quaking gene but do not exhibit the hypomyelination and tremor characteristic of the quaking mouse. Higher rates of incorporation of adenine and adenosine into intracellular nucleotides of the slice were observed in the quaking mouse and the heterozygous mouse as compared to the parent C57B1/6J strain. However, the increase in incorporation occurred in compartments not associated with adenylate cyclases. Thus, the percent conversion of radioactive nucleotides to cyclic AMP in cortical slices from the strains containing the mutant gene was markedly lower than that seen with the parent strain after stimulation with norepinephrine, adenosine, or veratridine, but not after an adenosine–norepinephrine combination. The absolute accumulations of both radioactive and endogenous cyclic AMP were similar in slices from quaking mice, heterozygous mice, and the parent strain except with adenosine as the stimulatory agent. In the latter case, the absolute accumulations were significantly lower in slices from the quaking and heterozygous mice. The ratio of conversions of [^{14}C]adenine- and [^{3}H]adenosine-labeled nucleotides to cyclic AMP in slices from quaking and heterozygous mice were, as in the parent strain, dependent upon the stimulatory agent. It would have been tempting to speculate that alterations in labeling with radioactive adenine and adenosine and in responses to adenosine were due to alterations in adenine or adenosine transport into brain tissue lacking normal myelination or that altered cerebral activity due to tremors in the quaking mouse have led to compensatory changes in adenine nucleotide metabolism. However, the data with heterozygous mice clearly demonstrated that the biochemical alterations in nucleotide metabolism were not directly due to the hypomyelination and tremor of the quaking mouse.

3.1.11 Release and Uptake of Cyclic AMP

Release of cyclic AMP to the medium did not appear to be a significant phenomenon with brain slices under a variety of conditions including electrical stimulation (Kakiuchi and Rall, 1968b; Sattin and Rall, 1970; Pull and McIlwain, 1972a,b). Release occurred from rabbit cortical slices under control and amine-stimulated conditions at a rate of approximately 10 to 20 pmol/mg protein/10 min. A lesser value (3 to 6 pmol/mg protein/10 min) for the efflux of cyclic AMP into the media was observed with guinea pig cortical slices under control and adenosine-stimulated conditions. Compound 48/80 increased the efflux of cyclic AMP from slices of rat cerebral cortex, brainstem, hypothalamus, and cerebellum (Lindl *et al.*, 1976). Neither diphenhydramine or propranolol blocked the drug-elicited increase in efflux. The effect of phosphodiesterase inhibitors on efflux of cyclic AMP has not been investigated in brain slices. In cultured cells, phosphodiesterase inhibitors tend to inhibit efflux (see Section 3.5.2).

The presence of a high-affinity uptake system for cyclic AMP (K_m, 0.14 μM) reported in rat cortical slices (Johnston and Balcar, 1973) would presumably reduce the net efflux of the cyclic nucleotide. Radioactivity in rat cerebral cortical slices after 8 min of incubation with 0.01 μM [8-^{3}H]-cyclic AMP was reported to be almost completely present as cyclic AMP. Dibutyryl cyclic AMP and cyclic GMP inhibited uptake of radioactive cyclic AMP, while 5'-AMP, adenosine, and ouabain were not effective inhibitors. The uptake system was most active in slices from cerebellum, cerebral cortex, and striatum, less active in midbrain and hypothalamus, and least active in medulla. The incorporation of radioactivity, derived from [8-^{3}H]cyclic AMP into mouse synaptosomes has been reported (Lee and Dubos, 1972). The effects of various treatments of synaptosomes on subsequent incorporation of radioactivity was assessed: Cycloheximide decreased incorporation, while adenine nucleotides increased it.

Axonal and dendritic transport of cyclic AMP to secondary sites of action after formation at cell bodies has been proposed (McIlwain, 1976). Axonal transport of radioactivity derived from adenosine has been reported in central neurons (Schubert and Kreutzberg, 1975a,b). Electrical stimulation of axonal tracts increased the transfer of radioactive compounds derived from adenosine to postsynaptic elements in granule cells of the dentate gyrus (Schubert *et al.*, 1976b).

3.1.12 Effects of Drug and Other Treatments of Animals on the Cyclic AMP-Generating Systems in Brain

Chronic or acute treatments of animals with drugs or protocols which interfere with or augment mechanisms involving putative neurotransmitters in the central nervous system might be expected to result in compensatory changes in the responsiveness of cyclic AMP-generating systems to these same neurotransmitters. Such changes have been extensively investigated in brain slices. Conversely, adaptive changes in the responsiveness of cyclic AMP-generating systems after drug or environmental manipulation of animals could provide valuable insights as to the effects of such manipulations on the function of various neurotransmitter systems. Adaptive changes in responsiveness of cyclic AMP-generating systems to alterations in synaptic input has been briefly reviewed (Dismukes and Daly, 1976b).

6-Hydroxydopamine

Treatment of rats with intraventricular 6-hydroxydopamine to destroy presynaptic noradrenergic nerve trerminals resulted in a long-term potentiation of norepinephrine- and isoproterenol-elicited accumulations of cyclic AMP in slices from cerebral cortex, hypothalamus, and brain stem (Palmer, 1972; Weiss and Strada, 1972; Huang *et al.,* 1973b; Kalisker *et al.,* 1973). Intraventricular 6-hydroxydopamine depleted norepinephrine in midbrain, but did not affect responses of cyclic AMP-generating systems to norepinephrine in this brain region (Dismukes and Daly, 1975b). Cerebellar levels of cyclic AMP were extremely high, and norepinephrine elicited a similar small increase in cyclic AMP levels in slices from both control and 6-hydroxydopamine-treated animals (Palmer, 1972). In strains of rats in which responses of norepinephrine-sensitive cyclic AMP-generating systems in cerebral cortical slices were relatively large (cf. Skolnick and Daly, 1974a), treatment with 6-hydroxydopamine did not further enhance the responsiveness (cited in Skolnick and Daly, 1976b). It would appear that in these rat strains, norepinephrine-sensitive cyclic AMP systems were already maximally responsive, perhaps because of a genetically low level of noradrenergic input to cerebral cortex.

Treatment of guinea pigs with 6-hydroxydopamine had no effect on responses of cyclic AMP-generating systems to norepinephrine–adenosine or norepinephrine–isobutylmethylxanthine in neocortical slices (Dismukes *et al.,* 1976a). Norepinephrine has virtually no effect on cyclic AMP levels in guinea pig cortical slices in the absence of either adenosine or isobutyl-methylxanthine. A greater accumulation of cyclic AMP was elicited by electrical stimulation in cerebellar slices from guinea pigs pretreated with 6-hydroxydopamine (Zanella and Rall, 1973). Responses to adenosine in cerebellar slices did not appear significantly enhanced.

Treatment of chicks with 6-hydroxydopamine resulted in an enhanced accumulation of cyclic AMP in cerebrum in response to intravenous isoproterenol, either in the presence or absence of a phosphodiesterase inhibitor, RO 20-1724 (Nahorski and Rogers, 1975). Responses to histamine were unaffected.

In rat cerebral cortical slices, loss of presynaptic uptake sites for norepinephrine was responsible for a shift in the dose–response curve for this catecholamine in cortical slices with the EC_{50} decreasing from 6 μM to

2 μM soon after 6-hydroxydopamine treatment (Kalisker *et al.*, 1973). Cocaine, an uptake inhibitor, had no effect on the norepinephrine dose–response curve in slices from 6-hydroxydopamine-treated animals but did decrease the EC_{50} in slices from control rats. The EC_{50} for isoproterenol was unchanged by 6-hydroxydopamine treatment. Approximately 4 days after treatment with 6-hydroxydopamine, postsynaptic changes occurred which appearred to be responsible for the increase in the magnitude of the maximal accumulations of cyclic AMP elicited by norepinephrine and isoproterenol. Accumulations of cyclic AMP elicited by interaction of catecholamines with either α- or β-receptors appeared to be approximately doubled in cortical slices from the 6-hydroxydopamine-treated rats (Huang *et al.*, 1973b: Kalisker *et al.*, 1973). The potentiation, however, appeared to involve β-adrenergic mechanisms to a somewhat greater extent than α-mechanisms. Responses to adenosine, dopamine, serotonin, veratridine, and combinations of adenosine with serotonin or histamine were not increased or were only marginally increased in cortical slices after 6-hydroxydopamine treatment. The maximal accumulation elicited by an adenosine–norepinephrine combination was, however, significantly increased. In the presence of phosphodiesterase inhibitors such as isobutyl-methylxanthine or papaverine, the accumulations of cyclic AMP elicited by norepinephrine and isoproterenol were still significantly greater in slices from 6-hydroxydopamine-treated rats, suggesting that the increase in maximal accumulations of cyclic AMP reflects changes in formation and not degradation of cyclic AMP. Total levels of adenylate cyclase and phospho-diesterase activity in homogenates of rat cerebral cortex were marginally decreased by the 6-hydroxydopamine treatment (Kalisker *et al.*, 1973), suggesting that measurement of total levels of these enzymes is of limited use in establishing the functional activity of specific cyclic AMP-generating systems in brain.

Treatment of neonatal rats for 4 days with subcutaneous 6-hydroxy-dopamine did not affect the time of development of sensitivity of cyclic AMP-generating systems to norepinephrine or a combination of adenosine–norepinephrine in rat cortical slices (cited in Perkins, 1975; cf. Perkins and Moore, 1973). At 12 days of age, however, the response of cyclic AMP-generating systems to norepinephrine was over threefold higher in cerebral cortical slices from the 6-hydroxydopamine-treated rats. Neither the time of development nor the responsiveness of adenosine-sensitive cyclic AMP-generating systems were altered by 6-hydroxydopamine.

Intracranial injection of 6-hydroxydopamine to rat neonates either at birth or on Day 5 or 8 resulted in enhanced responses of norepinephrine-sensitive cyclic AMP-generating systems in cortical slices prepared on Day 35 from the young adult rats (Palmer and Scott, 1975). Surprisingly, injec-tion of 6-hydroxydopamine on Day 14 did not result in enhanced responsiveness. Levels of norepinephrine in the young adult rats were not ascertained, so it remained unclear as to whether absence of hyperresponsive cyclic AMP systems was due to lack of destruction of developing noradrenergic terminals by 6-hydroxydopamine on Day 14 or to other factors.

Subcutaneous administration of 6-hydroxydopamine to neonatal rats led to enhanced responses of cyclic AMP-generating systems in slices from neocortex and midbrain of adult rats sacrificed at 4 to 5 months of age (Dismukes and Daly, 1975b). Enhanced responses in neocortical slices also pertained with isoproterenol, prostaglandin E_1, and an adenosine–norepinephrine combination, but not with adenosine. In slices from medulla-pons and cerebellum the response to norepinephrine was not significantly enhanced after neonatal 6-hydroxydopamine treatment. The enhanced response to norepinephrine in midbrain slices of adult rats was of interest, since adult levels of norepinephrine in this brain region were nearly doubled after neonatal treatment with 6-hydroxydopamine, presumably due to the proliferation of noradrenergic neuronal terminals. Treatment of adult rats with 6-hydroxydopamine destroyed noradrenergic terminals in the midbrain, but did not result in enhanced responses of norepinephrine-sensitive cyclic AMP-generating systems. It was proposed that the enhanced response to norepinephrine in midbrain slices after neonatal treatment with 6-hydroxydopamine was due to additional cyclic AMP-generating systems associated with new functional noradrenergic synapses.

Dihydroxytryptamines

Intraventricular administration of dihydroxytryptamines, agents which cause somewhat selective degeneration of serotonergic nerve terminals, had no significant or only marginal effects on accumulations of cyclic AMP elicited in rat cerebral cortical slices by norepinephrine, serotonin, adenosine, etc. (Huang *et al.*, 1973b). Intraventricular administration of 5,7-dihydroxytryptamine, an agent which destroys to some extent noradrenergic terminals, tended to increase responsiveness of cyclic AMP-generating systems of cortical slices to norepinephrine.

Reserpine

This *Rauwolfia* alkaloid depletes central levels of norepinephrine, serotonin, and dopamine and, thus, should reduce transynaptic input via these neurotransmitter systems. Prior treatment of rats with reserpine resulted in an increase in the magnitude of the accumulation of cyclic AMP elicited by norepinephrine in slices from cortex, hypothalamus, and hippocampus (Palmer *et al.*, 1973, 1976a; Dismukes and Daly, 1974). Significant potentiation of norepinephrine responses was not seen in slices from cerebellum, midbrain, or brain stem. In studies from one laboratory, reserpine pretreatment apparently enhanced responses to norepinephrine in rat cortical slices, but the results were cited as being quite variable (Perkins, 1975). Reserpine treatment enhanced norepinephrine responses in slices of rat limbic forebrain about 1.5-fold (Vetulani and Sulser, 1975). A 1.4- to 1.6-fold increase in the response of cyclic AMP-generating systems of rat cortical slices to norepinephrine was manifest within 2 days and disappeared between Days 9 and 16 after reserpine treatment (Dismukes and Daly, 1975). The EC_{50}, for norepinephrine did not appear to be significantly altered. The response to isoproterenol or to a norepinephrine– phentolamine combination was significantly enhanced after reserpinization, while the response to a norepinephrine–propranolol combination did not appear altered. In the presence of a phosphodiesterase inhibitor, the response to norepinephrine was still enhanced about 1.4-fold in cortical slices from the reserpinized rats, while responses to serotonin, dopamine, and histamine were unchanged from those in slices from control rats. The response to the depolarizing agent, veratridine, was not enhanced in rat cortical slices after reserpinization. The response to adenosine was, however, enhanced 1.4-fold after reserpine treatment.

In another study with treatment of rats for 4 days with reserpine the maximal responses to norepinephrine and isoproterenol in rat cerebral cortical slices were increased greater than twofold (Palmer *et al.*, 1976a). No clear change in the affinity of the catecholamines for the cyclic AMP-generating systems in slices from reserpinized rats was apparent. After reserpine treatment, the response to norepinephrine was virtually blocked completely by propranolol and was unaffected by phentolamine. Reserpine would, thus, appear to selectively increase β-responses in rat cortical slices (Dismukes and Daly, 1974; Palmer *et al.*, 1976a). In homogenates from reserpinized rats, stimulation of cortical cyclases by norepinephrine, iso-proterenol, and dopamine was slightly increased, while basal and fluoride-stimulated cyclase activities were unchanged (Palmer *et al.*, 1976a). In homogenates of neuronal enriched fractions of cerebral cortex from reser-pinized rats the activation of cyclases by norepinephrine and isoproterenol was significantly enhanced, while the dopamine activation was unaffected. In homogenates from glial enriched fractions activation of cyclases by norepinephrine, isoproterenol, and dopamine was either unaffected after reserpinization or was slightly reduced.

In contrast to results from other laboratories (see above) the maximal accumulation of cyclic AMP elicited by norepinephrine in thick cerebral cortical slices did not appear to be significantly increased in rats treated with reserpine for 4 days (Palmer *et al.*, 1976b). The EC_{50} for norepinephrine was, however, significantly reduced. One hour after treatment with reserpine, the cyclic AMP-generating systems in cortical slices were subresponsive to norepinephrine, but again the maximal response was not affected. Further studies will be required to define the reasons for such apparently discordant results.

Chronic treatment of rats with reserpine first decreases spontaneous motor activity and than after 8 to 12 days of treatment leads to a significant increase in motor activity above that of placebo controls. At the time of enhanced motor activity, the responses of cyclic AMP-generating systems in adenine-labeled rat brain slices to norepinephrine were twofold higher than in slices from control rats (Williams and Pirch, 1974). Incubations were in the presence of caffeine. Thus, hyperresponsiveness of central postsynaptic cyclic AMP-generating systems to norepinephrine would appear to play a role in the increased spontaneous motor activity observed during recovery of reserpinized rats (see p. 287).

Reserpine treatment of Sprague–Dawley rats which had already had noradrenergic terminals destroyed by neonatal treatment with 6-hydroxydopamine did not affect the responses of cyclic AMP-generating systems in cortical slices to norepinephrine (Dismukes and Daly, 1975b). In midbrain, neonatal treatment with 6-hydroxydopamine increases rather than decreases noradrenergic innervation, but reserpinization had no effect on responses to norepinephrine in midbrain slices from either control rats or in rats treated as neonates with 6-hydroxydopamine. The reasons for the lack of adaptive responses in cyclic AMP systems in midbrain to interruption of noradrenergic input are as yet unknown.

Treatment of guinea pigs with reserpine had no effect on responses of cyclic AMP-generating systems to norepinephrine–isobutylmethylxanthine or adenosine–norepinephrine in neocortical slices (Dismukes et al., 1976a). Serotonin had no significant effect on cyclic AMP levels in cortical slices of control or reserpinized guinea pigs, even in the presence of isobutylmethylxanthine. The response to adenosine and the synergistic response to adenosine–serotonin were enhanced in cortical slices from reserpinized rats. The adenosine response was nearly doubled and probably accounted from the modest enhancement of the response to adenosine–serotonin. A greater accumulation of cyclic AMP was elicited by electrical stimulation in guinea pig cortical and cerebellar slices from animals pretreated with reserpine (Kakiuchi et al., 1969; Zannella and Rall, 1973). Responses in cerebellar slices to adenosine did not appear to be significantly enhanced.

Pretreatment of rabbits with reserpine appeared to have little effect on accumulations of cyclic AMP elicited by serotonin, norepinephrine, or histamine in cortical, hypothalamic, or cerebellar slices (Kakiuchi and Rall, 1968b).

Prior treatment of cats with reserpine did not alter the response of brain cyclases to epinephrine in brain homogenates prepared 48 hr later (Klainer *et al.*, 1962).

Treatment of chicks with reserpine resulted in an enhanced accumulation of cyclic AMP in cerebrum in response to intravenous isoproterenol (Nahorski and Rogers, 1975).

Inhibitors of Synthesis of Neurotransmitters

No studies on the effects of treatments with α-methyl-p-tyrosine, an inhibitor of synthesis of catecholamines, p-chlorophenylalanine, an inhibitor of synthesis of serotonin, or other such inhibitors on responsiveness of norepinephrine- and serotonin-sensitive cyclic AMP-generating systems have been published. Treatment of rats with α-methyl-p-tyrosine led in some experiments to enhanced responsiveness of norepinephrine-sensitive cyclase systems in cortical slices, but the results were inconsistent (R. K. Dismukes, unpublished results, Perkins, 1975, unpublished results).

Lesions of the Medial Forebrain Bundle

The medial forebrain bundle contains ascending noradrenergic, serotonergic, and histaminergic tracts. After lesions of the medial forebrain bundle, responses of cyclic AMP-generating systems to norepinephrine and isoproterenol were enhanced in rat cerebral cortical slices (Dismukes *et al.*, 1975). Responses to norepinephrine–propranolol, adenosine, and prostaglandin E_1 were not affected. The enhanced response to norepinephrine occurred within 2 days and was maintained for at least 3 weeks. Responses to norepinephrine were also enhanced in hippocampal slices but were unchanged in slices from midbrain or cerebellum. Responses to either histamine and serotonin in the presence of a phosphodiesterase inhibitor, isobutylmethylxanthine, were enhanced in rat cortical slices after lesioning. The apparent enhancement in the response to serotonin was not, however, statistically significant. In hippocampal slices, the response to histamine was enhanced after lesioning. Phosphodiesterase activity in cerebral cortex was unaltered after lesions of the medial forebrain bundle (Breckenridge and Johnston, 1969).

Lesions of the medial forebrain bundle had no effect on the responses of cyclic AMP-generating systems in guinea pig neocortical slices to histamine, adenosine, histamine–adenosine, norepinephrine–adenosine, or serotonin–adenosine (Dismukes *et al.*, 1976a). The reason for lack of adaptive changes of amine-sensitive cyclic AMP-generating systems in guinea pig cerebral cortical slices after 6-hydroxydopamine, reserpine, or lesions of the medial forebrain bundle are unclear.

Phenothiazines, Antidepressants, and Other Psychoactive Drugs

Increased synaptic levels of biogenic amines elicited by agents which either release or inhibit reuptake and/or metabolism of the amines might be expected to result in adaptive reductions in the responsiveness of postsynaptic cyclic AMP-generating systems. Releasing agents (amphetamines), uptake inhibitors (phenothiazines and tricyclic antidepressants), and metabolic inhibitors (monoamine oxidase inhibitors) have been studied in this regard.

Chronic oral amphetamine, an amine-releasing agent, led to a reduced responsiveness of norepinephrine-sensitive cyclic AMP-generating systems in mouse cortical slices (Martres *et al.*, 1975). The maximal response to norepinephrine was reduced 20 to 30% during a period of 5 hr to 10 days after the beginning amphetamine treatment. No change in the EC_{50} for norepinephrine was detected. The responses of cortical cyclic AMP-generating systems to adenosine, dopamine, and serotonin were unaltered by amphetamine treatment. Pretreatment of rats with p-chloroamphetamine reduced both basal levels of cyclic AMP and norepinephrine-elicited accumulations of cyclic AMP in slices from hypothalamus and brain stem (Palmer *et al.*, 1972a).

Prior treatment of Sprague–Dawley rats with an uptake inhibitor, imipramine, for 5 days, led to a 40% decrease in responses of cyclic AMP-generating systems to norepinephrine in cerebral cortical slices (Frazer *et al.*, 1974). Prior administration of both imipramine and a thyroid hormone, triiodothyronine, also resulted in a decrease in responses to norepinephrine in cortical slices, but the reduction was less pronounced. Chronic treatment of rats with desipramine or iprindole reduced by 70% the responses of norepinephrine-sensitive cyclic AMP-generating systems in slices of limbic forebrain (Vetulani and Sulser, 1975). Treatment with the antidepressant for more than 2 weeks was required for a significant reduction in norepinephrine responses. Treatment of rats with either chlorpromazine or imipramine for 6 days resulted in a marked reduction in the response of norepinephrine-sensitive cyclic AMP-generating systems in rat cerebral cortical slices (Schultz, 1976). At least 6 days were required. Treatment with phenobarbital or diazepam had no effect on responses to norepinephrine. Pretreatment of rats with trifluoperazine tranquilizer resulted in a marked decrease in the accumulation of cyclic AMP elicited by N,N-dimethyltryptamine in slices from brain stem (Uzunov and Weiss, 1972).

Pretreatment of rats with the monoamine oxidase inhibitor, pargyline, increased basal levels of cyclic AMP in incubated slices of cortex, hypothalamus, brain stem, hippocampus, and cerebellum, but did not apparently alter responses to norepinephrine (Palmer et al., 1971, 1973). Chronic treatment of rats with monoamine oxidase inhibitors has been reported to reduce the responsiveness of norepinephrine-sensitve cyclic AMP-generating systems in slices of limbic forebrain (Vetulani et al., 1975).

Chronic subcutaneous administration of isoproterenol almost completely abolished the accumulation of cyclic AMP normally elicited in chick cerebrum by intravenous isoproterenol (Nahorski and Rogers, 1975). The response to isoproterenol was, however, nearly fully manifest in chicks treated with RO 20-1724, suggesting that increases in cerebral phosphodiesterase elicited by isoproterenol had been responsible for the subsensitivity. Histamine responses were unaffected by chronic treatment with isoproterenol. Others have reported significantly higher adenylate cyclase activity in cerebral cortical homogenates from rats sacrificed 24 hr after a single intracisternal injection of norepinephrine, serotonin, or histamine (Chou et al., 1971a,b). The "activation" of cyclase by intracisternal norepinephrine was maximal only after 20 hr and was not blocked by a protein synthesis inhibitor, cycloheximide.

Ethanol

Chronic treatment of rodents with ethanol enhances norepinephrine turnover in brain, while during withdrawal from ethanol turnover of norepinephrine is reduced. French et al. (1974) reported greatly decreased responses of cyclic AMP-generating systems in cortical slices to norepinephrine after chronic treatment of rats with ethanol. During ethanol withdrawal a combination of hyperresponsiveness of cyclase systems to norepinephrine and a reduction in norepinephrine "release" was proposed to be involved in withdrawal seizures. During ethanol withdrawal the accumulation of cyclic AMP elicited by norepinephrine was, indeed, enhanced in rat cerebral cortical slices, but not in slices from hypothalamus (French and Palmer, 1973). The increase appeared to involve primarily α-adrenergic mechanisms. Chronic treatment with alcohol decreased the EC_{50} for norepinephrine-stimulated accumulation of cyclic AMP in rat cerebral cortical slices, while having no effect on maximal accumulations (French et al., 1975a,b). During 3 days of withdrawal from alcohol, the EC_{50} for norepinephrine responses was significantly increased, but the maximal response was unaffected. Thus, during alcohol treatment norepinephrine-sensitive cyclic AMP-generating systems exhibited subsensitivity, while during withdrawal supersensitivity developed. The response to cyclic AMP-generating systems in rat cortical slices to submaximal concentrations of histamine was also enhanced during ethanol withdrawal (French et al., 1975a). Serotonin responses were detectable only in slices from ethanol-withdrawal rats. The response to histamine in slices from ethanol-withdrawal rats was blocked by an antihistamine, chlorpheniramine, by an α-antagonist, phenoxybenzamine, and by a β-antagonist, propranolol, while the response to serotonin was blocked by methysergide, phenoxybenzamine, and propranolol. Responses to histamine–norepinephrine combinations were no greater than that due to either amine alone. The nonspecific nature of the increase in amine responses during ethanol withdrawal clearly emphasizes the need for further research on the nature of ethanol-induced changes in cyclic AMP-generating systems.

Chronic treatment of mice with ethanol increased adenylate cyclase activity in cortical monogenates and basal levels of radioactive cyclic AMP in adenine-labeled cortical slices (Isräel et al., 1972; Kuriyama and Isräel, 1973). Acute ethanol treatment had no effect on adenylate cyclase activity. Phosphodiesterase activity was not altered by chronic ethanol treatment. A significant accumulation of cyclic AMP in cortical slices was no longer elicited by norepinephrine after chronic alcohol treatment, while histamine still had a marginal stimulatory effect.

Stress

A variety of stresses are known to increase turnover of central neurotransmitters. Virtually nothing is known about the effect of stress on responsiveness of cyclic AMP-generating systems. Preliminary data on isolation stress in rats indicated a slight reduction in responses of norepinephrine-sensitive cyclic AMP-generating systems in cortical slices (P. Skolnick and J. Daly, unpublished results). Electroconvulsive treatment of rats for 8 days reduced by 30 to 50% the responses of norepinephrine-sensitive cyclic AMP-generating systems in slices of limbic forebrain (Vetulani and Sulser, 1975). In reserpinized rats, electroconvulsive treatment reduced norepinephrine responses by about 20%. Interestingly, the handling associated with electroconvulsive treatments resulted in significantly enhanced basal levels of cyclic AMP in incubated slices of limbic forebrain.

Morphine

The effects of morphine and other narcotic analgesics on cyclic AMP-generating systems in brain tissue have been extensively studied. In spite of these efforts no clear conclusions are as yet warranted.

Chronic treatment of mice with morphine has been reported to either decrease or increase adenylate cyclase activity in cerebral homogenates, to have no effect on phosphodiesterase activity, and to reduce protein kinase activity (Chou et al., 1971a; Clark et al., 1972; Naito and Kuriyama, 1973).

Naito and Kuriyama (1973) reported slightly *enhanced* levels of adenylate cyclase in mouse cerebral cortex after chronic dietary administration of morphine for 7 to 28 days. Phosphodiesterase levels were unaffected. After an acute dose of morphine, these workers reported *no* change in either cyclase or phosphodiesterase activity. Chronic administration of morphine from a pellet implanted for 3 days was reported to *reduce* levels of adenylate cyclase in mouse cerebral cortex (Chou *et al.*, 1971a) but had no effect on phosphodiesterase. During a 26-hr withdrawal period after removal of the pellet, no changes in cyclase or phosphodiesterase were observed. After an acute dose of morphine adenylate cyclase levels were reported to be significantly enhanced in cerebral cortex and brain stem, but not in cerebellum or hypothalamus. The levels of cyclic AMP-dependent protein kinases in rat brain homogenates, reduced by chronic treatment with morphine, became elevated above levels in control rats after 18 hr of withdrawal (Clark *et al.*, 1972). Chronic administration of heroin to rats had no effect on levels of brain phosphodiesterase (Collier *et al.*, 1975). Another group (Singhal *et al.*, 1973) reported that acute or chronic treatment of rats with morphine had no effect on levels of adenylate cyclase or phosphodiesterase activity in cerebral cortex, thalamus–hypothalamus, or cerebellum. During withdrawal, adenylate cyclase levels in all brain regions were significantly reduced, and this reduction was prevented or antagonized by methadone. Acute or chronic treatment with morphine was stated to have no effect on basal or fluoride-stimulated levels of cyclase in cerebral cortex, cerebellum, or thalamus–hypothalamus of rat (Merali *et al.*, 1975). Phosphodiesterase activity was also unaffected. It was stated that cyclase levels declined during withdrawal, while phosphodiesterase remained unaffected. Replacement of morphine with methadone prevented the reduction in cyclase.

Chronic or acute treatment of rats with morphine did not appear to result in significant changes in the magnitude of the accumulation of cyclic AMP elicited in cortical slices by norepinephrine, adenosine, or veratridine, or in hypothalamic slices by norepinephrine (M. Huang, A. K. S. Ho, and J. W. Daly, unpublished results).

Effects of chronic heroin treatment on basal and prostaglandin-sensitive adenylate cyclase in rat brain were inconsistent (Collier *et al.*, 1975). Usually no effect was observed, but it was stated that basal levels of cyclase in brain homogenates were increased by heroin in two experiments and that the stimulatory effect of prostaglandin E_1 was greatly increased in one experiment.

Chronic treatment of rats with morphine has been reported either to have no effect (Kuschinsky, 1975; Van Inwegen *et al.*, 1975) or to enhance (Clouet and Iwatsubo, 1974; Clouet *et al.*, 1975) dopamine-sensitive adenylate cyclase activity in striatum. Acute treatment of rats with morphine was reported to increase both basal and dopamine-stimulated adenylate cyclases in particulate preparations from striatum (Clouet and Iwatsubo, 1974; Clouet et al., 1975). Basal levels of adenylate cyclase were increased in midbrain, but not in other brain regions, except perhaps medulla. Chronic treatment with morphine increased only the dopamine-sensitive component in striatal preparations. Admininstration of a large dose of morphine to chronically morphinized rats prior to sacrifice increased basal levels of adenylate cyclase in cortex and cerebellum. Another group (Puri et al., 1975) reported that an acute treatment of male hooded rats with high dosages of morphine slightly enhanced basal cyclase levels in homogenates of striatum, but did not affect dopamine or fluoride-stimulated activity. High K_m phosphodiesterase activity in striatal homogenates was decreased by the morphine pretreatment, while the low K_m activity was not significantly affected. A third group reported that acute or chronic morphine treatment, abstinence withdrawal, or withdrawal precipitated with naloxone had no significant effects on basal, fluoride-, or dopamine-stimulated activity of striatal cyclases from rat (Van Inwegen et al., 1975). Dopamine-stimulated cyclase activity did appear marginally reduced in chronically treated rats and in rats undergoing withdrawal. A fourth group reported that striatal levels of basal and dopamine-stimulated cyclase were slightly elevated in chronically morphinized rats and decreased during withdrawal (Merali et al., 1975). The dopamine response was actually not significantly different after chronic morphine, and no response to dopamine was seen with striatal cyclases from animals undergoing withdrawal. Adenylate cyclase, cyclic AMP, and protein kinase levels were, in addition, measured in striatal synaptosomes from control rats, chronically morphinized rats, and rats undergoing abstinence or naloxone withdrawal. Cyclase and cyclic AMP levels were increased by chronic morphinization and decreased during withdrawal. Methadone could not prevent the decrease elicited by withdrawal. Protein kinase levels were marginally increased by chronic morphinization and decreased during withdrawal. Methadone antagonized the withdrawal-elicited decrease in kinase activity.

Effects of Lesions and Psychoactive Agents on Dopamine-Sensitive Cyclic AMP-Generating Systems

Lesions of the nigro-striatal pathway, or treatment of animals with dopaminergic antagonists, reserpine, or α-methyl-p-tyrosine result in an apparent supersensitivity to dopaminergic agonists in vivo. Attempts to correlate the dopaminergic supersensitivity to alterations of responsiveness of dopamine-sensitive cyclic AMP systems in striatum have not been particularly successful.

Electrolytic or 6-hydroxydopamine lesions of the nigro-neostriatal dopaminergic pathway led in 3 days to a decrease in the EC_{50} for dopamine- or norepinephrine-elicited accumulation of cyclic AMP in slices of caudate nucleus (Krueger et al., 1976). Isobutylmethylxanthine was present in the incubations. The maximal accumulation of cyclic AMP elicited by catecholamines was not affected by lesioning. The accumulations of cyclic AMP elicited by apomorphine were not consistently greater in slices from the striatum from the lesioned hemisphere. In homogenates of caudate nucleus, dopamine-sensitive adenylate cyclase activity was not altered after electrolytic or 6-hydroxydopamine lesions (Krueger et al., 1976 and citations to unpublished results of M. Goldstein and U. Ungerstedt, J. W. Kebabian and co-workers, and L. L. Iversen). However, one group (Mishra et al., 1974) reported that after unilateral lesions of the substantia nigra in rats the maximal responses of adenylate cyclases to dopamine and dopaminergic agonists were significantly enhanced in homogenates of caudate nucleus, and the EC_{50} for dopamine was decreased. Lesions were made by radiofrequency irradiation or with 6-hydroxydopamine. The latter technique resulted in a more profound depletion of dopamine in the caudate and had no effect on basal levels of cyclase. In contrast, basal levels of cyclase in the caudate nucleus were greatly decreased after radio-frequency lesions. Animals were sacrificed 10 to 36 days after radiofrequency lesions and 100 to 120 days after 6-hydroxydopamine lesions.

Responses of dopamine-sensitive adenylate cyclases in striatal homogenates were not enhanced after prior treatment of mice with either intra-striatal 6-hydroxydopamine unilaterally or with chronic α-methyl-p-tyrosine (Von Voightlander et al., 1973). Indeed, the responses to dopamine appeared somewhat diminished after these treatments; i.e., 10 μM dopamine significantly enhanced cyclase activity in control but not in treated preparations. Treatment of rats with reserpine for 2 days had no significant effect on dopamine-sensitive adenyl cyclases of striatum (Rotrosen et al., 1975). It was stated that increases in striatal cyclic AMP elicited in vivo by apomorphine or amphetamine were unaltered after reserpine treatment and that mesolimbic and striatal levels of high K_m phosphodiesterase were also unaltered. Chronic treatment with haloperidol for 2 weeks had no effect on dopamine-sensitive adenylate cyclases from rat striatum (Von Voightlander et al., 1975). Apomorphine-elicited increases in cyclic AMP levels in striatum in vivo were also not affected by the prior chronic treatment with haloperidol. However, another group (Iwatsubo and Clouet, 1975) reported that acute treatment of rats with the dopaminergic antagonist, haloperidol, elicited a transient increase in dopamine-sensitive cyclase activity in caudate synaptosomal preparations. Chronic treatment with haloperidol also appeared to result in a compensatory increase in dopamine-sensitive cyclases in the caudate nucleus. Chronic treatment with chlorpromazine had no effect on dopamine-sensitive adenylate cyclases of rat striatum (Rotrosen *et al.*, 1975). It was stated that increases in striatal cyclic AMP elicited *in vivo* by apomorphine or amphetamine were unaltered by "chronic neuroleptic pretreatment" and that mesolimbic and striatal levels of high K_m phosphodiesterase were also unaltered. Prior administration of lysergic acid diethylamide to rats reduced the dopamine response of cyclases in striatal homogenates (Spano *et al.*, 1975b).

Hormones

Various endocrine hormones are considered to be involved in the development and control of central functions. A limited number of studies on the effect of hormones and/or removal of endocrine glands on central cyclic AMP systems have been reported.

Administration of triiodothyronine for 5 days had no effect on responses of cortical norepinephrine-sensitive cyclic AMP-generating systems (Frazer *et al.*, 1974). Neonatal thyroidectomy had little effect on the development of norepinephrine-sensitive cyclic AMP-generating systems in rat brain slices (Schmidt and Robison, 1972; Singhal *et al.*, 1973b). The development of rat brain adenylate cyclase, phosphodiesterase, and protein kinase was not significantly affected by thyroidectomy. Endogenous levels of cyclic AMP in brain, however, increased during development to a lesser extent in thyroidectomized rats. Thyroxine treatment of rat pups had no effect on basal levels of microsomal protein kinases or on cyclic AMP activation of brain microsomal protein kinase determined on postnatal Day 10 with histone as substrate (Schmidt, 1974). Thyroxine had no effect on adenylate cyclase in the mature brain (cited as J. Perkins, personal communication).

Insulin administration to elicit hypoglycemia in rats caused a slight increase in adenylate cyclase activity and a slight decrease in phosphodiesterase activity in brain homogenates (Hetenyi and Singhal, 1973). Evisceration-elicited hypoglycemia was accompanied by very slight increase in brain adenylate cyclase.

Adrenalectomy or treatment of rats with methylxanthines or hydrocortisone had no effect on phosphodiesterase levels in cerebral cortex (Vernikos-Danellis and Harris, 1968).

Pretreatment of rats with thyrotrophin-releasing hormone appeared to enhance *in vivo* dopaminergic mechanisms without affecting activity of basal or dopamine-sensitive cyclases from the caudate nucleus (Green *et al.*, 1975).

Other Treatments

Prostaglandin E_1 appeared to have a slightly greater stimulatory effect on adenylate cyclases from rat cerebral cortex in animals pretreated with indomethacin, an inhibitor of prostaglandin synthesis, but the activation was still only about 25% (Van Inwegen *et al.*, 1975). Indomethacin treatment appeared to have slightly decreased the response of cyclases to catecholamines.

Accumulations of cyclic AMP elicited by norepinephrine, isoproterenol, adenosine, prostaglandin E_1, and histamine were compared in cerebral slices from male rats raised from weaning in either impoverished or enriched environments (Dismukes and Daly, 1976a). The accumulation of cyclic AMP elicited by prostaglandin E_1 was significantly greater in slices from impoverished rats, while the response to histamine was marginally greater in slices from enriched rats. Responses to other agents were unaffected by the environmental manipulations.

Unilateral epileptogenic foci formed by freezing techniques in rat cerebral cortex elicited profound changes in levels of adenylate cyclase, phosphodiesterase, and cyclic AMP in both the lesioned and contralateral cortex (Walker *et al.*, 1973). Basal levels of adenylate cyclase in the lesioned cortex were increased threefold over a 24-hr period, while low K_m phosphodiesterase levels decreased within 4 hr to one-third their initial value followed by a slight increase over the following 4 to 20 hr. After 24 hr phosphodiesterase levels were still reduced nearly 50%. Adenylate cyclase increased less than threefold in the contralateral cortex 8 hr after lesioning, but had decreased by about 50 to 60% by 24 hr. Cyclic AMP levels had increased nearly fourfold in the lesioned cortex by 8 hr and were still slightly elevated at 24 hr. Cyclic AMP levels increased more slowly in the contralateral cortex, but by 8 hr had attained the same fourfold increase seen in the lesioned cortex. The mechanisms involved in these changes were unclear. Increases in cyclic AMP elicited by injury might be expected through feedback-control to increase phosphodiesterase activity, but instead a decrease in this enzyme was observed. At 24 hr when adenylate cyclase activity was maximally elevated, cyclic AMP levels were only slightly greater than in sham-operated animals.

Cycloheximide has effects on sensitivity of animals to various centrally active drugs (cf. Green *et al.*, 1975). Treatment of mice with inhibitors of protein synthesis such as chloramphenicol and cycloheximide resulted within a period of 5 hr in a reduction in both basal and dopamine-sensitive adenylate cyclases in homogenate of caudate nucleus (Tang *et al.*, 1974). Treatment with a stimulator of cerebral protein synthesis such as the double-stranded RNAs (polyinosinic acid and polycytosinic acid) had no effect on basal levels of cyclase but increased the dopamine-sensitive cyclases. Green *et al.* (1975), however, did *not* detect any effect of pretreatment of rats with cycloheximide on basal or dopamine-sensitive adenylate cyclase levels in homogenates of caudate nucleus.

The stimulatory effect of choleratoxin on adenylate cyclase activity in intact cells is known to involve activation of cyclases after a prior binding of the toxin to a cell surface ganglioside. Injection of choleratoxin into the nucleus accumbens resulted in a marked and long-term increase in adenylate cyclase activity in nucleus accumbens, striatum, and olfactory tubercle but not in cortex or hypothalamus (Miller and Kelly, 1975). Dopamine-sensitive adenylate cyclase was increased at 5 hr after choleratoxin treatment, but after 24 hr dopamine had no effect on the elevated basal levels of cyclase.

Undernourished rats (18 pups per mother) exhibited levels of brain adenylate cyclase and phosphodiesterase similar to those in normal rats during the period from 3 to 20 days after birth (Kauffman *et al.*, 1972). Neonatal infection of pathogen-free mice with an enterovirus or neonatal malnutrition of mice resulted in an apparent increase in phosphodiesterase activity in brain and a decrease in cyclic AMP levels at 3 to 4 months of age (Lee and Dubos, 1972). Levels of adenylate cyclase were not significantly altered by either of the neonatal treatments. Treatment of 5-week-old mice from control, neonatal infection, and neonatal malnutrition groups with theophylline 1 hr prior to sacrifice interestingly appeared to have reduced phosphodiesterase activity in homogenates from the latter two groups, but not in the control group. In addition, the treatment with theophylline elevated levels of cyclic AMP in brain of all three groups. The elevated levels of cyclic AMP were not significantly different in the three groups; i.e., theophylline caused a greater increase in the neonatal infection and neonatal malnutrition mice. Metabolism of intraperitoneal [8-^{14}C]cyclic AMP to radioactive CO_2 was significantly higher in mice from the neonatal malnutrition group and slightly higher in mice from the neonatal infection group as compared to control mice. Incorporation of radioactivity from intraperitoneal [8-^{14}C]cyclic AMP into brain and *in vitro* incorporation of radioactivity from [8-^{3}H]cyclic AMP into synaptosomes were, however, both significantly reduced in the neonatally treated groups.

Adaptation of Cyclic AMP Systems to Alterations in Synaptic Input in the Pineal Gland

The β-adrenergic-sensitive adenylate cyclases of secretory cells of the pineal gland provide a model for investigation of physiological and pharmacological alterations of postsynaptic cyclic AMP-generating systems in response to changes in presynaptic noradrenergic input. In pineal gland, elevations of cyclic AMP in secretory cells lead to an increase in levels of serotonin N-acetyltransferase, resulting thereby in reductions in serotonin levels and increases in melatonin formation. Protein synthesis appears involved in cyclic AMP-mediated increases in the transferase activity. Diurnal variations in the sensitivity of the cyclic AMP-generating systems to catecholamines were consonant with adaptive changes to alterations in noradrenergic input (Romero and Axelrod, 1975). Thus, during the day when sympathetic activity in the pineal is low, the cyclic AMP-generating system was "supersensitive" to stimulation with isoproterenol, while during the night when sympathetic activity is high in the pineal, a subsensitivity developed. In addition to the increase in the responsiveness of cyclic AMP-generating systems during the day, the efficacy with which dibutyryl cyclic AMP activated induction of serotonin N-acetyltransferase was also increased, indicative of adaptive control of the cyclic AMP-controlled system at two sites: (i) formation of cyclic AMP and (ii) action of cyclic AMP. In addition, phosphodiesterase activity was lower during the day (Minneman and Iversen, 1976a, see below). The adenylate cyclase in homogenates from "subsensitive" pineal glands exhibited a similar affinity for activation by isoproterenol and for binding of the β-antagonist, dihydroalprenolol (Kebabian *et al.,* 1975). Changes in number of binding sites for dihydroalprenolol correlated with changes in levels of pineal adenylate cyclase. Levels of basal, isoproterenol, and fluoride-stimulated adenylate cyclases were much higher in "supersensitive" pineals. Decreases in cyclases elicited *in vivo* by isoproterenol were not blocked by an inhibitor of protein synthesis, cycloheximide. Since isoproterenol was much more potent in eliciting increases in serotonin N-acetyltransferase in "supersensitive" pineals, but had no greater apparent affinity for the cyclase, it was proposed that the effectiveness with which cyclic AMP mediates responses was also increased in "supersensitive" pineals.

Earlier studies had established that postsynaptic cyclic AMP-generating systems in pineal glands became more responsive to norepinephrine or isoproterenol after 6-hydroxydopamine or reserpine treatment, after denervation, ganglionectomy, or after exposure of animals to continuous light (Weiss and Costa, 1967; Weiss, 1969, 1971; Weiss and Strada, 1972; Deguchi and Axelrod, 1973; Axelrod, 1974; Strada and Weiss, 1974). The development of hyperresponsiveness of the cyclic AMP-generating systems could be prevented in ganglionectomized animals by chronic administration of norepinephrine. In homogenates of pineal glands, both fluoride- and catecholamine-activated cyclase levels were enhanced by a prior *in vivo* reduction of adrenergic input into the pineal. The development of basal and fluoride-stimulated cyclase activity in the pineal gland, however, occurred to a similar extent in control rats and in rats ganglionectomized on Day 1 after birth (Weiss, 1971). Norepinephrine-stimulated cyclase measured 9 weeks later was slightly greater in the ganglionectomized rats.

Responses of cyclic AMP-generating systems in pineal glands to catecholamines were increased after artificial interruption in noradrenergic input, but in these early studies the affinity of catecholamines for the β-receptors modulating adenylate cyclase activity was apparently also increased (Deguchi and Axelrod, 1973). In denervated pineals it appeared probable that the superinduction of N-acetyltransferase elicited by isoproterenol was due only to the increased responsiveness of norepinephrine-sensitive cyclases. Dibutyryl cyclic AMP did not elicit superinduction of N-acetyltransferase in denervated pineals. These results contrast with physiological light–dark control of cyclic AMP mechanisms wherein only the maximal response of cyclic AMP systems to catecholamines was increased and where, in addition, dibutyryl cyclic AMP was more effective in eliciting increases in the transferase (Romero and Axelrod, 1975). Phosphodiesterase activity was not apparently altered in pineals under conditions of decreased sympathetic activity (Strada and Weiss, 1974). Others (Oleshansky and Neff, 1975) have reported that refractoriness of pineal cyclic AMP-generating systems to isoproterenol was due both to a decrease in isoproterenol-sensitive adenylate cyclases and to an increase in low K_m phosphodiesterase. During dark periods, when noradrenergic input to pineal is elevated, levels of cyclic AMP- and cyclic GMP-phosphodiesterases were significantly increased (Minneman and Iversen, 1976a). Ganglionectomy or propranolol blocked the dark-induced increase in phosphodiesterase, while a protein synthesis inhibitor, cycloheximide, only partially blocked the increase. Choleratoxin activated adenylate cyclases in cultured pineal glands and thereby elicited an increase in phosphodiesterase activity (Minneman and Iversen, 1976b). Cycloheximide blocked the increase in phosphodiesterase activity.

Denervation by ganglionectomy resulted in an increase in guanylate cyclase activity in rat pineal (Strada et al., 1976).

3.2 Cyclic GMP in Brain Slices

Cyclic GMP-generating systems in brain have been investigated in some detail in cerebellar slices and to a lesser extent in cerebral cortical slices of various mammalian species. After initial postdecapitation elevations in cyclic GMP (see Section 2.2.1) levels of cyclic GMP were reported to become stable in slices after 60 to 90 min of incubation (Ferrendelli et al., 1973b). Basal levels of cyclic GMP in brain slices stabilized at 0.2 to 4 pmol/mg protein except in cerebellar slices, where in rat levels as high as 20 to 70 pmol/mg protein have been observed (see Table 3). Initial levels of cyclic GMP in slices of mouse cerebellum were as high as 150 pmol/mg protein and then decreased to 4 to 18 pmol/mg protein after 30 to 60 min of incubation. Significant release of cyclic GMP from brain slices was not detectable (Ferrendelli *et al.*, 1973b). Norepinephrine, histamine, adenosine, muscarinic agonists, amino acids, and depolarizing agents have been reported to elicit accumulations of cyclic GMP in brain slices. The responses appear dependent on extracellular calcium ions and, indeed, incubation of cerebellar slices in calcium-free medium reduces levels of cyclic GMP (Ohga and Daly, 1976a). The extent of the reduction depends on the species and brain region. As was the case with cyclic AMP generation in brain slices, data on accumulations of cyclic GMP have not always been in agreement. The reasons for these inconsistencies are not apparent, but may at least in some cases be due to the rapid and often transient nature of elicited accumulations of cyclic GMP. The effects of various agents on levels of cyclic GMP in brain slices has been recently reviewed (Ferrendelli, 1975).

Interrelationships between levels of cyclic AMP and levels of cyclic GMP have been suggested in nonneuronal systems (cf. Goldberg *et al.*, 1973, 1975). In cerebellar slices of various species no relationships between basal levels of the two cyclic nucleotides were apparent (Ohga and Daly, 1976a). Ratios of cyclic AMP to cyclic GMP were 4.6 in rabbit, 0.5 in guinea pig, 2.1 in rat, and 1.0 in mouse cerebellar slices. Cyclic GMP levels in cerebellar slices could be reduced by incubation in calcium-free medium and then increased upon addition of calcium. Cyclic AMP levels were virtually unaffected under these conditions.

3.2.1 Rabbit

Norepinephrine had no effect on cyclic GMP levels in rabbit cortical slices and has been reported to either increase or reduce levels in cerebellar slices (Kuo *et al.*, 1972; Kinscherf *et al.*, 1976). Histamine increased cyclic GMP levels two to threefold in rabbit cerebral cortical slices but had no effect in cerebellar slices (Kuo *et al.*, 1972; Lee *et al.*, 1972). In cerebral cortical slices, acetylcholine and muscarinic agonists such as bethanechol and pilocarpine elicited a transient twofold increase in cyclic GMP levels. Maximal levels of less than 3 pmol/mg protein were attained in about 2 min. The responses were prevented by a muscarinic blocking agent, atropine, but not by a nicotinic blocking agent, hexamethonium. A nicotinic agonist, tetramethylammonium ion, had no effect on levels of cyclic GMP. In rabbit cerebellar slices, acetylcholine elicited a two- to threefold transient increase in cyclic GMP levels. This is surprising in view of the probable lack of cholinergic innervation in cerebellum. Maximal levels of less than 5 pmol/mg protein were attained in about 1 min in cerebellar slices. In another study, acetylcholine was stated to have no consistent effect in cortical or cerebellar slices (Kinscherf *et al.*, 1976). Glutamate increased levels of cyclic GMP in rabbit cerebral cortical slices, but had no significant effect on levels in cerebellar slices. γ-Aminobutyrate and glycine had no effect in either brain region, while high concentrations of potassium ions elevated cyclic GMP in both regions. After preincubation for an extended period in calcium-free medium, addition of calcium caused a twofold increase in basal levels of cyclic GMP in rabbit cerebellar slices (Ohga and Daly, 1976a).

3.2.2 Guinea Pig

Norepinephrine, histamine, and adenosine were reported to elicit calcium-dependent two- to threefold accumulations of cyclic GMP in guinea pig cerebral cortical slices (Ohga and Daly, 1976a; Schwabe et al., 1976b). In another study, norepinephrine had no significant effect (Kinscherf et al., 1976). Norepinephrine and in one study adenosine elicited accumulations of cyclic GMP in cerebellar slices (Kinscherf et al., 1976; Ohga and Daly, 1976a,b). Acetylcholine and carbamylcholine were cited to have no effect in guinea pig cortical and cerebellar slices (Kinscherf et al., 1976). Glutamate (10 mM) and high concentrations of potassium ions elevated levels of cyclic GMP in slices from cerebral cortex and cerebellum. γ-Aminobutyrate and glycine had no effect in either brain region. Veratridine elicited a two- to threefold increase in cyclic GMP levels in guinea pig cerebellar slices (Ohga and Daly, 1976a,b). The response to veratridine was calcium dependent and was partially antagonized by high concentrations of magnesium ions. The response was not significantly antagonized by antagonists of neuromodulators such as theophylline, atropine, strychnine, diethyl glutamate, picrotoxin, sotalol, or phentolamine. It was antagonized by chlorpromazine and promethazine, compounds which also antagonized calcium-elicited accumulation of cyclic AMP in guinea pig cerebellar slices. Isobutylmethylxanthine had little effect on the accumulation of cyclic GMP elicited by veratridine. It was suggested that about 100 pmol/mg protein of cyclic GMP in guinea pig cerebellar slices might be a maximal level.

In guinea pig cerebellar slices incubated for a prolonged period, readdition of calcium resulted in a rapid sevenfold increase in levels of cyclic GMP (Ohga and Daly, 1976a,b). Norepinephrine and adenosine augmented this calcium-elicited increase, while histamine, phenylephrine, glutamate, γ-aminobutyrate, glycine, prostaglandin E_1, and carbamylcholine had no effect. The norepinephrine effect was dependent on calcium ions and was antagonized by sotalol, but not by phentolamine. The response was potentiated by isobutylmethylxanthine. Isoproterenol also slightly augmented the calcium-elicited accumulation of cyclic GMP in cerebellar slices. The adenosine effect was antagonized by theophylline. In guinea pig cerebral cortical slices after a prolonged incubation in calcium-free medium, levels of cyclic GMP were not significantly altered by the addition of calcium ions.

The effects of various agents on calcium-elicited accumulations of cyclic GMP in guinea pig cerebellar slices have been studied in detail (Ohga and Daly, 1976b). Antagonists to acetylcholine, glycine, glutamate, γ-aminobutyrate, adenosine, or norepinephrine (see above) did not reduce the calcium-elicited accumulation of cyclic GMP. High concentrations of magnesium ions partially blocked the response to calcium. Various putative calcium antagonists such as tetracaine, cocaine, neomycin, ethanol, morphine, pentobarbital, and verapamil were relatively ineffective antagonists of calcium-elicited accumulations of cyclic GMP, as was dimethylsulfoxide. Verapamil actually potentiated the response to calcium ions. Promethazine (IC_{50} 100 μM) > l-brompheniramine > d-brompheniramine, diphenhydramine, chlorpromazine, and imipramine were the most effective antagonists of the calcium response. Other phenothiazines such as perphenazine, thioridazine, fluphenazine, and trifluoperazine were ineffective or only marginally effective antagonists of the calcium response. No clear correlations of the effectiveness of phenothiazines and imipramine as antagonists of the calcium response and as inhibitors of cerebellar guanylate cyclases were apparent (see Section 2.2.3). The calcium ionophores, A-23187 and X-537A, had a small and variable stimulatory effect and a marked inhibitory effect, respectively, on calcium-elicited accumulations of cyclic GMP in guinea pig cerebellar slices, but neither agent was studied in detail. The phosphodiesterase inhibitor, isobutylmethylxanthine, caused a fourfold potentiation of calcium-elicited accumulation of cyclic GMP, while diazepam, RO 20-1724, and papaverine caused a twofold potentiation. Theophylline had no effect, and SQ 20009 was slightly inhibitory. In calcium-free medium, all of the phosphodiesterase inhibitors except theophylline and SQ 20009 caused a threefold increase in levels of cyclic GMP.

3.2.3 Rat

Norepinephrine has been reported to either have no effect (Kinscherf *et al.,* 1976) or to elicit a threefold accumulation of cyclic GMP in rat cerebral cortical slices (Schwabe *et al.,* 1976b). Histamine and adenosine also elicited a threefold accumulation of cyclic GMP. In the presence of phosphodiesterase inhibitor, such as RO 20-1724 and ZK 62711, basal levels of cyclic GMP in cortical slices were increased and norepinephrine, histamine, and adenosine no longer had a stimulatory effect. Papaverine also increased basal levels of cyclic GMP in rat cortical slices (Palmer and Duszynski, 1975). Cyclic GMP levels in slices of rat brain were, after 30 min, high in cerebellum (27 pmol/mg protein) and hypothalamus (9 pmol/mg protein) and lower in slices from striatum, thalamus–midbrain, brain stem, hippocampus, and cerebral cortex (3.5 to 6 pmol/mg protein) (Palmer and Duszynski, 1975). Carbamylcholine increased cyclic GMP levels only in cerebral cortical slices. Acetylcholine, pilocarpine, or the cholinesterase inhibitor, physostigmine, increased cyclic GMP in cortical slices, while methacholine had no effect. Atropine partially antagonized the response to carbamylcholine. Glutamate, γ-aminobutyrate, glycine, and high concentrations of potassium ions had no effect on cyclic GMP levels in rat cortical slices (Kinscherf et al., 1976). Potassium ions did increase levels of cyclic GMP in cerebellar slices. In another study potassium ions did increase cyclic GMP in rat cortical slices (Kimura et al., 1975). The response was blocked in calcium-free medium. Veratridine elicited a twofold accumulation of cyclic GMP in rat cerebellar slices which was potentiated by the phosphodiesterase inhibitor, ZK 62711, and marginally increased by RO-1724 (Schwabe et al., 1976a). After a prolonged incubation in calcium-free medium, addition of calcium elicited only a small increase in levels of cyclic GMP in rat cerebellar slices in contrast to the marked increases which pertained with guinea pig, rabbit, and mouse (Ohga and Daly, 1976a).

It has been proposed (Laborit et al., 1974) that guanosine may augment the accumulation of cyclic GMP elicited by acetylcholine in brain slices. The proposal was based on the ability of guanosine to potentiate increases in oxygen consumption elicited in rat brain slices in high potassium media and by acetylcholine (see, however, Section 3.2.4). Guanosine also potentiated metabolic effects of insulin, both in brain slices and on levels of glycogen in whole brain in vivo. Guanosine alone had no effect on cyclic GMP levels in mouse cerebellar slices (see below).

Azide enhanced levels of cyclic GMP in slices of rat cerebral cortex and cerebellum (Kimura et al., 1975). Hydroxylamine also stimulated cyclic GMP accumulation in cortical slices, and its effects were additive with azide. Cyanide had no effect in cortical slices. Neither incubation with calcium-free EGTA-containing medium nor addition of atropine, propranolol, phenoxybenzamine, diphenhydramine, aminooxyacetic acid, or γ-aminobutyrate blocked the response to azide.

Acute treatment of rats with harmaline led to an increase in soluble but not particulate guanylate cyclase in rat cerebellum (Spano et al., 1975a).

3.2.4 Mouse

Norepinephrine had no effect on levels of cyclic GMP in cerebral cortical slices of Swiss-Webster mice (Kinscherf et al., 1976). Norepinephrine elicited a two- to fourfold increase in cyclic GMP levels in mouse cerebellar slices (Ferrendelli, 1975; Ferrendelli *et al.*, 1975; Kinscherf *et al.*, 1976). Both phentolamine and propranolol completely blocked the response to norepinephrine. Epinephrine elicited a response similar to that elicited by norepinephrine, while neither isoproterenol nor phenylephrine had any significant effect on cyclic GMP levels, although the latter α-agonist tended to reduce cyclic GMP levels as did dopamine at high concentrations. The response to norepinephrine was blocked in calcium-free medium and either reduced or unaffected by low sodium-medium. Theophylline greatly increased basal levels of cyclic GMP in mouse cerebellar slices, but had little effect on the norepinephrine response. Dopamine, histamine, and serotonin even at 1 mM concentrations had little or no effect on cyclic GMP levels.

Neither adenosine nor guanosine had any effect on cyclic GMP levels in mouse cerebellar slices, nor did adenosine have a significant effect on cyclic GMP accumulations elicited by norepinephrine (Ferrendelli *et al.*, 1973b, 1975). Prostaglandins at 3 μM concentrations had no effect in cerebellar slices (Ferrendelli, 1975).

Acetylcholine, methacholine, and carbamylcholine had no effect on levels of cyclic GMP in cortical or cerebellar slices (Ferrendelli *et al.*, 1973b; Kinscherf, 1976). Glutamate elevated levels of cyclic GMP in mouse cortical slices, while γ-aminobutyrate and glycine had no effect. Glutamate, a putative excitatory neurotransmitter, and γ-aminobutyrate and glycine, putative inhibitory neurotransmitters, elevated levels of cyclic GMP in mouse cerebellar slices (Ferrendelli *et al.*, 1974, 1975; Ferrendelli, 1975; Kinscherf *et al.*, 1976). Taurine had no significant effect. Glutamate (10 mM) caused a rapid tenfold increase in cyclic GMP levels. This increase was slightly potentiated by theophylline. Glycine (1 mM) and γ-aminobutyrate (5 mM) elicited a slower threefold and twofold increase, respectively, in levels of cyclic GMP. In both cases, the increase was further potentiated by the presence of theophylline. Theophylline also increased basal levels of cyclic GMP in cerebellar slices. The possible role of release of these amino acids in depolarization-evoked accumulation of cyclic GMP is uncertain. Maximal stimulatory concentrations of glutamate and high concentrations of potassium ions were no more effective than potassium ions alone. It should be pointed out that glutamate itself is considered a depolarizing agent in brain slices. The stimulatory effects of the amino acids on cyclic GMP accumulation in all cases required calcium ions in the medium. Sodium ions were required for glutamate- and probably for γ-aminobutyrate- and glycine-elicited accumulation of cyclic GMP in mouse cerebellar slices (Ferrendelli, 1975). The effects of glutamate and glycine were additive, while the effects of combinations of γ-aminobutyrate with either glutamate or glycine were not additive. Combinations of glutamate and norepinephrine had greater than additive effects on accumulations of cyclic GMP in mouse cerebellar slices, while combinations of glycine and norepinephrine had only additive effects. γ-Aminobutyrate appeared to inhibit the response to norepinephrine.

Depolarizing agents such as veratridine, ouabain, and high concentrations of potassium ions elevated cyclic GMP levels in mouse cerebellar slices about 30-fold (Ferrendelli et al., 1973b, 1974, 1975, 1976; Kinscherf et al., 1976). The effects of potassium ions were significant at 30 mM and increased up to 120 mM. The effects of submaximal stimulatory concentrations of the depolarizing agents were additive. Potassium ions increased cyclic GMP levels in mouse cortical slices 10-fold. In both brain regions, accumulation of cyclic GMP elicited by potassium ions or veratridine was maximal in about 6 min, while 15 min was required with ouabain. Atropine did not prevent the effects of depolarizing agents in cerebellar slices, nor did theophylline prevent the effects of potassium ions. The response to veratridine was dependent on sodium ions. Combinations of potassium ions and norepinephrine had effects on cyclic GMP levels in mouse cerebellar slices only somewhat greater than those due to potassium alone. Depolarizing agents did not have any effect on cyclic GMP levels in calcium-free media and the effects of potassium ions were partially blocked by high concentrations of magnesium ions. Barium and strontium, but not magnesium, manganese, or cobalt, could replace the requirement for calcium ions in potassium-elicited accumulation of cyclic GMP in mouse cerebellar slices. Cobalt antagonized the response to potassium ions in normal Krebs–Ringer medium. The results suggested that a calcium-mediated excitation–coupling process was responsible for the release of a stimulatory substance, which was neither adenosine nor acetylcholine. The released substance was then responsible at least in part for the elevation of cyclic GMP elicited by the depolarizing agents. Depolarizing agents might, however, directly activate cyclic GMP-generating systems by influx of calcium ions. After prolonged incubation in calcium-free medium, addition of calcium ions caused a 3-fold increase in levels of cyclic GMP in mouse cerebellar slices (Ohga and Daly, 1976a). Glutamate (1 mM) did not enhance the accumulation of cyclic GMP elicited by calcium ions. The calcium ionophore, A-23187, caused a marked increase in cyclic GMP levels in mouse cerebellar slices (Ferrendelli et al., 1976). The solvent, ethanol–acetone, used to add the ionophore to the medium, caused a reduction in levels of cyclic GMP and probably partially antagonized calcium or calcium plus ionophore-elicited accumulations of cyclic GMP.

Radioactive guanine, on incubation with mouse cerebral slices, was completely converted to xanthine (Wong and Henderson, 1972). Thus, it appears unlikely that a guanine-prelabeling technique will be useful in the study of formation of cyclic GMP in brain slices.

3.2.5 Cat

Norepinephrine had no effect on cyclic GMP levels in slices of cat cerebral cortex (Kinscherf *et al.*, 1976). Norepinephrine did elicit an accumulation of cyclic GMP in cerebellar slices. Glutamate elevated cyclic GMP in cortical slices, while γ-aminobutyrate and glycine had no effect. Potassium ions increased cyclic GMP in cortical and cerebellar slices. In one experiment, high potassium ions were reported to have elevated cyclic GMP 2.5- to 5-fold in slices of cat olfactory bulb, striatum, inferior and superior colliculi, hippocampus, thalamus, brain stem, and spinal cord.

3.3 Cyclic AMP in Ganglia and Peripheral Neurons

The effects of biogenic amines, acetylcholine, electrical stimulation, and depolarizing agents on cyclic AMP levels have been investigated in ganglion preparations from mammals and lower organisms. The results are consonant with stimulation of postsynaptic cyclic AMP-generating systems by biogenic amines. Release of endogenous amines appears to be elicited in ganglia by electrical stimulation or depolarizing agents and at least in some ganglia by interaction of cholinergic agents with muscarinic receptors. The sequence of (1) preganglionic nerve impulse, release of acetylcholine, and activation of muscarinic receptors on interneurons, (2) intraneuronal nerve impulse, release of a catecholamine, and activation of cyclic AMP-generating systems in postganglionic neurons appeared to be associated with inhibitory synaptic transmission (see Section 4.3.2).

3.3.1 Vertebrates

Sympathetic Ganglia

Preganglionic stimulation elicited a two- to fivefold increase in cyclic AMP levels in rabbit superior cervical ganglia (McAfee *et al.*, 1971; Greengard *et al.*, 1972; Kalix *et al.*, 1974), a fourfold increase in cat superior cervical ganglion (Chatzkel *et al.*, 1974), and an eightfold increase in bullfrog sympathetic ganglion (Weight *et al.*, 1974). Postganglionic stimulation of the rabbit superior cervical ganglion had no effect, nor did stimulation of the cervical vagus nerve have any effect on cyclic AMP levels in the nerve or in the nodose ganglion, a ganglion with nerve cell bodies but no synapses. The elevation of cyclic AMP elicited in rabbit superior cervical ganglion by preganglionic stimulation was blocked by a muscarinic antagonist, atropine, and by α-antagonists, but was not significantly affected by a nicotinic antagonist, hexamethonium, or by β-antagonists. The increases in cyclic AMP were potentiated by the phosphodiesterase inhibitors, theophylline and RO 20-1724. The results were consonant with the following interpretation: Preganglionic stimulation elicited a release of acetylcholine which in turn, by activation of muscarinic receptors on the interneurons, caused a depolarization and release of a catecholamine. The amine elicited an accumulation of cyclic AMP in the adrenergic cell body by interaction with a receptor that could be blocked by α-antagonists. Direct acetylcholine-mediated transmission which would be blocked by hexamethonium did not appear to be involved in the formation of cyclic AMP. In bullfrog ganglia, neither cholinergic nor adrenergic antagonists blocked the accumulation of cyclic AMP elicited by preganglionic stimulation (R. A. Lehne, A. Suria, and E. Costa, personal communication). Further studies on responses of cyclic AMP-generating systems in sympathetic ganglia have been conducted with incubated slices or whole ganglia from rabbit, rat, steer, and cat.

In the rabbit superior cervical ganglion, carbamylcholine and the muscarinic agonist, bethanechol, elicted about twofold accumulations of cyclic AMP (McAfee et al., 1971; Greengard, et al., 1972; Kalix et al., 1974). The elevation of cyclic AMP elicited by carbamylcholine was blocked by atropine, and by α-antagonists such as phentolamine, phenoxybenzamine, and thymoxamine, but not by a nicotinic antagonist, hexamethonium, or by β-antagonists. The response to carbamylcholine was blocked in calcium-free medium and in the presence of a local anesthetic, tetracaine, and was potentiated by theophylline and RO 20-1724. The latter compound elevated basal levels of cyclic AMP in ganglia. Adenosine had no effect either in the presence or absence of carbamylcholine. In rabbit superior cervical ganglia, dopamine increased cyclic AMP levels by only 15% (Kalix et al., 1974). Chlorpromazine, haloperidol, and various analogs were weak antagonists of dopamine-elicited accumulations of cyclic AMP.

In cultured rat superior cervical ganglia (nor)epinephrine and isoproterenol elicited a transient 6- to 20-fold increase in levels of cyclic AMP, while even much higher concentrations of dopamine or phenylephrine had only marginal, relatively slow effects on cyclic AMP levels (Cramer et al., 1973a; Cramer and Lindl, 1974; Lindl et al., 1974, 1975; Otten et al., 1974; Lindl and Cramer, 1975). The order of potency of the catecholamines was isoproterenol > epinephrine > norepinephrine. The response of cyclic AMP-generating systems to norepinephrine was partially blocked by either phentolamine or propranolol, with the β-antagonist more effective, and was completely blocked by a combination of α- and β-antagonists. The response to epinephrine was blocked by the β_1-antagonist, practolol. Theophylline had no effect on responses to catecholamines in cultured rat ganglia. Acetylcholine had no effect on basal levels of cyclic AMP or on the response to epinephrine. Potassium ions in combination with theophylline increased cyclic AMP levels in rat superior cervical ganglia (Webb *et al.,* 1975).

The accumulation of cyclic AMP elicited by (nor)epinephrine in rat superior cervical ganglia was accompanied by a marked efflux of cyclic AMP (Cramer and Lindl, 1974; Lindl and Cramer, 1974, 1975; Lindl *et al.,* 1975). Probenecid (*p*-(di-*n*-propylsulfanoyl)benzoic acid) had only a slight inhibitory effect on accumulations of cyclic AMP elicited by epinephrine and had no effect on efflux. Papaverine potentiated both the accumulation and efflux of cyclic AMP elicited by norepinephrine in rat superior cervical ganglia. However, although accumulations of cyclic AMP elicited by norepinephrine during a series of stimulations did not significantly decrease, the response to a norepinephrine–papaverine combination became undetectable by the fourth stimulation. Similarly, efflux of cyclic AMP remained constant during sequential stimulations with norepinephrine but declined to undetectable levels during sequential stimulations with norepinephrine–papaverine. It is possible that prolonged exposures to papaverine depleted ATP in ganglia (cf. Doore *et al.,* 1975). Prolonged incubation of ganglia with epinephrine did reduce ATP levels (Lindl *et al.,* 1975).

Both basal levels of cyclic AMP and responses to isoproterenol decreased markedly during culture of rat ganglia for 2 days (Cramer *et al.,* 1973a). It was stated that postsynaptic noradrenergic cells survived and developed sprouts, while presynaptic terminals and interstitial cells degenerated during culture of the ganglia, suggesting that the isoproterenol-sensitive cyclases were not uniquely located in noradrenergic cells but were perhaps associated with glial elements. However, the threefold increase in cyclic AMP levels that was elicited in rat superior cervical ganglion *in vivo* by isoproterenol was virtually lost when the noradrenergic cells had been destroyed by prior treatment with 6-hydroxydopamine or nerve growth factor antiserum (Otten *et al.,* 1974). Basal levels of cyclic AMP were only slightly reduced in the ganglia from the pretreated rats. Interestingly, more than 60 min was required in normal rats before a second injection of isoproterenol would elicit a transient accumulation of cyclic AMP in the superior cervical ganglion similar in magnitude to that of the first isoproterenol-elicited accumulation. Epinephrine, dopamine, and to a lesser extent norepinephrine when administered *in vivo* with phenoxybenzamine elicited accumulations of cyclic AMP in rat superior cervical ganglia (Hanbauer *et al.,* 1975a). Isoproterenol also elicited an accumulation of cyclic AMP, which was blocked by propranolol. Catecholamine-elicited accumulations of cyclic AMP were reduced in decentralized ganglia.

In cultured rat superior cervical ganglia, histamine (EC_{50}, 200 μM) elicited a two- to eightfold increase in cyclic AMP levels (Cramer and Lindl, 1974; Lindl and Cramer, 1974; Lindl *et al.*, 1974, 1975). Similar increases in levels of radioactive cyclic AMP were seen in adenine-labeled ganglia. The histamine–elicited increase in cyclic AMP levels was antagonized by both H_1-(diphenhydramine) and H_2-(burimamide) antagonists, but not by a β-antagonist. Burimamide alone elicited an increase in cyclic AMP levels. Efflux of cyclic AMP from incubated ganglia into the medium was slightly increased by histamine. The histamine–elicited increase in cyclic AMP levels in the ganglia was blocked by probenecid. The ratio of radioactive cyclic AMP in the medium to radioactive cyclic AMP in the ganglia was similar under control and histamine conditions, indicating that rates of efflux were directly proportional to intracellular levels of cyclic AMP. Probenecid had little independent effect on the efflux of radioactive cyclic AMP. Release of phosphodiesterase to the medium appeared to decrease during incubations with histamine, while release of the cytoplasmic enzyme, lactate dehydrogenase, was unaffected. The compound 48/80 caused degranulation of mast cells in rat superior cervical ganglia and increased release of ATP, histamine, and norepinephrine (Lindl *et al.*, 1974). Concomitantly, compound 48/80 elevated cyclic AMP levels in the tissue by as much as sevenfold and greatly increased efflux of cyclic AMP into the medium. Diphenhydramine nearly completely blocked the stimulatory effects of compound 48/80 on ganglionic levels and efflux of cyclic AMP. Propranolol slightly reduced the accumulation of cyclic AMP elicited by compound 48/80, but had no significant effect on the enhanced efflux of cyclic AMP. A combination of diphenhydramine and propranolol completely blocked the accumulation of cyclic AMP elicited by 48/80 in the ganglia, but the efflux rate now remained elevated.

In adenine-labeled rat superior cervical ganglia, only a very small percentage of the total radioactivity was present as ATP (6 to 10%) or cyclic AMP (0.6 to 1.6%) (Lindl *et al.*, 1975). The ratio of endogenous ATP to cyclic AMP was 800, while the ratio of radioactive ATP to cyclic AMP varied from 2 to 16 under control and histamine- or norepinephrine-stimulated conditions. It would appear that ATP serving as precursor of cyclic AMP had been selectively labeled during incubation with radioactive adenine, but the nature of the major portion of radioactivity in the adenine-labeled ganglia deserves further study. Antimycin A_1, an inhibitor of oxidative phosphorylation, inhibited incorporation of radioactive adenine into ATP in rat superior cervical ganglia, while having no effect on total levels of ATP (Lindl *et al.*, 1975).

Nerve growth factor elicited a transient increase in cyclic AMP levels in cultured rat superior cervical ganglia (Nikodijevic *et al.*, 1975). Others have reported that nerve growth factor had no effect on levels of cyclic

AMP in chick dorsal root ganglia, while theophylline did elicit an increase (Frazier *et al.,* 1973).

In adenine-labeled slices of bovine superior cervical ganglia, dopamine (EC$_{50}$, 9 μM) and at higher concentrations norepinephrine (EC$_{50}$, 40 μM) elicited about a fivefold increase in radioactive cyclic AMP (Kebabian and Greengard, 1971). Dopamine elicited a similar increase in endogenous cyclic AMP. Theophylline increased basal levels and potentiated the amine responses. Responses to dopamine were inhibited by α-antagonists but not by β-antagonists. β-Antagonists did, however, reduce the effects of norepinephrine. Chlorpromazine, haloperidol, and various analogs were weak antagonists of dopamine-elicited accumulations of cyclic AMP in bovine superior cervical ganglia (Kalix *et al.,* 1974). Others have reported a threefold increase in levels of cyclic AMP in bovine superior cervical ganglia elicited by dopamine in the presence of theophylline (Williams *et al.,* 1974). Dopamine-elicited accumulations of cyclic AMP in slices of bovine superior cervical ganglia were potentiated by the phosphodiesterase inhibitor, SQ 20006 (Kebabian *et al.,* 1975c). Acetylcholine slightly inhibited the dopamine response. Acetylcholine alone had no significant effect on levels of cyclic AMP in ganglia, but bethanechol had a marginal stimulatory effect. Another group confirmed that in the presence of theophylline, dopamine and norepinephrine elicited similar accumulations of cyclic AMP in slices of bovine superior cervical ganglia, with dopamine the more potent agonist (Roch and Kalix, 1975a,b). Both tyramine and serotonin had very small effects on cyclic AMP levels in ganglion slices which might have been due to release of endogenous catecholamines. A dopamine-β-hydroxylase inhibitor, diethyldithiocarbamate, had no effect on the response to dopamine. In the absence of phosphodiesterase inhibitor, either theophylline or RO 20-1724, the amines had no or only a small effect on cyclic AMP levels. Rates of disappearance of cyclic AMP after stimulation by norepinephrine were retarded by the continued presence of theophylline. Adenosine had no effect on cyclic AMP levels in ganglion slices, either alone or in the presence of theophylline or RO 20-1724. In the presence of theophylline, depolarizing agents, such as veratridine, ouabain, and high concentrations of potassium, cesium, or ammonium ions elicited a three- to fourfold increase in cyclic AMP levels in bovine ganglia (Kalix and Roch, 1975; Roch and Kalix, 1975b). Tetracaine and tetrodotoxin blocked the response to veratridine. Tetracaine at high concentrations antagonized responses to potassium ions. The presence of theophylline was in most experiments required for potassium-elicited accumulations of cyclic AMP. The response to potassium was not significantly affected by atropine, burimamide, and pyrilamine, but was partially antagonized by phentolamine and propranolol. The stimulatory effects of potassium ions and either norepinephrine or dopamine were less than additive. The results suggest that depolarizing agents in bovine ganglia elicit accumulations of cyclic AMP via release of catecholamines. Angiotensin, a ganglionic depolarizing agent, had no effect on levels of cyclic AMP in bovine superior cervical ganglia (Kebabian *et al.*, 1975c).

Immunofluorescent histochemical assay indicated that dopamine-elicited accumulations of cyclic AMP in bovine superior cervical ganglia occurred primarily in postganglionic neurons (Kebabian *et al.*, 1975a). Norepinephrine elicited accumulations of cyclic AMP in postganglionic neurons and, in addition, in fibroblast and blood vessel-like cells. The phosphodiesterase inhibitor, SQ 20006, was present in all incubations.

Histamine, in the presence of theophylline or SQ 20006 elicited a two- to threefold accumulation of cyclic AMP in slices of bovine superior cervical ganglion (Kebabian *et al.*, 1975c; Roch and Kalix, 1975a). The response to histamine was antagonized by burimamide, but not by combination of phentolamine and propranolol or by atropine, and appeared additive with the responses to norepinephrine and to dopamine.

The results with rabbit and bovine superior cervical ganglia indicate that dopamine is probably the catecholamine involved as a neurotransmitter in accumulation of cyclic AMP elicited in postganglionic noradrenergic neurons. In rat superior cervical ganglia, the results are not yet definitive as to whether dopamine or norepinephrine or both are involved as the neurotransmitter. Neither dopamine nor norepinephrine had significant effects on levels of cyclic AMP in cat superior cervical ganglia (Williams *et al.*, 1975).

Retina

Dopamine- and norepinephrine-sensitive cyclic AMP-generating systems would appear to occur in the ganglion cells of the retina. In incubated rabbit retina, dopamine (EC_{50}, 1 μM) and apomorphine, but not amantadine, mescaline, isoproterenol, or the catechol metabolite of piribedil, elicited accumulations of cyclic AMP (Bucher and Schorderet, 1974; Schorderet, 1975). The response to dopamine and apomorphine was blocked by haloperidol. In incubated bovine retina, dopamine, apomorphine, (nor)epinephrine, and the depolarizing agents, ouabain and high concentrations of potassium ions, elicited twofold increases in cyclic AMP levels (Brown and Makman, 1972, 1973; Makman *et al.*, 1975a,b). Adenosine, serotonin, and histamine had no effect. Fluphenazine, haloperidol, chlorpromazine, lysergic acid diethylamide, and ergotamine blocked dopamine responses, while phentolamine was much less effective. The effects of dopamine and the depolarizing agents on cyclic AMP levels were additive, suggesting that the response to depolarizing agents does not involve release of dopamine.

Peripheral Neurons

Electrical stimulation of the motor neurons innervating striated muscle of rat or frog had no effect on cyclic AMP levels in muscle, while epinephrine markedly elevated levels of cyclic AMP (Posner *et al.*, 1965). Neuronal terminals represent such a small amount of the total tissue that any effects of electrical stimulation or epinephrine on neuronal levels of cyclic AMP would probably have been undetectable. Stimulation of the rabbit cervical vagus nerve had no effects on levels of cyclic AMP in the nerve (McAfee *et al.*, 1971), nor did dopamine or acetylcholine affect levels of cyclic AMP in bovine lingual nerve (Kebabian *et al.*, 1975c). Isoproterenol or theophylline increased cyclic AMP levels in desheathed frog sciatic nerves two- to threefold (Horn and McAfee, 1976). Cyclic AMP levels in sciatic nerve of hypoactive (immobilized) and hyperactive (mobile) hind limbs of a rat oscillated with maxima reached at 36 and 64 days and minima at 12 and 50 days in the immobilized limb (Appenzeller *et al.*, 1976). In the mobile limb maxima were reached at 20 and 64 days, and a single minimum was reached at 44 days.

3.3.2 Invertebrates

Molluscs

In adenine-labeled abdominal ganglia of the marine mollusc, *Aplysia californica*, electrical stimulation of nerves led to a twofold increase in levels of radioactive cyclic AMP in the ganglion but not in the nerves (Cedar and Schwartz, 1972; Cedar *et al.*, 1972). There was, however, no increase in endogenous cyclic AMP levels. High concentrations of magnesium which prevent synaptic transmission prevented the increase in radioactive cyclic AMP, while depolarization of ganglionic neurons with ouabain or glutamate had no effect on cyclic AMP levels. Adenosine, carbamylcholine, glutamate, norepinephrine, and histamine had no significant effects on cyclic AMP levels in the ganglion and the adenosine antagonist, theophylline, had no effect on the elevations of cyclic AMP elicited by electrical stimulation. Serotonin and dopamine did cause a threefold increase in levels of radioactive cyclic AMP. In other experiments, serotonin (EC_{50}, 6 μM) caused an eightfold and dopamine a sixfold increase in endogenous levels of cyclic AMP. After one stimulation with serotonin, the ganglionic cyclic AMP systems were refractory to a restimulation with serotonin for 10 to 15 min. Serotonin antagonists, such as lysergic acid diethylamide and methysergide, were relatively ineffective against the serotonin-elicited accumulation of cyclic AMP. In subsequent studies octopamine-elicited accumulations of cyclic AMP in the ganglia were blocked by phentolamine, and serotonin-elicited accumulations were blocked by methysergide (Levitan *et al.,* 1974). Serotonin elicited accumulations of cyclic AMP in all regions of the *Aplysia* nervous system. The data suggest that serotonin and dopamine or octopamine released by electrical stimulation activated postsynaptic adenylate cyclases in the abdominal ganglion.

Insects

In cockroach thoracic ganglion, levels of cyclic AMP were increased by octopamine, dopamine, and serotonin (Nathanson and Greengard, 1973, 1974). Theophylline greatly potentiated the response to octopamine. In addition, these amines and relatively high concentrations of norepinephrine stimulated adenylate cyclase activity in homogenates. The EC_{50}'s for octopamine, serotonin, and dopamine were less than 2 μM, while the EC_{50} for norepinephrine was 30 μM. The stimulatory effects of combinations of octopamine, dopamine, and serotonin were additive in homogenates, suggesting the presence of separate receptors. The effects of octopamine and dopamine were antagonized by phentolamine, but not by propranolol. The effects of serotonin were effectively antagonized by lysergic acid diethylamide, 2-bromolysergic acid diethylamide, and cyproheptadine. Both of the lysergic acid derivatives at higher concentrations stimulated the cockroach adenylate cyclase. Catecholamines have also been reported to activate adenylate cyclases in homogenates from cockroach brain (Rojakovick and March, 1972). Isoproterenol had no effect. Formation of cyclic AMP and adenosine from ATP in homogenates of tobacco hornworm brains was stimulated in the presence of theophylline and fluoride by the insect hormone, β-ecdysone (Vedeckis and Gilbert, 1973).

3.4 Cyclic GMP in Ganglia and Peripheral Neurons

The effects of acetylcholine and electrical stimulation on levels of cyclic GMP in sympathetic ganglia have been investigated. Preganglionic stimulation appears to elicit release of acetylcholine which, on interaction with postsynaptic muscarinic receptors, activates postsynaptic cyclic GMP-generating systems. Activation of cyclic GMP systems appears to be associated with slow excitatory postsynaptic potentials (see Section 4.3.2). In bovine superior cervical ganglia, only slight cross-inhibitions between acetylcholine-elicited accumulation of cyclic GMP and dopamine-elicited accumulations of cyclic AMP were detected (Kebabian *et al.,* 1975c).

3.4.1 Vertebrates

Sympathetic Ganglia

Preganglionic stimulation elicited a twofold increase in levels of cyclic GMP in bullfrog sympathetic ganglia (Weight *et al.*, 1974). Elevated levels of cyclic GMP were maintained for at least 2 min. Blockage of transmitter release by high concentrations of magnesium ions prevented stimulus-evoked increases in cyclic GMP, as did the presence of the muscarinic antagonist, atropine.

Acetylcholine and the muscarinic agonist, bethanechol, but not the nicotinic agonist, N,N-dimethylphenylpiperazinium, elicited four- to five-fold accumulations of cyclic GMP in bovine superior cervical ganglia (Kebabian *et al.*, 1975c). Atropine, but not hexamethonium, blocked the response to acetylcholine and to bethanechol. The response to acetylcholine was greatly reduced in calcium-free medium. The phosphodiesterase inhibitor SQ 20006 slightly potentiated the response to acetylcholine. Dopamine had a marginal inhibitory effect on the response to acetylcholine. Histamine increased cyclic GMP levels twofold in the presence of SQ 20006. Angiotensin, a ganglionic depolarizing agent, had no effect on cyclic GMP levels in bovine superior cervical ganglia (Kebabian *et al.*, 1975c).

Immunofluorescent histochemical assay indicated that acetylcholine-elicited accumulations of cyclic GMP in bovine superior cervical ganglia occurred primarily in postganglionic neurons (Kebabian *et al.*, 1975a). A phosphodiesterase inhibitor, SQ 20006, was present in the incubations.

Carbamylcholine had no significant effect on levels of cyclic AMP or cyclic GMP *in vivo* in rat superior cervical ganglion (Hanbauer *et al.*, 1975a).

Retina

Levels of radioactive cyclic GMP derived from [^{3}H]hypoxanthine in bovine retina were reduced after illumination (Goridis and Virmaux, 1974). The light-induced reduction in cyclic GMP was prevented by the phosphodiesterase inhibitor, SQ 20009.

Peripheral Neurons

Acetylcholine elicited a twofold accumulation of cyclic GMP in bovine lingual nerve (Kebabian *et al.*, 1975c). Carbamylcholine or theophylline increased cyclic GMP levels in desheathed frog sciatic nerves twofold (Horn and McAfee, 1976).

3.4.2 Invertebrates

The control of cyclic GMP-generating systems in the ganglia of invertebrates has apparently not been investigated, although such studies would appear profitable in view of the simplicity of the neuronal systems.

3.5 Cyclic Nucleotides in Cells of Neuronal or Glial Origin

Cultured cells provide an excellent model system for the study of the factors controlling the *in vivo* formation and degradation of cyclic nucleotides. Such studies are relevant and complementary to studies on cyclic nucleotide-generating systems in the heterogenous brain slice preparations, but caution should be exercised in extrapolating results with cultured cells to the function of cyclic nucleotide-generating systems in the dynamic integrated complex of neurons, astrocytes, and oligodendrocytes that comprise the central nervous system.

3.5.1 Fetal Brain Cells

Reaggregation Cultures

Cells from fetal mouse brain in reaggregation cultures responded to norepinephrine or isoproterenol with a four- to sixfold increase in cyclic AMP levels (Seeds and Gilman, 1971). This response developed during culture and was manifest at 9 days but not at 15 hr. Theophylline did not further potentiate the catecholamine-elicited accumulation of cyclic AMP. Thus, with respect to cyclic AMP generation these cultures, which contain proportions of neurons and glia probably similar to those in the immature mouse brain, exhibited catecholamine responses similar in magnitude to those of brain slice preparations.

Surface Cultures

Cells from fetal rat brain in surface cultures responded to isoproterenol with a remarkable 60- to 100-fold increase in cyclic AMP levels (Gilman and Schrier, 1972; Sturgill *et al.*, 1975). The response to isoproterenol developed during culture and was maximal after about 14 days. In surface culture extensive multiplication of cells, presumably mainly glial cells, took place. The response to isoproterenol was blocked by β-antagonists such as sotalol and dichlorisoproterenol and was virtually unaffected by an α-antagonist, phentolamine. Theophylline had little effect on the response.

Norepinephrine appeared to elicit only a 17-fold increase in cyclic AMP levels, but a complete dose–response curve for norepinephrine was not reported. These results contrast to responses in rat brain slices, where both α- and β-receptors appear involved in norepinephrine-stimulated formation of cyclic AMP and where norepinephrine elicited a much greater accumulation of the cyclic nucleotide than did isoproterenol (see Section 3.1.3). Adenosine and prostaglandin E_1 elicited 12- and 30-fold increases, respectively in levels of cyclic AMP in the surface cultures of rat fetal brain cells. Radioactive 2-chloroadenosine was not significantly incorporated into confluent cultures of rat fetal brain cells either in the presence or absence of isoproterenol and no formation of 2-chloro cyclic AMP could be detected (Sturgill *et al.*, 1975). Thus, under conditions where the adenosine analog stimulated formation of cyclic AMP, it did not serve a precursor of a cyclic nucleotide. Adenosine–catecholamine combinations did not have synergistic effects on cyclic AMP formation. Histamine, serotonin, and high concentrations of potassium ions had no effect. Dopamine had only a marginal effect.

3.5.2 Neuroma Cells

Cultured cells derived from various neuromas of rat, mouse, or human origin have been investigated with regard to accumulations of cyclic AMP. The results primarily with neuroblastoma and astrocytoma cell lines are relevant to the role of neurons and glia, respectively, in responses of cyclic AMP-generating systems in brain slices to different agents, although it should be stressed that tumor cell lines may show greatly altered enzyme levels or hormone responsiveness compared to that of the parent tumor cells or to that of normal cells. For example, levels of adenylate cyclase in cultured hamster astrocytes were reduced 50% after virus-induced transformation (Weiss *et al.*, 1971) and clones of glioma cells often lost responses to various agents during subculturing (see Perkins, 1973). Cyclic AMP levels are usually low in rapidly proliferating cell cultures and are apparently further reduced during mitosis (see Section 4.2). Responses of cyclic AMP-generating systems to various agents also vary during culture. A critical review of the advantages and disadvantages of cultured tumor cells as models for the study of cyclic nucleotide roles has appeared (Chlapowski *et al.*, 1975).

Neuroblastoma Cells

In mouse neuroblastoma cell lines, prostaglandins E_1 (EC_{50}, 0.2 μM) and E_2 elicited a three- to tenfold increase in levels of cyclic AMP (Gilman and Nirenberg, 1971b; Gilman and Minna, 1973; Hamprecht and Schultz, 1973a,b; Prasad *et al.,* 1973a,c; Sheppard and Prasad, 1973; Matsazawa and Nirenberg, 1975; Prasad and Kumar, 1975; Simantov and Sachs, 1975b). Theophylline had no effect or only slightly potentiated the response to prostaglandin, while other phosphodiesterase inhibitors such as papaverine, RO 20-1724, isobutylmethylxanthine, and diazepam elevated basal levels of cyclic AMP in neuroblastoma cells and greatly potentiated the effects of prostaglandin (Blume *et al.,* 1973; Gilman and Minna, 1973; Hamprecht and Schultz, 1973a,b; Prasad *et al.,* 1973a,c; Schultz and Hamprecht, 1973; Sheppard and Prasad, 1973; Glazer and Schneider, 1975; Sahu and Prasad, 1975; Simantov and Sachs, 1975b). Repetitive stimulations of cyclic AMP accumulations could be elicited by prostaglandin E_1–phosphodiesterase combinations in neuroblastoma cells.

In studies with various neuroblastoma cell lines, isoproterenol, (nor)epinephrine, histamine, serotonin, dopamine, acetylcholine, carbamylcholine, and prostaglandins $F_{1\alpha}$, $F_{2\alpha}$, A_1, A_2, and B_2 had no significant effects either alone or in the presence of phosphodiesterase inhibitors (Gilman and Nirenberg, 1971b; Blume *et al.,* 1973; Matzazawa and Nirenberg, 1975; Prasad *et al.,* 1975b). Norepinephrine but not dopamine or dopa elicited an accumulation of cyclic AMP in certain neuroblastoma cell lines (Schubert *et al.,* 1976a). In the presence of the phosphodiesterase inhibitor, RO 20-1724, both dopamine and norepinephrine elevated cyclic AMP levels in certain neuroblastoma cell lines (Prasad, 1975; Sahu and Prasad, 1975). Acetylcholine was stated to decrease these responses. The presence of serum was postulated to be necessary to observe stimulatory effects of catecholamines in neuroblastoma cells.

Adenosine and 2-chloroadenosine elicited about a 2-fold increase in cyclic AMP levels in certain neuroblastoma cell lines (Blume *et al.,* 1973; Hamprecht and Schultz, 1973a,b; Schultz and Hamprecht, 1973; Blume and Foster, 1975; Maguire *et al.,* 1975; Matzawa and Nirenberg, 1975; Prasad *et al.,* 1973b). Theophylline was inhibitory to this response, while other phosphodiesterase inhibitors such as RO 20-1724, (EC_{50}, 30 μM), isobutylmethylxanthine, SQ 20009, diazepam, and papaverine greatly potentiated the response. In the presence of a phosphodiesterase inhibitor, adenosine (EC_{50}, 2 μM) and 2-chloroadenosine elicited a 20- to 40-fold accumulation of cyclic AMP, while 5'-AMP elicited only a 3-fold increase and ATP, ADP, guanosine, isoguanosine, 2'-, 3'-, and 5'-deoxyadenosines, and adenine arabinoside were virtually inactive (Blume *et al.,* 1973; Schultz and Hamprecht, 1973a,b; Blume and Foster, 1975). The response to adenosine in the presence of RO 20-1724 was competitively inhibited by theophylline. After one stimulation of neuroblastoma cells with adenosine and washing, readdition of adenosine elicited a second accumulation of cyclic AMP. Phosphodiesterase inhibitors were present in these restimulation experiments. Norepinephrine had no effect in these neuroblastoma cells, even in the presence of adenosine. Effects of adenosine and prostaglandin on cyclic AMP levels were less than additive, and adenosine thus appeared to slightly inhibit prostaglandin-elicited accumulations of cyclic AMP (Matsuzawa and Nirenberg, 1975).

Cyclic AMP levels within neuroblastoma cells have been reported to be elevated by butyric acid, by 5-bromodeoxyuridine, by dibutyryl cyclic AMP and cyclic AMP, and by the absence of serum in the culture medium (Sheppard and Prasad, 1973; Prasad *et al.*, 1973a; Glazer and Schneider, 1975). In some cell lines culture in serum-free medium had no effect on levels of cyclic AMP (Prasad and Kumar, 1975).

Acetylcholine through interaction with muscarinic receptors inhibited the response of cyclic AMP-generating systems to prostaglandin E_1 and adenosine in neuroblastoma cells (Prasad, 1975). Extracellular calcium ions were not required for this inhibitory effect. Acetylcholine in the presence of a phosphodiesterase inhibitor increased cyclic AMP levels in certain neuroblastoma clones and either had no effect or reduced cyclic AMP levels in other clones (Sahu and Prasad, 1975). Bethanechol, a muscarinic agonist, mimicked the stimulatory but not the inhibitory effects of acetylcholine. The inhibitory effect of acetylcholine on basal levels of cyclic AMP was stated to be unchanged in calcium-free medium and to be antagonized by atropine and hexamethonium.

Various volatile anesthetics such as halothane and methoxyhalothane caused nearly a twofold elevation of cyclic AMP levels in mouse neuroblastoma cells (Seager, 1975). This increase was not blocked by tetracaine or potentiated by theophylline, although 2 mM theophylline did increase basal levels of cyclic AMP nearly twofold.

In adenine-labeled neuroblastoma cells, prostaglandin E_1 either alone or with a phosphodiesterase inhibitor elicited accumulations of radioactive cyclic AMP (Hamprecht and Schultz, 1973a). However, the percent conversion of adenine-labeled nucleotides to cyclic AMP was markedly less than the percent conversion of total endogenous nucleotides to cyclic AMP.

Interrelationships of accumulations of cyclic AMP and cyclic GMP in neuroblastoma cells have been investigated with carbamylcholine, prostaglandin E_1, and adenosine (Matsuzawa and Nirenberg, 1975). Carbamylcholine (EC_{50}, 100 μM) elicited a rapid transient 40- to 200-fold increase in cyclic GMP levels in various mouse neuroblastoma cell lines, and in a neuroblastoma–L cell hybrid, but not in a rat glioma cell line. Phosphodiesterase inhibitors, such as isobutylmethylxanthine, RO 20-1724, and papaverine, did not increase, but did prolong the response to carbamylcholine. No changes in levels of cyclic AMP were observed. Atropine, a muscarinic antagonist, blocked the response of cyclic GMP-generating systems to carbamylcholine, while d-tubocurarine, a nicotinic antagonist, had no effect. Prostaglandin E_1 elicited a rapid but transient sixfold increase in cyclic GMP levels in neuroblastoma cells which preceded the slower sustained increase in cyclic AMP levels. Atropine had no effect on either response. The effects of carbamylcholine and prostaglandin on cyclic GMP levels were additive or greater than additive, while carbamylcholine inhibited the prostaglandin-elicited accumulation of cyclic AMP. The inhibitory effects of carbamylcholine were somewhat slow in onset and were prevented by atropine. Adenosine inhibited the carbamylcholine-elicited accumulations of cyclic GMP, and conversely carbamylcholine inhibited the adenosine-elicited accumulation of cyclic AMP. These results and data with hybrid cells (see below) indicate inhibitory interrelationships between cyclic AMP and cyclic GMP-generating systems in certain cultured cell lines.

Glioma Cells

In cell lines from rat, mouse, or human gliomas, the catecholamines, (nor)epinephrine and isoproterenol, elicited remarkable 30- to 4000-fold increases in levels of cyclic AMP (Clark and Perkins, 1971; Gilman and Nirenberg, 1971a; Schultz *et al.*, 1972; De Vellis and Kukes, 1973; Gilman and Minna, 1973; Perkins, 1973; Schwartz *et al.*, 1973; Browning *et al.*, 1974a,b; Clark *et al.*, 1974, 1975; Maguire *et al.*, 1974, 1976a; Penit *et al.*, 1974; Brostrom *et al.*, 1974; Traber *et al.*, 1974; Doore *et al.*, 1975; Edstrom *et al.*, 1975; Oey, 1975; Schlegel and Oey, 1975; Sundarraj *et al.*, 1975; Hsu and Brooker, 1976; Schubert *et al.*, 1976b). Although isoproterenol (EC_{50}, 0.3 μM) was a much more potent agonist than norepinephrine (EC_{50}, 5 μM) the maximal accumulations of cyclic AMP elicited by the two catecholamines were similar. Dopamine, epinine, octopamine, and phenylephrine elicited relatively small accumulations of cyclic AMP in rat glioma cells (Gilman and Nirenberg, 1971a; De Vellis and Kukes, 1973; Clark *et al.*, 1975; Schubert *et al.*, 1976a), except in one study in which 100 μM dopamine elicited a 35-fold accumulation of cyclic AMP (Schlegel and Oey, 1975). The responses to dopamine were blocked by propranolol. Responses to (nor)epinephrine and isoproterenol in glioma cells have in all studies been blocked by β-antagonists, while α-antagonists have had little or no effect. Hydroxybenzylpindolol was a very potent antagonist (Maguire *et al.*, 1976a,b). The β_1-antagonist, practolol, had relatively low activity as an antagonist (Gilman and Minna, 1973). The responses to isoproterenol in glioma cells have not been inhibited by prostaglandins or carbamylcholine. Theophylline had little effect on the magnitude of the accumulation of cyclic AMP elicited by norepinephrine or isoproterenol (Clark and Perkins, 1971; Gilman and Nirenberg, 1971a; Schultz *et al.*, 1972). The phosphodi-

esterase inhibitors, papaverine and isobutylmethylxanthine, greatly potentiated the effects of norepinephrine in rat glioma cells and retarded the
disappearance of cyclic AMP in cells previously incubated with norepinephrine (Schultz *et al.*, 1972; Browning *et al.*, 1974a,b; Hamprecht and
Schultz, 1973a,b). Phosphodiesterase inhibitors, such as RO 20-1724 and
papaverine, elevated basal levels of cyclic AMP in glioma cells (Edstrom *et
al.*, 1975). Papaverine was a potent inhibitor of oxidative metabolism in
glioma cells in addition to its effects on phosphodiesterase (Browning *et
al.*, 1974a). Lithium ions potentiated the epinephrine-elicited accumulation
of cyclic AMP in rat glioma cells (Schimmer, 1973). The magnitude of the
response of catecholamine-sensitive cyclic AMP-generating systems in
glioma cells was strongly dependent on the culture time and conditions. In
one study with rat glioma cells the maximal responses to norepinephrine
were not seen until many days after the cells had become confluent
(Schwartz *et al.*, 1973), while in another study with human glioma cells the
maximal responses to norepinephrine were attained before the cells had
formed a confluent monolayer and then declined markedly (Clark and
Perkins, 1971). Further studies with human glioma cells indicated that
maximal responsiveness was attained after 3 to 4 days of culture and then
declined and disappeared after 8 days (Clark *et al.*, 1975). The same pattern
of increase and subsequent loss of responsiveness was repeated when these
cells were trypsinized, transferred, and recultured. Isoproterenol-sensitive
adenylate cyclase activity assayed in homogenates of rat glioma cells
increased during culture until cells reached the stationary phase (Benda *et
al.*, 1972).

Histamine had nó effect on levels of cyclic AMP in rat glioma cells
(Gilman and Nirenberg, 1971a; Schultz *et al.*, 1972). Histamine (EC_{50}, 9
μM) elicited a 4- to 20-fold increase in cyclic AMP levels in certain clones
of a human glioma cell line (Clark and Perkins, 1971; Perkins, 1973). In
some experiments with confluent human glioma cells, histamine elicited a
significantly greater accumulation of cyclic AMP than did norepinephrine.
Propranolol did not prevent the effect of histamine. The magnitude of the
response to histamine increased only slightly after the cells had formed
monolayers. Combinations of histamine and norepinephrine did not appear
to have additive effects. Repeated subculturing of human glioma cells
resulted in a progressive loss of responsiveness to histamine (Clark *et al.*,
1975). Histamine at 100 μM was reported to elicit a 40-fold accumulation of
cyclic AMP in rat glioma cells (Schlegel and Oey, 1975). The response was
unexpectedly blocked by propranolol. Serotonin, carbamylcholine, γ-ami-
nobutyrate, and veratridine had either no or only marginal effects on cyclic
AMP levels in rat glioma cells (Gilman and Nirenberg, 1971a; Schultz *et
al.*, 1972).

Adenosine either alone or in combination with norepinephrine or histamine had no or only a marginal effect on cyclic AMP levels in various rat glioma cell lines (Gilman and Nirenberg, 1971a; Schultz et al., 1972). Adenosine (EC_{50}, 10 μM) did increase cyclic AMP levels in a human glioma cell line, and its effects were blocked by theophylline and potentiated by papaverine (Perkins, 1973; Clark et al., 1974, 1975). ATP, ADP, and AMP also elicited accumulations of cyclic AMP in the human glioma cells. AMP was hydrolyzed to adenosine relatively slowly in the presence of the cultured cells, suggesting a direct stimulation of cyclic AMP-generating systems by the adenine nucleotides. The response of cyclic AMP-generating systems to adenosine was potentiated by the phosphodiesterase inhibitor, papaverine, as had been the response to norepinephrine. Inhibition of uptake of adenosine into the cells by dipyridamole did not antagonize the adenosine-elicited accumulation of cyclic AMP, providing evidence for an extracellular site of adenosine action. Dipyridamole did not potentiate the effect of norepinephrine. Combinations of adenosine and norepinephrine had effects on cyclic AMP levels no greater than those due to norepinephrine alone.

Prostaglandins of the E series had no or only marginal effects, either alone or in the presence of potent phosphodiesterase inhibitor in some rat glioma cell lines (Gilman and Nirenberg, 1971a; Hamprecht and Schultz, 1973b), while in other cell lines prostaglandins of the E series elicited at least a twofold accumulation of cyclic AMP (Minna and Gilman, 1973; Traber et al., 1974; Edstrom et al., 1975). Theophylline had no effect on the prostaglandin-elicited accumulations of cyclic AMP in rat glioma cells. Prostaglandins E_1 and E_2 elicited a large accumulation of cyclic AMP in human glioma cells which was slightly enhanced by theophylline (Perkins, 1973; Clark et al., 1975). Prostaglandin A_1 elicited a small accumulation of cyclic AMP, while prostaglandin $F_{2\alpha}$ had neither agonist nor antagonist activity. The response to 10 μM prostaglandin E_1, but not the response to isoproterenol or adenosine, was blocked by 100 μM meclofenamic acid (Clark et al., 1975). Meclofenamic acid is not normally considered a prostaglandin antagonist, but rather an inhibitor of prostaglandin biosynthesis. The response to the prostaglandin was also blocked by the prostaglandin antagonist, 7-oxa-13-prostynoic acid. The effects of prostaglandin and norepinephrine on levels of cyclic AMP in human glioma cells were nearly additive.

In contrast to its stimulatory effects in neuroblastoma cells, 5-bromodeoxyuridine had little effect on cyclic AMP levels in glioma cells, but did cause a subsequent reduction in the magnitude of the accumulation of cyclic AMP elicited by norepinephrine (Schwartz et al., 1973). The latter effect may have been related to an increase in phosphodiesterase activity in cells cultured in the presence of the uridine derivative.

Rat glioma cells incorporated radioactive adenine into intracellular nucleotides which were converted to cyclic AMP during incubations of such labeled cells with norepinephrine or isoproterenol (Schultz *et al.,* 1972). However, the percent conversion of radioactive nucleotides to cyclic AMP appeared much lower than conversions of total endogenous nucleotides to cyclic AMP. Adenine was incorporated more rapidly into human glioma cells than was adenosine (Clark *et al.,* 1975). Varying the length of time of incorporation of radioactive adenine or adenosine from 5 to 60 min prior to stimulation with norepinephrine had no effect on the subsequent percent conversion of total labeled nucleotides to cyclic AMP, indicating that the pool of intracellular nucleotides labeled during a period of 5 to 60 min remained constant. The percent conversion of labeled nucleotides to cyclic AMP was not significantly different in adenosine- and adenine-labeled cells. The specific activities of cyclic AMP in control and norepinephrine- and prostaglandin-stimulated glioma cells were similar (Perkins, 1973; Clark *et al.,* 1975). The accumulation of cyclic AMP elicited by isoproterenol or norepinephrine in rat glioma cells was accompanied by a marked efflux of cyclic AMP into the media (Penit *et al.,* 1974; Schlaeger and Köhler, 1976). This efflux was inhibited by probenecid. Adenine-labeled human glioma cells incubated with norepinephrine or prostaglandin E_1 both accumulated intracellular radioactive cyclic AMP and lost radioactive cyclic AMP into the medium (Clark *et al.,* 1975). Excretion of radioactive cyclic AMP from stimulated cells was not altered by the presence of 1 mM cyclic AMP in the incubation medium but was markedly inhibited by dipyridamole. Rates of efflux of cyclic AMP in rat glioma cells were high when intracellular levels of cyclic AMP were elevated by norepinephrine (Browning *et al.,* 1976). Isobutylmethylxanthine caused a further increase in intracellular levels of cyclic AMP but decreased efflux. The efflux of cyclic AMP from isoproterenol-stimulated rat glioma cells was inhibited by inhibitors of oxidative phosphorylation, such as carbonyl cyanide *p*-trifluoromethoxyphenylhydrazone, and valinomycin, by probenecid, prostaglandin A_1, and papaverine (Doore *et al.,* 1975). Except for probenecid and prostaglandin A_1 these agents reduced intracellular levels of ATP. Propranolol antagonized intracellular accumulation of cyclic AMP and thereby reduced efflux. Neither chlorpromazine, prostaglandins of the E and F series, colchicine, vinblastine, cytochalasin, cycloheximide, calcium ions, nor the calcium ionophore, A 23187, greatly altered efflux of cyclic AMP. In all, the results are consonant with an ATP-dependent transport of cyclic AMP from glioma cells. It is of interest that three of the compounds, namely dipyridamole, papaverine, and isobutylmethylxanthine, which inhibited efflux of cyclic AMP are, in addition, potent inhibitors of phosphodiesterase.

Refractoriness of cyclic AMP-generating systems after a prior stimulation have been studied extensively in glioma cells. In human glioma cells after one stimulation with norepinephrine and washing, reintroduction of norepinephrine did not elicit another accumulation of cyclic AMP (Clark and Perkins, 1971), while introduction of histamine did elicit an accumulation of cyclic AMP. Such results were reminiscent of those seen with brain slices (see pp. 102, 103, 116, 149). With rat glioma cells norepinephrine did cause repetitive accumulations of cyclic AMP (Schultz *et al.*, 1972). The magnitude of the accumulations of cyclic AMP markedly declined during repetitive stimulations with norepinephrine, except when a phosphodiesterase inhibitor, papaverine, was present, suggesting that elevations of intracellular cyclic AMP resulted in an increase of an associated phosphodiesterase activity (see Section 4.1.4). Isobutylmethylxanthine, like papaverine, partially restored the response of glioma cells to restimulation with norepinephrine (Browning *et al.*, 1974a,b). An induction of phosphodiesterase was reported in rat glioma cell lines and the induction of phosphodiesterase activity by norepinephrine was proposed to be involved in refractoriness of cyclic AMP-generating systems to a second stimulation by norepinephrine (Schwartz and Passoneau, 1974). Indeed, if phosphodiesterase induction by norepinephrine was blocked by cycloheximide, the cyclic AMP-generating systems did not become refractory to a second stimulation by norepinephrine. The results did not exclude effects of cycloheximide on other cyclic AMP-dependent inductive effects unrelated to phosphodiesterase activity. In one rat glioma cell line, the refractoriness of cyclic AMP-generating systems to norepinephrine was shown to be due to both increases in cyclic AMP-phosphodiesterase and to decreases in norepinephrine-sensitive adenylate cyclases (Browning *et al.*, 1976). Refractoriness developed after (nor)epinephrine and isoproterenol but not after dopamine or phenylephrine and appeared dependent on activation of a β-sensitive cyclic AMP-generating system. A norepinephrine pretreatment greatly reduced a subsequent response of the cyclic AMP-generating systems to norepinephrine, both in the presence and absence of a phosphodiesterase inhibitor, isobutylmethylxanthine. The rate of hydrolysis of cyclic AMP after a norepinephrine stimulation and washing was significantly increased in refractory cells. A calcium-independent phosphodiesterase specific for cyclic AMP had been induced in the refractory cells by the pretreatment with norepinephrine. Cycloheximide, although nearly completely blocking protein synthesis, and increases in phosphodiesterase activity only partially prevented development of refractoriness of cyclic AMP-generating systems. An explanation was found in the fact that norepinephrine-sensitive adenylate cyclase activity had been greatly decreased in refractory cells. In another rat glioma cell line cyclic AMP-generating systems became refractory to norepinephrine in the absence of any apparent alteration in phosphodiesterase activity (De Vellis and Brooker, 1974).

In this instance, a cyclic AMP-mediated increase in levels of a protein inhibitory to cyclic AMP formation was proposed (see Section 4.1.4). In other cell lines phosphodiesterase activity did increase after exposure to catecholamines. In human glioma cells, neither levels of phosphodiesterase nor rates of degradation of cyclic AMP in experiments where propranolol was added to norepinephrine-stimulated cells were altered during development of refractoriness to norepinephrine (Perkins et al., 1975). Rates of incorporation of radioactive adenine into cyclic AMP rapidly decreased during development of refractoriness of norepinephrine-sensitive cyclic AMP-generating systems in these cells. Incorporation of adenine into intracellular ATP remained unchanged. Thus, in this human glioma cell line, refractoriness involved primarily alterations in responsiveness of adenylate cyclases. Refractoriness of cyclic AMP-generating systems in the glioma cells to the biogenic amine were likely to have been responsible for the marked decline in levels of cyclic AMP which occurred during the period following attainment of maximal levels of cyclic AMP at 1 min with norepinephrine and 5 min with histamine in human glioma cells (Clark and Perkins, 1971). Agonist-induced loss of responsiveness was observed in human glioma cells with both norepinephrine and prostaglandin (Clark et al., 1975; Perkins, 1976; Perkins et al., 1975). Cells pretreated with norepinephrine remained responsive to prostaglandin. However, after exposure to prostaglandin some loss of responsiveness to norepinephrine was observed. The half-time for recovery of responsiveness of norepinephrine-sensitive cyclic AMP-generating systems in human glioma cells after a 2-hr stimulation with norepinephrine was about 8 hr. In another study cyclic AMP-generating systems in rat glioma cells were stated to be refractory to stimulation by norepinephrine for at least 60 hr after an initial exposure to the amine (Oey, 1975).

Catecholamines elicited an accumulation of cyclic GMP in rat glioma cell lines (Hsu and Brooker, 1976). At least in part activation of a β-receptor appeared to be involved. After prolonged incubation with a catecholamine, both cyclic AMP- and cyclic GMP-generating systems became refractory to restimulation.

Incubation of a rat glioma cell line with low concentrations of glucocorticoids (corticosterone, hydrocortisone, triamcinolone) resulted in a marked increase in both basal levels of cyclic AMP and in the accumulation of cyclic AMP elicited by norepinephrine (Brostrom et al., 1974). The effect of corticosterone became maximal after about 48 hr. Other steroids such as cholic acid, estradiol, pregnenolone, progesterone, and testosterone had no effect. Studies with cell-free systems from these glioma cell lines indicated that the enhanced responsiveness of the cyclic AMP-generating systems in the corticosterone-treated cells was due to an increase in norepinephrine-sensitive adenylate cyclases rather than a change in properties of the cyclase or an increase in phosphodiesterases. After removal of corticosterone, adenylate cyclase returned to control levels within 72 hr.

Hybrid Cells

All hybrid clones derived from fusion of neuroblastoma and glioma cell lines responded to prostaglandin E_1, while the norepinephrine response of the parent glioma cells was not expressed in such hybrids, even in the presence of a phosphodiesterase inhibitor (Hamprecht and Schultz, 1973b; Traber et al., 1975d). Similar results were obtained with hybrids of glioma or neuroblastoma cells with other somatic cells (Gilman and Minna, 1973; Minna and Gilman, 1973). Responsiveness to prostaglandins appeared to be a dominant trait, while responsiveness to norepinephrine appeared to be a recessive trait in these hybrid cells. In glioma–fibroblast hybrids, levels of isoproterenol-sensitive adenylate cyclase rapidly increased during the first 3 days of culture, followed by a marked decrease (Benda et al., 1972). Fluoride-sensitive cyclase activity from hybrid cells reached a stable maximum level after 5 days. The inhibition of prostaglandin-stimulated formation of cyclic AMP in neuroblastoma–glioma hybrid cells by 7-oxa-13-prostynoic acid has been cited (Traber et al., 1975b). The response to 2-chloroadenosine was stated to be fully manifest in hybrids of neuroblastoma cells with a nonresponsive L cell line (Maguire et al., 1975).

Theophylline potentiated the response of cyclic AMP-generating systems to isoproterenol or prostaglandin E_1 only in certain cultured cell lines. When a neuroblastoma cell line in which theophylline potentiated the isoproterenol response was hybridized with a theophylline-insensitive somatic cell line, the response to isoproterenol was potentiated in the hybrid cells (Minna and Gilman, 1973). Similarly, when a theophylline-insensitive glioma cell and a theophylline-sensitive somatic cell line were hybridized, the response to prostaglandin was potentiated by theophylline in the hybrid cells; i.e., potentiation of hormone responses by theophylline appeared to be a dominant trait in hybrid cells.

The inhibition of prostaglandin-elicited increases in levels of cyclic AMP by morphine and other narcotic analgesics has been studied extensively with neuroblastoma–glioma hybrid cell lines (Traber et al., 1974, 1975b,c,d; Van Inwegen et al., 1975; Klee et al., 1975; Sharma et al., 1975a,b). Morphine has been demonstrated to antagonize the accumulation of cyclic AMP elicited by prostaglandin E_1 in neuroblastoma cells and in neuroblastoma–glioma hybrid cells, but to have no effect on prostaglandin- or norepinephrine-elicited accumulations of cyclic AMP in glioma cells. Morphine inhibited adenosine-elicited accumulations of cyclic AMP in hybrid cells, while usually lowering basal levels of cyclic AMP. The ability of morphine to inhibit responses of cyclic AMP-generating systems appeared to be directly correlated with the number of narcotic binding sites present in each cell type. Thus, morphine was most effective in hybrid cells which have large numbers of narcotic binding sites, less effective in neuroblastoma cells which have only small numbers of binding sites, and ineffective in glioma cells which have no detectable narcotic binding sites. The inhibition of the prostaglandin response by morphine appeared noncompetitive in nature and was prevented by the presence of the narcotic antagonist, naloxone. Morphine inhibited both basal and prostaglandin-stimulated adenylate cyclases in homogenates of hybrid cells (Klee *et al.*, 1975; Sharma *et al.*, 1975a). Naloxone prevented the effects of morphine, but at a high concentration also slightly inhibited adenylate cyclase. The relative potencies of etorphine > levorphan > morphine > 3-allylprodine for inhibition of prostaglandin-sensitive cyclase from hybrid cells and for binding at opiate receptors were quite similar. Nalorphine, a narcotic analgesic with mixed agonist–antagonist properties, inhibited prostaglandin-sensitive cyclases and competitively antagonized the inhibition by a more effective agonist, morphine. Dextrophan was virtually inactive. Although the potency of various narcotics towards inhibition of adenylate cyclase in homogenates and their affinity for narcotic binding sites in the same preparation were comparable, the results of kinetic analysis of narcotic binding was consonant with a simple noncooperative process, while data on inhibition of adenylate cyclases were consonant with a strongly cooperative process. The threshold for activation of adenylate cyclases by the stable GTP analog, guanylylimidodiphosphate, was reduced tenfold by the presence of morphine. No inhibition of cyclase activity by morphine could be observed if concentrations of guanylylimidodiphosphate above 10 μM were present. The data suggest that activation of opiate receptors causes a general inhibition of adenylate cyclases, which can be overcome by GTP.

Culture of neuroblastoma–glioma hybrid cells with morphine for 4 days resulted in an increase in levels of basal and prostaglandin-sensitive adenylate cyclases (Sharma *et al.*, 1975a). Naloxone prevented the increase in cyclase activity. After 1 day of withdrawal from morphine the levels of cyclase in the cells returned to control values. Basal levels of cyclic AMP were unaltered in morphine-cultured cells and responses of cyclic AMP-generating systems to prostaglandin and adenosine were reduced because of the continued presence of morphine. If naloxone was added to the final incubation medium, basal levels of cyclic AMP increased in morphine-cultured cells and enhanced responsiveness of prostaglandin- and adenosine-sensitive cyclic AMP-generating systems was revealed. In a similar experiment with RO 20-1724 present, responses to prostaglandin and adenosine were greater in the morphine-cultured cells. A prior incubation of hybrid cells with morphine or methadone resulted in an enhanced maximal response of cyclic AMP-generating systems to prostaglandin E_1 (Traber *et al.*, 1975c). Dextrophan, levorphan, and naloxone did not have this effect. Enhanced responsiveness developed maximally within 6 to 15 hr of incubation with morphine and was prevented by cycloheximide. The response to prostaglandin in cells previously cultured with morphine was sensitive to inhibition by morphine, while in cells previously cultured with methadone or levorphan the response was no longer sensitive to inhibition by morphine, but it was sensitive to inhibition by norepinephrine (see below).

Morphine elevated cyclic GMP levels and decreased cyclic AMP levels in neuroblastoma–glioma hybrid cells (Traber *et al.*, 1975b). Naloxone blocked these effects. Levorphan, but not its inactive enantiomer, dextrophan, had effects similar to morphine. At very high concentrations the narcotic analgesics and naxolone had the opposite effect, causing an increase in cyclic AMP and a decrease in cyclic GMP levels.

Carbamylcholine (EC_{50}, 0.1 μM) and acetylcholine elicited a transient fourfold accumulation of cyclic GMP in neuroblastoma–glioma hybrid cells which was accompanied by a transient decrease in levels of cyclic AMP (Gullis *et al.*, 1975a). The effects of carbamylcholine were reduced in low sodium medium. A nicotinic agonist, the tetramethylammonium ion, had smaller effects on cyclic GMP and cyclic AMP levels in the hybrid cell line and in neuroblastoma cell lines. At concentrations greater than 0.1 μM both tetramethylammonium and to a lesser extent carbamylcholine began to inhibit cyclic GMP accumulations. A muscarinic agonist, pilocarpine, elicited a small increase in levels of cyclic GMP and a small decrease in cyclic AMP. The effects of low concentration of pilocarpine on cyclic GMP and cyclic AMP levels were reversed in low sodium medium.

Norepinephrine elicited accumulations of cyclic GMP in neuroblastoma–glioma hybrid cells (cited in Traber *et al.*, 1975a,b). The nature of the receptor involved was not mentioned, but data on inhibition of cyclic AMP-generating systems by norepinephrine suggested the involvement of an α-adrenergic receptor (see below).

Three classes of compounds have been reported to elevate cyclic GMP levels in the hybrid cells and all three types of compounds, (i) narcotic analgesics such as morphine, (ii) cholinergic agonists, and (iii) norepinephrine inhibited responses of cyclic AMP-generating systems to prostaglandin E_1 (Traber *et al.*, 1975a,b,c,d) and adenosine (cited in Gullis *et al.*, 1975a). Antagonism of cyclic AMP-generating systems by narcotic analgesics has been discussed (see above). Carbamylcholine or an acetylcholine–physostigmine combination antagonized prostaglandin E_1, and RO 20-1724-elicited accumulations of cyclic AMP in hybrid cells (Traber *et al.*, 1975a). Carbamylcholine was many fold more active in reducing basal levels of cyclic

AMP than in reducing prostaglandin-elicited accumulations of cyclic AMP. The inhibitory effect of acetylcholine in the presence of the cholinesterase inhibitor, physostigmine, was blocked by atropine but not by nicotinic antagonists such as tubocurarine and α-bungarotoxin. Accumulations of cyclic AMP elicited by prostaglandin E_1 in neuroblastoma–glioma hybrid cells were antagonized by norepinephrine > phenylephrine, dopamine > isoproterenol (Traber *et al.*, 1975d). Phentolamine was much more effective than either haloperidol or propranolol in blocking the inhibition by catecholamines, indicated that an α-receptor was involved. The relationship of the increases in cyclic GMP levels elicited by morphine, carbamylcholine, and norepinephrine to the concomittant inhibition of cyclic AMP-generating systems is unclear. However, it should be noted that the inhibitions also pertained in homogenates. One highly speculative interpretation would be that inhibition of cyclic AMP-generating systems by these agents is dependent in intact cells both on reduction of GTP via formation of cyclic GMP and on a subsequent direct inhibition of GTP-free adenylate cyclase. A prior incubation of neuroblastoma–glioma hybrid cells with morphine (see above), isoproterenol, or carbamylcholine resulted in an increase in the responsiveness of cyclic AMP-generating systems to prostaglandin E_1 (Traber *et al.*, 1975c). The response to prostaglandin in cells pretreated with morphine, isoproterenol, or carbamylcholine was sensitive to inhibition by morphine, norepinephrine, and carbamylcholine. The mechanism involved in this induction of hyperresponsive cyclic AMP-generating systems is unclear, but at least for the morphine treatment it required protein synthesis. All three inducing agents share the ability to inhibit cyclic AMP-generating systems and to elevate cyclic GMP levels in the neuroblastoma–glioma hybrid cells.

4

Functional Role of Cyclic Nucleotides

Delineation of specific roles of cyclic nucleotides, in particular cyclic AMP, in the nervous system has been based primarily on attempts to correlate alterations of cyclic AMP and/or cyclic GMP levels in intact cells, tissues, or organs with alterations in (1) metabolic pathways, (2) cell differentiation, and growth and expression of the phenotype, (3) membrane function, and (4) central behavioral and vegetative effects. Enhanced intracellular levels of cyclic AMP or a functionally "equivalent" analog have been expected to pertain as a result of the following: (1) the presence of high concentrations of extracellular cyclic AMP, dibutyryl cyclic AMP, butyryl cyclic AMP, 8-benzylthio cyclic AMP, etc.; (2) the presence of a phosphodiesterase inhibitor such as theophylline, isobutylmethylxanthine, papaverine, or RO 20-1724; and/or (3) the presence of an agent that is a stimulant of cyclic AMP-generating systems in neuronal or glial cells i.e., biogenic amines, adenosine, prostaglandin, or depolarizing agents. Antagonists of the stimulatory agents have also been employed to advantage. Similar paradigms have been employed to alter cyclic GMP levels, for example, through the use of dibutyryl cyclic GMP* or agents such as acetylcholine that stimulate cyclic GMP-generating systems. The difficulties in establishing such correlations are apparent. Nonspecific or noncyclic nucleotide-related effects of the nonphysiological concentrations of cyclic nucleotide analogs, phosphodiesterase inhibitors or stimulatory agents, lack of effects of these agents on the relevant cyclic nucleotide-generating system, perhaps masked by pronounced effects on nonrelevant compartments or systems, requirements

---

*It should be noted that dibutyryl cyclic GMP is extremely weak as an activator of cyclic GMP-dependent protein kinases (see Section 2.4.2).

for only a virtually undetectable increase and/or a sustained increase in the cyclic nucleotide for a particular response, various feedback controls on cyclic nucleotide formation, and interrelationships between formation and function of cyclic AMP and cyclic GMP represent only a few of the problems in attempts to establish a role for cyclic nucleotides in intact cells or organisms. Such problems appear to be nearly insurmountable in the complex functionally integrated central nervous system.

4.1 Enzymatic Processes

The influence of cyclic AMP-dependent mechanisms on enzymatic processes involved in intermediary metabolism; formation and disposition of membrane constituents; levels and properties of cyclases, phosphodiesterases, and kinases; protein phosphorylation; and DNA, RNA, and protein synthesis have been investigated in cell-free systems, cultured cells, brain slices, and intact animals. In cultured fetal brain cells, apparent effects of cyclic AMP-dependent mechanisms on levels of enzymes or other processes could be direct, that is, on the rate of synthesis or activity of specific enzymes within certain cells, or indirect, for example, by preventing proliferation of cell types which either contain or do not contain high levels of the enzyme. In cultured neuroblastoma or glioma cells apparent effects of cyclic AMP-dependent mechanisms on enzymatic phenomena could be (1) direct, (2) due to an altered expression of the phenotype in cells in which cell division has been inhibited, or (3) a secondary effect dependent on differentiation of the neuroma cell. Cyclic AMP-dependent processes do in neuroma and other cells appear to lead to a blockade of the cell cycle in the G_1-phase, a point at which expression of the differentiated phenotype is thought to be allowed (see Section 4.2). In brain slices and brain of intact animals, the heterogeneous nature of the tissue makes difficult the correlation of cyclic AMP levels with alterations in enzymatic phenomena.

4.1.1 Intermediary Metabolism

Attempts to demonstrate correlations between alterations of metabolic parameters such as glycogen synthetase and phosphorylase activity, glycogen levels, glucose oxidation, lactate production, and oxygen consumption with levels of cyclic AMP in brain tissue have as yet not been completely successful, probably because of the heterogeneous nature of the brain slice preparation. Cyclic AMP would be expected to increase the proportion of glycogen synthetase D and phosphorylase a, while increasing glucose oxidation, lactate production, and oxygen consumption and decreasing glycogen levels.

Cell-Free Preparations

Phosphorylase-b kinase kinase and glycogen synthetase-I kinase activity were apparently present in brain homogenates, but cyclic AMP did not further activate phosphorylase in such homogenates (see Section 2.4.1). Cyclic AMP increased the rate of oxidation of glutamate by rat brain homogenates and mitochondrial fractions and with partially purified glutamate dehydrogenase (Erwin, 1969; Setchenska *et al.*, 1975). ADP and AMP had, however, similar effects. The adenine nucleotides reduced the K_m of the dehydrogenase for NAD.

Brain Slices

In some studies with brain slices, alterations of cyclic AMP levels in response to histamine, norepinephrine, adenosine, or combinations of these agents did not appear to have had significant effects on phosphorylase activity, glucose oxidation, lactate formation, and oxygen uptake (Rall and Gilman, 1970; Kakiuchi and Rall, 1968a). No correlations between phosphorylase-a levels in rabbit cortical and cerebellar slices and the elevation of cyclic AMP levels by norepinephrine and histamine were apparent. Phosphorylase-a activity decreased rapidly during incubation of brain slices and it would appear that phosphorylase activity in brain tissue after sacrifice was mainly present in the phosphorylated a form (cf. Drummond *et al.*, 1964b). The stimulatory effects of electrical pulsation of guinea pig cortical slices on glycolysis, lactate formation, and adenosine release (Heller and McIlwain, 1973; Pull and McIlwain, 1973, 1975) were accompanied by an accumulation of cyclic AMP (see Section 3.1). Similarly, other known stimulants of cyclic AMP-generating systems in brain slices, namely, histamine, glutamate, and adenosine, also increased lactate production in guinea pig cortical slices. In chick cerebral slices, elevation of cyclic AMP by epinephrine, isoproterenol, or histamine had no effect on levels of phosphorylase a or glycogen (Edwards *et al.*, 1974). A variety of biogenic amines, such as norepinephrine, dopamine, histamine, and serotonin, reduced glycogen levels in incubated rat brain slices from cortex, caudate, and thalamus (Mrsulja, 1972a,b). Dibutyryl cyclic AMP and cyclic AMP also reduced glycogen levels, with the dibutyryl analog eliciting the most profound reduction. Treatment of rats before sacrifice with a β-antagonist, propranolol, specifically blocked the reduction in glycogen levels elicited by norepinephrine and dopamine in brain slices from cortex, caudate, and thalamus. Treatment with an α-antagonist, phenoxybenzamine, had no effect on the reduction in glycogen levels elicited by the biogenic amines or the cyclic nucleotides. Thus, a β-receptor appeared to be involved in catecholamine-controlled glycogenolysis in rat brain. *In vivo* treatment of rats with the H_1-antihistamine, antazoline, prevented subsequent histamine-elicited reductions in glycogen in incubated slices of cortex, caudate or thalamus but had no effect on reductions in glycogen elicited by norepine-phrine, dopamine, serotonin, cyclic AMP, or dibutyryl cyclic AMP (Mrsulja, 1973). Relatively low concentrations of exogenous cyclic AMP inhibited aerobic glycolysis in rabbit forebrain slices, while 1 mM cyclic AMP stimulated aerobic glycolysis and to a lesser extent respiration (Dittmann and Herrmann, 1970). In another report, cyclic AMP was found to have no effect on glycolysis or lactate formation in guinea pig cortical slices (Takagaki, 1972). Cyclic AMP did increase levels of fructose diphos-phate and triose phosphates. Surprisingly, cyclic GMP, like cyclic AMP and dibutyryl cyclic AMP, decreased glycogen levels in brain slices from rat cortex, caudate, and cerebellum (Mrsulja, 1974). Prior treatment of rats with various drugs appeared to alter the effect of cyclic GMP, but not that of the cyclic adenine nucleotides, on glycogen levels in brain slices. Prior treatment with atropine was reported to prevent the response to cyclic GMP in slices of cortex and caudate, while prior treatment with propranolol, reserpine, or chlorpromazine blocked the cyclic GMP response in slices from all three brain regions. Cyclic IMP had no effect on glucose or oxygen consumption, or on lactate production in rat cortical slices (Laborit and Thuret, 1974).

Ganglia and Peripheral Neurons

High concentrations of potassium ions slightly increased levels of lactate dehydrogenase in rat superior cervical ganglia (Webb *et al.*, 1975). Octopamine increased phosphorylase-a levels in cockroach nerve cords and decreased glycogen levels (Robertson and Steele, 1972). Caffeine potentiated the effect of octopamine, and it was stated that cyclic AMP also increased levels of phosphorylase a.

Glutamine synthetase activity in cultured retina was enhanced by cyclic AMP and the dibutyryl derivative (Chader, 1971). The effect was inhibited by both actinomycin D and cycloheximide, suggesting that cyclic AMP elicits enhanced synthesis of the messenger RNA for *de novo* forma-tion of glutamine synthetase. In later studies, it was found that an unidenti-fied rather nonpolar contaminant had been responsible for the induction of retinal glutamine synthetase by one sample of dibutyryl cyclic AMP (Jones *et al.,* 1973). "Uncontaminated" dibutryl cyclic AMP, cyclic AMP, dibutyryl cyclic GMP, and (nor)epinephrine only occasionally caused small increases in glutamine synthetase.

Cultured Cells

Dibutyryl cyclic AMP, (nor)epinephrine, histamine, and papaverine stimulated glycogenolysis in rat glioma cells (Opler and Makman, 1972; Newburgh and Rosenberg, 1972; Browning *et al.,* 1974a,b). The effect of norepinephrine was blocked by propranolol. Presumably, the enhanced glycogenolysis in these cells was due to enhanced levels of phosphorylase a, although inactivation of glycogen synthetase might also have been involved. During restimulations of glioma cells with norepinephrine, the accumulation of cyclic AMP elicited by reintroduction of the catecholamine was greatly reduced, but the enhancement in rates of glycogenolysis was not reduced. Papaverine, although not significantly elevating cyclic AMP levels in glioma cells, caused a great increase in glycogenolysis and conversion of phosphorylase b to the a form. However, papaverine also greatly decreased respiration in these cells. Such an effect at the mitochondrial level would have been expected to result in an increase in efflux of calcium ions from the mitochondria into the cytoplasm. The results provide a cautionary note with regard to use of papaverine as a phosphodiesterase inhibitor in intact cell systems. Norepinephrine had no effect on glycolysis in neuroblastoma cells.

Norepinephrine elicited an increase in lactate dehydrogenase activity in rat glioma cells by a cyclic AMP-dependent mechanism (Schwartz *et al.,* 1973; De Vellis and Kukes, 1973). Dibutyryl cyclic AMP also increased levels of lactate dehydrogenase. Elevation of levels of cyclic AMP by norepinephrine for 2.5 hr. was sufficient to elicit a full induction of lactate dehydrogenase measured 24 hr. later. During first 2.5-hr. period RNA synthesis was required. Subsequently protein synthesis was essential. Transcription of RNA appeared to require RNA polymerase III. Induction of lactate dehydrogenase by norepinephrine did not occur in glioma–fibroblast hybrid cells in which the response of cyclic AMP systems to norepinephrine was absent.

Cyclic AMP mechanisms did not appear involved in the induction of glycerol phosphate dehydrogenase by glucocorticoids in glioma cells (De Vellis and Kukes, 1973). De Vellis and Kukes (1973) cite an inhibition of uptake of 2-deoxyglucose and a stimulation of uptake of 2-aminoisobutyric acid concomitant with norepinephrine-elicited accumulations of cyclic AMP in rat glioma cells. Levels of glutamate and ATP could be significantly increased in rat glioma cells by dibutyryl cyclic AMP under serum-free conditions (Schousboe *et al.,* 1975).

Dibutyryl cyclic AMP or agents that elevate cyclic AMP levels greatly increased ornithine decarboxylase activity in glioma and neuroblastoma cells (Bachrach, 1975). Induction of ornithine decarboxylase activity in neuroblastoma cells by isobutylmethylxanthine or an adenosine–isobutyl-methylxanthine combination was antagonized by carbamylcholine, an agent which decreases cyclic AMP levels and increases cyclic GMP levels in neuroblastoma cells (see Section 3.5.2). Actinomycin and cycloheximide prevented cyclic AMP-dependent increases in ornithine decarboxylase. The relationship of cyclic AMP-controlled levels of ornithine decarboxylase to cell proliferation was unclear: Decarboxylase levels were high in rapidly growing cultures and low in confluent cultures.

Intact Brain

Postdecapitation increases in levels of cyclic AMP in rabbit cortex were not reflected in parallel changes in phosphorylase a (Kakiuchi and Rall, 1968a), while in mouse both cyclic AMP and phosphorylase a did increase after decapitation (Breckenridge and Norman, 1962, 1965; Lust and Passonneau, 1976). Phosphorylase-a levels were increased after decapitation in the mouse cerebral cortex and in the molecular and granular layers of the cerebellum. The increases in cortex were inhibited in mice treated with reserpine or pentobarbital. Insulin, caffeine, cocaine, and amphetamine increased cortical levels of phosphorylase a in control mice, while a monoamine oxidase inhibitor, reserpine, chlorpromazine, pheno-barbital, and pentobarbital had no effect or slightly decreased cortical levels of phosphorylase a (Breckenridge and Norman, 1962, 1965; Drummond and Bellward, 1970). In part, difficulties in establishing correlations between postdecapitation increases in cyclic AMP and phosphorylase a, particularly in animals larger than mice, lie in problems inherent in measuring the true levels of phosphorylase a in brain. Thus, a small initial increase in cyclic AMP in brain tissue may be sufficient to completely activate phosphorylase a, and subsequent postdecapitation increases in cyclic AMP will appear to have no effect. Indeed, studies with hypothermic mice support this proposal (Lust and Passonneau, 1976, see below).

After decapitation or insulin-administration glycogenolysis and gly-colysis were increased in rat brain, but in spite of elevations in cyclic AMP, the proportion of glycogen synthetase in the active dephosphorylated glucose-6-phosphate-independent (I) form increased (Goldberg and O'Toole, 1969). The role of the two forms of glycogen synthetase in brain metabolism was not clear. The "active" I form apparently increased in brain under conditions where glycogen stores were depleted, while the "inactive" phosphorylated glucose-6-phosphate-dependent (D) form increased under conditions, such as administration of glucose to diabetic animals, where brain glycogen levels were increased.

In normal and hypothermic mice, increased levels of brain phosphorylase a following electroconvulsive shock correlated with increases in cyclic AMP (Lust and Passonneau, 1976). Postdecapitation increases in cyclic AMP and phosphorylase a and decreases in glycogen synthetase activity followed similar time courses in hypothermic mice, while in normal mice phosphorylase-a levels were initially very high. Thus, under hypothermic conditions correlations of levels of both phosphorylase a and glycogen synthetase with increases in cyclic AMP were excellent; while in normothermic mice, elevation of phosphorylase a and depression of glycogen synthetase had occurred very rapidly, probably triggered by initial small increases in cyclic AMP levels. Homocysteine-elicited convulsions resulted in increases in cyclic AMP in brain concomitant with an increase in phosphorylase a and a decrease in glycogen content (Folbergrova, 1975).

Stab wound trauma to mouse cerebral cortex resulted in a transient sevenfold increase in cyclic AMP, with a maximum reached at about 1 min (Watanabe and Passonneau, 1974). This transient rise in cyclic AMP was associated with a transient increase in phosphorylase-a content and decreases in glycogen content. However, conversion of glycogen synthetase to the inactive phosphorylated form was not apparent. Indeed, the amount of the active form increased after stab wound trauma, reaching a maximum within 1 to 10 min.

The transient increase in cortical cyclic AMP in the anoxic hemisphere of the gerbil brain was accompanied and followed by reductions in glycogen, glucose, and an increase in lactate (Watanabe and Ishii, 1976).

Intraventricular cyclic AMP, dibutyryl and monobutyryl cyclic AMP and biogenic amines affected mouse brain levels of glucose, glycogen and lactate (Leonard, 1972, 1975a,b). The cyclic nucleotides caused an initial increase in glycogen and lactate and a decrease in glucose followed by a decrease in lactate and an increase in glucose. These effects were blocked by propranolol which, however, did not affect the behavioral depression elicited by the cyclic nucleotides. Fluoride also altered glycolysis, but it should be noted that this ion has not been reported to alter adenylate cyclase activity in intact cells.

Ethimazole (N,N-dimethyl-imidazole-4,5-dicarboxamide) increased cyclic AMP levels in rat brain while decreasing glycogen (Zavodskaya *et al.*, 1975). It was stated that ethimazole markedly activated brain adenylate cyclase. Brain levels of cyclic AMP in fasted rats have been reported to be transiently elevated by an antilipolytic agent, β-pyridylcarbinol (Burkard *et al.*, 1971).

In chicks, elevation of *in vivo* levels of cyclic AMP in cerebrum by intravenous epinephrine, isoproterenol, or histamine was accompanied by conversion of phosphorylase b to the a form and a decrease in cerebral glycogen (Edwards *et al.*, 1974.) Norepinephrine had no effects on either cyclic AMP, phosphorylase, or glycogen. The activation of phosphorylase, the reduction of glycogen, and the increase in cyclic AMP elicited in chick cerebrum by parenteral isoproterenol were all blocked by propranolol (Nahorski *et al.*, 1975b). In contrast, metiamide blocked completely the increase in cyclic AMP elicited by histamine, but only partially blocked increases in phosphorylase a and glycogenolysis. Adrenergic and H_1-antagonists had no effect on the histamine response.

4.1.2 Membrane Metabolism

The *in vitro* activation of Na^+,K^+-ATPase from rat brain by catecholamines and serotonin has been reported (Yoshimura, 1973). Cyclic AMP had no effect. In certain neuroblastoma cell lines, differentiation elicited by dibutyryl cyclic AMP was accompanied by an increased activity of Na^+,K^+-ATPase and Mg^{2+}-ATPase (Ledig *et al.*, 1975).

The incorporation of radioactive acetate, glucose, or serine into neutral and polar lipids in brain slices from immature rats was reduced by the presence of dibutyryl cyclic AMP and theophylline (Weiss and Stiller, 1974). The hydrolysis of phosphatidylcholine by a phospholipase of synaptic membranes was stimulated by cyclic nucleotides with cyclic AMP > cyclic GMP > cyclic CMP, cyclic UMP, and by a variety of putative neurotransmitters (Gullis and Rowe, 1975a,b). Acylation of choline glycerophospholipids of the synaptic membranes with oleic acid, in the presence of cofactors and fluoride ion to inhibit phospholipases, was stimulated by cyclic AMP > cyclic GMP, a variety of putative neurotransmitters and adenosine. The effects of adenosine were antagonized by theophylline.

Intracellular levels and secretion of a plasminogen activator were markedly increased in neuroblastoma cells exposed to dibutyryl cyclic AMP, butyrate, or prostaglandin E_1, while theophylline had no effect (Laug *et al.*, 1976). Fibrinolytic activity was, however, totally dependent on addition of exogenous plasminogen.

4.1.3 Neurotransmitter Metabolism

Acetylcholine

Intraventricular dibutyryl cyclic AMP decreased release of acetylcholine guinea pig cortex, while cyclic GMP increased release (Beani *et al.*, 1975), presumably reflecting nucleotide-elicited central sedation and excitation, respectively (see p. 293). Intraventricular dibutyryl cyclic AMP in rats increased acetylcholine levels in both cortical and subcortical areas (Askew and Ho, 1975). Levels of choline acetyltransferase and acetylcholinesterase were unaffected except in subcortex where the level of acetylcholinesterase was somewhat decreased. Intravenous dibutyryl cyclic AMP had no effect on levels of acetylcholine in brain.

Cyclic AMP and analogs, prostaglandin, and phosphodiesterase inhibitors elicited increases in levels of acetylcholinesterase, choline acetyltransferase, and acetylcholine receptors in certain lines of cultured neuroblastoma cells (Furmanski et al., 1971; Prasad and Vernadakis, 1972; Simantov and Sachs, 1972; 1973, 1975a,b,c; Prasad et al., 1973c; Prasad and Mandal, 1973; Truding et al., 1974; Glazer and Schneider, 1975). Increases in acetylcholinesterase and choline acetyltransferase did not appear linked to morphological differentiation in neuroblastoma cells, since agents such as butyrate and cyclic AMP which inhibit growth, but do not cause morphological differentiation, increased levels of the enzymes. Treatment of neuroblastoma cells with 5-bromodeoxyuridine elevated cyclic AMP levels (see Section 3.5.2), elicited differentiation, and increased levels of acetylcholinesterase and choline acetyltransferase. X irradiation, a treatment that induces differentiation but does not cause elevations of intracellular cyclic AMP, caused increases in acetylcholinesterase and choline acetyltransferase. The data suggest that inhibition of cell division results in increases in enzyme levels and that cyclic AMP mechanisms may not be necessarily directly involved. Induction of acetylcholinesterase in neuroblastoma cells by dibutyryl cyclic AMP was not inhibited by actinomycin D, while induction by 5-bromodeoxyuridine was inhibited (Simantov and Sachs, 1975b). In a neuroblastoma cell line with temperature-sensitive cyclic AMP-dependent protein kinases, levels of acetylcholinesterase and acetylcholine receptors were not enhanced by low concentrations of prostaglandin or dibutyryl cyclic AMP (Simantov and Sachs, 1975a). Induction of acetylcholinesterase by dibutyryl cyclic AMP in "temperature-resistant" neuroblastoma cell lines was much greater at 40°C compared to induction at 37°C (Simantov and Sachs, 1975b). In contrast, 5-bromodeoxyuridine had lesser effects on acetylcholinesterase induction at the higher temperature. Inhibition of growth by both dibutyryl cyclic AMP and 5-bromodeoxyuridine was much greater at the higher temperature. In certain neuroblastoma clones, dibutyryl cyclic AMP and cyclic AMP increased acetylcholinesterase while decreasing choline acetyltransferase (Simantov and Sachs, 1972). 5-Bromodeoxyuridine increased both enzymes. In certain clones dibutyryl cyclic AMP caused parallel increases in acetylcholinesterase and acetylcholine receptors (Simantov and Sachs, 1973). Acetylcholine has been reported to induce acetylcholinesterase in mouse neuroblastoma cells concomitant with differentiation (Hawkins et al., 1972).

Cyclic AMP-linked increases in levels of acetylcholinesterase apparently occurred in cultured fetal chick and rat brain cells and at least one line of glioma cells (Werner *et al.,* 1971; Schrier and Shapiro, 1973; Shapiro, 1973). Choline acetyltransferase was increased in the chick brain cells but decreased in rat brain cells.

Biogenic Amines

Effects of cyclic AMP on activity and levels of tyrosine hydroxylase have been investigated with synaptosomes and with soluble enzyme, in brain slices, intact brain, ganglia, and cultured cells. The results clearly indicate an activation of tyrosine hydroxylase by a cyclic AMP-dependent mechanism. Since tyrosine hydroxylase is primarily a presynaptic enzyme, physiological control of this important enzyme by cyclic AMP would represent an example of a presynaptic role for cyclic AMP in nervous tissue.

In homogenates or synaptosomes from brain tissue or with soluble enzyme, cyclic AMP and various analogs elicited an activation of tyrosine hydroxylase (Ebstein *et al.,* 1974; Harris *et al.,* 1974, 1975; Morgenroth *et al.,* 1974; Goldstein *et al.,* 1975b; Lloyd and Kaufman, 1975; Lovenberg and Bruckwich, 1975; Lovenberg *et al.,* 1975; Roth *et al.,* 1975). ATP and magnesium ions were required for cyclic AMP-dependent activation of tyrosine hydroxylase. The activated enzyme had a higher affinity for the tetrahydropteridine cofactor, while the potency of inhibitory catechols such as norepinephrine, dopamine, and apomorphine was decreased. The affinity of the enzyme for tyrosine was either unaffected or increased. Agents known to inhibit cyclic AMP-dependent protein kinases, such as EDTA, ADP, adenosine, and protein kinase modulator protein, inhibited activation of tyrosine hydroxylase by cyclic nucleotides. Addition of exogenous protein kinases enhanced the activation. Dibutyryl cyclic AMP has been demonstrated to activate tyrosine hydroxylase in cell-free preparations from rat cerebral cortex, forebrain, hippocampus, striatum, mesolimbic brain, hypothalamus, septum, and brain stem. Calcium ions elicited a similar activation of tyrosine hydroxylase in hippocampal homogenates, but unlike the effect of cyclic AMP the calcium-elicited activation was reversed by EGTA (Roth *et al.,* 1975). Dibutyryl cyclic AMP, monobutyryl cyclic AMP, 8-bromo- and 8-methylthio cyclic AMP, but not cyclic AMP itself activated tyrosine hydroxylase in rat striatal synaptosomes (Harris *et al.,* 1975). Dibutyryl cyclic AMP increased rates of hydroxylation of both tyrosine and phenylalanine in synaptosomes from striatum, cerebral cortex, and brain stem. Hydroxylation of tryptophan and uptake of tryptyphan was slightly enhanced in striatal synaptosomes. The cyclic nucleotide had no effect on uptake of tyrosine or phenylalanine, disposition of dopamine, subcellular distribution of tyrosine hydroxylase, or on levels of dopa decarboxylase in synaptosomes. Rates of synthesis of dopamine were increased in rat striatal synaptosomes by dibutyryl cyclic AMP without any effect on release of dopamine (Patrick and Barchas, 1976). Prior treatment of rats with haloperidol enhanced striatal tyrosine hydroxylase activity, but dibutyryl cyclic AMP under phosphorylating conditions then still caused a further activation of the soluble tyrosine hydroxylase (Goldstein *et al.,* 1975b). Although the data clearly indicated that a cyclic AMP-dependent phosphorylation was involved in the activation of tyrosine hydroxylase no incorporation of phosphate into tyrosine hydroxylase could be detected (Lovenberg *et al.,* 1975; Lloyd and Kaufman, 1975). The activation of bovine caudate tyrosine hydroxylase by cyclic AMP–ATP–magnesium was mimicked by phosphatidylserine (Lloyd and Kaufman, 1975). The activations by cyclic AMP–ATP–magnesium and by phosphatidylserine were not additive. It was proposed that phosphorylating conditions produce a phosphorylated protein that activates tyrosine hydroxylase in a manner similar to phosphatidylserine.

In brain slices from rat cortex and striatum, dibutyryl cyclic AMP increased the rate of synthesis of dopamine from exogenous radioactive tyrosine but not from exogenous dopa (Goldstein *et al.,* 1973; Anagnoste *et al.,* 1974; Taneda *et al.,* 1974). Dibutyryl cyclic AMP had no effect on uptake of radioactive tyrosine into striatal slices, on the apparent K_m of tyrosine hydroxylase for tyrosine, or on the specific activity of tyrosine or dopamine in the slice. It would appear that the stimulatory effect of dibutyryl cyclic AMP on dopamine synthesis in brain slices occurred through an activation of tyrosine hydroxylase. Prior treatment of rats with haloperidol increased rates of conversion of radioactive tyrosine to dopamine in striatal slices, while a prior treatment with a dopaminergic agonist, apomorphine, reduced the conversion rates. The addition of dibutyryl cyclic AMP enhanced rates of conversion of tyrosine to dopamine in slices from haloperidol- and apomorphine-treated animals. High concentrations of potassium ions or the absence of calcium ions increased formation of dopamine from tyrosine in striatal slices. In the presence of dibutyryl cyclic AMP, only high potassium elicited a further increase in rates of formation of dopamine.

The cyclic AMP-dependent alterations in striatal tyrosine hydroxylase *in vitro* are similar to the alterations in the enzyme elicited *in vivo* by dopaminergic antagonists, that is an increase in affinity for tetrahydropteridine cofactor and a reduction in affinity for inhibitory catecholamines (Lovenberg and Bruckwick, 1975 and references therein). Stimulation of the locus coeruleus elicited this type of activation of tyrosine hydroxylase in rat hippocampus (Roth *et al.,* 1975). Transection of the nigro-striatal dopaminergic pathway resulted in a transient increase in striatal cyclic

AMP and a transient activation of tyrosine hydroxylase (Zivkovic *et al.*, 1975, 1976). Apomorphine enhanced cyclic AMP levels in both the intact and lesioned striata, while having no effect on the activation of tyrosine hydroxylase in the lesioned striatum or on levels in the intact striatum. Haloperidol caused an activation of tyrosine hydroxylase only in the intact striatum, while having no effect on cyclic AMP levels in either striatum. Lesions in haloperidol- or reserpine-treated animals had no effect on cyclic AMP levels and the drug-elicited activation of tyrosine hydroxylase was rapidly reduced after lesioning. The mechanisms involved in the control of tyrosine hydroxylase activity *in vivo* in brain were not resolved. Haloperidol and reserpine have no effects on striatal levels of cyclic AMP, but they do activate tyrosine hydroxylase. Apomorphine elicits an accumulation of cyclic AMP but has no effect or reduces activity of tyrosine hydroxylase and prevents the *in vivo* activation of tyrosine hydroxylase by dopaminergic antagonists or reserpine. Lesions increase both cyclic AMP and tyrosine hydroxylase. Regardless of the mechanisms involved in activation of tyrosine hydroxylase it would appear that apomorphine or haloperidol have effects only when the nigro-striatal pathway is intact.

In slices of rat brain stem, dibutyryl cyclic AMP, but not cyclic AMP, theophylline, or norepinephrine, increased uptake of radioactive tryptophan and conversion to serotonin and 5-hydroxyindole acetic acid (Forn *et al.*, 1972). Cycloheximide did not block the effect of dibutyryl cyclic AMP.

Intraventricular dibutyryl cyclic AMP increased the apparent rate of serotonin and dopamine synthesis in brain (Tagliamonte *et al.*, 1971a,b,c). Dibutyryl cyclic AMP increased levels of tryptophan, suggesting that this might be the mechanism, whereby it elicited enhanced synthesis of serotonin. Tryptophan levels in brain are below saturation values for tryptophan hydroxylase, the rate-limiting enzyme for the biosynthesis of serotonin. Dibutyryl cyclic AMP also increased brain levels of tyrosine. Tyrosine hydroxylase, important to the synthesis of catecholamines, is, however, fully saturated with respect to substrate in normal animals. Methylxanthines increased levels of serotonin in brain stem of rats and antagonized the decline in serotonin levels usually seen after administration of *p*-chlorophenylalanine, an inhibitor of serotonin biosynthesis (Berkowitz and Spector, 1971). Methylxanthines enhanced apparent turnover of norepinephrine *in vivo* in brain, perhaps due to an increased rate of release (Berkowitz *et al.*, 1970; Waldeck, 1971; Corrodi *et al.*, 1972). Turnover rates of dopamine and serotonin appeared to be decreased. It is uncertain whether these effects are related to the activity of methylxanthines as phosphodiesterase inhibitors.

Cyclic AMP-dependent mechanisms appear to control the synthesis of melatonin from serotonin in pineal gland by effects on levels of serotonin *N*-acetyltransferase activity (Klein *et al.*, 1973; and references therein).

Induction of serotonin N-acetyltransferase in pineal gland by isoproterenol or dibutyryl cyclic AMP appeared to involve stimulation of transcription and in addition a stimulation of posttranscriptional processes (Romero *et al.*, 1975).

Levels of tyrosine hydroxylase in cultured rat or mouse superior cervical ganglia were elevated by dibutyryl cyclic AMP, theophylline, and potassium ions (Keen and McLean, 1972a,b; Mackay and Iversen, 1972a,b; Keen and McLean, 1974). Theophylline, which by itself had only a slight stimulatory effect on tyrosine hydroxylase activity, significantly potentiated the response to potassium ions. Cycloheximide blocked increases in tyrosine hydroxylase in ganglia, indicating that the process does not involve a simple phosphorylation-dependent process (see above). With cultured ganglia neither acetylcholine nor carbamylcholine had any effect on tyrosine hydroxylase activity (cited in Goodman *et al.*, 1974). Levels of norepinephrine in cultured rat ganglia were increased by dibutyryl cyclic AMP, cyclic AMP, and theophylline. Papaverine caused a profound depletion of norepinephrine which was prevented by a monoamine oxidase inhibitor, pargyline. The turnover of norepinephrine in ganglion was unchanged by dibutyryl cyclic AMP, while the rate of synthesis from tyrosine, but not from dopa, was increased. Thus, the dibutyryl cyclic AMP-elicited increase in levels of norepinephrine appeared to be primarily due to activation of tyrosine hydroxylase. Elevation of tyrosine hydroxylase activity by potassium ions was observed in ganglia from both neonatal and adult mice (Mackay and Iversen, 1972b). Dibutyryl cyclic AMP and potassium ions have been reported not only to increase levels of tyrosine hydroxylase, but in addition levels of dopamine-β-hydroxylase, monoamine oxidase, and dopa decarboxylase in cultured superior cervical ganglia (Keen and McLean, 1972a, 1974; Mackay and Iversen, 1972a; Silberstein *et al.*, 1972; Goodman *et al.*, 1974; Webb *et al.*, 1975). Cycloheximide unexpectedly increased the activity of dopa decarboxylase and monoamine oxidase, but this protein-synthesis inhibitor did block further increases in all four enzyme activities elicited by potassium ions or dibutyryl cyclic AMP. Cycloheximide did not block the dibutyryl cyclic AMP-elicited elevation in levels of norepinephrine in cultured ganglia. Dibutyryl cyclic AMP increased levels of monoamine oxidase in chick embryo sympathetic ganglia, both in the presence and absence of nerve growth factor (Phillipson and Sandler, 1975a,b). Dibutyryl cyclic AMP increased levels of tyrosine hydroxylase in the presence of nerve growth factor. GDP increased levels of tyrosine hydroxylase and blocked the increase elicited by ACTH. The latter results were discussed in terms of possible facilitative effects of GDP (or GTP) on activation of adenylate cyclase.

Clearly, cyclic AMP-dependent mechanisms elicit increases in tyrosine hydroxylase and dopamine-β-hydroxylase in sympathetic ganglion.

The extent to which cyclic AMP-dependent mechanisms are involved in transsynaptic induction of tyrosine hydroxylase and dopamine-β-hydroxylase seen *in vivo* in sympathetic ganglia and in adrenal medulla under conditions of increased sympathetic activity such as reserpinization or cold stress has proven difficult to establish. Indeed, a role for cyclic AMP in the phenomenon of transsynaptic induction has been questioned (Goodman *et al.*, 1974; Otten *et al.*, 1973, 1974). *In vivo,* transsynaptic induction involves the interaction of acetylcholine with postsynaptic nicotinic receptors. *In vitro,* carbamylcholine elicits increases in cyclic AMP in ganglia, via interactions with muscarinic receptors (see Section 3.3.1). *In vitro* dibutyryl cyclic AMP elicits increases in a variety of ganglionic enzymes rather than just tyrosine hydroxylase and dopamine-β-hydroxylase. *In vivo* isoproterenol-elicited increases in cyclic AMP levels in adrenergic cell bodies of the rat superior cervical ganglion did not lead to increases in levels of tyrosine hydroxylase. Correlations between transient early increases in cyclic AMP levels and the much later elevations in tyrosine hydroxylase levels in rat superior cervical ganglion after reserpine or swimming stress were not apparent (Otten *et al.*, 1972). Subsequent studies indicated that β-agonists do elicit *in vivo* induction of tyrosine hydroxylase activity in rat superior cervical ganglion and that a low but sustained accumulation of cyclic AMP is necessary to initiate the induction process (Hanbauer *et al.*, 1975a,b). Induction of tyrosine hydroxylase occurred 48 hr after administration of β-agonists. A sustained accumulation of cyclic AMP for about 90 min was required for the induction of tyrosine hydroxylase. Epinephrine or repeated injections of isoproterenol elicited such a sustained accumulation of cyclic AMP and a subsequent induction of tyrosine hydroxylase, while dopamine and norepinephrine did not. Propranolol blocked the increase in tyrosine hydroxylase induced by epinephrine. *In vivo* experiments with various blocking agents provided evidence that reserpine-elicited increases in tyrosine hydroxylase in rat superior cervical ganglia involved stimulation of glucocorticoid and nicotinic but not β-adrenergic receptors.

Cyclic AMP-dependent mechanisms have been implicated in increases of tyrosine hydroxylase in neuroblastoma cells (Prasad *et al.*, 1972, 1973c; Waymire *et al.*, 1972; Richelson, 1973; Prasad and Kumar, 1975). Dibutyryl and monobutyryl cyclic AMP, other analogs of cyclic AMP, phosphodiesterase inhibitors, and prostaglandin E_1 greatly increased levels of tyrosine hydroxylase in neuroblastoma cells. Cyclic AMP was ineffective. Such treatments also caused differentiation of neuroblastoma cells. Differentiation of cells induced by X irradiation or serum-free medium did not result in changes in tyrosine hydroxylase activity. Levels of the hydroxylase could be increased in X-ray and serum-free differentiated cells by dibutyryl cyclic AMP. Butyrate, an agent known to increase cyclic AMP levels in neuroblastoma cells, elevated hydroxylase levels. The effect appeared to be linked to inhibition of cell growth since butyrate does not cause differentiation. Unlike the enzymes concerned with acetylcholine formation and degradation, increases in tyrosine hydroxylase in neuroblastoma cells thus appeared to be more directly linked to cyclic AMP-dependent mechanisms. Elevated levels of tyrosine hydroxylase reached a maximum 4 days after introduction of dibutyryl cyclic AMP and persisted after removal of the cyclic nucleotide for at least 2 days. The cyclic nucleotide-elicited increase in tyrosine hydroxylase was blocked by cycloheximide. The kinetic properties of the enzyme from treated cells did not appear to be altered in contrast to the cyclic AMP-induced changes in properties of tyrosine hydroxylase in brain preparations (see above). Dibutyryl cyclic AMP decreased levels of dopamine-β-hydroxylase in a neuroblastoma cell line, while having no effect or enhancing the activity of the enzyme in neuroblastoma–glioma hybrid cell lines (Hamprecht *et al.*, 1974). Hybrid cell lines underwent differentiation in the presence of dibutyryl cyclic AMP. Dibutyryl cyclic AMP-elicited differentiation of neuroblastoma cells was accompanied by an increase in uptake of radioactive tyrosine and a proportional increase in formation of dopamine, norepinephrine, and their metabolites (Wexler and Katzman, 1975). Catechol-*O*-methyltransferase levels were not affected in neuroblastoma cells by dibutyryl cyclic AMP or prostaglandin (Prasad and Mandal, 1972; Prasad *et al.*, 1973a).

Prostaglandins

Cyclic AMP increased prostaglandin E_2 synthesis in rat brain homogenates (Abdulla and McFarlane, 1972). Dibutyryl cyclic AMP increased prostaglandin synthesis in neuroblastoma and glioma cells (Hamprecht *et al.*, 1973). The major prostaglandins produced by these cells are of the E series. In the neuroblastoma cells the increased formation and efflux of prostaglandin was accompanied by an increase in intracellular levels. In the glioma cells the efflux into the medium greatly increased, while intracellular levels of prostaglandins remained constant.

Amino Acids

Dibutyryl cyclic AMP increased levels of glutamate decarboxylase in fetal rat brain cells, but not in glioma cells (Schrier and Shapiro, 1973). Glutamate decarboxylase levels were not altered in neuroblastoma cells (Prasad *et al.*, 1973c). Uptake of γ-aminobutyric acid by rat glioma cells was stated to be inhibited by cyclic AMP and norepinephrine (Hutchison *et al.*, 1973).

4.1.4 Cyclases, Phosphodiesterases, and Kinases

Cyclases

Differentiation of certain neuroblastoma cell lines elicited by culture with prostaglandin E_1, the phosphodiesterase inhibitor RO 20-1724, or butyrate resulted in enhanced cyclase activity and in altered responses of the cyclase to various agents (Prasad, 1974; Prasad and Gilmer, 1974; Kumar et al., 1975; Prasad et al., 1975c,d). Phosphodiesterase activity and cyclic AMP levels were also increased in the differentiated cells. After RO 20-1724-induced differentiation the cyclases in homogenates were more responsive to acetylcholine and dopamine, while responsiveness to prostaglandin E_1 and GTP were unaltered. However, in homogenates from differentiated cells, GTP now augmented prostaglandin activation of cyclases. After differentiation by X irradiation, the dopamine-sensitive cyclase was no longer detectable in homogenates. Manganese ions at 1 mM inhibited adenylate cyclase activity to a greater extent in RO 20-1724-differentiated neuroblastoma cells than in undifferentiated cells. Differentiation in serum-free medium did not result in any change in cyclase levels. Catecholamine-elicited accumulations of cyclic AMP resulted in reductions in norepinephrine-responsive adenylate cyclases in certain rat glioma cell lines (Browning et al., 1976) and in an apparent increase in a factor inhibitory to adenylate cyclase in another rat glioma cell line (De Vellis and Brooker, 1974) (see below).

Phosphodiesterases

Dibutyryl cyclic AMP or elevation of intracellular cyclic AMP by prostaglandin E_1 in neuroblastoma cells, by catecholamines in glioma cells, and by phosphodiesterase inhibitors in both cell types resulted in an increase in phosphodiesterase activity in certain neuroblastoma (Prasad and Kumar, 1973; Kumar et al., 1975; Prasad et al., 1975d) and glioma (Schwartz et al., 1973; Uzunov et al., 1973; De Vellis and Brooker, 1974; Schwartz and Passonneau, 1974; Browning et al., 1976) cell lines. Phosphodiesterase activity in neuroblastoma cells differentiated by culture with RO 20-1724 was slightly elevated and in the absence of magnesium appeared to be less susceptible to inhibition by calcium ions or imidazole than the activity in nondifferentiated cells. Manganese ions caused a greater activation of phosphodiesterases from the differentiated cells. In rat glioma cells norepinephrine, through interaction with a β-receptor, enhanced threefold the activity of only one of the two phosphodiesterases present in this cell line (Uzunov et al., 1973). The "inducible" diesterase apparently corresponded to peak IV of rat brain (cf. Figure 3) and after treatment with norepinephrine represented the major phosphodiesterase in the glioma cell homogenates. Cycloheximide prevented the norepinephrine-elicited increase in this phosphodiesterase in rat glioma cells and a dibutyryl cyclic AMP-elicited increase in phosphodiesterase in mouse neuroblastoma cells. Actinomycin did not prevent the increase in phosphodiesterase activity in neuroblastoma cells. A dibutyryl cyclic AMP–theophylline combination or norepinephrine elicited marked increases in both low K_m and high K_m phosphodiesterase activity in rat glioma cells (Schwartz and Passonneau, 1974). Cycloheximide or actinomycin D prevented these increases. The increase in phosphodiesterase elicited by norepinephrine was blocked by β-antagonists but not by an α-antagonist. The magnitude of the accumulation of cyclic AMP elicited during an initial 0.5- to 5-min incubation with norepinephrine correlated quite well with the magnitude of a subsequent induction of low K_m phosphodiesterase activity measured 3 hr later. Phosphodiesterase levels did not, however, increase in all glioma cell lines whose cyclic AMP-generating systems become refractory to stimulation by norepinephrine. Thus, norepinephrine elicited accumulation of cyclic AMP in two rat glioma clones, RGC6 and RGC6 2B, but induction of phosphodiesterase activity occurred only in the former clone (De Vellis and Brooker, 1974). Refractoriness to norepinephrine in the 2B clone appeared to involve a cyclic AMP-elicited increase in a protein or proteins that inhibited subsequent formation of cyclic AMP. Development of refractoriness of cyclic AMP-generating systems to norepinephrine could be largely prevented by acetoxycycloheximide or actinomycin. Actinomycin was effective only when added simultaneously with norepinephrine, while the cycloheximide could actually reverse refractoriness to norepinephrine. Thus, norepinephrine appeared to elicit via a cyclic AMP mechanism *de novo* synthesis of an RNA responsible for the synthesis of the inhibitory protein. Time-course studies indicated that the proposed inhibitory protein turned over very rapidly in glioma cells with a half-time of less than 1 hr. The nature of this protein and the generality of its involvement in refractoriness of cyclic AMP-generating systems warrant further investigation. Stimulation of cyclic AMP-generating systems by norepinephrine had no apparent effect on levels of phosphodiesterase in a human glioma cell line, although refractoriness to a restimulation did develop (Perkins *et al.*, 1975). Catecholamine-elicited accumulations of cyclic AMP resulted in an increase in a calcium-independent phosphodiesterase in rat glioma cell line, but also caused a reduction in norepinephrine-sensitive adenylate cyclases (Browning *et al.*, 1976). Calcium-dependent phosphodiesterase activity and cyclic GMP-phosphodiesterase activity were unaffected. Cycloheximide or actinomycin completely blocked the increase in phosphodiesterase activity but did not completely prevent the development of refractoriness of cyclic AMP-generating systems and thus probably had no effect on cyclic AMP-elicited reductions in adenylate cyclase. 5-Bromodeoxyuridine, an agent that had little effect on cyclic AMP levels in glioma cells, caused an increase in phosphodiesterase in cultures of dividing cells (Schwartz *et al.*, 1973).

Kinases

Differentiation of neuroblastoma cells elicited by prostaglandin E_1 or RO 20-1724 was accompanied by apparent increases in two cyclic AMP-binding sites in homogenates (Prasad *et al.*, 1975e). The increase was blocked by cycloheximide. X irradiation did not increase levels of binding sites. Treatment of glioma cells with prostaglandin E_1 or RO 20-1724 did not increase levels of cyclic AMP binding sites. Cyclic AMP-dependent protein kinase activity in neuroblastoma cells was unaltered in differentiated neuroblastoma cells, suggesting that measures of cyclic AMP binding do not provide an adequate means of assessing levels of cyclic AMP-dependent kinases (Prasad *et al.*, 1976). Factors related to function of kinases, such as rates of incorporation of radioactive phosphate into phosphoproteins, levels of cyclic AMP-dependent protein kinases assayed in homogenates with histone as substrate, and levels of ATP, were similar in suspension cultures of undifferentiated neuroblastoma cells and in monolayer cultures in which outgrowth of neuritic processes indicated some degree of differentiation (Casola *et al.*, 1974). Cyclic AMP-dependent translocation of protein kinase from cytoplasm to nuclei in a rat glioma cell line has been reported (Salem and De Vellis, 1976).

4.1.5 Protein Phosphorylation

The effects of agents that are known to enhance cyclic AMP levels in brain slices on the incorporation of radioactive phosphate into phosphoproteins of guinea pig cerebral cortical slices has been investigated in detail (Reddington *et al.*, 1973; Weller and Rodnight, 1973a,b; Williams *et al.*, 1974a,b; Williams and Rodnight, 1975, 1976). The protocol involved labeling of slices with radioactive phosphate followed by determination of the "specific activity" of protein (serine) phosphate. Total phosphoproteins in membrane fractions from rat forebrain decreased slightly after decapitation. The protein phosphate content of the membranes was increased on incubation with ATP, indicating that membrane protein is not completely phosphorylated *in situ* in rat brain. Incorporation of radioactive phosphate in proteins of guinea pig cortical slices was increased by norepinephrine (EC_{50}, 1.5 μM), isoproterenol (EC_{50}, 0.3 μM), histamine, serotonin, and electrical pulsation. High concentrations of potassium ions appeared to increase incorporation of phosphate into protein, but a decrease in the rate of incorporation of radioactive phosphate into intracellular ATP under these conditions complicated any interpretation of the results with potassium ions. Adenosine, another stimulant of cyclic AMP-generating systems in brain slices, had no effect on incorporation of radioactive phosphate. Adenosine antagonized the stimulatory effect of histamine, but not the increase in protein phosphorylation elicited by norepinephrine, serotonin, or electrical pulsation. Adenosine had been shown to inhibit cyclic AMP-dependent autophosphorylation of synaptosomal membrane fractions (see Section 2.4.1), but at much higher concentrations than those that blocked the effect of histamine on phosphorylation in slices. The effects of norepinephrine and pulsation were nonadditive, while the effects of serotonin or histamine and pulsation were additive. The effects of norepinephrine or of electrical pulsation on protein phosphorylation were blocked by β-antagonists such as propranolol, dichlorisoproterenol, and practolol, but not by α-antagonists, such as phentolamine and phenoxybenzamine. It should be noted that norepinephrine stimulated cyclic AMP formation in guinea pig cortical slices primarily through α-adrenergic receptors (see Section 3.1.2). Propranolol alone increased protein phosphorylation. Both d- and l-isomers of propranolol antagonized the effect of pulsation while, consonant with its greater activity as a β-antagonist, only the l-isomer was effective against norepinephrine. Low concentrations of trifluoperazine or prostaglandin E_1 antagonized the increase in protein phosphorylation elicited by norepinephrine or electrical pulsation. Tetrodotoxin blocked the increase in protein phosphorylation elicited by electrical pulsation in cortical slices, but not that due to histamine. Maximal increases in the stimulation of rates of incorporation of phosphate into brain slice proteins occurred within 2 sec of the electrical pulsation (Williams and Rodnight, 1975). A prior pulsation for 10 sec of unlabeled slices nearly completely prevented the stimulatory effect of pulses applied 4 min later. If a 10-min period was interposed between pulses, the second set was fully stimulatory. Thus, electrical pulsation appeared to elicit a rapid net phosphorylation of a limited number of serine residues whose turnover in brain slices was nearly complete within 10 min. The net incorporation of radioactive phosphate in such experiments would, of course, be dependent on the activity of both protein kinases and phosphatases. The stimulatory effects of electrical pulsation and of norepinephrine on phosphate incorporation in brain slices were localized to the neuronal fraction, while the effects of histamine and serotonin were localized to the glial fraction. The results suggest that norepinephrine released by electrical pulsation elicited an increase in incorporation of phosphate into neuronal phosphoproteins of guinea pig cerebral cortical slices, while histamine and serotonin have effects on glial sites. Direct comparisons of cyclic AMP levels and changes in phosphate incorporation in brain slices should provide a further delineation of the relationship of the increase in phosphorylation to cyclic AMP-dependent mechanisms.

In slices of rat caudate nucleus both 8-bromo cyclic AMP and the phosphodiesterase inhibitor, isobutylmethylxanthine, selectively stimulated the phosphorylation of three proteins with molecular weights of 85,000, 80,000, and 49,000 (Krueger *et al.*, 1975). Cyclic AMP and its butyryl derivatives were ineffective in the slice preparation. The two higher molecular weight proteins appeared to be associated with synaptosomal membranes, while the lower molecular weight protein appeared to represent the regulatory unit of cyclic AMP-dependent protein kinases (see Section 2.4.1).

Radioactive phosphate was incorporated into microtubular protein in guinea pig cerebral cortical slices (Reddington and Lagnado, 1973; Lagnado *et al.*, 1975). The more recent studies indicated that β-tubulin incorporated nearly twofold more radioactivity than γ-tubulin, but that minor high molecular weight microtubular proteins contained nearly two-thirds of the total microtubular radioactivity. Effects of agents which elevate cyclic AMP levels in brain slices on labeling of microtubular protein were not ascertained. Microtubular protein isolated from rat brain slices in which cyclic AMP levels were elevated threefold by incubation with adenosine–histamine had not incorporated significant amounts of radioactive phosphate (Murray and Froscio, 1971). Microtubules isolated from chick brain slices after incubation with radioactive phosphate had significant associated radioactivity (Piras and Piras, 1974). No incorporation of radioactive phosphate into tubulin of control and differentiated neuroblastoma cells was detected (Soloman *et al.*, 1976).

It is not yet known whether the demonstrated *in vivo* phosphorylation of myelin basic protein of oligodendroglial cells was dependent on cyclic AMP (Miyamoto and Kakiuchi, 1973). *In vitro* myelin basic protein was an excellent substrate for cyclic AMP-dependent protein kinase.

Dibutyryl cyclic AMP enhanced the phosphorylation of a protein with an apparent molecular weight of 118,000 in *Aplysia* abdominal ganglia (Levitan and Barondes, 1974; Levitan *et al.*, 1974). Long incubations of 15 hr with radioactive phosphate were required to generate stable patterns of phosphoproteins. Octopamine and serotonin also enhanced phosphorylation of the protein with a molecular weight of 118,000. Phentolamine blocked the effect of octopamine, while methysergide blocked the effect of serotonin. The protein had a half-life of 4 to 5 hr, markedly lower than the 90-hr half-life of total incorporated protein phosphate. The protein whose phosphorylation appeared dependent on cyclic AMP-dependent mechanisms was not associated with large neurons, connective nerves, or bag cell clusters and it was suggested that it was associated with the neuropil which contains virtually all the synapses of the ganglion. The protein was associated with crude "mitochondrial" fractions from ganglia. Cyclic AMP-dependent phosphorylation of proteins corresponding in molecular weight to protein II (cf. Figure 14) was not detected in intact *Aplysia* abdominal ganglion.

4.1.6 DNA, RNA, and Protein Synthesis

Cyclic AMP-dependent phosphorylation of histones might result in altered DNA–histone interactions, derepression of template activity, and increased synthesis of specific messenger RNA (see Langan, 1970). Effects of cyclic AMP mechanisms on incorporation of precursors into DNA, RNA, and protein have been examined in brain tissue and in cultured cells. Apparent cyclic AMP-dependent alterations in turnover of DNA, RNA, and protein may, however, not reflect direct effects of cyclic AMP in cultured cells, but may be secondary to inhibition of growth and/or differentiation.

Brain

During incubation of rat brain slices with depolarizing agents such as high concentrations of potassium ions, glutamate, and veratridine alkaloids, conditions under which cyclic AMP levels are elevated, the rate of incorporation of radioactive adenine into RNA was reduced (Glick and Quastel, 1972). Except in the case of high potassium, the reduction in adenine incorporation into RNA probably merely reflected reduced rates of incorporation of adenine into adenine nucleotides and decreases in ATP content of the slice.

Intraventricular administration of dibutyryl cyclic AMP to goldfish altered the composition of brain RNA newly synthesized from radioactive precursors (Shashoua, 1971). Thus, the dibutyryl derivative elicited an increase in the uridine to cytidine ratio in RNA derived from radioactive orotic acid and increased the amount of radioactive nuclear RNA and cytoplasmic RNA derived from radioactive uridine. Incorporation of uridine into nuclear RNA was increased four- to sixfold over a 2-hr period, while incorporation into polysomal RNA was increased by 40 to 50%. Labeling of ribosomal and transfer RNA did not appear altered. The results suggest a cyclic AMP-evoked increase in formation of messenger RNA in goldfish brain.

Ganglia

In *Aplysia* abdominal ganglion, stimulation of cyclic AMP formation by serotonin did not alter rates of incorporation of radioactive uridine into RNA (Cedar and Schwartz, 1972).

Cultured Cells

Differentiation of neuroblastoma cells by dibutyryl cyclic AMP resulted in a marked decrease in incorporation of thymidine into DNA (Lin and Mitsunobu, 1972; Prasad *et al.*, 1972). Differentiation of neuroblastoma cells by dibutyryl cyclic AMP, prostaglandin E_1, or RO 20-1724 resulted in a 50% decrease in DNA content, suggesting that a larger proportion of the asynchronous cell population was present in the post-cell division G_1 phase (Prasad *et al.*, 1973b). Cells inhibited by butyrate also had a decreased content of DNA. In earlier studies dibutyryl cyclic AMP appeared to have caused a marginal decrease in DNA content of neuroblastoma cells (Prasad and Vernadakis, 1972). Differentiation of neuroblastoma cells by dibutyryl cyclic AMP either increased (Prasad *et al.*, 1973b) or decreased (Lim and Mitsunobu, 1972; Glazer and Schneider, 1975) rates of incorporation of uridine into RNA. RNA content of differentiated cells and butyrate-inhibited cells was higher than in untreated cells (Prasad *et al.*, 1972). Differentiation of neuroblastoma cells by dibutyryl cyclic AMP or papaverine was accompanied by a decrease in rates of incorporation of radioactive uridine into ribosomal and heterogeneous RNA (Glazer and Schneider, 1975). In contrast, cyclic AMP stimulated incorporation of uridine and butyrate had no effect. The effects appeared primarily to be due to alterations in rates of uptake of uridine and levels of UTP. Incorporation of adenosine into total and cytoplasmic RNA was decreased during short incubations (Bondy *et al.*, 1974) and increased during long incubations (Prasad *et al.*, 1975b) in differentiated neuroblastoma cells as compared to control cells. The proportion of radioactivity associated with cytoplasmic RNA was significantly greater in differentiated cells, in particular in cells differentiated by prostaglandin E_1 or RO 20-1724. Since polyadenylic sequences are typical of messenger RNA but not of ribosomal and transfer RNA it was proposed that the data indicated enhanced synthesis of messenger RNA in differentiated cells. DNA template activity measured by binding of actinomycin was similar in undifferentiated and RO 20-1724-differentiated neuroblastoma cells. Adenine phosphoribosyl transferase activity in neuroblastoma cells was unaffected by dibutyryl cyclic AMP and slightly increased by papaverine (Glazer and Schneider, 1975).

Dibutyryl cyclic AMP increased incorporation of leucine and proline into protein of neuroblastoma cells (Lim and Mitsunobu, 1972; Prasad *et al.*, 1972). The profile of proline-labeled proteins in undifferentiated neuroblastoma cells and in cells differentiated by culture in serum-free media were quite similar (Morgan and Seeds, 1975).

The effect of differentiation of neuroblastoma cells on template activity of chromatin for RNA synthesis in a DNA-dependent cell-free system and on the composition of histone and nonhistone chromosomal proteins has been investigated (Zornetzer and Stein, 1975). The template activity was reduced threefold in cells differentiated by culture in serum-free media. Histone profiles were unaltered, but incorporation of tryptophan into nonhistone chromosomal proteins of molecular weight 120,000–140,000 was markedly decreased and profiles of certain other nonhistone chromosomal protein appeared to be altered. Similar changes in tryptophan incorporation were manifest in cells differentiated by dibutyryl cyclic AMP.

Treatment of rat glioma cells with dibutyryl cyclic AMP reduced rates of incorporation of radioactive uridine into RNA and of thymidine into DNA (Lim and Mitsunobu, 1972; Gibson *et al.*, 1974). The phosphodiesterase inhibitor, papaverine, had even greater inhibitory effects on uridine incorporation but was very toxic to the cells. Incorporation of proline into protein was increased in dibutyryl cyclic AMP-treated cells.

4.2 Cell Morphology, Differentiation, and Growth

Cyclic AMP-dependent mechanisms have been strongly implicated in inhibition of growth of neuroblastoma and glioma cells. Such inhibited cells often undergo morphological differentiation, the extent of which appears to be strongly dependent on many variables, including the cell line and culture conditions. Embryonic cells from brain, ganglia, and ectoderm also undergo differentiation when exposed to analogs of cyclic AMP. Cyclic AMP appears to inhibit cell division and cause blockage of cells in the G_1 phase of the cell cycle. Blockage of cell division at this phase has been thought to allow expression of the differentiated phenotype, so it remains unclear as to what extent cyclic AMP is directly involved in differentiation. Cyclic GMP levels often increase early in the G_1 phase, and elevations of cyclic GMP have been proposed to be a positive signal and elevations of cyclic AMP a negative signal in controlling cell division and growth of cultured cells (cf. Rudland *et al.*, 1974; Strada and Pledger, 1975).

Morphological differentiation of neuroma and neuronal cells appears to be dependent on synthesis of new protein and presence of microtubules and microfilaments. Cyclic AMP-dependent mechanisms have been proposed to stabilize microtubules and thereby favor morphological differentiation (see Section 4.2.6). The differentiation of neuroblastoma cells as affected by cyclic AMP mechanisms and other factors has been reviewed in detail (Prasad and Kumar, 1974; Prasad, 1975; Prasad *et al.*, 1975d). Prasad (1975) has proposed that a mutation leading to increases in phosphodiesterase activity in neurons is a primary event in development of neuroblastoma cells.

Studies on differentiation in the various cultured cells provide evidence suggestive of a role for cyclic AMP in the process of maturation and assembly of the central nervous system. These studies, however, appear less relevant to the role of cyclic AMP in the mature, fully developed brain unless such cyclic AMP-dependent mechanisms are involved in the formation of new intracellular connections or in regenerative processes after trauma.

4.2.1 Neuroblastoma Cells

Analogs of cyclic AMP such as dibutyryl cyclic AMP and 8-benzylthio cyclic AMP, prostaglandin E_1, high concentrations of prostaglandin A_1, and phosphodiesterase inhibitors inhibit growth (cell division) in neuroblastoma cells and cause morphological differentiation consisting primarily of the extension of medium to long neuritic processes (Furmanski *et al.*, 1971; Prasad and Hsie, 1971; Lim and Mitsunobu, 1972; Prasad, 1972a,b; Prasad and Sheppard, 1972b; Prasad and Vernadakis, 1972; Monard *et al.*, 1973; Prasad *et al.*, 1972, 1973a,b; Prasad and Mandal, 1973; Sheppard and Prasad, 1973; Adolphe *et al.*, 1974; Bondy *et al.*, 1974; Chalazonitis and Greene, 1974; Schubert *et al.*, 1974; Truding *et al.*, 1974; Glazer and Schneider, 1975; Ledig *et al.*, 1975; Prasad, 1975; Prasad and Kumar, 1975; Steinbach and Schubert, 1975; Zornetzer and Stein, 1975; Laug *et al.*, 1976). Cyclic AMP, cyclic GMP, dibutyryl cyclic GMP, ATP, ADP, AMP, and butyrate inhibited cell growth but were ineffective in eliciting differentiation. Butyrate did elevate cyclic AMP levels in neuroblastoma cells. Cyclic GMP did not prevent the differentiation elicited by cyclic AMP (Miller and Ruddle, 1974). The phosphodiesterase inhibitors, papaverine and RO 20-1724, were generally effective in eliciting differentiation, while theophylline was not particularly effective. It should be noted that papaverine inhibits both cyclic AMP- and cyclic GMP-phosphodiesterases, while RO 20-1724 inhibits effectively only cyclic AMP-phosphodiesterases (see Section 2.3.11). Acetylcholine, an agent which in neuroblastoma cells often depresses cyclic AMP levels and elevates cyclic GMP, has been reported to elicit neuritic outgrowths in mouse neuroblastoma cells (Harkins *et al.*, 1972). Most studies on differentiation of neuroblastoma cells have been with lines from mouse tumors. Dibutyryl cyclic AMP was reported to cause differentiation of human neuroblastoma cells (MacIntyre *et al.*, 1972).

Differentiation was reported to be elicited in human neuroblastoma cells by dibutyryl cyclic AMP, prostaglandin E_1, and phosphodiesterase inhibitors (Prasad and Kumar, 1975; Prasad et al., 1975d). In addition to causing differentiation, papaverine and RO 20-1724 had toxic effects. Cyclic AMP, cyclic GMP, and adenosine had no effect on growth or morphology of human glioma cells. Butyrate had mainly toxic effects, but it did cause morphological differentiation.

Various neuroblastoma cell lines showed differing degrees of differentiation in response to the presence of dibutyryl cyclic AMP, prostaglandin E_1, or RO 20-1724: Four cell lines differentiated readily in response to all three agents; one cell line responded only to dibutyryl cyclic AMP and RO 20-1724, another only to prostaglandin and RO 20-1724; two cell lines responded only to prostaglandin and one line only to RO 20-1724 (Prasad, 1972; Prasad et al., 1973c). Certain neuroblastoma cell lines, resistant to the differentiating effects of dibutyryl cyclic AMP or prostaglandin E_1, have been investigated in detail (Simantov and Sachs, 1975a,c). Increases in intracellular cyclic AMP elicited by prostaglandin or dibutyryl cyclic AMP were similar in resistant and nonresistant cells. The levels of cyclic AMP-dependent protein kinases and cyclic AMP binding proteins were not significantly less in the resistant cells. The binding proteins and cyclic AMP dependency of protein kinases from resistant cells were much more sensitive to heat inactivation.

Dibutyryl cyclic AMP did not elicit neuritic outgrowths in cultures of neuroblastoma cells attached to collagen (Miller and Levine, 1972). Rapid synchronized neuritic outgrowths occurred in these cells after treatment with collagenase. Various other treatments of neuroblastoma cells caused differentiation without, in some cases, having any apparent effect on cyclic AMP levels. X irradiation or the presence of factors released from glial or glioma cells elicited differentiation of neuroblastoma cells but did not measurably increase levels of cyclic AMP (Prasad and Vernadakis, 1972; Prasad et al., 1973a; Monard et al., 1973). Serum-free media elicited differentiation of neuroblastoma cells while elevating cyclic AMP levels in mouse neuroblastoma cells about twofold. Serum-free media did not increase cyclic AMP levels in human neuroblastoma cells (Prasad and Kumar, 1975). Lack of nutrients in serum-free medium presumably is responsible for inhibition of growth of cells under such conditions. 5-Bromodeoxyuridine caused differentiation of neuroblastoma cells, but its effect on cyclic AMP levels was not assessed (Schubert and Jacob, 1970). A later study demonstrated a twofold increase in cyclic AMP levels in neuroblastoma cells in the presence of the uridine derivative (Prasad et al., 1973a). Nerve growth factor elicited differentiation of neuroblastoma cells (Waris et al., 1973). Dimethylsulfoxide caused differentiation of neuroblastoma cells without increasing cyclic AMP levels (Kimhi et al., 1976).

Morphological differentiation of neuroblastoma cells elicited by dibutyryl cyclic AMP appeared irreversible, since such differentiated cells did not renew cell division or retract processes in the absence of the cyclic nucleotides (MacIntyre *et al.*, 1972; Prasad and Vernadakis, 1972). Within 1 day of drug-elicited differentiation the process was, however, reversible. Others have also reported that after a 1-day exposure dibutyryl cyclic AMP-elicited differentiation of neuroblastoma cells was reversible (Zornetzer and Stein, 1975). It appears likely that only during the initial stages of morphological differentiation is the process reversible in neuroblastoma cells.

Dibutyryl cyclic AMP enhanced neuritic outgrowth in enucleated neuroblastoma cells (Miller and Ruddle, 1974). The results clearly indicate that dibutyryl cyclic AMP has an effect on neuritic outgrowth independent of any effects on nuclear activity. Cycloheximide, an inhibitor of protein synthesis, prevented both neuritic outgrowths and long-term elevations of cyclic AMP elicited by prostaglandin E_1 or RO 20-1724 in neuroblastoma cells while actinomycin, an inhibitor of RNA synthesis, had no effect (Lim and Mitsunobu, 1972; Prasad *et al.*, 1972; Sheppard and Prasad, 1973).

Neuroblastoma cells transplanted into denervated gastrocnemius muscles multiplied less rapidly than in innervated muscles, suggesting the release of trophic factors from the nerves that increase growth rate of these tumor cells or perhaps prevent differentiation (Batkia and Rayner, 1976).

4.2.2 Glioma Cells

Dibutyryl cyclic AMP, catecholamines, prostaglandin E_1, and phosphodiesterase inhibitors such as papaverine and RO 20-1724 have been reported to inhibit growth and elicit morphological changes in glioma cells (Lim and Mitsunobu, 1972; Schwartz *et al.*, 1973; Hamprecht *et al.*, 1973; Daniels and Hamprecht, 1974; Edstrom *et al.*, 1974, 1975; Gibson *et al.*, 1974; Schubert *et al.*, 1974; Oey, 1975; Steinbach and Schubert, 1975; Sundarraj *et al.*, 1975; Thust and Warzok, 1975). The cells first became spindle shaped and then extended processes resulting in a star-shaped or stellate appearance. Process formation elicited by dibutyryl cyclic AMP in glioma cells appeared to involve "shrinkage" of cytoplasm, while process formation in neuroblastoma cells had occurred mainly by "extension" (Steinbach and Schubert, 1975). Butyrate and theophylline had little or no effect on morphology of the glioma cells. These studies have been mainly with rat glioma cells, but dibutyryl cyclic AMP has been reported to elicit morphological differentiation in mouse glioma cells (Sundarraj *et al.*, 1975). Dibutyryl cyclic AMP and theophylline had mainly toxic effects on human glioma cells (MacIntyre *et al.*, 1972). In rat glioma cells the morphological differentiation elicited by (nor)epinephrine, dopamine, and histamine was blocked by propranolol (Oey, 1975; Schlegel and Oey, 1975). The blockade by the β-antagonist suggests that all of these diverse amines at the concentration tested, 100 μM, activated a β-adrenergic receptor.

Dibutyryl cyclic AMP and papaverine have in one study been reported to elicit morphological changes in rat glioma cells only with low density cultures (Gibson *et al.*, 1974). Papaverine was relatively toxic. Dibutyryl cyclic AMP or prostaglandin E_1 elicited a star-shaped morphology and formation of long processes within 1 hr on glioma cells already spindle shaped after culture in serum-free medium (Edstrom *et al.*, 1974). These morphological changes occurred much more slowly in normal glioma cells.

Certain agents elicited differentiation of glioma cells without apparently altering cyclic AMP levels. Thus, 5-bromodeoxyuridine had little effect on cyclic AMP levels in glioma cells but did cause differentiation of cells, both in nonconfluent and confluent cultures (Schwartz *et al.*, 1973). The phosphodiesterase inhibitor, isobutylmethylxanthine (referred to as RO 20-7222), and N^6-substituted adenines caused differentiation of glioma cells but had no apparent effect on levels of cyclic AMP (Edstrom *et al.*, 1975). Incubation in serum-free medium resulted in a spindle-shaped or star-shaped morphology in glioma cells (Edstrom *et al.*, 1974; Thust and Warzok, 1975) but had no effect on cyclic AMP levels (see Section 3.5.2). Absence of magnesium ions in the medium elicited differentiation of glioma cells (cited in Edstrom *et al.*, 1975).

The morphological differentiation elicited by catecholamines and phosphodiesterase inhibitors reversed within about 24 hr, while that elicited by prostaglandin did not reverse appreciably until after 72 hr (Edstrom *et al.*, 1975). In another study the norepinephrine-elicited morphological changes in rat glioma cells were also reported to be reversible; all of the cells having regained a normal flattened shape within 8 hr after exposure to the amine (Oey, 1975). After one treatment with norepinephrine the cells were refractory to norepinephrine-elicited differentiation for at least 60 hr.

Norepinephrine elicited morphological differentiation of both normal and enucleated glioma cells (Oey, 1975). As had been the case with neuroblastoma cells, cycloheximide inhibited the induced outgrowth of processes in glioma cells, while actinomycin had no effect (Edstrom *et al.*, 1974).

4.2.3 Hybrid Cells

Neuroblastoma–glioma hybrid cells developed in the presence of dibutyryl cyclic AMP remarkable neuritic processes and clear and dense core vesicles similar to those seen, respectively, in cholinergic and adrenergic cells (Daniels and Hamprecht, 1974; Hamprecht *et al.*, 1974).

4.2.4 Fetal Cells

Cultured fetal rat brain cells underwent morphological differentiation into multipolar cells which resemble mature astrocytes when exposed to mono- or dibutyryl cyclic AMP or to a dialyzed soluble protein from brain homogenates (Lim et al., 1973; Shapiro, 1973). Prostaglandin E_1 had no effect, and norepinephrine was not tested. Dibutyryl cyclic AMP, serum-free conditions, and to a lesser extent theophylline elicited morphological differentiation of cultured glial cells from newborn rats (Moonen et al., 1975, 1976). The effects were markedly dependent on the composition of the culture media. Cells differentiated by exposure to dibutyryl cyclic AMP resembled mature astrocytes with star-shaped morphology and long processes. The processes contained a highly ordered system of microfilaments. Differentiation by dibutyryl cyclic AMP was only partially reversible.

The effect of dibutyryl cyclic AMP on neural differentiation of explants of chick ectoderm was ascertained using as immunofluorescent assay with antisera specific to antigens from chick brain (Bjerre, 1974). The cyclic AMP derivative significantly increased the fraction of explants yielding neural antigens. Theophylline had primarily toxic effects. Neural differentiation was increased in explants of amphibian ectoderm during culture in the presence of dibutyryl cyclic AMP, 8-bromo cyclic AMP, and a combination of theophylline and cyclic AMP (Wahn et al., 1975a). Differentiation was assessed by microscopic examination of the cultured explants. The cyclic AMP analogs increased the extent of differentiation of cells to neurons, melanophores, and glia. Identification of neurons in these dibutyryl cyclic AMP-differentiated cultures has been discussed (Dichter, 1975, Wahn et al., 1975b).

4.2.5 Ganglia and Peripheral Neurons

Dibutyryl cyclic AMP elicited formation and growth of neuritic processes in cultured dorsal root ganglion cells from rat or mouse (Haas et al., 1972). Cycloheximide inhibited neurite elongation. Butyrate stimulated neurite extension while theophylline did not, though the latter agent did increase intracellular levels of cyclic AMP.

Cyclic AMP and various analogs increased neuritic outgrowths in cultured dorsal root sensory ganglion cells from chick embryos (Hier et al., 1972, 1973; Roisen et al., 1972b,c,d,e, 1975; Frazier et al., 1973; Roisen and Murphy, 1973). Cyclic GMP inhibited neuritic outgrowths. Butyrate stimulated neuritic outgrowths while theophylline had no effect. Cyclic AMP mechanisms did not appear to be involved in the neurite extension elicited in chick ganglia by nerve growth factor (Hier et al., 1972, 1973;

Frazier *et al.*, 1973). Thus, nerve growth factor did not at any time elevate cyclic AMP levels in the cultured ganglia and did not activate adenylate cyclases in homogenates. The outgrowth of neuritic processes by nerve growth factor was not potentiated by theophylline. In rat superior cervical ganglia nerve growth factor did elicit an accumulation of cyclic AMP (Nikodijevic *et al.*, 1975). Dibutyryl cyclic AMP did not stimulate neurite extension in chick sympathetic ganglia (Frazier *et al.*, 1973), in contrast to its stimulatory effect on chick sensory ganglia.

After crushing or hemisection of rat sciatic nerve, dibutyryl cyclic AMP, injected intramuscularly near the site of the lesion, greatly accelerated restoration of muscle innervation by this nerve as measured by return of sensorimotor function (Pichichero *et al.*, 1973). The large increase in cyclic AMP observed near the site of crushing of rabbit sciatic nerve (Appenzeller and Palmer, 1972) might possibly serve a function in the normal regenerative processes. Cyclic AMP levels increased distal to the crush at a time prior to Schwann cell proliferation.

4.2.6 Role of Microtubules

A unifying theory on the mechanisms involved in cyclic AMP-elicited changes in cell morphology is that the cyclic nucleotide either enhances formation of microtubules or stabilizes microtubules. Evidence for stabilization of microtubule systems in tissue slices by cyclic AMP has been reported (Gillespie, 1971). Thus, a cyclic AMP–dibutyryl cyclic AMP combination appeared to inhibit binding of colchicine to subunits of microtubules, suggesting that the cyclic nucleotides had shifted the equilibrium between subunits and microtubules by stabilizing the microtubules. The technique, using radioactive colchicine and rat pancreatic, splenic, and liver slices, was based on measurement of the extent of binding of colchicine to soluble protein, presumably depolymerized subunits of the microtubules. Calcium ions greatly decreased the extent of binding. Cyclic AMP and the dibutyryl derivative decreased binding, particularly in the absence of calcium ions. The observation that dibutyryl cyclic AMP reversed the inhibition of the neurite extension of chick embryo sensory ganglia elicited by a colchicine derivative that interacts with microtubule subunits (Roisen *et al.*, 1972c) is compatible with the hypothesis of a cyclic AMP-dependent formation or stabilization of microtubules. Conversely, agents such as vinblastine and colchicine which destabilize microtubules prevented cyclic AMP-dependent differentiation of neuroblastoma cells (Sheppard and Prasad, 1973). Colchicine, vinblastine, and concanavalin A both inhibited and reversed the neuritic extension elicited by dibutyryl cyclic AMP in neuroblastoma cells (Simantov *et al.*, 1975). It was proposed that concanavalin A, on binding to the surface of neuroblastoma cells, interfered with assembly of cytoplasmic microtubules. Vinblastine completely prevented and reversed morphological changes elicited in glioma cells by dibutyryl cyclic AMP or prostaglandin E_1 (Edstrom *et al.*, 1974), while colchicine both inhibited and reversed norepinephrine-elicited differentiation of glioma cells (Oey, 1975). Dibutyryl cyclic AMP was unable to reverse the inhibitory effects of cytochalasin, an agent which interacts with the small microfilaments rather than the microtubule subunits (Roisen and Murphy, 1973). Cytochalasin B did, however, prevent cyclic AMP dependent differentiation of neuroblastoma cells (Sheppard and Prasad, 1973).

Differentiated neuroblastoma cells no longer retracted neuritic processes in the cold after exposure to dibutyryl cyclic AMP (Kirkland and Burton, 1972). This result is also compatible with stabilization of microtubules by the cyclic AMP analog. Variation in concentrations of extracellular calcium ions had no effect on the stabilization of neuritic processes by dibutyryl cyclic AMP.

Levels of tubulin in neuroblastoma cells were similar in undifferentiated cells and in cells differentiated by culture in serum-free media (Morgan and Seeds, 1975). Thus, neither differentiation nor the increase in cyclic AMP levels under the latter conditions had any effect on levels of tubulin. Glioma cells contained much less tubulin than neuroblastoma cells. Nerve growth factor but not dibutyryl cyclic AMP stimulated synthesis of tubulin in cultured chick dorsal root ganglion cells (Hier *et al.*, 1972). Presumably, nerve growth factor elicited neuritic outgrowths at least in part by such an enhancement in synthesis of microtubule protein. These results are at least consonant with the proposal that dibutyryl cyclic AMP elicited neuritic outgrowths by effects on stability rather than on levels of microtubules. The effects of dibutyryl cyclic AMP and theophylline on levels of microtubules and of microfilaments in cultured sympathetic ganglia have been investigated (Leonetti and Seite, 1975).

4.2.7 Trophic Factors

A role for cyclic AMP in trophic effects of glia on neurons (see Section 4.2.1) or neurons on glia, other neurons, or muscle has not been established. Dibutyryl cyclic AMP, theophylline, or extracts of sympathetic ganglia delayed reversal of differentiation and the subsequent increase in rates of multiplication of cultured smooth muscle cells (Chamley and Campbell, 1975). Muscle cells which were sympathetically innervated also remained differentiated for relatively long periods. It was proposed that trophic factors released from sympathetic neurons activated adenylate cyclase in muscle cells and thereby repressed differentiation. A combination of cyclic AMP and theophylline had an effect similar to nerve explants or homogenates in maintaining cholinesterase levels and end plate structure of newt muscles in organ culture (Lentz, 1972). The results suggested a role for cyclic AMP in trophic effects of nerves on muscle.

4.3 Membrane Phenomena

Putative neurotransmitters and neuromodulators that enhance levels of either cyclic AMP or cyclic GMP in brain tissue often have profound depressant or stimulatory effects on spontaneous firing rates of central neurons. A variety of studies have implicated formation of cyclic AMP in the depression of central neuronal firing, in particular by norepinephrine but also by dopamine, serotonin, histamine, and adenosine. Depression of firing of central neurons by cyclic AMP-dependent mechanisms is accompanied by a hyperpolarization of the membrane. The biogenic amines often, however, have stimulatory effects on firing of certain neurons. Thus, identification of discrete populations of neurons is fundamental to any study of the function of a particular amine. This is a difficult task in many brain regions. Cerebellar Purkinje cells are readily identified by their firing pattern and receive a well-defined noradrenergic input, and cyclic AMP-mechanisms have, therefore, been studied in detail in these cells. Formation of cyclic GMP has been implicated in the stimulatory effects of acetylcholine on central neurons. Evidence for the involvement of cyclic AMP in the neuronal hyperpolarization elicited by biogenic amines in sympathetic ganglia has been provided. Although cyclic AMP has been very strongly implicated in the electrophysiological responses of neurons to norepinephrine and other amines, it is difficult to preclude other mechanisms such as a calcium-dependent hyperpolarization resulting from stimulation of calcium translocation by the biogenic amine. In cultured cells, effects of cyclic AMP on membrane properties and membrane constituents can be studied, but with neuroma cells, it is often difficult to delineate whether cyclic AMP mechanisms are directly involved or whether observed changes result from cyclic AMP-elicited differentiation. Although roles for cyclic AMP and cyclic GMP as the inhibitory and stimulatory "second messengers" which regulate firing rates and excitability of neurons have been proposed, certainly other effects of cyclic nucleotides on membranal properties and events probably pertain. The apparent involvement of cyclic AMP in transmitter–release phenomena in motor neurons and sympathetic neurons and in mobilization of calcium ions opens up the possibility that similar phenomena in the central nervous system may involve cyclic AMP. Cyclic nucleotides have also been reported to affect membrane phenomena in a variety of nonneuronal cells (cf. review by Greengard, 1976).

4.3.1 Central Neurons

Cerebellar Purkinje Cells

A role for norepinephrine-elicited increases in cyclic AMP levels in the modulation of spontaneous electrical activity in cerebellar Purkinje cells has been firmly established by the extensive studies of Bloom, Hoffer, Siggins, and co-workers with rat, rabbit, and other species (Hoffer *et al.,* 1969, 1970, 1971a,b,c, 1972; Siggins *et al.,* 1969, 1971a,b,c,d,e, 1973; Woodward *et al.,* 1971; Bloom *et al.,* 1972a,b,c; Bloom *et al.,* 1975). These and other studies on control of neuronal activity by neuromodulators and cyclic AMP have been comprehensively reviewed (Bloom, 1975). The cerebellar Purkinje cells of rat and other species normally exhibit (1) irregular high-frequency bursts of electrical spike activity due to excitation by climbing fibers, (2) rapid irregular single action potentials, and (3) long pauses of nonspike activity. A variety of agents slow the discharge rates in these cells when administered microiontophoretically. These include tyramine, amphetamine, histamine, serotonin, γ-aminobutyrate, glycine, and the catecholamines, (nor)epinephrine and isoproterenol (Hoffer *et al.,* 1971a; Siggins *et al.,* 1971b; Bloom *et al.,* 1972a). The inhibitory effects of norepinephrine on discharge rates were prevented by the β-antagonist, sotalol, but not by another β-antagonist, nifenalol (IPNEA), or by lysergic acid diethylamide. Fluphenazine and α-flupenthixol were potent antagonists of norepinephrine and isoproterenol-elicited inhibition of Purkinje neurons (Freedman and Hoffer, 1975; Skolnick *et al.,* 1976; Hoffer *et al.,* 1976). Fluphenazine did not affect the inhibition elicited by cyclic AMP or by γ-aminobutyrate. Dibutyryl cyclic AMP and cyclic AMP had inhibitory effects similar to those of norepinephrine, but more rapid in onset. Both the cyclic AMP derivatives and the catecholamines increased the frequency of long pauses in spike activity (Hoffer *et al.,* 1970). Surprisingly, cyclic GMP had a similar inhibitory effect (Hoffer *et al.,* 1971b). ATP was excitatory, while 5'-AMP had no effect (see p. 248). After norepinephrine there was a delay of from 5 to 30 sec, while with the cyclic nucleotides the rate of response and the recovery latencies were usually faster. Cyclic AMP inhibited discharge of about 50 to 70% of Purkinje cells in cerebellum of rat, rabbit, cat, pigeon, and frog. γ-Aminobutyrate, another depressant of Purkinje cell activity, randomized the single-spike discharges and often abolished the climbing fiber bursts in marked contrast to the effects of amines and cyclic AMP.

Serotoninergic innervation of cerebellar Purkinje cells has not been demonstrated, yet serotonin had an inhibitory effect on firing of such cells in rat cerebellum (Bloom *et al.,* 1972c). Cerebellar granule cells for which tentative evidence indicative of serotoninergic innervation has been obtained were excited rather than inhibited by serotonin.

The inhibitory effects of cyclic AMP, cyclic GMP, and norepinephrine were potentiated by theophylline and its ethylenediamine salt, aminophylline, and by papaverine (Siggins *et al.*, 1971e). The methylxanthines, either on parenteral or iontophoretic application, had modest inhibitory effects on discharge rates of Purkinje cells. Nicotinate, an agent which in some systems appears to activate phosphodiesterases, reduced on iontophoretic administration the inhibitory effects of norepinephrine and cyclic AMP (Hoffer *et al.*, 1971b; Siggins *et al.*, 1971b).

Prostaglandin E_1 had effects opposite to those of norepinephrine and cyclic AMP. Thus it increased the rate of spontaneous discharge of Purkinje cells by reducing the frequency of long pauses in spike activity. Prostaglandins of the E series reversed the inhibitory effects of norepinephrine and methylxanthines but did not prevent the inhibitory effects of γ-aminobutyrate or cyclic AMP (Hoffer *et al.*, 1969; Siggins *et al.*, 1969, 1971b,c) (Figure 17). Prostaglandin $F_{2\alpha}$ did not antagonize the inhibitory effect of norepinephrine. The mechanism whereby prostaglandins inhibit the norepinephrine response is uncertain; direct effects on adenylate cyclases, phosphodiesterase, or membrane permeability cannot be excluded.

Electrical stimulation of the locus coeruleus in the dorsal medullary brain stem with its afferent tracts to the cerebellum resulted in a decrease in the discharge rates of Purkinje cells (Siggins *et al.*, 1971d; Bloom *et al.*, 1972b; Hoffer *et al.*, 1972). The phosphodiesterase inhibitor, papaverine, potentiated the inhibitory effects of locus coeruleus stimulation. Parenteral fluphenazine and α-flupenthixol antagonized the inhibition of Purkinje cells elicited by stimulation of the locus coeruleus, but not the inhibition elicited by stimulation of basket and stellate cell parallel fibers (Freedman and Hoffer, 1975). Locus coeruleus stimulation was not effective in rats that have been pretreated either with agents such as reserpine or α-methyl-*p*-tyrosine which will deplete norepinephrine in presynaptic terminals of brain, or with 6-hydroxydopamine, an agent which destroys noradrenergic terminals. Administration of dopa to bypass the blockade of norepinephrine synthesis in α-methyl-*p*-tyrosine-treated rats restored the inhibitory effects of locus coeruleus stimulation (Bloom *et al.*, 1972b). After 6-hydroxydopamine treatment, the spontaneous discharge rate of Purkinje cells was increased due to reductions in the frequency of long pauses in electrical activity (Hoffer *et al.*, 1971c). The results strongly suggest that norepinephrine, released from noradrenergic terminals originating from neurons in the locus coeruleus, regulates spontaneous electrical activity in Purkinje cells by a mechanism involving norepinephrine-elicited accumulation of cyclic AMP within the Purkinje cell. Other results were consonant with this interpretation. Thus, desipramine, which inhibits presynaptic uptake of catecholamines, potentiated the inhibitory effect of norepinephrine on Purkinje cells but had no effect in 6-hydroxydopamine-treated rats (Hoffer

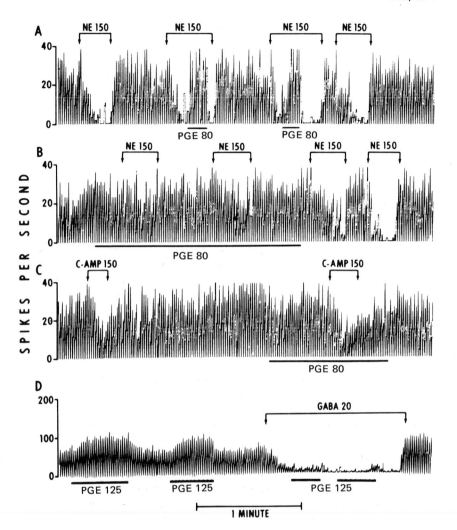

Figure 17. Effect of norepinephrine (NE), cyclic AMP (C-AMP), γ-aminobutyrate (GABA), and prostaglandins of the E series (PGE) on rates of spontaneous discharge of rat cerebellar Purkinje cells. Numbers represent the ejection current in nanoamperes. Duration of drug application is indicated by arrows; for prostaglandin, by lines beneath the records. (Modified from Hoffer *et al.*, 1969, *Science,* copyright American Association for the Advancement of Science.)

et al., 1971a). Norepinephrine, tyramine, amphetamine, cyclic AMP, and methylxanthines had inhibitory effects in 6-hydroxydopamine-treated rats. Amphetamine at high ejection currents has significant local anesthetic activity which might cause direct depression of neurons (see Bunney and Aghajanian, 1976, and references therein). Prostaglandin E_1 no longer increased spontaneous discharge rates in 6-hydroxydopamine-treated rats but still antagonized the effect of norepinephrine (Hoffer *et al.*, 1969; Siggins *et al.*, 1971c).

In neonatal rats which have not yet established synaptic innervation of Purkinje cells, glutamate had excitatory effects on such cells, while norepinephrine, serotonin, cyclic AMP, and γ-aminobutyrate had inhibitory effects (Woodward *et al.*, 1971). Prostaglandin antagonized the response of Purkinje cells to norepinephrine in the neonatal rat. Purkinje cells in neonatal rats appeared to be much more sensitive to the inhibitory effects of norepinephrine and cyclic AMP (Woodward *et al.*, 1971). Any of a number of factors might be responsible for the heightened sensitivity in neonates, and no conclusions as to the presence or absence of hyperresponsive cyclic AMP-generating systems in Purkinje cells prior to synaptic innervation are warranted.

Purkinje cells in cerebella of rats of which granule, basket, and stellate interneurons have been eliminated by neonatal X irradiation showed normal chemosensitivity, that is, inhibition by norepinephrine, cyclic AMP, serotonin, and γ-aminobutyrate and excitation by glutamate (Woodward *et al.*, 1974). Inhibitory effects of norepinephrine were blocked by sotalol; excitatory effects of acetylcholine by atropine.

With an immunofluorescent technique for the histological detection of cyclic AMP it was shown that either topical application of norepinephrine to cerebellum or electrical stimulation of the locus coeruleus elicited a striking increase in fluorescence of the cerebellar Purkinje cells (Siggins *et al.*, 1973). Fluorescence of the granule cell layer was unchanged. Other inhibitory agents such as glycine, serotonin, histamine, and γ-aminobutyrate had no effect on fluorescence of Purkinje cells. It was not ascertained whether prostaglandin E_1 prevented the norepinephrine-elicited increase in fluorescence of Purkinje cells. In 6-hydroxydopamine-treated rats, stimulation of the locus coeruleus did not elicit an increase in Purkinje cell fluorescence.

Inhibitory agents such as γ-aminobutyrate, norepinephrine, cyclic AMP, and dibutyryl cyclic AMP and stimulation of locus coeruleus all elicited hyperpolarization of Purkinje cells (Hoffer *et al.*, 1971b; Siggins *et al.*, 1971d,e). Except for γ-aminobutyrate, this hyperpolarization was accompanied by an increase in membrane resistance; γ-aminobutyrate caused a decrease in resistance (Figure 18). The mechanism of the change in membrane conductance elicited by cyclic AMP-dependent mechanisms is unknown. Changes in chloride ion conductances did not appear to be involved. A specific phosphorylation of membrane proteins associated with ionic channels catalyzed by cyclic AMP-dependent protein kinases is an attractive hypothesis. Such phosphorylations might result in activation of Na^+,K^+-ATPase (see p. 255) or a decrease in resting conductance for sodium or calcium ions. It should be noted that calcium ions slowed

MEMBRANE POTENTIAL CHANGE   RESISTANCE CHANGE

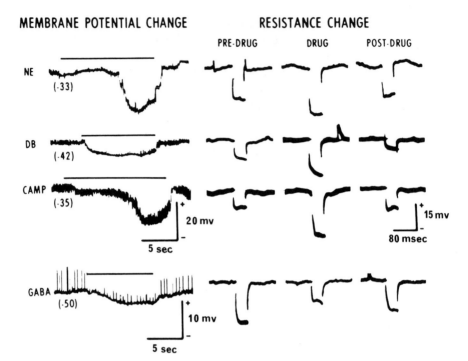

Figure 18. Effect of norepinephrine (NE), dibutyryl cyclic AMP (DB), cyclic AMP (CAMP), and γ-aminobutyrate (GABA) on membrane potential and membrane resistance of rat cerebellar Purkinje cells. Numbers in parentheses are resting membrane potential in millivolts. Solid lines above recording indicate the duration of drug application by ejection currents of 100 to 150 nA. Input resistance was measured with brief 1-nA current (1 mV = MΩ). (Modified from Siggins et al., 1971, Science, copyright American Association for the Advancement of Science.)

spontaneous discharge rates in Purkinje cells, while metal chelators increased discharge rates (Hoffer et al., 1971b; Siggins et al., 1971b, see pp. 256–258).

Another laboratory, in studies with perhaps less definitive identification of Purkinje cells and with pentobarbital instead of halothane anesthesia (cf. Siggins et al., 1971a, and discussion in Siggins et al., 1971c, and Bloom et al., 1974) demonstrated inhibitory effects of norepinephrine, but not of cyclic AMP or the dibutyryl derivative on cerebellar Purkinje cells (Godfraind and Pumain, 1971, 1972). Parenteral administration of aminophylline did not appear to potentiate the effectiveness of norepinephrine or cyclic AMP. In these studies, glutamate was frequently used to increase spontaneous discharge rates of the Purkinje cells. A third laboratory also could not confirm an effective inhibition of Purkinje cells by cyclic AMP (Lake and Jordan, 1974). In these studies with spontaneously firing Purkinje cells, cyclic AMP depressed only 20% of the tested cells, while exciting a slightly larger percentage. Cyclic AMP has a rather low transfer number for microinotophoretic release as the anion and, in addition, large variations in amount of release both with one pipette and with different pipettes have been observed (Bloom et al., 1974; Shoemaker et al., 1975). Such variations and low or zero rates of release from micropipettes might have contributed to frequent absence of effects of cyclic AMP in some microiontophoretic studies of central neurons. In addition, both permeability and rapid metabolism by phosphodiesterase represent large barriers to the intracellular action of iontophoretic cyclic AMP. Bloom (1974, 1975) has provided detailed critiques on biological, pharmacological, and technical problems inherent to microiontophoretic studies of central neurons, with particular emphasis on studies concerned with the role of cyclic AMP in the norepinephrine-elicited inhibition of central neurons. These include, from a biological standpoint, the positive identification of neurons and their study under conditions as nearly physiological as possible; that is, not excited by another agent and fully recovered from prior microiontophoretic applications of other drugs. Pharmacologically, the interpretation of the effects of so-called specific agents should not be done without consideration of possible indirect or nonspecific effects either directly on the neuron or more generally on other inputs to the test neuron. Technically, the effects of transport constants, pH, stability, metabolic and physical barriers, and variability in pipettes both in initial, sustained, or repeated ejection periods on the observed responses to each individual agent should be considered.

The ability of cyclic AMP and eleven derivatives to inhibit firing of cerebellar Purkinje cells has been assessed using both microiontophoresis and electroosmosis (Siggins and Henriksen, 1975). The three most active derivatives, 8-amino, 8-benzylthio and 8-p-chlorophenylthio cyclic AMP, inhibited 80 to 92% of the tested cells. The activities of the other cyclic nucleotides were as follows: cyclic AMP, N^6-monobutyryl > 8-bromo, 8-isopropylthio > 8-methylthio, dibutyryl >> 8-methylamino, 2'-O-monobutyryl, 2'-deoxy. The last three least active derivatives actually excited over 50% of the tested cells. The ability of the various cyclic nucleotides to inhibit Purkinje cells correlated with their potency as activators of brain cyclic AMP-dependent protein kinases. Clearly, in spite of other factors such as microiontophoretic transfer numbers, membrane permeability, and activity as substrates for phosphodiesterases, cyclic AMP analogs which are potent activators of protein kinase were very effective inhibitors of Purkinje cells. Analogs with very low activity towards protein kinase tended to excite cells, suggesting that for any analog its effect is a result of both inhibition through activation of cyclic AMP-dependent kinases and excitation through some other mechanism. Studies from another laboratory indicated that Purkinje cells were depressed by 5'-AMP, ADP, ATP, 2',3'-cyclic AMP, 2'-AMP, 3'-AMP, and adenosine (Kostopoulos *et al.,* 1975). 3',5'-Cyclic AMP was less effective as a depressant. The low efficacy of cyclic AMP relative to 2',3'-cyclic AMP is difficult to rationalize in terms of low transfer numbers or lack of release or uptake of only one of the two cyclic nucleotides. Metabolic differences might, however, still pertain. Most of these adenine nucleotides including cyclic AMP stimulate accumulation of intracellular cyclic AMP in brain slices, presumably after hydrolysis to adenosine (see Section 3.1.2).

Norepinephrine, cyclic AMP, and the phosphodiesterase inhibitors, papaverine > aminophylline and caffeine, decreased firing rates of Purkinje cells in explants of rat cerebellum by increasing the number of long interspike intervals (Gahwiler, 1976). Combinations of these agents had synergistic inhibitory effects on cell firing. Butyrate derivatives of cyclic AMP had no effect even at 1 mM. Lead ions, which are known to inhibit adenylate cyclases, had inconsistent effects on norepinephrine-elicited depression of firing rates (cf. Nathanson and Bloom, 1975).

Cerebrum

Norepinephrine inhibits the firing of certain neurons in most brain regions, but it is as yet unclear as to whether these inhibitory effects are uniformly mediated by cyclic AMP-dependent mechanisms. Norepinephrine, serotonin, and histamine can have either inhibitory or stimulatory effects on firing of central neurons, thus making identification of neuronal cell types of great importance. It appears not unlikely that cyclic AMP-dependent mechanisms will be found to be involved in many inhibitory responses of central neurons to neurotransmitters and cyclic GMP-dependent mechanisms in excitatory responses (see below).

Cyclic AMP or dibutyryl cyclic AMP has been reported as inhibiting firing of central neurons from a variety of species including rat, cat, pigeon, and frog (see Bloom *et al.,* 1975). Norepinephrine inhibited the firing rate of a high percentage of cerebral cortical neurons in rat, cat, and guinea pig (Jordan *et al.,* 1972a; Lake *et al.,* 1972, 1973). Octopamine has been stated to have only weak depressant activity on cortical neurons sensitive to inhibition by norepinephrine (Phyllis, 1974a). Dibutyryl cyclic AMP had inhibitory effects in only a rather small percentage of cortical neurons of rat, cat, and guinea pig and this was interpreted as indicative of a lack of involvement of cyclic AMP in the response to norepinephrine. Studies on potentiation of norepinephrine effects by phosphodiesterase inhibitors were difficult because of the intrinsic depressant activity of aminophylline and to a lesser extent of papaverine. The inhibitory effects of aminophylline were undiminished in 6-hydroxydopamine-treated rats, indicating that a methylxanthine-induced release of norepinephrine was not involved. Papaverine potentiated the inhibitory effects of norepinephrine in a high percentage of cells. The inhibitory effects of aminophylline were blocked in all cat cortical neurons and in the majority of rat and guinea pig neurons by prostaglandin. Indeed, prostaglandin in these studies appeared to be a more effective antagonist of aminophylline than of norepinephrine. In cat, prostaglandin antagonized the inhibitory effect of norepinephrine in less than one-half of the cells and was an even less effective antagonist in cortical cells of rat or guinea pig. In rat cerebral cortex or hippocampus, the inhibitory effects of norepinephrine on discharge rates of various neurons were antagonized by prostaglandin E_1 (Siggins *et al.,* 1971c). A β-antagonist, dichlorisoproterenol, very effectively antagonized the inhibitory effects of norepinephrine on cerebral neurons (Freedman *et al.,* 1975).

Imidazoles inhibit firing of cortical neurons and are known to activate phosphodiesterases, a process that should *decrease* cyclic AMP levels. The inhibitory effects of a variety of imidazoles on central neurons were, however, not at all related to the potency of such compounds as *in vitro* activators of phosphodiesterases (Godfraind *et al.,* 1973).

A variety of compounds such as norepinephrine, serotonin, dopamine, amphetamine, tyramine, and γ-aminobutyrate were found to inhibit the spontaneous firing of hippocampal pyramidal cells (Segal and Bloom, 1974a). The inhibitory effect of norepinephrine was antagonized by a β-adrenergic blocker, sotalol, but not by an α-blocker, dibenamine. Phentolamine and dichlorisoproterenol had direct depressant effects. Cyclic AMP and its butyryl derivatives consistently inhibited firing of hippocampal pyramidal cells. The phosphodiesterase inhibitor, papaverine, potentiated the inhibitory effect of norepinephrine. At higher ejection currents, papaverine had direct depressant effects on the neurons as did the less potent phosphodiesterase inhibitor, aminophylline. Prostaglandins of the E series antagonized the effects of norepinephrine in less than half the cells tested. In this regard, the hippocampal pyramidal cells differ from the cerebellar Purkinje cells, where prostaglandins were effective antagonists of norepinephrine. Desipramine, an inhibitor of norepinephrine uptake, potentiated the effect of norepinephrine in normal, but not in 6-hydroxydopamine-treated rats. At higher ejection currents, desipramine had direct depressant effects on hippocampal neurons. In 6-hydroxydopamine-treated rats, the hippocampal cells fired more rapidly and both their sensitivity to norepinephrine and the duration of inhibition by norepinephrine were increased. The inhibitory effects of serotonin were not altered and surprisingly amphetamine, a norepinephrine-releasing agent, was still effective in 6-hydroxydopamine-treated rats. Electrical stimulation of the dorsal locus coeruleus with its efferent tracts to the hippocampus resulted in a decrease in firing of the pyramidal cells (Segal and Bloom, 1974b). The inhibitory effect of locus coeruleus stimulation on hippocampal cells was potentiated by a phospho-diesterase inhibitor, papaverine, and by an inhibitor of norepinephrine reuptake, desipramine, was blocked by sotalol, and was absent in reserpine plus α-methyl-p-tyrosine- or 6-hydroxydopamine-treated animals. Prosta-glandin E_1 antagonized the response to locus coeruleus stimulation in about one-half the cells. Bicuculline, an effective antagonist of the inhibitory effects of γ-aminobutyrate in hippocampal neurons, did not alter the inhibitory effects of locus coeruleus stimulation. The results in these pyramidal neurons were clearly consonant with a role of cyclic AMP in the inhibitory effects of norepinephrine.

Pyramidal tract neurons of the rat cerebral cortex have recently been shown to be inhibited by cyclic AMP and butyryl derivatives and to be excited by cyclic GMP (Stone *et al.*, 1975, Figure 19). Norepinephrine inhibited the firing of these neurons, while acetylcholine via a muscarinic receptor enhanced their firing. It was proposed that cyclic AMP and cyclic GMP mediated the responses to norepinephrine and acetylcholine, respectively. The response to norepinephrine was stated to be potentiated by a phosphodiesterase inhibitor, papaverine, and to be blocked by prostaglandin E_1. Cyclic GMP excited about 50% of rat cerebral cortical neurons. Another group reported that cyclic AMP and cyclic GMP inhibited about 50% of rat cortical neurons (Phyllis *et al.*, 1974).

Involvement of cyclic AMP mechanisms in the inhibitory effects of serotonin and histamine have not been established. The depressant effects of serotonin on central neurons have been reported to be antagonized by methysergide and sotalol, while excitatory effects of serotonin have been reported to be antagonized by methysergide and lysergic acid diethylamide (cf. Bloom *et al.*, 1972c). The latter compounds have direct depressant activity. The depressant effects of histamine on cerebral cortical neurons were antagonized by metiamide (Phillis *et al.*, 1975b). Metiamide did not antagonize the depressant effects of norepinephrine, dopamine, serotonin, or AMP (Phillis *et al.*, 1975b). Burimamide was less selective, and both of the H_2-antagonists blocked the excitatory effects of acetylcholine. H_1-Antagonists were relatively nonspecific antagonists of various inhibitors of neuronal firing (Phillis *et al.*, 1968).

Adenosine depressed the firing of various cerebral cortical neurons including corticospinal Betz cells (Phillis *et al.*, 1974, 1975a; Phillis and Kostopoulous, 1975). ATP, ADP, adenosine 5′-imidodiphosphate, 2′,3′-cyclic AMP, 2′-AMP, 3′-AMP, and 5′-AMP were also very effective depressants, as were the adenosine analogs, 2-chloroadenosine, 2′-deoxy-adenosine, and adenosine 5′-mononicotinate. Both control and glutamate-excited cortical neurons were inhibited by adenosine, ATP, ADP, AMP, and 2′,3′-cyclic AMP. In some instances, ATP had an initial excitatory effect on certain unidentified cortical neurons. 3′,5′-Cyclic AMP, cyclic

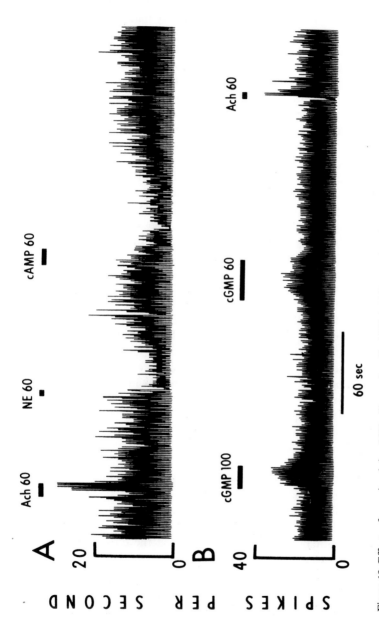

Figure 19. Effects of norepinephrine (NE), dibutyryl cyclic AMP (cAMP), cyclic GMP (cGMP), and acetylcholine (Ach) on rates of spontaneous discharge of rat cerebral cortical pyramidal tract neurons. Numbers represent the ejection current in nanoamperes. (Modified from Stone *et al.*, 1975), *Science*, copyright American Association for the Advancement of Science.)

GMP, GMP, GDP, GTP, IMP, ITP, 2'-deoxyadenosine 5'-phosphate, 8-bromoadenosine, inosine, guanosine, and adenine were much less effective depressants. Adenosine 5'-sulfate was completely inactive. The depressant activity of adenosine and 5'-AMP was potentiated by adenosine uptake inhibitors such as hexobendine and papaverine and antagonized by theophylline and caffeine. Hexobendine and papaverine had intrinsic depressant activity. Of the various compounds, 2-chloroadenosine appeared to be the most potent depressant and had a long duration of action. Although many of the adenine derivatives depressed cortical neurons and elevated cyclic AMP levels in cerebral cortical slices (see Table 5) there are a number of compounds for which this correlation does not pertain. Thus, 2'-deoxyadenosine, adenosine 5'-imidodiphosphate, and adenosine 5'-mononicotinate were effective depressants but had little effect on levels of cyclic AMP, while the converse is true for 3',5'-cyclic AMP, which was an ineffective depressant but did effectively elevate levels of cyclic AMP in brain slices, apparently after a prior hydrolysis to adenosine. Differences in rates of metabolic conversion of adenine nucleotides to adenosine or to inactive substances in the different experimental paradigms might explain some of these apparent inconsistencies. Furthermore, a slight partial agonist activity towards cyclic AMP-generating systems as observed in brain slices may still generate sufficient cyclic AMP to activate kinases in the intact neuron. Nonetheless, the potent depressant activity of 2',3'-cyclic AMP and the weak activity of 3',5'-cyclic AMP warrants further study.

Adenosine, AMP, ADP, and ATP inhibited the slow postsynaptic potential generated in a slice of guinea pig olfactory cortex upon stimulation of the innervating lateral olfactory tract fibers (Okada and Kuroda, 1975; Kuroda and Kobayashi, 1975; Kuroda *et al.*, 1976; Figure 20). Adenosine had no effect on the amplitude of the potential in presynaptic fibers. Cyclic AMP did not consistently inhibit postsynaptic potentials in the olfactory cortex, while inosine, guanosine, and GMP had no effect. The inhibition of postsynaptic potentials by adenosine was accompanied by an accumulation of cyclic AMP. ATP, ADP, and AMP also elicited accumulations of cyclic AMP. Theophylline blocked both the inhibition of postsynaptic potentials and the accumulation of cyclic AMP elicited by adenosine or adenine nucleotides. High concentrations of calcium ions antagonized adenosine-elicited inhibition of postsynaptic potentials and the concomitant accumulation of cyclic AMP. High concentrations of magnesium tended to antagonize the adenosine effects, but the inhibitions were not significant. Cysteate, a stimulant of cyclic AMP systems in cortical slices (Shimizu *et al.*, 1974) completely supressed the postsynaptic potentials elicited in olfactory cortex by stimulation of olfactory tract (Yamamoto and Matsui, 1976). It was suggested that this blockage was due to depolarization of postsynaptic neurons by the high concentrations of the excitatory amino acid, but the

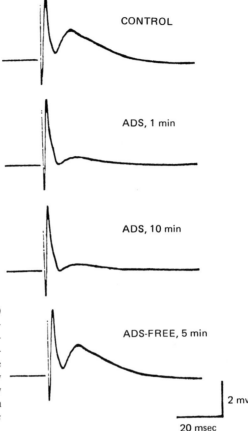

Figure 20. Effect of adenosine (ADS) on pre- and postsynaptic action potentials in olfactory tract fibers and olfactory cortical slices. Presynaptic potential was unaffected, while the postsynaptic N-wave was virtually completely and reversibly blocked by 100 μM adenosine. (Modified from Okada and Kuroda, 1975, *Proceedings of the Japanese Academy*.)

blockade might also have been due to "release" of adenosine (see Section 3.1.2).

In a slice of guinea pig superior colliculus, postsynaptic potentials elicited by stimulation of the innervating optic tract were not inhibited by adenosine or adenine nucleotides (Kuroda and Kobayshi, 1975). Serotonin and γ-aminobutyrate did inhibit postsynaptic potentials in the superior colliculus, but not in the olfactory cortex. Serotonin does markedly activate adenylate cyclases from superior colliculus (see Section 2.1.7).

Striatum

Dopamine released from terminals originating in the substantia nigra appears to act as an inhibitory neurotransmitter in the caudate nucleus

(Bloom *et al.*, 1965; Connor, 1970; York, 1972). Norepinephrine was, however, usually more effective than dopamine in reducing discharge rates of caudate neurons (Bloom *et al.*, 1965). α-Methyldopamine, a very weak dopamine agonist with respect to stimulation of adenylate cyclases from the caudate nucleus (see Section 2.1.7), blocked the inhibitory effects of both substantia nigra-stimulation and microiontophoretic dopamine on firing rates of caudate neurons (Connor, 1972). The β-antagonist, nifenalol (IPNEA), was ineffective as a blocker, while experiments with other catecholamine antagonists such as phentolamine, phenoxybenzamine, chlorpromazine, dichlorisoproterenol and propranolol were not definitive because of either low solubility, ionization, or local anesthetic activity of these compounds. The antagonist activity of compounds such as chlorpromazine which have intrinsic depressant activity can now be studied through the use of automated microiontophoresis and computer-generated histograms (cf. Freedman *et al.*, 1975).

Dopamine, apomorphine, cyclic AMP, and its butyryl derivatives inhibited firing of control striatal (caudate) neurons and of neurons excited by glutamate or homocysteate (Siggins *et al.*, 1974; Bunney and Aghajanian, cited in Bloom *et al.*, 1974; Bloom, 1975; Spehlman, 1975; Ungerstedt *et al.*, 1975; Yarbrough, 1975). Effective ejection currents for cyclic AMP were much lower for caudate neurons than for cerebellar Purkinje neurons. The inhibitory effects of dopamine were antagonized by chlorpromazine, fluphenazine, and α-flupenthixol, but not by a β-blocker, sotalol. Chlorpromazine had, surprisingly, little direct depressant activity on caudate neurons. It did not antagonize the inhibitory effect of cyclic AMP. Prostaglandin E_1 had either no effect or potentiated the dopamine response. Of the phosphodiesterase inhibitors tested, parenteral aminophylline potentiated dopamine responses, while iontophoretically neither theophylline nor papaverine greatly potentiated the dopamine-elicited inhibition of firing of caudate neurons. Isobutylmethylxanthine, however, effectively potentiated dopamine responses and, in contrast to aminophylline and papaverine, had little direct depressive effect on caudate neurons. The effectiveness of dopamine and apomorphine for inhibition of striatal (caudate) neurons was increased after focal 6-hydroxydopamine lesions of the nigrastriatal dopaminergic tracts (Siggins *et al.*, 1974; Ungerstedt *et al.*, 1975). The threshold for cyclic AMP was not altered by such lesions. Spontaneous firing rates of striatal neurons increased after lesions. Dopamine and apomorphine were also more effective inhibitors of caudate neurons in rats treated chronically with a dopaminergic blocking agent, haloperidol (Yarbrough, 1975). Supersensitivity to dopaminergic agonists after dopamine-blocking agents and lesions of nigra-striatal pathways contrasts with inconsistent reports of supersensitive cyclic AMP-generating systems in the striatum after similar treatments (see Section 3.1.13). One group has reported that dopamine was less effective in depressing firing of caudate neurons after ventromedial segmental lesions (Spehlmann, 1975).

Cyclic AMP, norepinephrine, dopamine, γ-aminobutyrate, and glycine had inhibitory effects on pallidal neurons of the entopeduncular nucleus (Obata and Yoshida, 1973). Stimulation of the caudate also inhibited these neurons through what appeared to be γ-aminobutyrate neuronal innervation.

Medulla-Pons–Brain Stem

In neurons of cat medulla oblongata, discharge rates were frequently depressed not only by norepinephrine and histamine, but also by cyclic AMP (Anderson et al., 1973). Cells that were excited by norepinephrine were not affected by cyclic AMP. Prostaglandin E_1 and nicotinate reduced the inhibitory effects of norepinephrine in about half the cells. Nicotinate also, however, often reduced the inhibitory effect of glycine. Prostaglandin E_1 usually failed to reduce the inhibitory effect of histamine. Both the ethylenediamine salt of theophylline (aminophylline) and ethylenediamine itself were potent inhibitory agents, suggesting that effects of this salt of theophylline may not always be related to phosphodiesterase inhibition. Inhibitory effects of norepinephrine on neurons of the medullary reticular formation were only infrequently antagonized by prostaglandin E_1 (Siggins et al., 1971c). Depressant effects of norepinephrine on spinal motor neurons were accompanied by hyperpolarizations and increases in membrane resistance (Engberg and Marshall, 1971), as has been the case for other central neurons.

In toto, the various results suggest that, at least in some central pathways norepinephrine or dopamine-elicited accumulations of cyclic AMP and resultant hyperpolarizations are involved in the inhibitory postsynaptic effects. Further studies on serotonin, histamine, and adenosine will be required to establish the mechanism and function of their inhibitory effects. It has been proposed that the inhibitory effects of biogenic amines on central neurons are due to activation of an electrogenic sodium pump (see Phillis, 1976, and references therein). Such an effect would be expected to result in membrane hyperpolarization and an increase in membrane resistance. Ouabain, which inhibits the activity of Na^+,K^+-ATPases antagonized norepinephrine-elicited depression of cerebral cortical neurons (Phillis, 1974b) and dopamine-elicited depression of caudate neurons (Yarbrough, 1976). Other agents which might interfere with the activity of the Na^+,K^+-ATPase such as ethanol and barbiturates, lithium ions, and fluoride antagonized norepinephrine and serotonin-elicited depression of cerebral cortical neurons (Phillis et al., 1974b; Phillis, 1976). Glutamate, an agent which enhances rather than inhibits sodium uptake, potentiated norepinephrine-elicited depression of cortical neurons. Calcium-elicited depression and hyperpolarization of neurons was proposed (Phillis, 1976) to perhaps occur by some other mechanism, since calcium ions are inhibitory to Na^+,K^+-ATPase. Alternatively, calcium ions might be involved in activation of a protein kinase, competition with sodium ions, or stimulation of Ca^{2+}-ATPases.

Calcium Ions

The depressant actions of calcium and magnesium ions on central neurons have been well documented (cf. Kato and Somjen, 1969; Phillis and Limacher, 1974; Phillis, 1976, and references therein). Other divalent cations such as nickel, cobalt, barium, manganese, zinc, and iron also inhibit central neurons. In motor neurons, calcium has been stated to cause a hyperpolarization and an increase in membrane resistance similar to that elicited by biogenic amines (Engberg *et al.*, 1974). The inhibitory effects of norepinephrine, dopamine, histamine, and serotonin in cerebral cortical neurons were frequently prevented by "calcium antagonists" such as manganese, lanthanum, nickel and cobalt ions, ethanol, verapamil, cocaine, procaine amide, other local anesthetics, strychnine, neomycin, and ruthenium red (Lake *et al.*, 1973b; Phillis *et al.*, 1973; Phillis, 1974a,b, 1976; Phillis and Limacher, 1974; Yarbrough *et al.*, 1974). Many of these "calcium antagonists" had, however, intrinsic depressant activity making their direct evaluation as amine antagonists difficult. Indeed, in most instances, the inhibitory effects of amines were compared only before and then after depression of the cell by the "calcium antagonist." A prior treatment with a calcium antagonist also antagonized inhibitory responses to acetylcholine and glycine in cat cortical neurons, but had no effect on excitatory responses to acetylcholine, or on inhibitory responses to γ-aminobutyrate. The direct depressant effect of calcium antagonists such as lanthanum, cobalt and nickel ions, and verapamil on cerebral cortical neurons could be blocked by a prior application of a different calcium antagonist. Ruthenium red and neomycin frequently excited cerebral cortical neurons (Phillis, 1976). EGTA and EDTA at iontophoretic dosages which did not directly excite cerebral cortical neurons did prevent norepinephrine-elicited depressions. Magnesium ions had no effect on norepinephrine or serotonin-elicited depression of cerebral cortical neurons. The results were proposed to indicate that inhibitory responses to amines were due to amine-elicited influx of calcium ions. The results do suggest that calcium ions are in some way involved in amine-elicited inhibition of neuronal firing, but further studies are clearly needed to define the interrelationship of calcium, cyclic AMP, and membrane properties in central neurons.

The assessment of antagonism of amine-elicited inhibition of firing rates of central neurons by agents possessing intrinsic depressant activity has been difficult with the usual microiontophoretic techniques. Through the use of automated microiontophoresis and computer-generated histograms, it has now proven possible to directly assess the effects of calcium antagonists on norepinephrine-elicited inhibition of rat cerebellar Purkinje neurons and cerebral cortical neurons (Freedman et al., 1975). Verapamil, manganese, and cobalt were ineffective as antagonists of norepinephrine. Lathanum effectively blocked norepinephrine- but not cyclic AMP-elicited inhibition of Purkinje cells and directly inhibited adenylate cyclase (Nathanson et al., 1976).

Possible interrelationships between calcium ions and cyclic AMP as "second messengers" in a variety of tissues have been discussed (Rasmussen, 1970; Rasmussen and Goodman, 1975; Berridge, 1975). Calcium ions are known to be involved in a variety of neuronal functions including excitation–secretion coupling at nerve endings. Calcium translocation has been proposed to be vital to membrane permeability, being able to control interconversions of membranes from a resting, calcium-associated state to an active, calcium-dissociated state. Membrane permeability to sodium, potassium, and calcium ions increases in the "active state," and it is this phenomenon that has been proposed to trigger action potential generation. Levels of free calcium ions are very low (0.1 μM) within cells and quite high (1 mM) in mammalian extracellular fluid, resulting in a continual passive influx of calcium. Ca^{2+},Mg^{2+}-Dependent ATPases at plasma membrane remove calcium from the cell, while various subcellular entities, such as mitochrondria and microsomes, accumulate calcium from the cytoplasm of the cell in energy-dependent processes. Sequestration of calcium at membrane sites is a well-known phenomenon. It has as yet been impossible to study in any satisfactory manner the levels and distribution of calcium ions within the cytoplasm, membranes, and subcellular entities of cells, although the influx and efflux and total binding of radioactive calcium in intact tissues and cells and with subcellular particles and membranes can be studied. Cyclic AMP, dibutyryl cyclic AMP, or methylxanthines did not have significant effects on ATP-dependent uptake of calcium ions into rat brain microsomes or on efflux of calcium from microsomes (Diamond and Goldberg, 1971). It is obvious that delineation of roles for calcium in modulating enzyme and membrane function in whole cells is difficult. All of the enzymes involved in cyclic nucleotide formation, degradation, and action have to greater or lesser degrees dependencies on the concentration of calcium ions. Thus, it is not surprising that alterations in levels and gradients of calcium which occur in intact cells after removal of calcium from the medium or after both removal of calcium and addition of the calcium chelator, EGTA, often have profound effects on generation of cyclic AMP and on its proposed physiological sequelae. It should be noted that the extent and rate of depletion of intracellular calcium elicited by incubation in calcium-free medium varies considerably with different types of cells. In many cell types, a hormone or other stimulus can activate cyclic AMP formation in the absence of extracellular calcium, but no physiological sequelae ensues. In other cases, accumulation of cyclic AMP is greatly reduced in the absence of extracellular calcium ions. Formation of cyclic GMP appears in many systems to be wholly dependent on a source of extracellular calcium ions. Evidence linking accumulations of cyclic AMP to changes in calcium ion mobilization, binding, and uptake has been obtained with various types of cells or cellular entities (cf. Rasmussen, 1970). It is obvious that there are a plethora of possible ways in which a hormonal response can involve interactions between calcium and cyclic nucleotides as "second messengers." As yet, such interactions cannot be defined in neuronal systems.

Brain Electrical Activity

Dibutyryl cyclic AMP and adenosine caused repetitive paroxysmal activity when applied topically to the rat cerebral cortex (Walker *et al.*, 1974). Fluoride, an agent which probably has no effect on adenylate cyclase in intact cells, elicited similar epileptiform discharges. Topical application of dibutyryl cyclic AMP to one hemisphere of kitten cerebral cortex elicited paroxysmal and convulsive activity and caused the appearance of transcallosally evoked responses at nonhomotopic sites, suggestive of facilitation of superficial synaptic pathways (Purpura and Shofer, 1972). Topical unilateral application of potassium ions to rat cerebral cortex resulted in the phenomenon referred to as cortical spreading depression of brain activity and was accompanied by a marked increase in cyclic AMP levels (Krivanek, 1976).

In explants of fetal or newborn mouse spinal cord and cerebral cortex, cyclic AMP, its dibutyryl derivative, and caffeine temporarily restored slow wave and repetitive spike discharges that were abolished in calcium-free medium (Crain and Pollock, 1973). The phosphodiesterase inhibitor, SQ 65442, an analog of SQ 20009, also restored complex bioelectrical activity. It is noteworthy that the cyclic AMP analogs were effective in these explants at micromolar concentrations and that AMP and ATP were ineffective. It was suggested that cyclic AMP is capable of mobilizing functional pools of membrane-bound calcium ions necessary in the absence of external calcium for synaptic transmission. After blockage under calcium-free conditions, cyclic AMP restored transganglionic transmission in the abdominal ganglion of the cockroach and in the paravertebral chain of the frog (Torda, 1974). The postganglionic neuron appeared to be depolarized under calcium-free conditions, but transmembrane potential was restored with cyclic AMP.

4.3.2 Ganglionic Neurons

Sympathetic Ganglia

Preganglionic stimulation of innervating cholinergic fibers elicited a postsynaptic action potential and in addition a prolonged postsynaptic hyperpolarization. The latter phenomenon is inhibitory to neuronal transmission and appears to be mediated by release of catecholamines from interneurons, followed by catecholamine-elicited accumulation of cyclic AMP in the postsynaptic neuron. The postsynaptic action potential in the rabbit superior cervical ganglion can be blocked by nicotinic antagonists such as hexamethonium or d-tubocurarine. Preganglionic stimulation under these conditions elicited a hyperpolarization of the postsynaptic ganglionic neuron which was potentiated by theophylline and blocked by prostaglandin E_1 or α-antagonists (McAfee and Greengard, 1972; Greengard and Kebabian, 1974; Kalix $et\ al.$, 1974; Kebabian $et\ al.$, 1975b; Figure 21). Carbamylcholine elicited a hyperpolarization but had no effect in the absence of calcium ions. Dopamine elicited a similar hyperpolarization which was blocked by prostaglandin E_1 and potentiated by theophylline (Figure 21). Cyclic AMP and its butyryl derivatives elicited a hyperpolarization. Excitability of the ganglionic neuron was reduced during the period of hyperpolarization. In addition to its effects on interneurons, it appeared that acetylcholine, released as a result of preganglionic stimulation, activated muscarinic receptors on postsynaptic neurons, thereby increasing levels of cyclic GMP. Cyclic GMP would appear to be involved in the slow excitatory postsynaptic potentials which result from preganglionic stimulation. Dibutyryl cyclic GMP did elicit a transient hyperpolarization followed by a depolarization of rabbit (McAfee and Greengard, 1972; Figure 21) and bullfrog sympathetic ganglia (cited in Weight $et\ al.$, 1974). Cyclic GMP had no effect. The results are consonant with the following interpretation: Stimulation of preganglionic fibers causes release of acetylcholine which (1) activates nicotinic receptors on the postganglionic neuron to elicit fast excitatory postsynaptic potential (f-EPSP); (2) activates muscarinic receptors on the postganglionic neuron to cause the accumulation of cyclic GMP which elicits the slow excitatory postsynaptic potential (s-EPSP), and (3) activates muscarinic receptors on the interneurons causing release of dopamine, which in turn activates adenylate cyclase receptors on

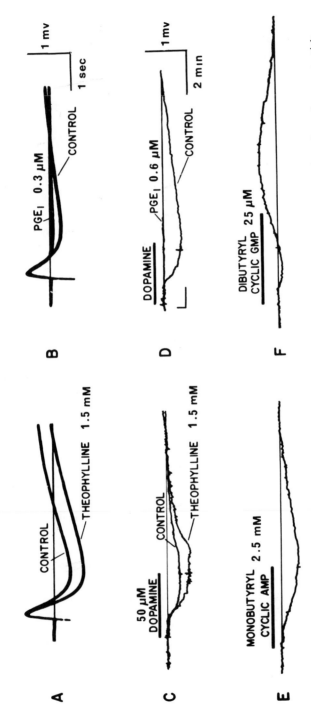

Figure 21. Effect of preganglionic stimulation (A,B), dopamine (C,D), and cyclic nucleotides (E,F) on synaptic and membrane potentials in postganglionic neurons of rabbit superior cervical ganglion. Hexamethonium (600 µM) was present in A and B to block propagated impulses. The duration of superfusion with dopamine or cyclic nucleotides is indicated by bars. Prostaglandin E₁ (PGE₁) or theophylline were present in superfusates for 15–30 min. (Modified from McAfee and Greengard, 1972, *Science*, copyright American Association for the Advancement of Science.)

the postganglionic neuron to thereby cause an accumulation of cyclic AMP, which elicits membrane hyperpolarization and the slow inhibitory postsynaptic potential (s-IPSP) (Greengard and Kebabian, 1974; Figure 22). Both dibutyryl cyclic AMP and dopamine have prolonged facilatory effects on the muscarinic slow excitatory postsynaptic potentials (Libet and Tosaka, 1970; Libet *et al.*, 1976). This facilitation thus appears to represent a long-term effect of cyclic AMP-dependent neurotransmission on the responsiveness of a cyclic GMP-dependent neurotransmission. During the initial period after dopamine or dibutyryl cyclic AMP, addition of cyclic GMP prevented the development of the long-term facilitation of slow excitatory postsynaptic potentials. In addition to dopamine, norepinephrine has been reported to elicit a hyperpolarization of ganglionic neurons of the rabbit superior cervical ganglion (Libet and Kobayashi, 1969). Dibutyryl cyclic GMP was in one study reported to have no effect on membrane potential of postganglionic neurons of bullfrog superior cervical ganglion (Suria, 1976).

Dopamine and dibutyryl cyclic AMP elicited hyperpolarization and a partial antagonism of transmission in the cat superior cervical ganglion (Machova and Kristofova, 1973). In the cat ganglion, aminophylline elicited an initial depolarization, followed by hyperpolarization and a late depolarization. In contrast, another group reported no consistent effect for dibutyryl cyclic AMP, a depressant effect for aminophylline and papaverine, and a facilatory effect for imidazole on ganglionic transmission in the cat superior cervical ganglion (Varagic and Zugic, 1973). Papaverine was more potent as a depressant than aminophylline. Imidazole potentiated and aminophylline antagonized the depolarization elicited by a nicotinic agonist, 1,1-dimethyl-4-phenylpiperazinium iodide.

Sodium-free medium which should reduce activity of Na^+,K^+-ATPase prevented catecholamine- or serotonin-elicited hyperpolarization and/or slow inhibitory postsynaptic potentials in postsynaptic neurons of rat superior cervical ganglia, as did an inhibitor of Na^+,K^+-ATPase, ouabain, and metabolic inhibitors such as cyanide and 2,4-dinitrophenol (Nishi and Koketsu, 1967; Nakamura and Koketsu, 1972; Koketsu *et al.*, 1973; Koketsu and Shirasawa, 1974). These results are consonant with a proposal by Phillis (1976) that amine-elicited inhibition and hyperpolarization of neurons involves an activation of Na^+,K^+-ATPase (see pp. 225–256). However, in the rabbit superior cervical ganglion, inhibition of Na^+,K^+-ATPase by ouabain did not block the hyperpolarizing effect of norepinephrine (Libet and Kobayashi, 1969).

Activation of a cyclic AMP-dependent diphosphoinositide kinase has been proposed to be responsible for the neuronal hyperpolarization elicited by cyclic AMP (Torda, 1972b). Intracellular microinjection of the catalytic unit of this enzyme along with its substrate produced an inhibitory hyperpolarization of neurons in rabbit sympathetic ganglia. The inhibitory hyper-

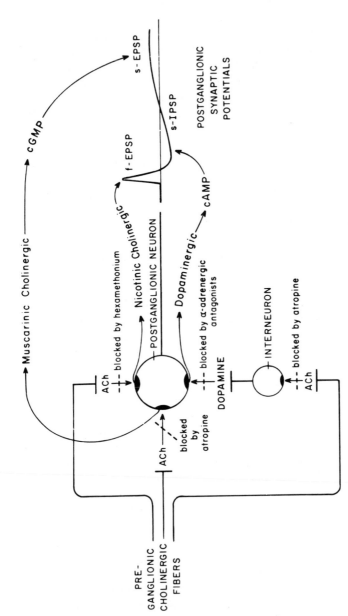

Figure 22. Schematic representation of synaptic connections in mammalian superior cervical ganglion and proposed role of acetylcholine (ACh), dopamine, cyclic AMP (cAMP), and cyclic GMP (cGMP). The postsynaptic action potential consists of a fast excitatory postsynaptic potential, f-EPSP; a slow excitatory postsynaptic potential, s-EPSP; and a slow inhibitory postsynaptic potential, s-IPSP. The nature of the catecholamine transmitters of interneurons of various species has been reviewed (Bloom, 1975). (Modified from Greengard and Kebabian, 1974; *Federation Proceedings*, copyright Federation of American Society for Experimental Biology.)

polarization, regardless of whether it was generated electrically or by injection of enzyme, was reversed by injection of the regulatory unit. Microinjection of cyclic AMP and diphosphoinositide produced an inhibitory hyperpolarization in the presence of theophylline.

Cyclic GMP has been proposed to be involved in the inhibition of posttetanic potentiation of fast excitatory postsynaptic potentials in bullfrog sympathetic ganglia by prostaglandins, diazepam, and isobutylmethylxanthine (Suria and Costa, 1973, 1974, 1975a,b; Suria, 1976). The posttetanic potentiation of postsynaptic potentials has been interpreted to be due to facilitation of acetylcholine release by increased calcium ion levels at presynaptic terminals after a train of impulses. Diazepam had no inhibitory effect on postsynaptic potentials except after a prior conditioning train of impulses. Dibutyryl cyclic GMP but not cyclic GMP, cyclic AMP, or dibutyryl cyclic AMP had an inhibitory effect on posttetanic potentiation. Dibutyryl cyclic GMP, diazepam, and γ-aminobutyrate caused depolarization of presynaptic nerve terminals in bullfrog ganglia. Such depolarizations were blocked by a γ-aminobutyrate antagonist, picrotoxin. The depolarizing effects of dibutyryl cyclic GMP and diazepam were blocked by pretreatment with agents, such as isoniazid and thiosemicarbazide, which block synthesis of γ-aminobutyrate. Cyclic AMP, dibutyryl cyclic AMP, and cyclic GMP had no effect on membrane potentials in presynaptic terminals. Dibutyryl cyclic GMP and diazepam had no effect on membrane potential of postganglionic neurons or on presynaptic action potentials, nor did dibutyryl cyclic GMP antagonize acetylcholine-elicited depolarization of the postganglionic neurons. Dibutyryl cyclic GMP, high concentrations of potassium, or electrical stimulation caused an enhanced efflux of radioactive γ-aminobutyrate from rat superior cervical ganglia, while carbamylcholine had little effect. A model was proposed by Suria (1976) in which release of γ-aminobutyrate from glial cells inhibits release of acetylcholine by causing depolarization of presynaptic terminals (cf. Koketsu *et al.,* 1974). During tetanic stimulation, release of potassium ions from nerves were proposed to activate cyclic GMP accumulation and release of γ-aminobutyrate from glial cells. After a tetanic stimulation release of γ-aminobutyrate presumably decreased and the system became hyperresponsive with respect to stimulation-evoked release of acetylcholine. At this point, the presence of dibutyryl cyclic GMP presumably would cause continued release of γ-aminobutyrate from the glial cells. Diazepam and isobutylmethylxanthine as phosphodiesterase inhibitors would presumably in this model lead to intraglial accumulation of cyclic GMP and a continued release of γ-aminobutyrate. It has, however, also been proposed that the inhibition of posttetanic potentiation by diazepam involves activation of prostaglandin synthesis (Suria and Costa, 1974) or a presynaptic accumulation of cyclic AMP (R. A. Lehne and A. Suria, personal communication).

Further study of this system is clearly needed to define the role of cyclic nucleotides in inhibition of posttetanic potentiation.

Intracellular injection of cyclic AMP into neurons of the gastropod *Helix pomatia* caused depolarization and increased spontaneous activity (Liberman *et al.*, 1975). Exogenous cyclic AMP or injection of 5'-AMP or ATP had no effect.

Retina

Dopamine and norepinephrine which activate retinal adenylate cyclases (see Section 3.3) inhibited electrical activity in retinal ganglion cells (Straschill and Perwein, 1969). Dopamine is known to be released on illumination of retina (Kramer, 1971).

The light-inhibited cyclic AMP- and cyclic GMP-generating systems in outer segments of photoreceptor cells, the light- and ATP-dependent formation of a heat-labile activator of rod outer segment phosphodiesterase, and the relationship of these observations to the light-elicited hyperpolarization of photoreceptor cells has been the subject of active research (Bitensky *et al.*, 1971, 1972, 1973, 1975; Bitensky and Gorman, 1972; Chader *et al.*, 1973, 1974a,b; Goridis *et al.*, 1973; Hendriks *et al.*, 1973; Miki *et al.*, 1973, 1974, 1975; Miller, 1973; Pannbacker, 1973; Bensinger *et al.*, 1974; Goridis and Virmaux, 1974; Keirns *et al.*, 1975; Manthorpe and McConnell, 1975). The photoreceptor cell represents an extremely specialized neuron. It contains in most vertebrates a rod outer segment comprised of many discs, stacked within the outer segment membrane. The discs may be isolated as discrete saccules after rupture of the outer segment membrane. This portion of the cell contains the light-sensitive pigment, rhodopsin. Photocapture by rhodopsin results in conversion of the protein to a bleached form. Even a fractional conversion by light of rhodopsin to bleached rhodopsin is accompanied in the rod outer segments by a decrease in sodium permeability and hyperpolarization. This light-sensitive portion of the photoreceptor cell is connected to the cell body by a fragile cilium. The photoreceptor cell then synapses upon cells of the bipolar layer of the retina. This layer consists primarily of nerve cells of three types; the prominent bipolar cells, the outer amichron cells, and the inner horizontal cells. Interconnections between these cells, the photoreceptor cells, and the final inner layer of cells, the ganglion cells with their efferent tracts to the optic centers and the superior colliculus, are under active study. A variety of neurotransmitters are probably involved in synaptic transmission within the retina. Adenylate cyclase, phosphodiesterase, and protein kinase have been found to be associated with the disc membranes of the rod outer segments (see Section 2).

Evidence suggestive for a role of cyclic nucleotides in the sequence involved in light-induced hyperpolarization of rod outer segments initially stemmed from studies on the light-sensitive cyclic AMP- and later cyclic GMP-generating systems in membranes from rod outer segments. These systems appeared to be strongly inhibited by light, and first adenylate and then guanylate cyclase activity in rod outer segments was reported to be inhibited by light. The mechanism was later found to involve the light- and ATP-dependent formation of an activator of phosphodiesterase (see Section 2.3.10). Thus, light via formation of bleached rhodopsin elicited an ATP-dependent formation of an activator of phosphodiesterase, thereby reducing levels of cyclic AMP and cyclic GMP in rod outer segments. Light-induced activation of cyclic GMP hydrolysis has appeared to be more important than activation of cyclic AMP hydrolysis. It has been proposed, based on a calculated ratio of rhodopsin to phosphodiesterase of 900:1 and the complete activation of all phosphodiesterases upon bleaching of only 0.1% of the rhodopsin, that in the presence of ATP one bleached rhodopsin molecule activates one phosphodiesterase (Miki *et al.*, 1975). Others (Manthorpe and McConnell, 1975) have reported a stoichiometric relationship between reduction of rhodopsin and activation of cyclic GMP hydrolysis with bovine preparations. The relationship of light-induced reduction in cyclic nucleotide levels in rod outer segments to the concomitant hyperpolarization of this neuronal cell is as yet unclear. It has been proposed that phosphorylation of bleached rhodopsin by a very specific protein kinase of rod outer segments leads to a release of calcium ions which decrease the outer membrane's sodium ion permeability, resulting in a hyperpolarization (Bitensky *et al.*, 1975; Weller *et al.*, 1975a,b,c). The activity of the protein kinase did not appear to be affected by cyclic nucleotides, but it was inhibited by theophylline. Calcium binding to disc membranes was not affected by cyclic AMP (Neufeld *et al.*, 1972).

In the photoreceptor (retinular) cell of the horseshoe crab, light elicits a depolarization rather than a hyperpolarization. Light-induced depolarization of retinular cells was antagonized by cyclic AMP (Wulff, 1971). Cyclic AMP was reported to reduce the magnitude of the light-induced receptor potential, to increase the latent period, and to decrease membrane resistance. Cyclic AMP was also cited as causing depolarization of the retinular cell. Miller *et al.* (1971) reported that cyclic AMP, theophylline, or light all caused depolarization of retinular cells and an increase in the firing of an associated neuron, the eccentric cell.

4.3.3 Peripheral Neurons

Axons

Dopamine, theophylline, cyclic AMP and its butyryl derivatives and cyclic GMP had no effect on membrane potentials of axons of the cervical vagus nerve (Greengard and Kebabian, 1974). Dibutyryl cyclic GMP, however, depolarized the vagus nerve. Dibutyryl cyclic GMP had no effect on membrane potentials of intraganglionic axons of the bullfrog superior cervical ganglia (Suria and Costa, 1974; Suria, 1976). Cyclic AMP and to a lesser extent dibutyryl cyclic AMP increased thresholds for initiation of action potentials, reduced spike amplitude and decreased conduction velocity in frog sciatic nerve (Van de Berg, 1974). Theophylline had similar effects and greatly potentiated the effect of cyclic AMP. In the absence of calcium ions, cyclic AMP was stated to have no effect on spike amplitudes. In a recent study with desheathed frog sciatic nerves, cyclic AMP, cyclic GMP, dibutyryl derivatives, phosphodiesterase inhibitors such as theophylline, or agents such as isoproterenol and carbamylcholine which elevate axonal levels of cyclic AMP and cyclic GMP, respectively, had no detectable effects on membrane potentials or action potentials (Horn and McAfee, 1976).

Sensory Neurons

The role of cyclic AMP in the stimulation of gustatory cells by bitter tasting substances has been investigated (Kurihara, 1972; Kurihara and Koyama, 1972; Price, 1973). Levels of adenylate cyclase and phosphodiesterase were relatively high in regions of bovine tongue containing gustatory cells. Various bitter tasting substances such as (thio)acetamide, (thio)urea, propylthiouracil, and quinine have been reported to activate cyclic AMP phosphodiesterases in homogenates from tongue epithelium. High levels of adenylate cyclase have been reported in rabbit olfactory epithelium (Bitensky et al., 1972).

Release of Neurotransmitters

A role for cyclic AMP in mechanisms involved in release of acetylcholine from presynaptic terminals of neuromuscular preparations has been proposed. Thus, (nor)epinephrine, dibutyryl cyclic AMP, and phosphodiesterase inhibitors such as methylxanthines, papaverine, a benzothiadiazine, hydrochlorothiazide, and a dialkoxybenzyl-2-imidazolidinone, RO 72956, appeared to increase the release of acetylcholine from the presynaptic neuronal terminal (Breckenridge et al., 1967; Goldberg and Singer, 1969; Varagic and Zugic, 1971; Varagic et al., 1972; Vapaatalo, 1974; Wilson, 1974). These compounds enhanced the magnitude of end plate potential and the force of the contracture of muscle elicited by stimulation of the motor nerve. Cyclic AMP, in contrast to the dibutyryl derivative, was ineffective, but dibutyryl cyclic GMP and monobutyryl cyclic UMP did increase the force of muscle contracture. Epinephrine, the methylxanthines, and dibutyryl cyclic AMP increased the rate of spontaneous release of acetylcholine as evidenced by an increase in the frequency of miniature end plate potentials. The evidence for a presynaptic involvement of cyclic AMP in these effects remains far from conclusive. Thus, although methylxanthines potentiated indirectly elicited muscle twitch and interacted additively in this regard with catecholamines, they also potentiated directly elicited twitch (Varagic and Zugic, 1971). No effects of cyclic AMP on responses of the diaphragm preparation were observed even in the presence of theophylline. Glucose-6-phosphate, a normal product of glycogenolysis, had effects on muscle twitch similar to those elicited by catecholamines or methylxanthines. The potent phosphodiesterase inhibitor, SQ 20009, has recently been reported to facilitate neuromuscular transmission (McNiece and Jacobs, 1976). Adenosine, another agent which might elevate cyclic AMP levels, appeared, however, to decrease release of acetylcholine in a neuromuscular preparation (Ginsborg and Hirst, 1972; Miyamoto and Breckenridge, 1974). The adenosine-elicited decrease in the frequency of miniature end plate potentials (spontaneous release of acetylcholine) and in the amplitude of end plate potentials (evoked release) could be antagonized by theophylline.

It has been proposed that the reduction in toxicity of d-tubocurarine by phosphodiesterase inhibitors such as papaverine and theophylline, by an α-agonist, ephedrine, and by dibutyryl cyclic AMP and cyclic GMP might also be related to a cyclic AMP-dependent increase in release of acetylcholine (Anttila and Vapaatalo, 1972; Vapaatalo, 1974). Various phosphodiesterase inhibitors did partially reverse the tubocurarine-induced blockade of muscle twitch in an indirectly stimulated rat phrenic nerve–diaphragm preparation (Varagic and Zugic, 1971; Vapaatalo and Anttila, 1972; Vapaatalo, 1974). Beneficial effects of theophylline and papaverine in the treatment of myasthenia gravis might be related to such phenomena. Calcium ions, epinephrine, and methylxanthines alleviated a neuromuscular disorder, the Eaton–Lambert syndrome, in which release of acetylcholine is defective (Takamori *et al.*, 1973). The effect of epinephrine appeared to be due to activation of an α-receptor. Phenylephrine was effective, while isoproterenol was ineffective. Involvement of cyclic AMP in these effects was not investigated.

In a recent study using drug perfusion techniques neither (nor)epinephrine, histamine, dibutyryl cyclic AMP, butyrate, nor cyclic AMP had any significant effect on spontaneous release of acetylcholine in resting rat phrenic nerve–diaphragm preparations (Miyamoto and Breckenridge, 1974). Direct injection of dibutyryl cyclic AMP did, as previously reported, increase transmitter release, presumably through osmotic effects. In preparations depolarized with 15 mM potassium ion, (nor)epinephrine and dibutyryl cyclic AMP increased rates of transmitter release, while monobutyryl cyclic AMP, cyclic AMP, and butyrate had no significant effect. Theophylline enhanced transmitter release in both resting and potassium-depolarized preparations. It was proposed that cyclic AMP-dependent mechanisms may increase presynaptic calcium conductances and thereby enhance calcium-dependent release of acetylcholine in stimulated preparations. Effects of theophylline on calcium may be due only in part to inhibition of phosphodiesterase. Dibutyryl cyclic AMP had no effect on the spontaneous release of radioactive acetylcholine from guinea pig cortical slices (Shimizu *et al.*, 1970a). Methylxanthines may, however, increase release of biogenic amines in brain (see Section 4.1.3).

Dibutyryl cyclic AMP and other analogs of cyclic AMP, and phosphodiesterase inhibitors such as theophylline, isobutylmethylxanthine, papaverine, and RO 20-1724 enhanced the stimulus-evoked release of norepinephrine from sympathetic neurons in spleen (Cubeddu *et al.*, 1974, 1975) and vas deferens (Wooten *et al.*, 1973). Dibutyryl cyclic AMP also enhanced spontaneous release of norepinephrine from vas deferens. Calcium ions were required for stimulus-evoked release of norepinephrine in control vas deferens but were not required in the presence of dibutyryl cyclic AMP or theophylline. At concentrations judged to be equipotent with respect to inhibition of splenic phosphodiesterase, papaverine was much more effective in enhancing evoked release of norepinephrine in spleen than either isobutylmethylxanthine or RO 20-1724. Indeed papaverine, both in the presence and absence of calcium, even increased spontaneous release of norepinephrine in spleen. Nerve stimulation did not evoke further release of norepinephrine in calcium-free medium in the presence of the phosphodiesterase inhibitor, papaverine. A direct effect of papaverine on synaptic vesicles, in addition to effects on phosphodiesterase, was suggested. RO 20-1724 also appeared to increase spontaneous release of norepinephrine, perhaps due to its activity as a monoamine oxidase inhibitor. The ability of an α-adrenergic antagonist, phentolamine, to enhance electrically elicited release of norepinephrine was not affected by phosphodiesterase inhibitors, suggesting that this effect was not mediated by a cyclic AMP-dependent mechanism.

A discussion of the role of cyclic AMP in release phenomena in nonneuronal preparations is beyond the scope of the present review. Cyclic AMP has been implicated in release phenomena for amylase, insulin, norepinephrine, thyrocalcitonin, and gastric HCl in a variety of cells of both neuronal and nonneuronal origin. Interactions of cyclic nucleotides and mobilization of calcium appear fundamental to such phenomena (cf. Berridge, 1975.)

4.3.4 Cultured Cells

Differentiation of mouse neuroblastoma cells with dibutyryl cyclic AMP is accompanied by an increase in the proportion of electrically excitable cells, and the rate of rise and amplitudes of evoked spikes and resting membrane potential were greater than in nondifferentiated cells (Chalazonitis and Greene, 1974). Butyric acid had similar effects, while in preliminary experiments N^6-monobutyryl cyclic AMP and 8-methylthio cyclic AMP had no effect on differentiation or on electrical properties of neuroblastoma cells. The electrophoretic mobility, and hence probably the total negative surface charge of undifferentiated neuroblastoma cells, was significantly less than for spontaneously differentiated neuroblastoma cells present in the same culture (Elul *et al.*, 1975). It was suggested that a high rate of cell division will be found to be associated with increased negativity of cell surfaces. No studies on cyclic AMP-differentiated cells were reported. It has been noted that agents such as prostaglandin E_1 which increased cyclic AMP levels caused hyperpolarization of neuroblastoma–glioma hybrid cells, while agents such as acetylcholine, α-adrenergic agonists, and morphine that antagonize accumulations of cyclic AMP caused depolarizations (Traber *et al.*, 1975d).

Neuroblastoma cells differentiated by culture with the phosphodiesterase inhibitor, RO 20-1724, no longer retained tumorigenic potency, and they did not react as readily with cancer cell agglutinins such as concanavalin A (Prasad, 1972c; Prasad and Sheppard, 1972a). Cells which had differentiated in response to dibutyryl cyclic AMP or prostaglandin E_1, however, still agglutinated with concanavalin A. Dibutyryl cyclic AMP-differentiated neuroblastoma cells had enhanced levels of a surface membrane glycoprotein (mol wt 105,000) (Truding *et al.*, 1974). Another membrane glycoprotein (mol wt 78,000) became exposed on surfaces of differentiated cells, but not in suspension culture cells, in which only growth inhibition was elicited by dibutyryl cyclic AMP.

Levels of a nervous system surface antigen I detected with a cytotoxicity assay were slightly decreased in glioma cells by dibutyryl cyclic AMP, while levels of a major surface histocompatibility antigen, H-2, were unaffected (Sundarraj *et al.*, 1975).

4.4 Levels of Cyclic Nucleotides in Brain

Effects of centrally active drugs on levels of cyclic nucleotides in different brain regions have been investigated in hopes that correlations or lack of correlations between such effects and the pharmacological activity of the compounds would provide insights into roles of cyclic nucleotides in the central nervous system. Levels of cyclic nucleotides have been measured in brain tissue, in cerebrospinal fluid, and in urine after drug treatments and environmental manipulations in humans and strains of animals exhibiting different behavioral profiles. Increases in cyclic AMP and cyclic GMP occur in brain tissue after decapitation and during anoxia, and a variety of studies with different antagonists have been employed in attempts to delineate the factors involved in postdecapitation changes, particularly with respect to cyclic AMP. As yet conclusions as to definitive roles for cyclic AMP and cyclic GMP in drug effects and in control of behavioral and vegetative functions of brain have not been obtained, but the data have provided many insights into potential interactions and roles for drug-elicited alterations in cyclic nucleotide generation. Further studies on the influence of various factors on brain levels of cyclic AMP and cyclic GMP may lead to significant findings. However, important changes in cyclic nucleotide levels in specific brain regions or cell types might easily be insignificant with respect to total levels of the nucleotide.

4.4.1 Postdecapitation Changes in Cyclic AMP in Brain

After sacrifice of animals, cyclic AMP levels rose rapidly in brain tissue (Breckenridge, 1964; Goldberg *et al.*, 1967, 1970; Kakiuchi and Rall, 1968a; Ditzion *et al.*, 1970; Steiner *et al.*, 1970, 1972; Schmidt *et al.*, 1970, 1971; Ebadi *et al.*, 1971a; Sattin, 1971; Burkard, 1972; Uzunov and Weiss, 1971, 1972b; Weiss and Strada, 1972; Dolby and Kleinsmith, 1974; Guidotti *et al.*, 1974; Jones *et al.*, 1974; Kimura *et al.*, 1974). During this initial period ATP levels in brain tissue fell rapidly, while levels of ADP and adenosine increased. The increase in levels of cyclic AMP was particularly large in cerebellum. In mouse, however, increases in cyclic AMP levels after decapitation were similar in cerebral cortex and cerebellum (Steiner *et al.*, 1972). Hypothermia somewhat delayed and reduced postdecapitation-elicited increases of cyclic AMP in cerebral cortex of mice (Lust and Passonneau, 1976). Postdecapitation increases in cyclic AMP complicate any study on the effect of psychoactive agents on levels of cyclic AMP in whole brain or in specific brain regions. Rapid freezing of the animal heads partially circumvents this problem, but it is not really rapid enough for animals larger than mice. Two other rapid methods of fixing brain have been described; microwave irradiation (Schmidt *et al.*, 1972) and freeze blowing of either forebrain (Nahorski and Rogers, 1973) or whole brain (Lust *et al.*, 1973) (see Section 2.1.3).

Methylxanthines, which have been shown to have activities as central stimulants, as phosphodiesterase inhibitors, and as antagonists of adenosine-sensitive cyclases in brain slices, reduced postdecapitation increases in cyclic AMP (Goldberg *et al.*, 1970; Paul *et al.*, 1970d; Sattin, 1971). Presumably, activity of methylxanthines as adenosine antagonists was primarily responsible for reductions in postdecapitation increases in cyclic AMP by theophylline and caffeine.

Various compounds which should either reduce or enhance the extent of activation of biogenic amine-dependent mechanisms either had no effect or antagonized postdecapitation increases in cyclic AMP. Many of these compounds have "nonspecific" local anesthetic activity. The results from different laboratories have not been completely consistent, probably due to different drug regimens and the use of different species or strains. Pretreatment of adult rabbits with chlorpromazine reduced the postdecapitation increase in cyclic AMP in cerebral cortex, while pretreatment with reserprine to deplete norepinephrine or with an antihistamine, diphenhydramine, had no effect (Kakiuchi and Rall, 1968a). Trifluoperazine, diphenhydramine, and a central stimulant, amphetamine, have been reported to slightly antagonize postdecapitation increases in cerebellar cyclic AMP in mice (Lust et al., 1976). Amphetamine had no effect on postdecapitation increases of cyclic AMP in rat brain (Paul et al., 1970d). Prior treatment of adult rats with dopa plus a monoamine oxidase inhibitor reduced postdecapitation increases in cyclic AMP. The cerebellar increase in cyclic AMP was blocked by prior treatment of rats with phenothiazines, chlorprothixene, haloperidol, and lithium salts (Uzunov and Weiss, 1971, 1972b). Trifluoperazine was a more effective antagonist than chlorpromazine.

Central depressants such as barbiturates, ethanol, papaverine, and, to a lesser degree, ether and halothane blocked the postdecapitation increase in brain cyclic AMP to varying extents in a variety of species and brain regions (Kakiuchi and Rall, 1968a; Dizion et al., 1970; Goldberg et al., 1970; Paul et al., 1970d; Volicer and Gold, 1973; Kimura et al., 1974). Ethanol in low concentrations enhanced the postdecapitation increases in cyclic AMP in pons and medulla. Pentylenetetrazole, a central convulsant, had no effect on postdecapitation increases of cyclic AMP in rat brain (Paul et al., 1970d). Diphenylhydantoin, an anticonvulsant, slightly antagonized increases in cyclic AMP in mouse cerebellum (Lust et al., 1976).

Postdecapitation increases in cyclic AMP levels occurred in developing rat brain at a time (3 days postpartum) when a norepinephrine-sensitive cyclase could not be detected with 5 μM norepinephrine in brain slices (Schmidt et al., 1970). A small response to 50 μM norepinephrine was manifest at this time. Responses to adenosine–norepinephrine combinations, to adenosine, but not to norepinephrine were observed in rat cortical slices at this time (3–5 days postpartum) by Perkins and Moore (1973b). Postdecapitation increases in rat cerebellar cyclic AMP levels were lower after a 12-hr dark period as compared to the increases seen after 12 hr of light (Weiss and Strada, 1972). In mouse forebrain postdecapitation increases in cyclic AMP were significantly greater during the middle of the night, the time of peak diurnal activity (Nahorski and Rogers, 1973).

Clearly, the factors involved in postdecapitation increases in cyclic AMP levels of brain are not established. Release of norepinephrine or histamine do not appear to be of prime importance. Instead, the data suggest that intense electrical activity and anoxia following decapitation lead to a decrease in ATP and an increase in adenosine in brain. The accumulation of adenosine within the tissue results in adenosine-mediated increases of cyclic AMP.

4.4.2 Effects of Drugs and Other Treatments on Levels of Cyclic AMP in Brain

Adenosine

Decreasing cerebral blood flow, oxygen tension, or carbon dioxide tension resulted in accumulation of adenosine in rat brain (Rubio *et al.*, 1975). Increases in adenosine correlated well with increases in cyclic AMP levels. A tenfold increase in adenosine was associated with only a twofold increase in cyclic AMP. Brief anoxia *in vivo* greatly increased cerebral levels of cyclic AMP in Wistar rats (Stefanovich and John, 1974). Unilateral ischemia produced in gerbils by ligation of a carotid artery resulted in a pronounced but transient increase in cortical levels of cyclic AMP in the ischemic hemisphere (Lust *et al.*, 1975; Watanabe and Ishii, 1976). Central hypoxia in dog resulted in an initial increase in levels of cyclic AMP in cerebral cortex followed by a decrease below control levels (Benzi and Villa, 1976). Adenylate cyclase activity measured in homogenates appeared to also increase and then decrease below control levels. Neither a β-agonist, N-butyl-p-octopamine (bamethan), a β-antagonist, dichlorisopro-terenol, nor papaverine had any effect on cyclic AMP levels under severe hypoxia, but both the β-agonist and papaverine increased the rate of recovery of cyclic AMP and adenylate cyclase during a posthypoxia period. Papaverine may have functioned only as a vasodilator. Glycogen levels greatly decreased and lactate increased during hypoxia.

A stab wound to one of the cerebral hemispheres in a mouse results in a transient sevenfold increase of cortical levels of cyclic AMP in this hemisphere and a small increase in the contralateral hemisphere (Watanabe and Passonneau, 1974, 1975). Hypothermia or theophylline administered to the mouse was effective in reducing the *in vivo* increase in cyclic AMP levels after injury. Compounds with local anesthetic activity such as the antihistamine, diphenhydramine, and the phenothiazines, chlorpromazine and trifluoperazine, also reduced the injury-elicited increase in cyclic AMP. The β-antagonists, dichlorisoproterenol and pronethalol, and the norepi-nephrine-depleting agent, reserpine, only marginally reduced the response to injury. The results suggest that neuronal depolarization and resultant increase in adenosine levels play a major role in the increase in cyclic AMP after stab wound injury. After stab wound injury, postdecapitation increases in cyclic AMP were less pronounced, and in some instances cyclic AMP actually decreased after decapitation.

Although these studies clearly implicate adenosine-elicited activation of cyclic AMP systems under certain extreme conditions in brain, the role of adenosine in the physiological function of brain is less clear. Adenosine may be involved in increases in levels of cyclic AMP in brain during convulsions (see p. 278).

Biogenic Amines and Related Drugs

Intraventricular epinephrine elicited a two- to threefold transient increase in rat brain cyclic AMP (Burkard, 1972). Norepinephrine and isoproterenol were much less effective and dopamine had only a marginal effect. Another group found no significant effect of smaller amounts of intraventricular norepinephrine on levels of cyclic AMP in rat brain (Schmidt *et al.*, 1972). Intravenous injection of epinephrine, isoproterenol, and histamine elicited a rapid increase in cyclic AMP levels in chick cerebral hemispheres (Edwards *et al.*, 1974; Nahorski *et al.*, 1974, 1975b,c). Noradrenaline, dopamine, adenosine, serotonin, and acetylcholine had no effect. One injection of propranolol reduced accumulations of cyclic AMP elicited by isoproterenol in chick cerebrum for at least 12 hr. Phentolamine had no effect. H_2-Antagonists such as metiamide, but not H_1-antagonists, blocked histamine-elicited increases in cyclic AMP in chick cerebrum. Intravenous isoproterenol had very small effects on levels of cerebral cyclic AMP in 28-day-old chicks, presumably due to development of the blood brain barrier (Nahorski *et al.*, 1975a). Lysergic acid diethylamide and *N,N*-dimethyltryptamine increased levels of cyclic AMP in rat cerebrum and brain stem, but not in cerebellum (Uzunov and Weiss, 1971, 1972b). Trifluoperazine antagonized the effect of both compounds.

Amine antagonists or depletion of amines had little or no effect on levels of cyclic AMP in brain. Thus the β-antagonists, dichlorisoproterenol or pronethalol, and the antihistamine, diphenhydramine, had little or no effect on levels of cyclic AMP in mouse cortex (Watanabe and Passonneau, 1975). Propranolol had been cited as reducing brain levels of cyclic AMP (unpublished results of A. R. Somerville in Leonard, 1975b). Reserpine, trifluoperazine, chlorpromazine, *p*-chlorophenylalanine methyl ester, and 6-hydroxydopamine had little or no effect on levels of cyclic AMP in brain or cerebellum (Uzunov and Weiss, 1971; Ferrendelli *et al.*, 1972; Mao *et al.*, 1974b; Watanabe and Passonneau, 1975). Chlorpromazine and haloperidol have been reported by another group to transiently increase levels of cyclic AMP in rat forebrain (Berndt and Schwabe, 1973). This increase was antagonized by theophylline. Theophylline did not, however, prevent the sedation induced by chlorpromazine.

Agents which should increase functional levels of amines by serving as either precursor or agonist, by releasing amines, or by inhibiting inactivation of amines have little or no effect on levels of cyclic AMP in whole brain, but in certain instances they have affected levels of the cyclic nucleotide in particular brain regions. Amphetamine and combinations of a monoamine oxidase inhibitor with dopa had little effect on levels of brain cyclic AMP (Paul *et al.*, 1970d; Ferrendelli *et al.*, 1972; Palmer *et al.*, 1972a; Schmidt *et al.*, 1972). *p*-Chloroamphetamine appeared to reduce levels of cyclic AMP as measured in hypothalamic and brain stem slices. The monoamine oxidase inhibitors, harmaline, pargyline and deprenyl (*N*-methyl-*N*-propynylphenylisopropylamine), had no effect on cerebellar levels of cyclic AMP (Mao *et al.*, 1974a,b; Opmeer *et al.*, 1976). Desipramine transiently increased cyclic AMP in rat forebrain (Berndt and Schwabe, 1973). The central stimulant, nomifensine (8-amino-1,2,3,4-tetrahydro-2-methyl-4-phenylisoquinoline), increased levels of cyclic AMP in rat striatum but not in hypothalamus or cerebellum (Gerhards *et al.*, 1974). Amphetamine, apomorphine, amantadine, nomifensine, and L-dopa had no effect on cyclic AMP levels in forebrain or cerebellum of mice (Gumulka *et al.*, 1976). Dopa caused an increase in levels of cyclic AMP in rat caudate nucleus but did not affect levels of cyclic AMP in the cerebellum (Garelis and Neff, 1974). The increase in the caudate was prevented by prior administration of a dopa decarboxylase inhibitor. Amphetamine and apomorphine increased levels of cyclic AMP in rat striatum and nucleus accumbens, but not in hypothalamus or cerebellum (Gerhards *et al.*, 1974; Carenzi *et al.*, 1975a; Costa *et al.*, 1975; Von Voightlander *et al.*, 1975; Spano *et al.*, 1976). Haloperidol blocked the drug-elicited increases, while morphine had no effect. Amphetamine and apomorphine increased cyclic levels in striatum of 6-hydroxydopamine-treated rats, while only apomorphine was effective in reserpinized rats. Lesions of the substantia nigra did not alter levels of cyclic AMP in rat striatum (Spano *et al.*, 1976). Such lesions would be expected to abolish dopaminergic input to the striatum. Intraventricular dopamine or 2-amino-6,7-dihydroxytetrahydronaphthalene caused increases in levels of cyclic AMP in striatum (Elkhawad *et al.*, 1975). The ergot alkaloid, ergonovine, caused a smaller increase.

Effects of biogenic amines and related drugs on levels of cyclic AMP in cerebrospinal fluid have been investigated. Probenecid markedly increased cerebrospinal levels of cyclic AMP in humans and rabbits, while having little effect on brain levels in rats (Cramer *et al.*, 1972a; Sebens and Korf, 1975). Presumably, the effects of probenecid on cyclic AMP levels in cerebrospinal fluid are due to interference with active translocation of the cyclic nucleotide from this physiological compartment. Intracisternal norepinephrine, isoproterenol, dopamine, and histamine elevated cyclic AMP levels in rabbit cerebrospinal fluid (Sebens and Korf, 1975). Intravenous isoproterenol also elevated cerebrospinal fluid levels of cyclic AMP. Dopa, haloperidol, and a tricyclic anti-depressant, indiomil, had no effect, nor did dopa, haloperidol, reserpine, desipramine, imipramine, clomipramine (chlorimpramine), or isoproterenol significantly reduce probenecid-elicited accumulation of cyclic AMP in the cerebrospinal fluid. One tricyclic antidepressant, maprotiline, did significantly reduce probenecid-elicited accumulations of cyclic AMP, and intracisternal histamine augmented the probenecid effect. Intraperitoneal administration of dopa caused a transient increase in levels of cyclic AMP in cisternal cerebrospinal fluid of rats (Kiessling *et al.*, 1975). An inhibitor of dopamine-β-hydroxylase antagonized the dopa-elicited increase in cerebrospinal cyclic AMP, as did propranolol. Phentolamine alone increased levels of cyclic AMP. Combinations of phentolamine and dopa had no greater effect than either agent alone. Piribedil, a compound with dopaminergic activity *in vivo*, had no effect on levels of cyclic AMP in cerebrospinal fluid.

The effect of administration of drugs known to affect central noradrenergic or dopaminergic mechanism on urinary excretion of cyclic AMP has been investigated in rats (Palmer and Evans, 1974). Reserpine caused an initial great decrease in urinary volume and in excretion of cyclic AMP followed by an increase in cyclic AMP excretion above control values. α-Methyl-p-tyrosine caused an initial decrease followed by elevated excretion of cyclic AMP. Intracranial 6-hydroxydopamine had no effect on urinary cyclic AMP. Chlorpromazine caused a slight increase in excretion of cyclic AMP. Amphetamine had no effect. Chronic administration of lithium carbonate increased excretion of cyclic AMP. Cyclic AMP excretion decreased when daily lithium injections were terminated. Another group reported that reserpine in rats decreased urinary excretion of cyclic AMP, while the tricyclic antidepressants, imipramine and amitryptyline, increased excretion (Keatinge *et al.*, 1975). Chlorpromazine had no effect.

Acetylcholine

Arecoline, a muscarinic agonist, and the cholinesterase inhibitors, paraoxon and physostigmine, had no effect on cyclic AMP levels in mouse cerebrum or cerebellum (Dinnendahl and Stock, 1975). Atropine, a muscarinic antagonist, increased levels of cyclic AMP in rat cerebellum while having no effect on cortical levels (Kimura *et al.*, 1974). Cortical and cerebellar levels of cyclic AMP were decreased in mice by oxotremorine and were unaffected by atropine (Ferrendelli *et al.*, 1970; Mao *et al.*, 1975b). The ganglionic nicotinic antagonists, chlorisondamine and mecamylamine, had no effect on cyclic AMP levels. Oxotremorine in another study was reported to have no effect on levels of cyclic AMP in mouse brain (Opmeer *et al.*, 1976).

Amino Acids

Intraventricular injection of either γ-aminobutyrate, glutamate, or glycine had no effect on levels of cyclic AMP in rat cerebellum (Mao *et al.*, 1974a). Picrotoxin, isoniazid, or strychnine had no effect on cerebellar levels of cyclic AMP. Reductions of central levels of γ-aminobutyrate by hydroxylamine, hydrazine, or aminooxyacetic acid had no effect on levels of cyclic AMP in rat brain (Mao *et al.*, 1975a).

Prostaglandins

Intravenous prostaglandin E_1 in rats caused a transient 30 to 80% elevation of cyclic AMP in cerebral cortex, hypothalamus, thalamus, hippocampus, striatum, cerebellum, and brain stem (Wellmann and Schwabe, 1973). The percentage increase was greatest in cerebral cortex and least in cerebellum and brain stem. Prostaglandins E_1 and E_2 transiently increased levels of cyclic AMP in mouse brain, while $PGF_{2\alpha}$ was virtually ineffective. The transient increase of cyclic AMP certainly did not correlate with the long-lasting sedative effect of prostaglandins. Treatment of rats with an inhibitor of prostaglandin synthesis, indomethacin, had no effect on brain levels of cyclic AMP (Mao *et al.*, 1974a).

Steroids

In vivo administration of estradiol benzoate evoked a transient increase in cyclic AMP levels in hypothalami of young female Holtzman rats (Gunaga *et al.*, 1974). A microwave technique was used to sacrifice the rats. Prior administration of either an estrogenic antagonist, clomiphene, an α-adrenergic antagonist, phentolamine, or a β-adrenergic antagonist, propranolol, prevented the estradiol-elicited increase in hypothalamic levels of cyclic AMP. Testosterone significantly decreased levels of cyclic AMP in brain of young male rats (Zimmerman and Isaacs, 1975).

Phosphodiesterase Inhibitors

Certain phosphodiesterase inhibitors such as theophylline and caffeine are central stimulants, while most others including papaverine, chlordiazepoxide, SQ 20009, ICI 63197, RO 20-1724, ZK 62711, and diazepam are central depressants (cf. Beer *et al.*, 1972). Theophylline, caffeine, papaverine, and ICI 63197 have been reported to increase levels of brain cyclic AMP (Breckenridge, 1964; Paul *et al.*, 1970d; Goldberg *et al.*, 1970; Lee and Dubos, 1972; Arbuthnott *et al.*, 1974; Watanabe and Passonneau,

1975). Diazepam had no effect on cyclic AMP in mouse cerebrum or cerebellum (Dinnendahl and Stock, 1975; Mao *et al.*, 1975a). Theophylline, but not papaverine, increased cyclic AMP in cisternal cerebrospinal fluid of rat (Kiessling *et al.*, 1975). Peripheral 8-bromo cyclic GMP increased brain levels of cyclic AMP (Fernandez-Pol and Hays, 1976).

Morphine

Effects of morphine, chronic morphinization, and withdrawal on levels of cyclic AMP in various brain regions have been investigated. The results from different laboratories are not completely in accord, probably due to differences in dosages, schedules, and strains of experimental animals. Acute treatment of rats with morphine had no significant effect on levels of cyclic AMP in cortex, thalamus–hypothalamus, or cerebellum (Singhal *et al.*, 1973a). Morphine in high dosage was reported to increase levels of cyclic AMP in rat brain (Biebuyck *et al.*, 1975). Acute administration of morphine has been reported to transiently elevate cyclic AMP levels in rat striatum (caudate) (Clouet and Iwatsubo, 1975; Bonnet, 1975; Couet *et al.*, 1975) or to have no effect in either striatum or nucleus accumbens (Carenzi *et al.*, 1975a, b; Racagni *et al.*, 1976). Viminol, another analgesic, also had no effect on striatal levels of cyclic AMP. High acute doses of morphine elevated cyclic AMP levels transiently, not only in striatum but also in midbrain, cortex, and cerebellum, and decreased levels in medulla and hypothalamus (Clouet and Iwatsubo, 1974; Clouet *et al.*, 1975). Acute administration of morphine transiently elevated cyclic AMP levels in rat caudate and subsequently lowered levels in substantia nigra and hypothalamus, while having no effect on levels in thalamus (Bonnet, 1975).

Cyclic AMP levels have been reported by a number of groups to be increased in striatum of chronically morphinized rats. Cyclic AMP levels were increased by chronic morphine in striatum and cortex, but not in other brain regions (Singhal *et al.*, 1973a; Clouet and Iwatsubo, 1974; Clouet *et al.*, 1975) or were increased in caudate, substantia nigra, and thalamus but not in hypothalamus (Bonnet, 1975). In the latter study acute administration of morphine to these animals transiently increased levels in substantia nigra and lowered levels in hypothalamus. Cyclic AMP levels in striatum of chronically morphinized rats and of rats undergoing withdrawal were reported to be slightly elevated (Merali *et al.*, 1975). One group, however, reported little effect of chronic morphinization on striatal and cerebellar levels of cyclic AMP (Mehta and Johnson, 1975). After 1 week of morphinization, but not later, cerebellar levels of cyclic AMP appeared to be reduced. During naloxone-precipitated withdrawal, levels of cyclic AMP increased significantly in cerebellum, while levels in striatum were unaffected.

Other Centrally Active Agents

Ethanol, a central depressant, decreased whole brain and cerebellar levels of cyclic AMP in rats (Volicer and Gold, 1973) or had no effect (Hunt *et al.*, 1976). Chronic treatment of mice with ethanol increased cerebral levels of cyclic AMP (Kuriyama and Isräel, 1973). Other central depressants such as diethyl ether and barbiturates had no effect on levels of cyclic AMP in brain (Kimura *et al.*, 1974); in some cases, barbiturates reduced levels of brain cyclic AMP (Paul *et al.*, 1970d; Schmidt *et al.*, 1972). Cyclic AMP levels in rat brain were reported to be greatly increased by anesthesia with halothane and ketamine (Biebuyck *et al.*, 1975). Phenobarbital and diphenylhydantoin had no effect on cerebellar levels of cyclic AMP (Costa *et al.*, 1975c).

Intraperitoneal injections of tetrahydrocannabinol to mice increased levels of cyclic AMP in whole brain, cerebellum, and medulla (Dolby and Kleinsmeith, 1974). The greatest increases were elicited by 0.1 and 1.0 mg/kg of the cannabinol. Higher dosages had no effect or decreased cyclic AMP levels. Injection of 2.0 mg/kg of the cannabinol caused a decrease in cyclic AMP levels in hypothalamus.

Convulsants

Electroconvulsive shocks caused transient large increases in cyclic AMP levels in rodent brain (Goldberg *et al.*, 1970; Sattin, 1971; Lust and Passonneau, 1976; Lust *et al.*, 1976). Methylxanthines or an increased supply of oxygen to the animals antagonized the increase in cyclic AMP. Electroconvulsive shock caused a very rapid fivefold increase in cyclic AMP levels in mouse cerebral cortex and a twofold increase in cerebellum (Watanabe and Passonneau, 1975; Lust and Passonneau, 1976; Lust *et al.*, 1976). Hypothermia delayed and prolonged the increase in cortical cyclic AMP elicited by electroconvulsive shock and reduced levels in control mice. Trifluoperazine, amphetamine, diphenylhydantoin, and diphenhydramine partially antagonized the increase in cyclic AMP elicited by electroconvulsive shock in cerebral cortex. Amphetamine potentiated the increase in cerebellar levels of cyclic AMP, while phenobarbital had a marginal inhibitory effect. The increase in cyclic AMP in mouse forebrain elicited by electroconvulsive shocks or by hexafluorodiethyl ether in convulsant dosages was antagonized by theophylline (Sattin, 1971). Convulsant levels of another methylxanthine, caffeine, did not elicit a significant increase in cyclic AMP in mouse forebrain. The convulsant, pentylenetetrazole, had no effect on levels of cyclic AMP in rat brain (Paul *et al.*, 1970d). Pentylenetetrazole and picrotoxin were stated to have no effect on cyclic AMP levels in mouse brain (Opmeer *et al.*, 1976). Homocysteine-elicited convulsions in mice elevated cortical levels of cyclic AMP (Folbergrova, 1975). When convulsions were prevented by phenobarbital, cyclic AMP levels were not elevated by homocysteine.

Stress

Stress is well known to increase turnover of central amines and might thus be expected to influence levels of cyclic AMP. The effect of the stress of electric foot shock or of restraint on levels of cyclic AMP in different brain regions of Sprague–Dawley rats has been examined (De La Paz *et al.*, 1975). Shock treatment resulted in significant increases in hippocampus, septum, and brain stem and marginal increases in most other brain regions and in whole brain. Restraint led to significant increases only in septum. Cyclic AMP levels were not altered in any rat brain region by cold stress but were greatly increased in the pituitary gland (Mao *et al.*, 1974b). Stress elicited by exposure of rats to loud bells ringing for 2 to 4 min either once or repeatedly had no significant effect on hypothalamic levels of cyclic AMP, while stress elicited by nitrogen anoxia significantly reduced hypothalamic levels (Siegel *et al.*, 1974). Cyclic AMP levels in mouse cerebrum and cerebellum were unaffected by heat stress, cold stress, or fighting (Dinnendahl, 1975). Effects of various stresses on levels of ATP, ADP, and AMP in brain have been investigated (Dickman *et al.*, 1973 and references therein). Levels of ATP tend to be decreased.

Neither heat nor cold stress had any effect on levels of cyclic AMP in cerebrospinal fluid of cats (Dascombe and Milton, 1975b). Neonatal malnutrition or neonatal infection with a pathogen resulted in a decrease in levels of cyclic AMP in brain of mice at 3 to 4 months of age (Lee and Dubos, 1972, see Section 3.1.13).

4.4.3 Effects of Drugs and Other Treatments on Levels of Cyclic GMP in Brain

Cyclic GMP levels in brain are altered by agents which either depress or stimulate central activity. Central depressants tend to lower levels of cyclic GMP, while central stimulants, tremorigenic agents, or convulsions tend to increase levels. In cerebellum the excitatory amino acid, glutamate, appears involved in maintaining high levels of cyclic GMP, while the inhibitory amino acid, γ-aminobutyrate has the opposite role (see reviews by Costa *et al.*, 1975b,c). It is tempting to speculate that excitatory neurotransmitters such as acetylcholine and glutamate activate cyclic

GMP-generating systems and that cyclic GMP is then responsible for neuronal excitation (cf. Stone *et al.*, 1975). No definite conclusions as to the effects of inhibitory biogenic amine or glycine systems on cyclic GMP levels are presently possible.

Levels of cyclic GMP in brain tissue increase after decapitation, but these increases have not been studied extensively. In rat cerebral cortex only a marginal increase in cyclic GMP occurred after decapitation, while the more profound postdecapitation increase in levels of cyclic GMP in cerebellum was antagonized by pentobarbital and to a lesser extent by ether (Kimura *et al.*, 1974). The factors involved in postdecapitation changes in levels of cyclic GMP in brain tissue are as yet undefined. Unilateral ischemia of gerbil brain elicited by ligation of one carotid artery resulted in a progressive decline in cerebral cortical levels of cyclic GMP over a 6-hr period (Lust *et al.*, 1975).

Central Depressants

Ethanol greatly decreased cyclic GMP levels in rat cerebellum (Hunt *et al.*, 1976; Volicer *et al.*, 1976). During withdrawal cyclic GMP levels increased to control levels. γ-Aminobutyrate levels were decreased during ethanol treatment (see below). Various other central depressants such as magnesium sulfate, diethyl ether, phenobarbital, and papaverine markedly decreased cerebellar levels of cyclic GMP in mice (Lust *et al.*, 1976). Pentobarbital reduced cerebral and cerebellar levels of cyclic GMP in mice (Opmeer *et al.*, 1976) and appeared to reduce cyclic GMP levels in rat cerebral cortex and cerebellum (Kimura *et al.*, 1974). Phenobarbital at high concentrations reduced cerebellar levels of cyclic GMP in rat (Costa *et al.*, 1975c). Reserpine and chlorpromazine decreased levels of cyclic GMP in mouse cerebellum (Ferrendelli *et al.*, 1972), while reserpine had no effect on levels in rat striatum (Racagni *et al.*, 1976). Morphine caused only a marginal reduction in levels of cyclic GMP in mouse cerebellum (Lust *et al.*, 1976). Acute administration of morphine decreased levels of cyclic GMP in rat caudate, substantia nigra, hypothalamus, and thalamus; this perhaps being associated with central depression (Bonnet, 1975). In chronically morphinized rats, levels of cyclic GMP were reduced in the four brain regions and acute administration of morphine had no effect, except for a transient increase in cyclic GMP levels in substantia nigra. In another study analgesic dosages of morphine, viminol, and azidomorphine were found to increase cyclic GMP levels in rat striatum (Racagni *et al.*, 1976). A morphine antagonist, naltrexone. (*N*-cyclopropylmethylnoroxymorphone), blocked the response to morphine. Rapid microwave fixation of rat brain was used in this study. Haloperidol had no effect on basal or morphine-stimulated levels of cyclic AMP in striatum.

Central Stimulants

Amphetamine increased levels of cyclic GMP in mouse cerebellum (Ferrendelli *et al.*, 1972; Lust *et al.*, 1976). Chlorpromazine but not atropine blocked the amphetamine-elicited increase in cerebellar cyclic GMP. Chlorpromazine concomitantly blocked the hyperactivity usually elicited by amphetamine. Amphetamine, apomorphine, amantadine, nomifensine, and dopa increased cyclic GMP levels in mouse forebrain and cerebellum (Gumulka *et al.*, 1976). Amphetamine and apomorphine increased cyclic GMP in rat striatum (Spano *et al.*, 1976). Lesions of the substantia nigra also increased levels of cyclic GMP in the striatum. Such lesions would abolish inhibitory dopaminergic input to striatal neurons.

Tremorigenic Agents

Oxotremorine, a muscarinic agonist, increased levels of cyclic GMP in mouse cortex and cerebellum (Ferrendelli *et al.*, 1970; Opmeer *et al.*, 1976). The time of maximal tremor associated with oxotremorine coincided with the maxima for cortical and cerebellar cyclic GMP. This tremor was blocked by atropine as were the rapid increases in cortical and cerebellar cyclic GMP. Diazepam and pentobarbital reduced the oxotremorine-elicited increase in cortical and cerebellar cyclic GMP. Dinnendahl and Stock (1975) state that oxotremorine increased cyclic GMP levels in mouse brain and that the response was not blocked by melanotropin-release inhibiting factor. Chlorpromazine did not block the oxotremorine-induced increase in levels of cyclic GMP in mouse cerebellum (Ferrendelli *et al.*, 1972). Presumably, oxotremorine, by interaction with extracerebellar cholinergic neurons, increases excitatory input to cerebellum, resulting in an increase in cyclic GMP levels. Harmaline, an agent which induces tremor and increases excitatory climbing fiber input to cerebellar Purkinje cells, greatly increased levels of cyclic GMP in rat cerebellum (Mao *et al.*, 1975a; Spano *et al.*, 1975a). Harmaline is a potent monoamine oxidase inhibitor, but two other inhibitors, pargyline and deprenyl, had no effect on cerebellar levels of cyclic GMP (Mao *et al.*, 1974a). Benztropine, an acetylcholine antagonist, had no effect on harmaline-elicited elevation of cyclic GMP in cerebellum. Diazepam inhibited harmaline-induced elevation of cerebellar cyclic GMP and tremor. Diazepam elicited a marked reduction of cerebellar levels of cyclic GMP in control animals. It was proposed that diazepam may release γ-aminobutyrate from presynaptic terminals on Purkinje cells, resulting in an inhibition of burst discharges from Purkinje cells and a reduction in levels of cyclic GMP (see p. 282). Harmaline increased levels of cyclic GMP in mouse cerebrum and cerebellum (Opmeer *et al.*, 1976). Diazepam and pentobarbital but not atropine antagonized the increase in cyclic GMP elicited by harmaline. Acute treatment of rats with harmaline led to an increase in soluble, but not particulate, guanylate cyclase in rat cerebellum (Spano *et al.*, 1975a). In newborn rats, neither harmaline nor diazepam had any effect on cerebellar levels of cyclic GMP, in contrast to the marked effects of those drugs in adult rats where synaptogenesis to Purkinje cells has been completed (Spano *et al.*, 1975a). 3-Acetylpyridine causes degeneration of the olivocerebellar climbing fiber pathway, and consonant with this degeneration the tremor and the increase in cerebellar cyclic GMP levels elicited by harmaline were blocked in rats treated with 3-acetylpyridine (Guidotti *et al.*, 1975). Basal levels of cyclic GMP were reduced in cerebellum of treated rats. Glutamate, the presumed neurotransmitter of the excitatory climbing fiber pathway, elicited convulsions and increased cerebellar levels of cyclic GMP in both normal and 3-acetylpyridine-treated rats.

Amino Acids

Intraventricular glutamate or glycine markedly increased cerebellar levels of cyclic GMP, while γ-aminobutyrate reduced cyclic GMP (Mao *et al.*, 1974a; Guidotti *et al.*, 1975). Picrotoxin, a γ-aminobutyrate antagonist, elevated cerebellar levels of cyclic GMP in rats as did isoniazid, an inhibitor of synthesis of γ-aminobutyrate (Mao *et al.*, 1974a). Strychnine, a glycine antagonist, had no effect on cerebellar cyclic GMP. Diazepam, a phosphodiesterase inhibitor and anticonvulsant, markedly decreased levels of cyclic GMP and levels of γ-aminobutyrate in rat cerebellum (Mao *et al.*, 1975a,b). It has been proposed that glutamate released from climbing fibers normally activates cyclic GMP formation in Purkinje cells, while γ-aminobutyrate released from basket cell input counteracts glutamate and reduces cyclic GMP levels in Purkinje cells (Mao *et al.*, 1974a). Diazepam has been proposed to affect cyclic GMP levels by mobilizing presynaptic γ-aminobutyrate (Costa *et al.*, 1975c). Diazepam did reduce firing of Purkinje cells (cited in Costa *et al.*, 1975c). A recent electrophysiological study on Purkinje cells and Deiters neurons, however, demonstrated an antagonism by diazepam and chlordiazepoxide of the inhibitory effects of γ-aminobutyrate and its pathways (Steiner and Felix, 1976).

In nervous mutant mice in which cerebellar Purkinje cells are virtually absent, cyclic GMP levels in cerebellum were greatly reduced (Mao *et al.*, 1975b). Diazepam, an agent which normally reduces cyclic GMP levels in cerebellum, had no effect on cerebellar cyclic GMP in "nervous" mutant mice. Diazepam reduced levels of cyclic GMP in both cerebral cortex and cerebellum of mice, suggesting γ-aminobutyrate mechanisms controlling cyclic GMP levels in both brain regions (Dinnendahl and Stock, 1975; Opmeer *et al.*, 1976).

Acetylcholine

Arecoline, a muscarinic agonist, increased cyclic GMP levels in mouse cerebrum and cerebellum (Dinnendahl and Stock, 1975). Atropine slightly increased cerebral and cerebellar levels of cyclic GMP, while combinations of arecoline and atropine now had virtually no effect on cyclic GMP. Others have reported a relatively slow increase in levels of cortical cyclic GMP and a concomitant decrease in cerebellar levels after atropine (Ferrendelli *et al.*, 1970). In rat, atropine increased levels of cyclic GMP in cerebral cortex, while having no effect on cerebellar levels (Kimura *et al.*, 1974). Cerebellum probably does not contain muscarinic synapses, so that the effects of arecoline or atropine on cyclic GMP levels in this brain region are likely to be indirect and due to interaction with extracerebellar muscarinic synapses modulating input to the cerebellum. Arecoline had no stimulatory effect on levels of cyclic GMP in the presence of diazepam (Dinnendahl and Stock, 1975). This is reminiscent of the inhibition of harmaline-elicited increases in cerebellar cyclic GMP by diazepam (see p. 281).

The cholinesterase inhibitors, paraoxon and physostigmine, reduced cyclic GMP levels in mouse cerebellum and slightly increased levels in cerebrum (Dinnendahl and Stock, 1975). Paraoxon had no effect on cyclic GMP levels in the presence of either atropine or diazepam. Another inhibitor, malaoxone, was reported to increase cyclic GMP levels in mouse cerebellum (Goldberg *et al.*, 1973).

Convulsants

Convulsant activity in brain leads to an increase in levels of cyclic GMP, and a variety of evidence with convulsant agents suggests that γ-aminobutyrate pathways may normally modulate in an inhibitory manner levels of cyclic GMP in brain. Many convulsants do either inhibit γ-aminobutyrate synthesis or are antagonists of γ-aminobutyrate receptors. These include thiosemicarbazide, isoniazid, picrotoxin, biccuculine, and pentylenetetrazole. γ-Aminobutyrate at postsynaptic sites such as the Purkinje cell causes an inhibitory hyperpolarization, while at presynaptic terminals of bullfrog sympathetic ganglion γ-aminobutyrate causes a depolarization (Koketsu *et al.*, 1974). Depolarization at a presynaptic terminal will be an inhibitory phenomenon if, as in sympathetic ganglia, it prevents functional release of an excitatory neurotransmitter.

Electroconvulsive shocks increased cyclic GMP levels in mouse cerebellum (Lust and Passonneau, 1976; Lust *et al.*, 1976). Levels of cyclic GMP in cerebellum increased more slowly than levels of cyclic AMP so that maximal levels of cyclic GMP were attained after the early excitatory phase of the convulsion and indeed occurred during the initial part of the depressive phase. Amphetamine potentiated the shock-elicited increase in cerebellar cyclic GMP, while phenobarbital slightly inhibited the increase. In early studies no change in levels of cyclic GMP in mouse cerebrum after electroconvulsive shock was detected (Goldberg *et al.*, 1970). Pentylenetetrazole increased levels of cyclic GMP in mouse cerebrum and cerebellum (Opmeer *et al.*, 1976). Diazepam and pentobarbital but not atropine antagonized the pentylenetetrazole-elicited increases in cyclic GMP.

Convulsant agents such as isoniazid, an inhibitor of glutamate decarboxylase, and picrotoxin, a γ-aminobutyrate antagonist, increased rat cerebellar levels of cyclic GMP in both convulsant and subconvulsant dosages (Mao *et al.*, 1975a). Levels of γ-aminobutyrate in cerebellum were decreased by those treatments. Diazepam inhibited convulsions and antagonized increases in cyclic GMP elicited in cerebellum by isoniazid and picrotoxin. Diazepam was more effective in inhibiting the effects of isoniazid. Picrotoxin increased cerebral and cerebellar levels of cyclic GMP in mice and diazepam, pentobarbital, and atropine antagonized the increases (Opmeer *et al.*, 1976). Glutamate elicited convulsions and increased levels of cerebellar cyclic GMP in rats (Guidotti *et al.*, 1975).

Stress

Heat stress, cold stress, or fighting increased cerebral and cerebellar levels of cyclic GMP in mice (Dinnendahl, 1975). The increase in cerebellar levels was maximal within the first few minutes after stress. Exposure of rats to cold stress resulted in a transient twofold increase in levels of cerebellar cyclic GMP (Mao *et al.*, 1974b). Levels of cyclic GMP were also significantly increased in hypothalamus and brain stem, but not in cerebral cortex or caudate nucleus. A wide variety of drugs including atropine, chlorisondamine, mecamylamine, *p*-chlorophenylalanine methyl ester, indomethacin, pargyline, reserpine, and intraventricular 6-hydroxydopamine had no effect on levels of cerebellar cyclic GMP in either control or cold-stressed animals. Levels of γ-aminobutyrate in cerebellum were increased by treatment of rats with drugs such as hydroxylamine, hydrazine, and aminooxyacetic acid which decrease metabolism of γ-aminobutyrate by decreasing activity of the enzyme, γ-aminobutyrate transaminase; the resultant elevation of γ-aminobutyrate showed an excellent inverse correlation with the magnitude of cold-stress-elicited increase in cerebellar cyclic GMP. Hydrazine decreased control levels of cerebellar cyclic GMP and caused a profound increase in levels of γ-aminobutyrate and profound inhibition of the increase in the cyclic GMP elicited by cold stress. Reduction of cerebellar levels of γ-aminobutyrate with subconvulsive and convulsive dosages of isoniazid resulted in a marked increase in cerebellar cyclic GMP levels in control and cold-stressed animals. However, there was no significant difference between the elevated levels in the control and cold-stressed animals. The results clearly indicate that stress-elicited increases in cyclic GMP in brain were under inhibitory control by γ-aminobutyrate.

4.4.4 Behavioral Correlations

Cyclic AMP levels in mouse forebrain were similar at low and high points of diurnal behavioral activity (Nahorski and Rogers, 1973). Levels of cyclic AMP in whole rat brain did not undergo significant diurnal fluctuations (Burkard et al., 1971).

Cyclic AMP levels in mouse brain were highest in two mouse strains, C57B1/6J and BALB/CJ, with a tendency toward aggression and were lower in three more passive mouse strains, CAF, A/J, and CBA/J (Barchas et al., 1974; Orenberg et al., 1975). In hybrids of BALB–A/J mice, levels of cyclic AMP were low, as was aggression, indicating that both characteristics were transmitted as recessive traits. In F_2 mice, a classical Mendelian 3:1 (nonfighter:fighter) ratio pertained, and the aggressive mice had higher levels of brain cyclic AMP than the nonaggressive mice.

In four strains of rat, high spontaneous behavioral activity (Segal et al., 1972) correlated with high responses of a norepinephrine-sensitive cyclic AMP-generating system in slices from midbrain-striatum and with low responses of such systems in cerebral cortical slices (Skolnick and Daly, 1974a, Figure 23, see Section 3.1.3). Correlations did not pertain between spontaneous behavioral activity and accumulations of cyclic AMP elicited in cortical or midbrain-striatal slices by isoproterenol, adenosine, adenosine-norepinephrine, or veratridine. The responses to the α-agonist, methoxamine, in cortical slices were, like responses to norepinephrine, inversely correlated with spontaneous behavioral activity (Skolnick and Daly, 1975b). It would appear that correlations of spontaneous activity and responsiveness of catecholamine-sensitive cyclic AMP-generating systems in cortex reflect mainly the α-adrenergic component. Intraventricular norepinephrine was more effective in increasing spontaneous motor activity (Segal et al., 1975) in BUF rats, a strain with more responsive norepinephrine-sensitive cyclic AMP systems in midbrain-striatum than in F-344 rats, a strain with less responsive midbrain-striatal systems (Skolnick and Daly, 1974a).

At the time of enhanced motor activity, which occurs after about 8 to 12 days of reserpine treatment, the responses of cyclic AMP-generating systems to norepinephrine in rat brain slices were significantly enhanced (Williams and Pirch, 1974). The magnitude of the response to norepineph-

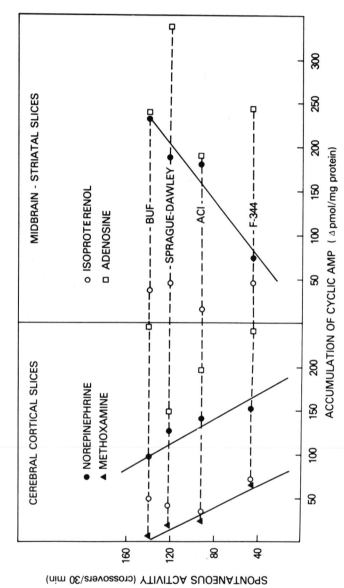

Figure 23. Correlations between spontaneous behavior activity and accumulations of cyclic AMP elicited by norepinephrine and methoxamine in brain slices from four rat strains. All agents were 100 μM and incubation with slices was for 9 to 15 min. The accumulation of cyclic AMP above basal values is plotted for each agent versus spontaneous activity. (Data from Skolnick and Daly, 1974a, 1975b.)

rine in brain slices from each reserpinized rat exhibited a positive correlation with the magnitude of the increase in motor activity of that rat above the average control activity (Figure 24; see p. 168).

The magnitude of accumulations of cyclic AMP elicited by adenosine in cerebral cortical slices from mice of C57, SEC, and DBA strains and in hybrids of C57–SEC and C57–DBA appeared to be inversely correlated with rates of active avoidance learning in these mice (Sattin, 1975, Figure 25, see Section 3.1.4). The C57B1/6J mice which exhibited lower responses to norepinephrine and adenosine-sensitive cyclic AMP-generating systems are much less susceptible to pentylenetetrazole and electroconvulsive and audiogenic seizures than DBA mice (Fuller and Sjursen, 1967; Schlesinger et al., 1968). Adenosine-elicited accumulations of cyclic AMP occur during convulsions and because of inhibitory effects on neuronal activity might protect against convulsions. Adenosine did protect mice against audiogenic seizures (Maitre et al., 1974). The responsiveness of the adenosine-sensitive cyclase systems in cerebral slices of the C57 and DBA mice does not, however, appear correlated with strain differences in sensitivity to convulsions.

Recent studies with eight inbred strains of mice did not provide any clear correlations between accumulations of cyclic AMP elicited by norepinephrine or adenosine in cerebral slices and rates of active avoidance learning (Stalvey et al., 1976). Adenosine- but not norepinephrine-elicited accumulations of cyclic AMP were correlated with spontaneous activity in five inbred strains and with active avoidance learning in individuals of an outbred strain.

Bilateral injections of choleratoxin into the rat nucleus accumbens caused a gradual, but long-lasting activation of adenylate cyclases and a concomitant increase in locomotor activity (Miller and Kelly, 1975; Iversen et al., 1975a). A similar increase in locomotor activity was elicited in 6-hydroxydopamine-treated animals. Injection of dopamine into this brain region is known to elicit a short-lasting increase in locomotor activity.

4.4.5 Clinical Correlations

Electroconvulsive therapy of depressed patients increased urinary cyclic AMP (Hamadah et al., 1972). Whether urinary levels reflect changes in cyclic AMP metabolism in the central nervous system is, however, not certain. A number of papers have provided data that appeared to correlate low amounts of urinary cyclic AMP with depression in humans (Abdulla and Hamadah, 1970; Paul et al., 1970b,c,d, 1971a,b; Cramer et al., 1972a,b). Manic patients appeared to excrete significantly more cyclic AMP than normal controls. In manic-depressive patients a large increase in

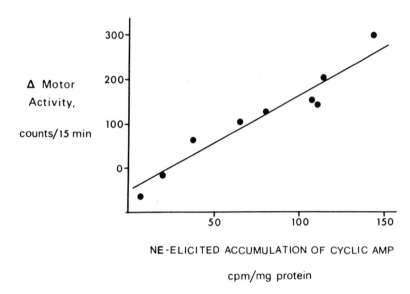

Figure 24. Correlation of reserpine-induced hyperactivity and enhanced responsiveness of cyclic AMP-generating systems to norepinephrine (NE) in rat brain slices. The increase in spontaneous motor activity of each individual rat above the average of controls is plotted against the norepinephrine (100 μM)-elicited increase in accumulations of radioactive cyclic AMP in adenine-labeled brain slices. Data were obtained after 8 to 12 days of chronic re-serpine treatment in Harvard Press slices incubated with caffeine. (Modified from Williams and Pirch, 1974, *Brain Research,* copyright Elsevier Publishing Co.)

urinary cyclic AMP occurred on the day of transition from the depressed to manic state. Excretion of urinary cyclic AMP reflected the extent of depression and was increased during successful therapy by electroshock treatment, antidepressants, dopa, and lithium ions. Urinary cyclic AMP was not significantly different in normal controls and in patients with neurotic depression. Other groups saw no correlations of urinary cyclic AMP levels with the affective state of manic-depressive patients (Brown *et al.,* 1972; Jenner *et al.,* 1972; Somerville, 1973) or of two patients with periodic catatonia (Perry *et al.,* 1973). However, in one patient decreases in cyclic AMP excretion over a period of 4 days correlated with periods of depression (Jenner *et al.,* 1972). It is possible that urinary changes in cyclic AMP reflected primarily increases in the physical activity of patients (cf. Robison *et al.,* 1970a). Exercise in normal controls has been reported to increase urinary cyclic AMP (Eccleston *et al.,* 1970), but another group reported no change in urinary cyclic AMP with exercise (Paul *et al.,*

1971a). Urinary excretion of cyclic AMP was significantly lower in controls than in patients suffering from either "neurotic" or "endogenous" depression (Sinanan *et al.*, 1974, 1975). Exercise did not increase urinary excretion of cyclic AMP during a subsequent 4-hr period. It was stated that as depression responded to therapy the urinary excretion of cyclic AMP increased to control values. Epinephrine did not elicit an increase in urinary cyclic AMP in lithium-treated humans, but did in normal controls (Ebstein *et al.*, 1976). No differences in responses of cyclic AMP-generating systems in platelets from depressed patients and normal controls were observed (Wang *et al.*, 1974). The phosphodiesterase inhibitor, ICI 63197, had no effect on urinary cyclic AMP (Somerville, 1973). Cyclic AMP and cyclic GMP levels in urine under various conditions has been reviewed (Murad, 1973; Moyes and Moyes, 1976).

Correlations between levels of cyclic AMP in cerebrospinal fluid and disease states have been attempted. The concentration of cyclic AMP in

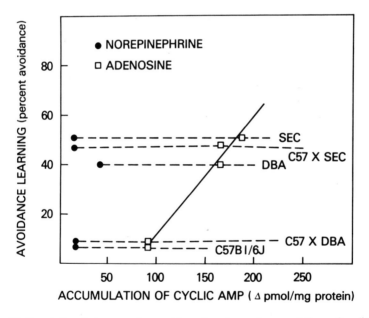

Figure 25. Correlations between active avoidance learning and accumulations of cyclic AMP elicited by norepinephrine (100 μM) and adenosine (200 μM) in cerebral cortical slices from three mice strains and hybrid mice. Incubations with agents were for 10 min. The accumulation of cyclic AMP above basal values is plotted versus percentage avoidances of electric shock in a shuttle box paradigm. (Data from Sattin, 1971, and Oliverio *et al.*, 1972.)

human cerebrospinal fluid is 10 to 40 μM (Murad *et al.*, 1969; Robison *et al.*, 1971; Broadus *et al.*, 1970), while the concentration of cyclic GMP is lower at 0 to 7 μM. No pronounced differences in levels of cyclic AMP pertained in cerebral spinal fluid from manic or depressed patients, from epileptics, or from other neurological patients (Robison *et al.*, 1970a; Cramer *et al.*, 1972a,b, 1973b). Manic and neurological patients had somewhat lower levels than depressed patients. Probenecid caused an increase in cerebrospinal cyclic AMP which was greatest in manic patients. Exercise had no effect on cyclic AMP in cerebrospinal fluid, and no diurnal variations were observed. In another study no clear correlations of levels of cyclic AMP in cerebrospinal fluid or of urinary excretion of cyclic AMP with neurological disease states were detected (Heikkinen *et al.*, 1974). Ingestion of papaverine, theophylline, phenothiazines, benzodiazepines, or anticonvulsants had no significant effect on cyclic AMP in cerebrospinal fluid or urine. Levels of cyclic AMP in cerebrospinal fluid were similar in untreated patients with Parkinson's disease, Huntington chorea, dystonia and dyskinesia, and spinocerebellar degeneration and in patients with peripheral neuro- or myopathic disorders (Cramer *et al.*, 1973b). Neither acute nor chronic treatment of patients with dopa altered the level of cyclic AMP. Levels of cyclic AMP in cerebrospinal fluid were somewhat lower in neurological patients with significant cerebral atrophy (Myllyla *et al.*, 1974b). Pneumonencephalography, the injection of air into the ventricular system, causes many central alterations, presumably due to temporary ischemia, but had no effect on levels of cyclic AMP in cerebrospinal fluid. Patients with acute or rapidly progressing brain damage had higher levels of cyclic AMP in cerebrospinal fluid than patients with chronic or slowly progressing brain damage (Myllyla *et al.*, 1975). Levels of cyclic AMP in cerebrospinal fluid of epileptics were lower than those in controls and they increased after convulsive attacks (Vapaatalo, 1974; Myllyla *et al.*, 1975). After cerebral infarction, cyclic AMP levels were increased in cerebrospinal fluid and in systemic venous blood (Welch *et al.*, 1975). Urinary excretion of cyclic AMP was not altered. Administration of glycerol to these patients decreased cerebrospinal levels of cyclic AMP and appeared to decrease "release" of cyclic AMP into cerebral venous blood. Levels of cyclic AMP in cerebrospinal fluid of children tended to be lower than those in adults (Myllyla *et al.*, 1975). Levels appeared to be higher in cerebrospinal fluid of individual children with cerebellar medulloblastoma, bacterial meningitis, Cushing's disease, and hypothalamic precocious puberty (Heikkinen *et al.*, 1975; Myllyla *et al.*, 1974a). Bacterial pyrogenic substances elicited hyperthermia in cats and an elevation of levels of cyclic AMP in cerebrospinal fluid (Dascombe and Milton, 1975a,b). 4-Acetamidophenol reduced the hyperthermia but had no effect on elevation of levels of cyclic AMP in cerebrospinal fluid. Cyclic AMP levels in cerebrospinal fluid increased twofold during fever elicited in rabbits by *Escherichia coli* endotoxin (Phillip-Dormston and Siegert, 1975a).

4.5 Central Behavioral and Vegetative Functions

Roles of cyclic nucleotides in the integrated function of the central nervous system have been probed primarily by administration of analogs of cyclic nucleotides. Possible correlations of alterations in central function after treatment with phosphodiesterase inhibitors or drugs or environmental manipulations that affect central levels of nucleotides are also relevant (see Section 4.4). Cyclic AMP, cyclic GMP, and analogs have been administered peripherally, intraventricularly, or directly into specific brain regions by intracerebral injections and effects on behavior, vegetative function, and interactions with drugs, particularly barbiturates and morphine, have then been assessed. The results of such studies must be considered to represent a pharmacological summation of both the specific and nonspecific effects of a cyclic nucleotide on a variety of systems and cell types and probably bear little relationship to the effects of physiological generation of cyclic AMP or cyclic GMP in specific cells of the functioning central nervous system. In particular, peripherally administered cyclic AMP, cyclic GMP, or analogs would not be expected to penetrate into the brain. However, incorporation of radioactivity from intraperitoneal [8-^{14}C]cyclic AMP into mouse brain has been reported (Lee and Dubos, 1972), and intravenous administration of cyclic AMP rapidly elevated levels of cyclic AMP in cat cerebrospinal fluid (Dascombe and Milton, 1975b,c). Intravenous cyclic AMP did not, however, increase levels of the cyclic nucleotide in rabbit cerebrospinal fluid (Sebens and Korf, 1975). Intravenous dibutyryl cyclic AMP increased permeability of brain capillaries as evidenced by increased permeation of intravenous ferretin into astrocytes (Joo *et al.*, 1975a). Thus, cyclic AMP mechanisms may be important to the control of the blood brain barrier (cf. Joo *et al.*, 1972). Peripherally administered cyclic AMP does appear to affect central function, but to what extent this represents direct effects in brain remains uncertain. Similarly, cyclic nucleotides administered intraventricularly will have greater effects on more accessible brain regions and lesser effects on regions distant from the ventricular space. Osmotic and toxic effects of the injection of relatively large amounts of the cyclic nucleotide cannot be ignored. Degradation by phosphodiesterases and penetration of the cyclic nucleotides will, of course, limit their sphere of action. Roles of cyclic AMP-generating systems in central function would appear to be profitably studied by injection of choleratoxin into specific brain regions (cf. Miller and Kelly, 1975). This toxin activates adenylate cyclases and should therefore result in a more physiological generation of elevated levels of cyclic AMP than injection of large amounts of cyclic AMP analogs.

4.5.1 Behavioral Effects

Effects of central administration of cyclic AMP or its dibutyryl derivative in whole animals have been studied by a number of groups. In rats (Gessa et al., 1970; Herman, 1973; Brus et al., 1974; Cohn, 1975), cats (Gessa et al., 1970; Clark et al., 1974b), chickens (Asakawa and Yoshida, 1971), rabbits (Phillip-Dormston and Siegert, 1975b), and goldfish (Shashoua, 1971), intraventricular or intracerebral injection of dibutyryl cyclic AMP and less effectively of cyclic AMP elicited an increase in spontaneous motor and exploratory activity. Episodes of catatonia, aggressive behavior, and convulsions were observed after intraventricular injection in mammals. N^6-Butyryl, N^6-octanoyl, and N^6-dansyl cyclic AMP had effects like those of the dibutyryl derivative. In most studies the effects of dibutyryl cyclic AMP occurred with a latency of 10 to 15 min and then persisted for several hours. Intracerebral injection of cyclic AMP or the dibutyryl derivative in chicken cortex elicited locomotor and vocal activity (Asakawa and Yoshida, 1971). This enhancement in locomotor activity could be blocked by high doses of intracerebral prostaglandin E_1. Central excitatory effects of histamine were also blocked by prostaglandin. Similar excitatory effects were observed in mammals or chickens after intracerebral injection of dibutyryl cyclic AMP into the hypothalamus (Breckenridge and Lisk, 1969; Gessa et al., 1970; Booth, 1972; Marley and Nistico, 1972; Dascombe and Milton, 1975a) or the mesencephalic reticular formation (Gessa et al., 1970). Surprisingly, intrahypothalamic administration of cyclic AMP to chickens induced behavioral and electrocortical sleep rather than the excitation, contralateral turning, convulsions, and bursts of electrocortical spike activity elicited by the dibutyryl derivative (Marley and Nistico, 1972). Cyclic AMP had effects only in chickens pretreated with aminophylline. Intrahypothalamic or intraventricular adenosine in aminophylline-treated chickens also elicited sleep. Intraperitoneal adenosine had sedative effects in mice (Maitre et al., 1974), and intraventricular adenosine had hypogenic effects in dog (Haulica et al., 1973). Catatonia elicited by dibutyryl cyclic AMP was pronounced in cats only after intracerebral injections into the reticular formation (Gessa et al., 1970). Injection of dibutyryl cyclic AMP into cat amygdala elicited convulsions and circling movements. Cerebellar injection elicited sleep without rapid eye movements, while no effects were seen after injection into caudate nucleus, putamen, or pallidum. Cyclic AMP itself, although ineffective in most brain regions, was effective in cerebellum, a brain region where levels of phosphodiesterase are relatively low. The effects of dibutyryl cyclic AMP in rats were not prevented by prior administration of chlorpromazine or reserpine. The increase in locomotor activity, irritability, and convulsions elicited by intraventricular dibutyryl cyclic AMP was intensified in rats previously treated with intraventricular 6-hydroxydopamine (Brus *et al.*, 1974). Intraventricular injection of subthreshold amounts of dibutyryl cyclic AMP in rats potentiated the excitatory effects of intraventricular norepinephrine (Herman, 1973). Conversely, norepinephrine prevented the convulsions normally elicited by the cyclic nucleotide. Behavioral effects of cyclic AMP itself were manifest only in animals treated with dimethylsulfoxide and/or theophylline. It has been claimed that cyclic AMP or the dibutyryl derivative would reverse reserpine-elicited ptosis in rodents, but no details were reported (Abdulla and Hamadah, 1970). In mice, dibutyryl cyclic AMP had no significant effect on reserpine-induced ptosis or behavioral depression (Doggett and Spencer, 1973). Dibutyryl cyclic AMP in mice has, in a number of investigations, been reported to cause sedation rather than excitation (see below). Dibutyryl cyclic GMP had no effect on the sedation followed by hyperactivity and convulsions elicited by intraventricular dibutyryl cyclic AMP in rats (Cohn, 1975). Topical application of dibutyryl cyclic AMP to kitten cerebral cortex resulted in convulsions (Purpura and Shoffer, 1972).

Although in most studies dibutyryl cyclic AMP elicited central excitation, a transient initial sedation was sometimes observed, and in mice sedation has been the usual effect. In one study intraventricular dibutyryl cyclic AMP was reported to cause sedation in cats (Varagic and Beleslin, 1973). In guinea pig, intraventricular dibutyryl cyclic AMP and cyclic AMP elicited sedation and synchronization of electroencephalographic patterns similar to that seen under barbiturate narcosis (Beani *et al.*, 1975). Adenosine, guanosine, and AMP had little or no effect. Cyclic GMP increased locomotor and exploratory behavior and desynchronized the electroencephalographic patterns. In mice, dibutyryl cyclic AMP and cyclic AMP have been reported to cause transient reductions in locomotor activity (Leonard, 1972) and sedation (Henion *et al.*, 1967) or to have little effect on behavior (Doggett and Spencer, 1971). The depressant effects of centrally administered ouabain were antagonized by dibutyryl cyclic AMP.

Preliminary findings indicated that unilateral injections of dibutyryl cyclic AMP into striatum induced contralateral turning similar to that seen after injections of dopamine or apomorphine (cited in Iversen *et al.*, 1975a).

Dibutyryl cyclic AMP injected into the rat nucleus accumbens elicited sniffing, salivation, and intermittent "leaps and jerks" and in some animals convulsions (Jackson *et al.*, 1975). These behavioral effects were quite unlike the increase in coordinated locomotor activity elicited by injection of dopamine and were more reminiscent of the convulsions elicited by norepinephrine. Theophylline, a central stimulant, potentiated apomorphine-induced turning in rats unilaterally lesioned by 6-hydroxydopamine (Fuxe and Ungerstedt, 1974; Arbuthnott *et al.*, 1974). It appeared unlikely that this potentiation of a dopaminergic mechanism by theophylline was due to inhibition of phosphodiesterase, since a variety of more potent phosphodiesterase inhibitors, such as papaverine, chlordiazepoxide, diazepam, and ICI 63197, which have central sedative properties, did not potentiate the apomorphine effect, but instead tended to reduce it. Theophylline and caffeine potentiated the stimulation of locomotor activity elicited by dopamine agonists (Fuxe and Ungerstedt, 1974; Anden and Jackson, 1975; Waldeck, 1975, and references therein). Caffeine potentiated amphetamine- and apomorphine-induced stereotyped behavior in guinea pigs (Klawans *et al.*, 1974). Enhanced toxic effects of methylxanthines in animals treated with monoamine oxidase inhibitors were reduced by *p*-chlorophenylalanine, a compound which reduces serotonin levels, but not by α-methyl-*p*-tyrosine, a compound which reduces catecholamine levels (Berkowitz *et al.*, 1971). It remains unclear as to whether inhibition of phosphodiesterases has any relevance to central actions of methylxanthines.

In contrast to the usual excitatory effects of intraventricular dibutyryl cyclic AMP and cyclic AMP, parentally administered cyclic AMP or dibutyryl cyclic AMP usually depressed activity and caused sedation. After intraperitoneal injection, dibutyryl cyclic AMP reduced spontaneous and exploratory motor activity (Henion *et al.*, 1967; Weiner and Olson, 1973; Pichichero *et al.*, 1973) and had antianxiety properties as measured in a behavioral conflict test (Beer *et al.*, 1972; Horovitz *et al.*, 1972). Intraperitoneal administration of the 6-piperidyl analog of cyclic AMP, but not dibutyryl cyclic AMP, was reported to cause sedation in rats (Vargui and Spano, 1971). Parenteral dibutyryl cyclic AMP decreased spontaneous behavioral activity in mice (Weiner and Olson, 1973, 1975). Dibutyryl cyclic AMP had no effect on rotarod performance except in combination with prostaglandin. A second treatment 24 hr later with the cyclic nucleotide had no effect on spontaneous behavioral activity.

Intraventricular, intrahypothalamic, or intrastriatal choleratoxin in chicken elicited an increase in motor activity (Nistico *et al.*, 1976). After intraventricular administration desynchronization of electrocortical activity was observed.

4.5.2 Vegetative Effects

Intraventricular or intracerebral dibutyryl cyclic AMP have been reported to elicit hyperthermia and in some instances hypothermia in various mammals. Intraventricular dibutyryl cyclic AMP elicited hyperthermia in cats (Gessa et al., 1970; Clark et al., 1974b). Antipyretics inhibited the hyperthermic response to dibutyryl cyclic AMP and to cholera enterotoxin but not to prostaglandin E_1. It was proposed that choleratoxin but not prostaglandin elicits fever by a cyclic AMP mechanism. Intraventricular or intrahypothalamic but not intrastriatal choleratoxin caused hyperthermia in chicken (Nistico et al., 1976). Another group reported that intraventricular dibutyryl cyclic AMP elicited a prolonged hyperthermia in cats (Varagic and Beleslin, 1973). A biphasic response, hypothermia followed by hyperthermia, was observed in about one-third of the cats after dibutyryl cyclic AMP administration. Such a biphasic response was not observed after administration of ATP or butyrate, both of which elicited only the hyperthermia. Intraventricular dibutyryl cyclic AMP but not cyclic AMP elicited a pronounced hyperthermia in rabbits (Phillipp-Dormston and Siegert, 1975b). Dibutyryl cyclic AMP did not elicit hyperthermia in squirrel monkey (Lipton and Fessler, 1974). High doses of cyclic AMP and dibutyryl cyclic AMP elicited hypothermia in guinea pigs (Beani et al., 1975). Cyclic GMP had no effect, but high doses were not studied. In mice, dibutyryl cyclic AMP antagonized ouabain- and reserpine-induced hypothermia (Doggett and Spencer, 1971; 1973). Dibutyryl cyclic AMP in control mice had little effect on body temperature. Dibutyryl cyclic AMP did not reduce the hypothermia associated with barbiturate treatment (Cohn et al., 1973a). Implantation of dibutyryl cyclic AMP or cyclic AMP in the anterior hypothalamus or arcuate nucleus of rats resulted in hyperthermia (Breckenridge and Lisk, 1969). Intrahypothalamic dibutyryl cyclic AMP or prostaglandin E_1 caused hyperthermia in rabbits (Laburn et al., 1974; Woolf et al., 1975, 1976). Theophylline increased and nicotinic acid decreased the hyperthermia elicited by intrahypothalamic prostaglandin E_1. Salicylate failed to antagonize hyperthermia elicited by injection of dibutyryl cyclic AMP into anterior hypothalamus of rabbits (Willies et al., 1976). The hyperthermia elicited by intrahypothalamic injection of a bacterial pyrogen or prostaglandin E_1 was antagonized by an exotoxin of Bacillus thuringiensis (Woolf et al., 1976). The hyperthermia elicited by dibutyryl cyclic AMP was not antagonized by this exotoxin, which in vitro inhibits adenylate cyclases. Cyclic AMP, dibutyryl cyclic AMP, AMP, ADP, and ATP injected into cat anterior hypothalamus elicited hypothermia (Dascombe and Milton, 1975a). High doses of dibutyryl cyclic AMP caused a transient hyperthermia. Intravenous administration of dibutyryl cyclic AMP had no effect on temperature in rabbit (Phillipp-Dormston and Siegert, 1975b), while intravenous cyclic AMP elicited hypothermia in cats (Dascombe and Milton, 1975b).

Intracerebral injection of dibutyryl cyclic AMP has been reported to have effects on food and water intake. Implantation of dibutyryl cyclic AMP in the mammilary body of the hypothalamus caused an increase in food intake and growth in rats (Breckenridge and Lisk, 1969). Intrahypothalamic injections of dibutyryl cyclic AMP had effects on both food intake and on preferential intake of salt- and saccharin-flavored food in rats (Booth *et al.*, 1972). Intraamygdaloid injections or intraperitoneal administration of the dibutyryl derivative had no significant effect on these parameters. Dibutyryl cyclic AMP was effective in increasing water intake only when injected in specific sites of the lateral hypothalamus (Rindi *et al.*, 1972; Sciorelli *et al.*, 1972). Effects of intrahypothalamic dibutyryl cyclic AMP on food intake were less pronounced and tended to be inhibitory. However, in combination with physostigmine, an inhibitor of acetylcholine esterase, dibutyryl cyclic AMP had a stimulatory effect on food intake when injected in the lateral hypothalamus. In combination with intraperitoneal atropine, a muscarinic antagonist, or with intrahypothalamic hemicholinium, an agent which might deplete acetylcholine by preventing reuptake of choline, dibutyryl cyclic AMP in the lateral hypothalamus now exhibited *inhibitory* effects on both water and food intake. The results clearly suggest an interrelationship between cholinergic mechanisms and the effects of intrahypothalamic dibutyryl cyclic AMP on ingestive responses.

Intraventricular dibutyryl cyclic AMP increased blood pressure and heart rate in cats (Saxena and Bahargava, 1974; Walland, 1975). Theophylline had similar effects and potentiated the central effects of ouabain. Intraventricular imidazole-4-acetic acid, an agent which might activate phosphodiesterases, reduced blood pressure and heart rate. High doses of intraventricular cyclic AMP and dibutyryl cyclic AMP reduced blood pressure and heart rate in guinea pigs (Beani *et al.*, 1975).

Implantation of dibutyryl cyclic AMP in the arcuate nucleus of the hypothalamus prolonged estrus cycles and resulted in pseudopregnancy in female rats (Breckenridge and Lisk, 1969). In spayed rats, intrahypothalamic dibutyryl cyclic AMP could not substitute for an estrogen in the induction of lordosis.

Microinjections of dibutyryl cyclic AMP into the median eminance of the hypothalamus, but not injections into the lateral hypothalamus, resulted in a significant increase in plasma levels of corticosterone, presumably via an increased release of corticotropin-releasing factor from the hypothalamus and a resultant increase in ACTH release from the pituitary (Hedge,

1971). The effect was blocked by dexamethasone. Injection of cyclic AMP and theophylline into the third ventricle elevated circulating levels of luteinizing hormone in rat (S. R. Ojeda and S. M. McCann, cited in Gunaga *et al.*, 1974). Intraventricular cyclic AMP had no effect on accumulation of iodide into the thyroid (Knopp and Mitro, 1973).

4.5.3 Centrally Active Drugs

Central Depressants

Intraventricular administration of dibutyryl cyclic AMP to rats shortened the narcosis elicited by amobarbital and a variety of other soporifics such as diazepam, ketamine, halothane, ethanol, methanol, paraldehyde, and chloral hydrate (Cohn *et al.*, 1973a,b, 1975a,b, 1976; Cohn, 1975). Dibutyryl cyclic AMP also significantly reduced the toxicity of amobarbital and other soporifics. No behavioral changes were observed after administration of dibutyryl cyclic AMP to amobarbital-treated rats. Dibutyryl cyclic AMP had no effect on levels of amobarbital in brain. Cyclic AMP and cyclic GMP had no effect on amobarbital narcosis, and dibutyryl cyclic GMP did not prevent the dibutyryl cyclic AMP-elicited shortening of amobarbital narcosis. Another group reported that high doses of intraventricular cyclic GMP in guinea pigs reversed pentobarbital narcosis and desynchronized the slow wave encephalographic pattern (Beani *et al.*, 1975). An α-adrenergic blocker, phentolamine, antagonized the effect of dibutyryl cyclic AMP on amobarbital narcosis. Propranolol did not antagonize the effect. In contrast to the shortening effect of dibutyryl cyclic AMP on amobarbital narcosis, intraventricular norepinephrine prolonged it. Intraperitoneal dibutyryl cyclic AMP reduced sleeping times in rats administered both amobarbital and norepinephrine. Toxic effects of intraventricular norepinephrine were not reduced by dibutyryl cyclic AMP. Intraperitoneal administration of a 6-piperidyl analog of cyclic AMP was reported by another group to prolong hexobarbital sleeping time in rats (Vargui and Spano, 1971). Brain levels of hexobarbital were increased by this cyclic AMP analog. Parenteral dibutyryl cyclic AMP had apparently no effect in hexobarbital sleeping time.

Ethanol

Cyclic AMP appeared to increase the rate of development of acute tolerance to ethanol in rats (Wahlstrom, 1975). Tolerance to ethanol was assessed by changes in threshold to hexobarbital anesthesia, 0.5 and 3 hr after ethanol. In cyclic AMP-treated animals rather high doses of hexobarbital were needed to supress electroencephalographic activity at both 0.5 and 3 hr, while in controls, tolerance had not developed at 0.5 hr and a lower dose of hexobarbital sufficed. Blood levels of alcohol were similar at 0.5 and 3 hr.

Morphine

Cyclic AMP and dibutyryl cyclic AMP on intravenous or intracerebral administration antagonized morphine analgesia and accelerated the development of tolerance of and dependence on morphine in rats (Ho *et al.*, 1972, 1973a,b, 1975a,b). 2′,3′-Cyclic AMP and cyclic GMP were ineffective. Chronic administration of theophylline had similar stimulatory effects on rate of development of tolerance and dependence. Withdrawal symptoms were much more pronounced in cyclic AMP-treated animals. The antagonism of the analgesic effects of morphine by an injection of cyclic nucleotide persisted for at least 24 hr. Cyclic AMP did not antagonize morphine analgesia in mice in which levels of biogenic amines had been increased by prior treatment with a monoamine oxidase inhibitor, pargyline. Increases in norepinephrine levels appeared to be responsible for the prevention of the antagonistic effect of cyclic AMP, since pretreatment with dihydroxyphenylserine to selectively increase norepinephrine levels prevented cyclic AMP action, while pretreatment with dopa to selectively increase dopamine or with tryptophan to selectively increase serotonin did not prevent the antagonism of morphine analgesia by cyclic AMP. Prior administration of a β-adrenergic antagonist such as propranolol, pronethalol, or dichlorisoproterenol or an inhibitor of protein synthesis such as cycloheximide greatly reduced the cyclic AMP-elicited acceleration of the rate of the development of tolerance and dependence on morphine. Repeated administration of dichlorisoproterenol was required in order to inhibit the development of dependence and tolerance in control animals. Clearly, biogenic amines are involved in both the antagonism of morphine analgesia by cyclic AMP and in the acceleration of the development of tolerance and dependence on morphine by cyclic AMP. For both effects norepinephrine appeared to be required. Another group reported that after intraperitoneal administration to mice cyclic AMP antagonized morphine analgesia measured 18 hr later (Gourley and Bechner, 1973). However, adenosine, ATP, AMP, and adenine also antagonized morphine analgesia.

Drugs which might be expected to alter central levels of cyclic AMP slightly antagonized (theophylline) or potentiated (imidazole) morphine analgesia (Ho *et al.*, 1973b; Contreras *et al.*, 1972). Theophylline and caffeine have intrinsic central analgesic activity (Paalzow and Paalzow, 1973). The phosphodiesterase inhibitors, isobutylmethylxanthine and theophylline, exacerbated many aspects of the morphine-withdrawal syndrome in rat (Collier and Francis, 1975). Imidazole, a substance known to activate brain phosphodiesterases, reduced the jumping normally associated with morphine withdrawal. Intraventricular cyclic AMP and dibutyryl cyclic AMP increased jumping, while cyclic GMP and dibutyryl cyclic GMP did not have a significant effect on jumping. Dibutyryl cyclic GMP reduced two other morphine-withdrawal symptoms, teeth chattering and chewing. Isobutylmethylxanthine had also reduced these symptoms. Phosphodiesterase inhibitors, such as isobutylmethylxanthine $>>$ theophylline $>$ caffeine $>$ RO 20-1724, potentiated a naloxone-elicited abstinence syndrome in morphine-dependent rats and caused a quasiabstinence syndrome in naloxone-treated control rats (Francis *et al.*, 1975). Headache was a common symptom in humans after intravenous administration of cyclic AMP and dibutyryl cyclic AMP (Levine, 1970). Methylxanthines antagonized this and other symptoms.

Conclusion

Further studies are obviously necessary for a better understanding of the role of cyclic AMP- and cyclic GMP-dependent mechanisms in the central nervous system. The present, already voluminous literature provides many indications of important roles for cyclic AMP in (1) establishment of the synaptically integrated central nervous system, (2) inhibitory regulation of membrane properties and hence of neuronal activity and responsiveness, (3) control of synthesis and release of neurotransmitter substances and mediation of their effects, (4) regulation of metabolic function, (5) feedback control of its own formation and action through alterations in adenylate cyclase, phosphodiesterase, and kinase activity, and (6) interactions with calcium ions. Alterations of cyclic AMP-generating systems in response to changes in synaptic input would appear to be fundamental to one aspect of adaptation in the central nervous system. Roles for cyclic GMP in the stimulatory regulation of neuronal activity and responsiveness have been indicated. Little evidence for interrelationships between cyclic AMP and cyclic GMP mechanisms have been provided in brain tissue. Further insights into the precise nature and role of cyclic nucleotide mechanisms and correlations with physiological functions and with the relevant morphological entities in which cyclic AMP or cyclic GMP serve as regulatory messengers of such functions in the central nervous system remain a challenge for the future.

References

Abdulla, Y. H., and Hamadah, K., 1970, 3',5'-Cyclic adenosine monophosphate in depression and mania, *Lancet* **i**:378–381.

Abdulla, Y. H., and McFarlane, E., 1972, Control of prostaglandin biosynthesis in rat brain homogenates by adenine nucleotides, *Biochem. Pharmacol.* **21**:2841–2847.

Adinolfi, A. M., and Schmidt, S. Y., 1974, Cytochemical localization of cyclic nucleotide phosphodiesterase activity of developing synapses, *Brain Res.* **76**:21–31.

Adolphe, M., Giroud, J. P., Timsit, J., Fontagne, J., and Lechat, P., 1974, Action de la prostaglandin A_2 sur la prolifération et la différenciation morphologique d'une lignée cellulaire de neuroblastoma murin, *C. R. Séances Soc. Biol.* **168**:694–699.

Agren, G., and Ronquist, G., 1974, (^{32}P)Phosphoryl transfer by endogenous protein kinase at the glia and glioma cell membranes, *Acta Physiol. Scand.* **92**:430–432.

Albin, E. E., and Newburgh, R. W., 1975a, Cyclic nucleotide-stimulable protein kinases in the central nervous system of *Manduca sexta, Biochim. Biophys. Acta* **377**:389–401.

Albin, E. E., and Newburgh, R. W., 1975b, Phosphoprotein phosphatase in the central nervous system of *Manduca sexta, Biochim. Biophys. Acta* **377**:381–388.

Alexander, R. W., Davis, J. N., and Lefkowitz, R. J., 1975, Direct identification and characterization of α-adrenergic receptors in rat brain, *Nature (London)* **258**:437–440.

Amer, M. S., and Browder, H. P., 1971, Effect of quazodine on phosphodiesterase, *Proc. Soc. Exp. Biol. Med.* **136**:750–752.

Amer, M. S., and Kreighbaum, W. E., 1975, Cyclic nucleotide phosphodiesterases: Properties, activators, inhibitors, structure–activity relationships, and possible role in drug development, *J. Pharmaceut Sci.* **64**:1–37.

Amer, M. S., Gomoll, A. W., and McKinney, G. R., 1972, Phosphodiesterase inhibition as a mechanism for the diuretic activity of 1-[*tert*-butylimino)methyl]-2-(3-indolyl)indoline hydrochloride (MI-8592-1), *Res. Commun. Chem. Pathol. Pharmacol.* **4**:467–476.

Anagnoste, B., Shirron, C., Friedman, E., and Goldstein, M., 1974, Effect of dibutyryl cyclic adenosine monophosphate on ^{14}C-dopamine biosynthesis in rat brain striatal slices. *J. Pharmacol. Exp. Ther.* **191**:370–376.

Anden, N- E., and Jackson, D. M., 1975, Locomotor activity stimulation in rats produced by dopamine in the nucleus accumbens: Potentiation by caffeine, *J. Pharm. Pharmacol.* **27**:666–670.

Anderson, E. G., Haas, H. L., and Hosli, L., 1973, Comparison of effects of noradrenaline and histamine with cyclic AMP on brain stem neurones, *Brain Res.* **49**:471–475.

Anttila, P., and Vapaatalo, H., 1972, Decreased toxicity of d-tubocurarine after pretreatment with drugs elevating the intracellular level of c-AMP in mice, *Naunyn-Schmiedebergs Arch. Pharmacol.* **273**:175–178.

Appel, S. H., and Locher, C., 1973, Changes in synapse membrane protein phosphorylation following electroconvulsive shock, *Neurology* **23**:41 Abs.

Appenzeller, O., and Palmer, G., 1972, The cyclic AMP (adenosine 3′,5′-phosphate) content of sciatic nerve: Changes after nerve crush, *Brain Res.* **42**:521–524.

Appenzeller, O., Ogin, G., and Palmer, G., 1976, Fiber size spectra and cyclic AMP content of sciatic nerves: Effect of muscle hypoactivity and hyperactivity, *Exp. Neurol.* **50**:595–604.

Appleman, M. M., Thompson, W. J., and Russell, T. R., 1973, Cyclic nucleotide phosphodies-terases, *Advan. Cyclic Nucleotide Res.* **3**:66–98.

Arbuthnott, G. W., Attree, T. J. Eccleston, D., Loose, R. W., and Martin, M. J., 1974, Is adenylate cyclase the dopamine receptor? *Med. Biol.* **52**:350–353.

Asakawa, T., and Yoshida, H., 1971, Studies on the functional role of adenosine 3′,5′-monophosphate, histamine and prostaglandin E_1 in the central nervous system, *Jap. J. Pharmacol.* **21**:569–583.

Askew, W. E., and Ho, B. T., 1975, Effects of intraventricular injections of N^6, $O^{2′}$-dibutyryl adenosine-3′, 5′-monophosphate on the rat brain cholinergic systems, *Canad. J. Biochem.* **53**:634–635.

Axelrod, J., 1974, The pineal gland: A neurochemical transducer, *Science* **184**:1341–1348.

Bachrach, U., 1975, Cyclic AMP-mediated induction of ornithine decarboxylase of glioma and neuroblastoma cells, *Proc. Nat. Acad. Sci. USA* **72**:3087–3091.

Banay-Schwartz, M., Teller, D. N., Gergely, A., and Lajtha, A., 1974, The effects of metabolic inhibitors on amino acid uptake and levels of ATP, Na^+, and K^+ in incubated slices of mouse brain, *Brain Res.* **71**:117–131.

Barchas, J. D., Ciaranello, R. D., Dominic, J. A., Deguchi, T., Orenberg, E., Renson, J., and Kessler, S., 1974, Genetic aspects of monoamine mechanisms, *Advan. Biochem. Psychopharmacol.* **12**:195–215.

Batkia, S., and Rayner, M. D., 1976, Mitotic changes in neuroblastoma transplanted into denervated host tissue, *Res. Commun. Chem. Pathol. Pharmacol.* **13**:145–148.

Baudry, M., Martres, M. P., and Schwartz, J. C., 1975, H_1- and H_2-receptors in the histamine-induced accumulation of cyclic AMP in guinea pig brain slices, *Nature (London)* **253**:362–363.

Bauer, R. J., Swiatek, K. R., Robins, R. K., and Simon, L. N., 1971, Adenosine 3′,5′-cyclic monophosphate derivatives. II. Biological activity of some 8-substituted analogs, *Biochem. Biophys. Res. Commun.* **45**:526–531.

Beani, L., Bianchi, C., and Bertelli, A., 1975, Effects of cyclic nucleotides on behavior, electrocorticogram and cortical acetylcholine release, *Pharmacol. Res. Commun.* **7**:347–360.

Beavo, J. A., Hardman, J. G., and Sutherland, E. W., 1970, Hydrolysis of cyclic guanosine and adenosine 3′,5′-monophosphate by rat and bovine tissues, *J. Biol. Chem.* **245**:5649–5655.

Beavo, J. A., Hardman, J. G., and Sutherland, E. W., 1971, Stimulation of adenosine 3′,5′-monophosphate hydrolysis by guanosine 3′,5′-monophosphate, *J. Biol. Chem.* **246**:3841–3846.

Beer, B., Chasin, M., Clody, D. E., Vogel, J. R., and Horovitz, Z. P., 1972, Cyclic adenosine monophosphate phosphodiesterase in brain: Effect on anxiety, *Science* **176**:428–430.

Benda, P., Premont, J., and Jard, S., 1972, Adénylate cyclase et phosphodiestérases dans les hybrides somatiques des cellules gliales, *C. R. Acad. Sci.* **275D**:1303–1306.

Bensinger, R. E., Fletcher, R. T., and Chader, G. J., 1974, Guanylate cyclase: Inhibition by light in retinal photoreceptors, *Science* **183**:86–87.

Benzi, G., and Villa, R. F., 1976, Adenyl cyclase system and cerebral energy state, *J. Neurol. Neurosurg. Psychiat.* **39**:77–83.

Berkowitz, B., and Spector, S., 1971, The effect of caffeine and theophylline on the disposition of brain serotonin in the rat, *Eur. J. Pharmacol.* **16**:322–325.

Berkowitz, B. A., Spector, S., and Pool, W., 1971, The interaction of caffeine, theophylline and theobromine with monoamine oxidase inhibitors, *Eur. J. Pharmacol.* **16**:315–321.

Berkowitz, B. A., Tarver, J. H., and Spector, S., 1970, Release of norepinephrine in the central nervous system by theophylline and caffeine, *Eur. J. Pharmacol.* **10**:64–71.

Berndt, S., and Schwabe, U., 1973, Effect of psychotropic drugs on phosphodiesterase and cyclic AMP level in rat brain *in vivo*, *Brain Res.* **63**:303–312.

Berridge, M. J., 1975, The interaction of cyclic nucleotides and calcium in the control of cellular activity, *Advan. Cyclic Nucleotide Res.* **6**:1–98.

Berti, F., Trabbucchi, M., Bernareggi, V., and Fumagalli, R., 1972, The effects of prostaglandins on cyclic-AMP formation in cerebral cortex of different mammalian species, *Pharmacol. Res. Commun.* **4**:253–259.

Biebuyck, J. F., Dedrick, D. F., and Scherer, Y. D., 1975, Brain cyclic AMP and putative transmitter amino acids during anesthesia, in *Molecular Mechanisms of Anesthesia* (B. R. Fink, ed.), Vol. I, pp. 451–470, Raven Press, New York.

Bitensky, M. W., and Gorman, R. E., 1972, Digitonin effects on photoreceptor adenylate cyclase, *Science* **175**:1363–1364.

Bitensky, M. W., Gorman, R. E., and Miller, W. H., 1971, Adenyl cyclase as a link between photon capture and changes in membrane permeability of frog photoreceptors, *Proc. Nat. Acad. Sci USA* **68**:561–562.

Bitensky, M. W., Miki, N., Keirns, J. J., Keirns, M., Baraban, J. M., Freeman, J., Wheeler, M. A., Lacy, J., and Marens, F. R., 1975, Activation of photoreceptor disk membrane phosphodiesterase by light and ATP, *Advan. Cyclic Nucleotide Res.* **5**:213–240.

Bitensky, M. W., Miki, N., Marcus, F. R., and Keirns, J. J., 1973, The role of cyclic nucleotides in visual excitation, *Life Sci.* **13**:1451–1472.

Bitensky, M. W., Miller, W. H., Gorman, R. E., Neufeld, A. H., and Robinson, R., 1972, The role of cyclic AMP in visual excitation, *Advan. Cyclic Nucleotide Res.* **1**:317–335.

Bjerre, J., 1974, A neuralizing influence of dibutyryl cyclic AMP on competent chick ectoderm, *Experientia* **30**:534–535.

Bloom, F. E., 1974, To spritz or not to spritz: The doubtful value of aimless iontophoresis, *Life Sci.* **14**:1819–1834.

Bloom, F., 1975, The role of cyclic nucleotides in central synaptic function, *Rev. Physiol. Biochem. Pharmacol.* **74**:1–104.

Bloom, F. E., Costa, E., and Salmoiraghi, G. C., 1965, Anesthesia and the responsiveness of individual neurons of the caudate nucleus of the cat to acetylcholine, norepinephrine and dopamine administered by microelectrophoresis, *J. Pharmacol. Exp. Ther.* **150**:244–252.

Bloom, F. E., Hoffer, B. J., Battenberg, E. R., Siggins, G. R., Steiner, A. L., Parker, C. W., and Wedner, H. J., 1972a, Adenosine 3',5'-monophosphate is localized in cerebellar neurons: Immunofluorescence evidence, *Science* **177**:436–438.

Bloom, F. E., Hoffer, B. J., and Siggins, G. R., 1972b, Norepinephrine mediated cerebellar synapses: A model system for neuropsychopharmacology, *Biol. Psychiat.* **4**:157–177.

Bloom, F. E., Hoffer, B. J., Siggins, G. R., Burker, J. L., and Nicoll, R. A., 1972c, Effects of serotonin on central neurons: Microiontophoretic administration. *Fed. Proc.* **31**:97–106.

Bloom, F. E., Siggins, G. R., and Hoffer, B. J., 1974, Interpreting the failures to confirm the depression of cerebellar Purkinje cells by cyclic AMP. *Science* **185**:627–628.

Bloom, F. E., Siggins, G. R., Hoffer, B. J., Segal, M., and Oliver, A. P., 1975, Cyclic nucleotides in the central synaptic actions of catecholamines, *Advan. Cyclic Nucleotide Res.* **5**:603–618.

Blumberg, J. B., Taylor, R. E., and Sulser, F., 1975, Blockade by pimozide of a noradrenaline sensitive adenylate cyclase in the limbic forebrain: Possible role of limbic noradrenergic mechanisms in the mode of action of antipsychotics, *J. Pharm. Pharmacol.* **27**:125–128.

Blume, A. J., and Foster, C. J., 1975, Mouse neuroblastoma adenylate cyclase, adenosine and adenosine analogues as potent effectors of adenylate cyclase activity, *J. Biol. Chem.* **250**:5003–5008.

Blume, A. J., and Foster, C. J., 1976a, Mouse neuroblastoma cell adenylate cyclase: Regulation by 2-chloroadenosine, prostaglandin E_1 and the cations Mg^{2+}, Ca^{2+} and Mn^{2+}, *J. Neurochem.* **26**:305–312.

Blume, A. J., and Foster, C. J., 1976b, Neuroblastoma adenylate cyclase. Role of 2-chloroadenosine, prostaglandin E_1, and guanine nucleotides in regulation of activity, *J. Biol. Chem.* **251**: 3399–3404.

Blume, A. J., Dalton, C., and Sheppard, H., 1973, Adenosine-mediated elevation of cyclic $3':5'$-adenosine monophosphate concentrations in cultured mouse neuroblastoma cells, *Proc. Nat. Acad. Sci. USA* **70**:3099–3102.

Boehme, E., 1970, Guanyl Cyclase Bildung von Guanosine-$3',5'$-monophosphat in Niere und anderen Geweben der Ratte, *Eur. J. Biochem.* **14**:422–429.

Bondy, S. C., Prasad, K. N., and Prudy, J. L., 1974, Neuroblastoma: Drug-induced differentiation increase proportion of cytoplasmic RNA that contains polyadenylic acid, *Science* **186**:359–361.

Bonnet, K. A., 1975, Regional alterations in cyclic nucleotide levels with acute and chronic morphine treatment, *Life Sci.* **16**:1877–1882.

Booth, D. A., 1972, Unlearned and learned effects of intrahypothalamic cyclic AMP injection on feeding, *Nature New Biol.* **237**:222–224.

Borgeat, P., Labrie, F., and Garneau, P., 1974, Characteristics of the action of prostaglandins on cyclic AMP accumulation in rat anterior pituitary gland, *Canad. J. Biochem.* **53**:455–460.

Boudreau, R. J., and Drummond, G. I., 1975, The effect of Ca^{++} on cyclic nucleotide phosphodiesterases of superior cervical ganglion, *J. Cyclic Nucleotide Res.* **1**:219–228.

Bradham, L. S., 1972, Comparison of the effects of Ca^{2+} and Mg^{2+} on the adenyl cyclase of beef brain, *Biochim. Biophys. Acta* **276**:434–443.

Bradham, L. S., Holt, D. A., and Sims, M., 1970, The effect of Ca^{2+} on the adenyl cyclase of calf brain, *Biochim. Biophys. Acta* **201**:250–260.

Brandt, H., Killilea, S. D., and Lee, E. Y. C., 1974, Activation of phosphorylase phosphatase by a novel procedure: Evidence for a regulatory mechanism involving the release of a catalytic subunit from enzyme-inhibitor complex(es) of higher molecular weight, *Biochem. Biophys. Res. Commun.* **61**:548–554.

Bray, J. J., Kon, C. M., and Breckenridge, B. M., 1971, Adenyl cyclase cyclic nucleotide phosphodiesterase and axoplasmic flow, *Brain Res.* **26**:385–394.

Breckenridge, B. M., 1964, The measurement of cyclic adenylate in tissues, *Proc. Nat. Acad. Sci. USA* **52**:1580–1586.

Breckenridge, B. M., and Johnston, R. E., 1969, Cyclic $3',5'$-nucleotide phosphodiesterase in brain, *J. Histochem. Cytochem.* **17**:505–511.

Breckenridge, B. M., and Lisk, R. D., 1969, Cyclic adenylate and hypothalamic regulatory functions, *Proc. Soc. Exp. Biol. Med.* **131**:934–935.

Breckenridge, B. M., and Norman, J. H., 1962, Glycogen phosphorylase in brain, *J. Neurochem.* **9**:383–392.

Breckenridge, B. M., and Norman, J. H., 1965, The conversion of phosphorylase b to phosphorylase a in brain, *J. Neurochem.* **12**:51–57.

Breckenridge, B. M., Burn, J. H., and Matschinsky, F. M., 1967, Theophylline, epinephrine, and neostigmine facilitation of neuromuscular transmission, *Proc. Nat. Acad. Sci. USA* **57**:1893–1897.

Broadus, A. E., Kaminsky, N. I., Hardman, J. G., Sutherland, E. W., and Liddle, G. W., 1970, Kinetic parameters and renal clearances of plasma adenosine $3', 5'$-monophosphate and guanosine $3',5'$-monophosphate in man, *J. Clin. Invest.* **49**:2222–2236.

Brooker, G., Thomas, L. J., Jr., and Appleman, M. M., 1968, The assay of adenosine 3',5'-cyclic monophosphate and guanosine 3',5'-cyclic monophosphate in biological materials by enzymatic radioisotopic displacement, *Biochemistry* **7**:4177–4181.

Brostrom, C. O., and Wolff, D. J., 1974, Calcium-dependent cyclic nucleotide phosphodiesterase from glial tumor cells, *Arch. Biochem. Biophys.* **165**:715–727.

Brostrom, C. O., and Wolff, D. J., 1976, Calcium-dependent cyclic nucleotide phosphodiesterase from brain: Comparison of adenosine 3',5'-monophosphate and guanosine 3',5'-monophosphate as substrates, *Arch. Biochem. Biophys.* **172**:301–311.

Brostrom, C. O., Huang, Y-C., Breckenridge, B. M., and Wolff, D. J., 1975, Identification of a calcium-binding protein as a calcium-dependent regulator of brain adenylate cyclase, *Proc. Nat. Acad. Sci. USA* **72**:64–68.

Brostrom, M. A., Kon, C., Olson, D. R., and Breckenridge, B. M., 1974, Adenosine 3',5'-monophosphate in glial tumor cells treated with glucocorticoids, *Mol. Pharmacol.* **10**:711–720.

Brown, B. L., Salway, J. G., Albano, J. D. M., Hullin, R. P., and Ekins, R. P., 1972, Urinary excretion of cyclic AMP and manic-depressive psychosis, *Brit. J. Psychiat.* **120**:405–408.

Brown, J. H., and Makman, M. H., 1972, Stimulation by dopamine of adenylate cyclase in retinal homogenates and of adenosine-3':5'-cyclic monophosphate formation in intact retina, *Proc. Nat. Acad. Sci. USA* **69**:539–543.

Brown, J. H., and Makman, M. H., 1973, Influence of neuroleptic drugs and apomorphine on the dopamine-sensitive adenylate cyclase of retina, *J. Neurochem.* **21**:477–479.

Browning, E. T., Brostrom, C. O., and Groppi, V. E., 1976, Altered adenosine cyclic 3',5'-monophosphate synthesis and degradation by C-6 astrocytoma cells following prolonged exposure to norepinephrine. *Mol. Pharmacol.* **12**:32–40.

Browning, E. T., Gropp, V. E., Jr., and Kon, C., 1974a, Papaverine, a potent inhibitor of respiration in C-6 astrocytoma cells, *Mol. Pharmacol.* **10**:175–181.

Browning, E. T., Schwartz, J. P., and Breckenridge, B. M., 1974b, Norepinephrine-sensitive properties of C-6 astrocytoma cells, *Mol. Pharmacol.* **10**:162–174.

Brus, R., Herman, Z. S., and Kostman, F., 1974, Behavioral effects of norepinephrine and dibutryl cyclic 3',5'-AMP in centrally sympathectomized rats, *Pharmacol. Biochem. Behav.* **2**:719–724.

Bublitz, C., 1973, Effects of lipids on cyclic-nucleotide phosphodiesterases, *Biochem. Biophys. Res. Commun.* **52**:173–180.

Bucher, M.-B., and Schorderet, M., 1974, Apomorphine-induced accumulation of cyclic AMP in isolated retinas of the rabbit, *Biochem. Pharmacol.* **23**:3079–3082.

Bucher, M. B., and Schorderet, M., 1975, Dopamine and apomorphine-sensitive adenylate cyclase in homogenates of rabbit retina, *Naunyn-Schmiedeberg's Arch. Pharmacol.* **288**:103–107.

Bunney, B. S., and Aghajanian, G. K., 1976, d-Amphetamine-induced inhibition of central dopaminergic neurons: Mediation by a striato-nigral feedback pathway, *Science* **192**:391–393.

Burkard, W. P., 1972, Catecholamine induced increase of cyclic adenosine 3',5'-monophosphate in rat brain *in vivo, J. Neurochem.* **19**:2615–2619.

Burkard, W. P., 1975, Adenylate cyclase in the central nervous system, in *Progress in Neurobiology,* (G. A. Kerkut and J. W. Phillis, eds.), Vol. 4, pp. 241–267, Pergamon Press, New York.

Burkard, W. P., and Gey, K. F., 1968, Adenyl Cyclase in Rattenhirn, *Helv. Physiol. Acta* **26**:197–198.

Burkard, W. P., Lengsfeld, H., and Gey, K. F., 1971, Cyclic adenosine 3',5'-monophosphate and adenylcyclase in liver, adipose tissue and brain of rats treated with β-pyridylcarbinol, *Biochem. Pharmacol.* **20**:23–28.

Butcher, R. W., and Sutherland, E. W., 1962, Adenosine 3′,5′-phosphate in biological materials. I. Purification and properties of cyclic 3′,5′-nucleotide phosphodiesterase and use of this enzyme to characterize adenosine 3′,5′-phosphate in human urine, *J. Biol. Chem.* **237**:1244–1250.

Cailla, H. L., Vannier, C. J., and Delaage, M. A., 1976, Guanosine 3′,5′-cyclic monophosphate assay at the 10^{-15} mole level, *Anal. Biochem.* **70**:195–202.

Campbell, M. T., and Oliver, I. T., 1972, 3′:5′-Cyclic nucleotide phosphodiesterases in rat tissue, *Eur. J. Biochem.* **28**:30–37.

Carenzi, A., Cheney, D. L., Costa, E., Guidotti, A., and Racagni, G., 1975a, Action of opiates, antipsychotics, amphetamine, and apomorphine on dopamine receptors in rat striatum: *In vivo* changes of 3′,5′-cyclic AMP content and acetylcholine turnover rate, *Neuropharmacol.* **14**:927–940.

Carenzi, A., Guidotti, A., Revuelta, A., and Costa, E., 1975b, Molecular mechanisms in the action of morphine and viminol (R_2) on rat striatum, *J. Pharmacol. Exp. Ther.* **194**:311–318.

Casnellie, J. E., and Greengard, P., 1974, Guanosine 3′,5′-cyclic monophosphate-dependent phosphorylation of endogeneous substrate proteins in membranes of mammalian smooth muscle, *Proc. Nat. Acad. Sci USA* **71**:1891–1895.

Casola, L., Di Matteo, G., and Augusti-Tocco, G., 1974, Neuroblastoma cells in culture: ^{32}P-phosphoprotein labeling and protein kinase activity, *Exp. Neurol.*, **44**:417–423.

Cedar, H., and Schwartz, J. H., 1972, Cyclic adenosine monophosphate in the nervous system of *Aplysia californica*. II. Effect of serotonin and dopamine, *J. Gen. Physiol.* **60**:570–587.

Cedar, H., Kandel, E. R., and Schwartz, J. H., 1972, Cyclic adenosine monophosphate in the nervous system of *Aplysia californica*. I. Increased synthesis in response to synaptic stimulation, *J. Gen. Physiol.* **60**:558–569.

Cehovic, G., Posternak, T., and Charollais, E., 1972, A study of the biological activity and resistance to phosphodiesterase of some derivatives and analogues of cyclic AMP, *Advan. Cyclic Nucleotide Res.* **1**:521–546.

Chader, G. J., 1971, Hormonal effects on the neural retina: Induction of glutamine synthetase by cyclic-3′,5′-AMP, *Biochem. Biophys. Res. Commun.* **43**:1102–1105.

Chader, G. J., Bensinger, R., Johnson, M., and Fletcher, R. T., 1973, Phosphodiesterase: An important role in cyclic nucleotide regulation in the retina, *Exp. Eye Res.* **17**:483–486.

Chader, G., Fletcher, R., Johnson, M., and Bensinger, R., 1974a, Rod outer segment phosphodiesterase: Factors affecting the hydrolysis of cyclic AMP and cyclic GMP, *Exp. Eye Res.* **18**:509–515.

Chader, G. J., Herz, L. W., and Fletcher, R. T., 1974b, Light activation of phosphodiesterase activity in retinal rod outer segments, *Biochim. Biophys. Acta* **347**:491–493.

Chader, G. J., Fletcher, R. T., O'Brien, P. J., and Krishna, G., 1976, Differential phosphorylation by GTP and ATP in isolate rod outer segments of the retina, *Biochemistry* **15**:1615–1620.

Chalazonitis, A., and Greene, L. A., 1974, Enhancement in excitability properties of mouse neuroblastoma cells cultured in the presence of dibutyryl cyclic AMP, *Brain Res.* **72**:340–345.

Chamley, J. H., and Campbell, G. R., 1975, Trophic influences of sympathetic nerves and cyclic AMP on differentiation and proliferation of isolated smooth muscle cells in culture, *Cell Tissue Res.* **161**:497–516.

Chasin, M., Harris, D. W., Phillips, M. B., and Hess, S. M., 1972, 1-Ethyl-4(isopropylidenehydrazino)pyrazolo-(3,4b)-pyridine-5-carboxylic acid, ethyl ester, hydrochloride (SQ20009)-A potent new inhibitor of cyclic 3′,5′-nucleotide phosphodiesterases, *Biochem. Pharmacol.* **21**:2443–2450.

Chasin, M., Mamrak, F., and Samaniego, S. G., 1974, Preparation and properties of a cell-free, hormonally responsive adenylate cyclase from guinea pig brain, *J. Neurochem.* **22:**1031–1038.

Chasin, M., Mamrak, F., Samaniego, S. G., and Hess, S. M., 1973, Characteristics of the catecholamine and histamine receptor sites mediating accumulation of cyclic adenosine 3′,5′-monophosphate in guinea pig brain, *J. Neurochem.* **21:**1415–1427.

Chasin, M., Rivkin, I., Mamrak, F., Samaniego, G., and Hess, S. M., 1971,α- and β-Adrenergic receptors as mediators of accumulation of cyclic adenosine 3′,5′-monophosphate in specific areas of guinea pig brain, *J. Biol. Chem.* **246:**3037–3041.

Chatzkel, S., Zimmerman, I., and Berg, A., 1974, Modulation of cyclic-AMP synthesis in the cat superior cervical ganglion by short term presynaptic stimulation, *Brain Res.* **80:**523–526.

Cheung, W. Y., 1966, Inhibition of cyclic nucleotide phosphodiesterase by adenosine 5′-triphosphate and inorganic pyrophosphate, *Biochem. Biophys. Res. Commun.* **23:**214–219.

Cheung, W. Y., 1967a, Properties of cyclic 3′,5′-nucleotide phosphodiesterase from rat brain, *Biochemistry* **6:**1079–1087.

Cheung, W. Y., 1967b, Cyclic 3′,5′-nucleotide phosphodiesterase: Pronounced stimulation by snake venom, *Biochem. Biophys. Res. Commun.* **29:**478–482.

Cheung, W. Y., 1969, Cyclic 3′,5′-nucleotide phosphodiesterase preparation of a partially inactive enzyme and its subsequent stimulation by snake venom, *Biochem. Biophys. Acta* **191:**303–315.

Cheung, W. Y., 1970, Cyclic nucleotide phosphodiesterase, *Advan. Biochem. Psychopharmacol.* **3:**51–65.

Cheung, W. Y., 1971a, Cyclic 3′,5′-nucleotide phosphodiesterase effect of divalent cations, *Biochim. Biophys. Acta* **242:**395–409.

Cheung, W. Y., 1971b, Cyclic 3′,5′-nucleotide phosphodiesterase: Evidence for and properties of a protein activator, *J. Biol. Chem.* **246:**2859–2869.

Cheung, W. Y., and Salganicoff, L., 1967, Cyclic 3′,5′-nucleotide phosphodiesterase: Localization and latent activity in rat brain, *Nature (London)* **214:**90–91.

Cheung, W. Y., Bradham, L. S., Lynch, T. J., Lin, Y. M., and Tallant, E. A., 1975a, Protein activator of cyclic 3′-5′-nucleotide phosphodiesterase of bovine or rat brain also activates its adenylate cyclase, *Biochem. Biophys. Res. Commun.* **66:**1055–1062.

Cheung, W. Y., Lin, Y. M., Liu, Y. P., and Smoake, J. A., 1975b, Regulation of bovine brain cyclic 3′,5′-nucleotide phosphodiesterase by its protein activator in *Cyclic Nucleotides in Disease* (B. Weiss, ed.), pp. 321–350, University Park Press, Baltimore.

Childers, S. R., and Siegel, F. L., 1975, Isolation and purification of a calcium-binding protein from electroplax of *Electrophorus electricus*, *Biochim. Biophys. Acta* **405:**99–108.

Chlapowski, F. J., Kelly, L. A., and Butcher, R. W., 1975, Cyclic nucleotides in cultured cells, *Advan. Cyclic Nucleotide Res.* **6:**245–338.

Chou, W. S., Ho, A. K. S., and Loh, H. H., 1971a, Effect of acute and chronic morphine and norepinephrine on brain adenyl cyclase activity, *Proc. West. Pharmacol. Soc.* **14:**42–46.

Chou, W. S., Ho, A. K. S., and Loh, H. H., 1971b, Neurohormones on brain adenyl cyclase activity *in vivo*, *Nature New Biol.* **233:**280–281.

Chrisman, T. D., Garbers, D., Parks, M. A., and Hardman, J. G., 1975, Characterization of particulate and soluble guanylate cyclases from rat lung, *J. Biol. Chem.* **250:**374–381.

Christensen, L. F., Meyer, Jr., R. B., Miller, J. P., Simon, L. N., and Robins, R. K., 1975, Synthesis and enzymic activity of 8-acyl and 8-alkyl derivatives of guanosine 3′5′-cyclic phosphate, *Biochemistry* **14:**1490–1495.

Clark, A. G., Jovic, R., Ornellas, M. R., and Weller, M., 1972, Brain microsomal protein kinase in the chronically morphinized rat, *Biochem. Pharmacol.* **21:**1989–1990.

Clark, R. B., and Perkins, J. P., 1971, Regulation of adenosine 3′:5′-cyclic monophosphate concentration in cultured human astrocytoma cells by catecholamines and histamine, *Proc. Nat. Acad. Sci USA* **68**:2757–2760.

Clark, R. B., Su, Y.-F., Gross, R., and Perkins, J. P., 1974a, Regulation of adenosine 3'-5'-monophosphate content in human astrocytoma cells by adenosine and the adenine nucleotides, *J. Biol. Chem.* **249**:5296–5303.

Clark, W. G., Cumby, H. R., and Davis, H. R., 1974b, The hyperthermic effect of intraventricular cholera enterotoxin in the unanaesthetized cat, *J. Physiol.* **240**:493–504.

Clark, R. B., Su, Y-F., Ortmann, R., Cubeddu, L., Johnson, G. L., and Perkins, J. P., 1975, Factors influencing the effect of hormones on the accumulation of cyclic AMP in cultured human astrocytoma cells, *Metabolism* **24**:343–358.

Clement-Cormier, Y. C., Kebabian, J. W., Petzold, G. L., and Greengard, P., 1974, Dopamine-sensitive adenylate cyclase in mammalian brain: A possible site of action of antipsychotic drugs, *Proc. Nat. Acad. Sci. USA* **17**:1113–1117.

Clement-Cormier, Y. C., Parrish, R. G., Petzold, G. L., Kebabian, J. W., and Greengard, P., 1975, Characterization of a dopamine-sensitive adenylate cyclase in the rat caudate nucleus, *J. Neurochem.* **25**:143–149.

Clouet, D. H., and Iwatsubo, K., 1975, Dopamine-sensitive adenylate cyclase of the caudate nucleus of rats treated with morphine, *Life Sci.* **17**:35–40.

Clouet, D. H., Gold, G. J., and Iwatsubo, K., 1975, Effects of narcotic analgesic drugs on the cyclic adenosine 3'5'-monophosphate–adenylate cyclase system in rat brain, *Brit. J. Pharmacol.* **54**:541–548.

Cohen, K. L., and Bitensky, M. W., 1969, Inhibitory effects of alloxan on mammalian adenyl cyclase, *J. Pharmacol. Exp. Ther.* **169**:80–86.

Cohn, M. L., 1975, Cyclic AMP, thyrotropin releasing factor and somatostatin: Key factors in the regulation of the duration of narcosis, in *Molecular Mechanisms of Anesthesia* (B. R. Fink, ed.), Vol. I, pp. 485–499, Raven Press, New York.

Cohn, M. L., Taylor, F., Cohn, M., and Yamaoka, H., 1973a, Dibutyryl cyclic AMP—an effective antidote against lethal amounts of amobarbital in the rat, *Res. Commun. Chem. Pathol. Pharmacol.* **6**:435–446.

Cohn, M. L., Yamaoka, H., Taylor, F. H., and Kraynack, B., 1973b, Action of intracerebroventricular dibutyryl cyclic AMP on amobarbital anaesthesia in rats, *Neuropharmacology* **12**:401–405.

Cohn, M. L., Cohn, M., and Taylor, F. H., 1974, Norepinephrine—an antagonist of dibutyryl cyclic AMP in the regulation of narcosis in the rat, *Res. Commun. Chem. Path. Pharmacol.* **7**:687–699.

Cohn, M. L., Cohn, M., and Taylor, F. H., 1975a, Effects of phentolamine on dibutyryl cyclic AMP and norepinephrine in rats anaesthetized with amobarbital. *Arch. Int. Pharmacodyn. Ther.* **217**:80–85.

Cohn, M. L., Cohn, M., Taylor, F. H., and Scattaregia, F., 1975b, A direct effect of dibutyryl cyclic AMP on the duration of narcosis induced by sedative, hypnotic, tranquiliser, and anaesthetic drugs in the rat, *Neuropharmacology* **14**:483–487.

Cohn, M. L., Cohn, M., and Taylor, F. H., 1976, Measurements of brain amobarbital concentrations in rats anaesthetized and overdosed with amobarbital and treated centrally with dibutyryl cyclic AMP, *Life Sci.* **18**:261–266.

Collier, H. O. J., and Francis, D. L., 1975, Morphine abstinence is associated with increased brain cyclic AMP, *Nature (London)* **225**:159–161.

Collier, H. O. J., and Roy, A. C., 1974a, Morphine-like drugs inhibit the stimulation by E prostaglandins of cyclic AMP formation by rat brain homogenates, *Nature (London)* **248**:24–27.

Collier, H. O. J., and Roy, A. C., 1974b, Hypothesis inhibition of E-prostaglandin-sensitive adenyl cyclase as the mechanism of morphine analgesia, *Prostaglandins* **7**:361–376.

Collier, H. O. J., Francis, D. L., McDonald-Gibson, W. J., Roy, A. C., and Saeed, S. A., 1975, Prostaglandins, cyclic AMP and the mechanism of opiate dependence, *Life Sci.* 17:85–90.

Connor, J. D., 1970, Caudate nucleus neurones; correlation of the effects of substantia nigra stimulation with iontophoretic dopamine, *J. Physiol.* 208:691–703.

Contreras, E., Castillo, S., and Quijada, L., 1972, Effect of drugs that modify 3',5'-AMP concentrations on morphine analgesia, *J. Pharm. Pharmacol.* 24:65–66.

Coquil, J. F., Virmaux, N., Mandel, P., and Goridis, C., 1975, Cyclic nucleotide phosphodiesterase of retinal photoreceptors. Partial purification and some properties of the enzyme, *Biochim. Biophys. Acta* 403:425–437.

Corbin, J. D., Keely, S. L., and Park, C. R., 1975, The distribution and dissociation of cyclic adenosine 3',5'-monophosphate-dependent protein kinases in adipose, cardiac, and other tissues, *J. Biol. Chem.* 250:218–225.

Corrodi, H., Fuxé, K., and Jonsson, G., 1972, Effects of caffeine on central monoamine neurons, *J. Pharm. Pharmacol.* 24:155–158.

Costa, E., Cheney, D. L., Racagni, G., and Zsilla, G., 1975a, An analysis at synaptic level of the morphine action in striatum and n. accumbens: Dopamine and acetylcholine interactions, *Life Sci.* 17:1–8.

Costa, E., Guidotti, A., and Mao, C. C., 1975b, Evidence for the involvement of GABA in the action of benzodiazepines: Studies on rat cerebellum, *Advan. Biochem. Psychopharmacol.* 14:113–130.

Costa, E., Guidotti, A., Mao, C. C., and Suria, A., 1975c, New concepts on the mechanism of action of benzodiazepines, *Life Sci.* 17:167–186.

Crain, S. M., and Pollock, E. D., 1973, Restorative effects of cyclic AMP on complex bioelectric activities of cultured fetal rodent CNS tissues after acute Ca^{++} deprivation, *J. Neurobiol.* 4:321–342.

Cramer, H., and Lindl, T., 1974, Release of cyclic AMP from rat superior cervical ganglia after stimulation of synthesis *in vitro*, *Nature (London)* 249:380–382.

Cramer, H., Paul, M. I., Silbergeld, S., and Forn, J., 1971, Determination of regional distribution of adenosine 3',5'-monophosphate in rat brain, *J. Neurochem.* 18:1605–1608.

Cramer, H., Goodwin, F. K., Post, R. M., and Bunney, W. E., Jr., 1972a, Effects of probenecid and exercise on cerebrospinal-fluid cyclic AMP in affective illness, *Lancet* i:1346–1347.

Cramer, H., Ng, L. K. Y., and Chase, T. N., 1972b, Effect of probenecid on levels of cyclic AMP in human cerebrospinal fluid, *J. Neurochem.* 19:1601–1602.

Cramer, H., Johnson, D. G., Hanbauer, I., Silberstein, S. D., and Kopin, I. J., 1973a, Accumulation of adenosine 3',5'-monophosphate induced by catecholamines in the rat superior cervical ganglion *in vitro*, *Brain Res.* 53:97–104.

Cramer, H., Ng, L. K. Y., and Chase, T. N., 1973b, Adenosine 3',5'-monophosphate in cerebrospinal fluid. Effect of drugs and neurologic disease, *Arch. Neurol.* 29:197–199.

Cubeddu, L., Barnes, E., and Weiner, N., 1974, Release of norepinephrine and dopamine-β-hydroxylase by nerve stimulation. II. Effects of papaverine, *J. Pharmacol. Exp. Ther.* 191:444–457.

Cubeddu, L., Barnes, E., and Weiner, N., 1975, Release of norepinephrine and dopamine hydroxylase by nerve stimulation. IV. An evaluation of a role for cyclic adenosine monophosphate, *J. Pharmacol. Exp. Ther.* 193:105–127.

Daile, P., Carnegie, P. R., and Young, J. D., 1975, Synthetic substrate for cyclic AMP-dependent protein kinase, *Nature (London)* 257:416–418.

Dalton, C., Crowley, H. J., Sheppard, H., and Schallek, W., 1974, Regional cyclic nucleotide phosphodiesterase activity in cat central nervous system: Effects of benzodiazepines, *Proc. Soc. Exp. Biol. Med.* 145:407–410.

Daly, J., 1972, Accumulation of cyclic AMP in tissue slices and intact cells: Prelabeling of intracellular pools of ATP, in *Methods in Molecular Biology* (M. Chasin, ed.), Vol. III, pp. 255–299, Marcel Dekker, New York.

Daly, J. W., 1975a, Cyclic adenosine 3′,5′-monophosphate role in the physiology and pharmacology of the central nervous system, *Biochem. Pharmacol.* **24:**159–164.

Daly, J. W., 1975b, Role of cyclic nucleotides in the nervous system, in *Handbook of Psychopharmacology* (L. L. Iversen, S. D. Iversen, and S. H. Snyder, ed.), Vol. 5, pp. 47–130, Plenum Publishing Corp., New York.

Daly, J. W., 1976, The nature of receptors regulating the formation of cyclic AMP in brain tissue, *Life Sci.* **18:**1349–1358.

Daniels, M. P., and Hamprecht, B., 1974, The ultrastructure of neuroblastoma glioma somatic cell hybrids: Expression of neuronal characteristics stimulated by dibutyryl adenosine 3′,5′-cyclic monophosphate, *J. Cell Biology* **63:**691–699.

Da Prada, M., Saner, A., Burkard, W. P., Bartholini, G., and Pletscher, A., 1975, Lysergic acid diethylamide: Evidence for stimulation of cerebral dopamine receptors, *Brain Res.* **94:**67–74.

Dascombe, M. J., and Milton, A. S., 1975a, The effects of cyclic adenosine 3′,5′-monophosphate and other adenine nucleotides on body temperature, *J. Physiol.* **250:**143–160.

Dascombe, M. J., and Milton, A. S., 1975b, Cyclic adenosine-3′,5′-monophosphate in cerebrospinal fluid, *Brit. J. Pharmacol.* **54:**254P–255P.

Dascombe, M. J., and Milton, A. S., 1975c, Cyclic adenosine-3′,5′-monophosphate in cerebrospinal fluid during fever and antipyresis, *J. Physiol.* **247:**29P–31P.

De Belleroche, J. S., Das, I., and Bradford, H. F., 1974, Absence of an effect of histamine, noradrenaline and depolarizing agents on levels of adenosine-3′,5′-monophosphate in nerve endings isolated from cerebral cortex, *Biochem. Pharmacol.* **23:**835–843.

Deguchi, T., and Axelrod, J., 1973, Superinduction of serotonin N-acetyltransferase and supersensitivity of adenyl cyclase to catecholamines in denervated pineal gland, *Mol. Pharmacol.* **9:**612–618.

De La Paz, R. L., Dickman, S. R., and Grosser, B. J., 1975, Effects of stress on rat brain adenosine 3′,5′-monophosphate *in vivo*, *Brain Res.* **85:**171–176.

De Robertis, E., Arnaiz, G. R. D.-L., Butcher, R. W., and Sutherland, E. W., 1967, Subcellular distribution of adenyl cyclase and cyclic phosphodiesterase in rat brain cortex, *J. Biol. Chem.* **242:**3487–3493.

De Vellis, J., and Brooker, G., 1974, Reversal of catecholamine refractoriness by inhibitors of RNA and protein synthesis, *Science* **186:**1221–1223.

De Vellis, J., and Kukes, G., 1973, Regulation of glial cell functions by hormones and ions: A review, *Texas Rep. Biol. Med.* **31:**271–293.

Dewar, A. J., Barron, G., and Richmond, J., 1975. Retinal cyclic-AMP phosphodiesterase activity in two strains of dystrophic rat, *Exp. Eye Res.* **21:**299–306.

Diamond, I., and Goldberg, A. L., 1971, Uptake and release of ^{45}Ca by brain microsomes, synaptosomes and synaptic vesicles, *J. Neurochem.* **18:**1419–1431.

Dichter, M. A., 1975, Identification of neurons in cultures, *Science* **190:**489.

Dickman, S., Harrison, J., and Grosser, B., 1973, Decrease in adenyl nucleotide concentrations in rat brain components after footshock stress, *Brain Res.* **53:**483–487.

Dinnendahl, V., 1975, Effects of stress on mouse brain cyclic nucleotide levels *in vivo*, *Brain Res.* **100:**716–719.

Dinnendahl, V., and Stock, K., 1975, Effects of arecoline and cholinesterase inhibitors on cyclic guanosine 3′,5′-monophosphate and adenosine 3′,5′-monophosphate in mouse brain, *Naunyn-Schmiedeberg's Arch. Pharmacol.* **290:**297–306.

Dismukes, K., and Daly, J. W., 1974, Norepinephrine-sensitive systems generating adenosine

3′,5′-monophosphate: Increased responses in cerebral cortical slices from reserpine-treated rats, *Mol. Pharmacol.* **10:**933–940.

Dismukes, K., and Daly, J. W., 1975a, Accumulation of adenosine 3′,5′-monophosphate in rat brain slices: Effects of prostaglandins, *Life Sci.* **17:**199–210.

Dismukes, R. K., and Daly, J. W., 1975b, Altered responsiveness of adenosine 3′,5′-monophosphate generating systems in brain slices from adult rats after neonatal treatment with 6-hydroxydopamine, *Exp. Neurol.* **49:**150–160.

Dismukes, R. K., and Daly, J. W., 1976a, Altered brain cyclic AMP responses in rats reared in enriched or impoverished environments, *Experientia* **32:**730–731.

Dismukes, R. K., and Daly, J. W., 1976b, Adaptive responses of brain cyclic AMP-generating systems to alterations in synaptic input, *J. Cyclic Nucleotide Res.* **2:**321–336.

Dismukes, R. K., Ghosh, P., Creveling, C. R., and Daly, J. W., 1975, Altered responsiveness of adenosine 3′,5′-monophosphate-generating systems in rat cortical slices after lesions of the medial forebrain bundle, *Exp. Neurol.* **49:**725–735.

Dismukes, R. K., Ghosh, P., Creveling, C. R., and Daly, J. W., 1976a, Norepinephrine depletion and responsiveness of norepinephrine-sensitive cortical cyclic AMP-generating systems in guinea pig brain, *Exp. Neurol.* **52:**206–215.

Dismukes, K., Rogers, M., and Daly, J. W., 1976b, Cyclic adenosine 3′,5′-monophosphate formation in guinea pig brain slices: Effect of H_1- and H_2-histaminergic agonists, *J. Neurochem.* **26:**785–790.

Dittmann, J., and Herrmann, H.-D., 1970, An action of adenosine 3′,5′-monophosphate on glucose metabolism of rabbit brain slices, *Experientia* **26:**133–134.

Ditzion, B. R., Paul, M. I., and Pauk, G. L., 1970, Measurement of adenosine 3′,5′-monophosphate (cyclic AMP) in brain, *Pharmacology* **3:**25–31.

Doggett, N. S., and Spencer, P. S. J., 1971, Pharmacological properties of centrally administered ouabain and their modification by other drugs, *Brit. J. Pharmacol.* **42:**242–253.

Doggett, N. S., and Spencer, P. S. J., 1973, Pharmacological properties of centrally administered agents which interfere with neurotransmitter function: A comparison with the central depressant effects of ouabain, *Brit. J. Pharmacol.* **47:**26–38.

Dolby, T. W., and Kleinsmeith, L. J., 1974, Effects of Δ^9-tetrahydrocannabinol on the levels of cyclic adenosine 3′,5′-monophosphate in mouse brain, *Biochem. Pharmacol.* **23:**1817–1825.

Donnelly, T. E., Jr., Kuo, J. F., Miyamoto, E., and Greengard, P., 1973a, Protein kinase modulator from lobster tail muscle. II. Effects of the modulator on holoenzyme and catalytic subunit of guanosine 3′, 5′-monophosphate-dependent and adenosine 3′,5′-monophosphate-dependent protein kinases, *J. Biol. Chem.* **248:**199–203.

Donnelly, T. E., Jr., Kuo, J. F., Reyes, P. L., Liu, Y. P., and Greengard, P., 1973b, Protein kinase modulator from lobster tail muscle. I. Stimulatory and inhibitory effects of the modulator on the phosphorylation of substrate proteins by guanosine 3′,5′-monophosphate-dependent and adenosine 3′,5′-monophosphate-dependent protein kinases, *J. Biol. Chem.* **248:**190–198.

Doore, B. J., Basor, M. M., Spitzer, N., Mawe, R. C., and Saier, M. H., 1975, Regulation of adenosine 3′,5′-monophosphate efflux from rat glioma cells in culture, *J. Biol. Chem.* **250:**4371–4372.

Dousa, T., and Hechter, O., 1970, Lithium and brain adenyl cyclase, *Lancet* **i:**834–835.

Dowd, F., and Schwartz, A., 1975, The presence of cyclic AMP-stimulated protein kinase substrates and evidence for endogenous protein kinase activity in various Na^+, K^+-ATPase preparations from brain, heart and kidney, *J. Mol. Cell. Cardiol.* **7:**483–497.

Drummond, G. I., and Bellward, G., 1970, Studies on phosphorylase b kinase from neural tissues, *J. Neurochem.* **17:**475–482.

Drummond, G. I., and Duncan, L., 1968, On the mechanisms of activation of phosphorylase b kinase by calcium, *J. Biol. Chem.* **243**:5532–5538.

Drummond, G. I., and Ma, Y., 1973, Metabolism and functions of cyclic AMP in nerve, in *Progress in Neurobiology* (G. W. Kerkut and J. W. Phillis, eds.), pp. 119–176, Pergamon Press, Oxford/New York.

Drummond, G. I., and Perrott-Yee, S., 1961, Enzymatic hydrolysis of adenosine 3',5'-phosphoric acid, *J. Biol. Chem.* **236**:1126–1129.

Drummond, G. I., and Powell, C. A., 1970, Analogues of adenosine 3',5'-cyclic phosphate as activators of phosphorylase b kinase and as substrates for cyclic 3',5'-nucleotide phosphodiesterase, *Mol. Pharmacol.* **6**:24–30.

Drummond, G. I., Gilgan, M. W., Reiner, E. J., and Smith, M., 1964a, Deoxyribonucleoside-3',5'-cyclic phosphates. Synthesis and acid catalyzed and enzymic hydrolysis, *J. Amer. Chem. Soc.* **86**:1626–1630.

Drummond, G. I., Keith, J., and Gilgan, M. W., 1964b, Brain glycogen phosphorylase, *Arch. Biochem. Biophys.* **105**:156–162.

Drummond, G. I., Severson, D. L., and Duncan, L., 1971, Adenyl cyclase: Kinetic properties and fluoride and hormone stimulation, *J. Biol. Chem.* **246**:4166–4173.

Duffy, M. J., and Powell, D., 1975, Stimulation of brain adenylate cyclase activity by the undecapeptide substance P and its modulation by the calcium ion, *Biochim. Biophys. Acta* **385**:275–280.

Duffy, M. J., Wong, J., and Powell, D., 1975, Stimulation of adenylate cyclase activity in different areas of human brain by substance P, *Neuropharmacology* **14**:615–618.

Dumler, I. L., and Etingof, R. H., 1976, Protein inhibitor in cyclic adenosine 3':5'-monophosphate phosphodiesterase in retina, *Biochim. Biophys. Acta* **429**:474–484.

Du Moulin, A., and Schultz, J., 1975, Effect of some phosphodiesterase inhibitors on two different preparations of adenosine 3',5'-monophosphate phosphodiesterase, *Experientia* **31**:883–884.

Ebadi, M. S., Weiss, B., and Costa, E., 1971a, Microassay of adenosine 3',5'-monophosphate (cyclic AMP) in brain and other tissues by the luciferin-luciferase system, *J. Neurochem.* **18**:183–192.

Ebadi, M. S., Weiss, B., and Costa, E., 1971b, Distribution of cyclic adenosine monophosphate in rat brain, *Arch. Neurol.* **24**:353–357.

Ebert, R., and Schwabe, U., 1973, Studies on the antipolytic effect of adenosine and related compounds in isolated fat cells, *Naunyn-Schmiedeberg's Arch. Pharmacol.* **278**:247–259.

Ebstein, B., Roberge, C., Tabachnick, J., and Goldstein, M., 1974, The effect of dopamine and of apomorphine on dB-cAMP-induced stimulation of synaptosomal tyrosine hydroxylase, *J. Pharm. Pharmacol.* **26**:975–978.

Ebstein, R., Belmaker, R., Grunhaus, L., and Rimon, R., 1976, Lithium inhibition of adrenaline-stimulated adenylate cyclase in humans, *Nature (London)* **259**:411–412.

Eccleston, D., Loose, R., Pullar, I. A., and Sugden, R. F., 1970, Excercise and urinary excretion of cyclic AMP, *Lancet* **ii**: 612–613.

Edstrom, A., Kanje, M., Lofgren, P., and Walum, E., 1975, Drug-induced alterations in morphology and level of cAMP in cultured human glioma cells, *Exp. Cell Res.* **95**:359–364.

Edstrom, A., Kanje, M., and Walum, E., 1974, Effects of dibutyryl cyclic AMP and prostaglandin E₁ on cultured human glioma cells, *Exp. Cell Res.* **85**:217–223.

Edwards, C., Nahorski, S. R., and Rogers, K. J., 1974, *In vivo* changes in cerebral cyclic adenosine 3',5'-monophosphate induced by biogenic amines: Association with phosphorylase activation, *J. Neurochem.* **22**:565–572.

Egrie, J. C., and Siegel, F. L., 1975, Adrenal medullary cyclic nucleotide phosphodiesterase: Lack of activation by the calcium-dependent regulator, *Biochem. Biophys. Res. Commun.* **67**:662–669.

Ehrlich, Y. H., and Routtenberg, A., 1974, Cyclic AMP regulates phosphorylation of three protein components of rat cerebral cortex membranes for thirty minutes, *FEBS Lett.* **45**:237–243.

Eipper, B. A., 1974a, Rat brain tubulin and protein kinase activity, *J. Biol. Chem.* **249**:1398–1406.

Eipper, B. A., 1974b, Properties of rat brain tubulin, *J. Biol. Chem.* **249**:1407–1416.

Elkhawad, A. O., Munday, K. A., Pont, J. A., and Woodruff, G. N., 1975, The effect of dopamine receptor stimulants on locomotor activity and cyclic AMP levels in the rat striatum, *Brit. J. Pharmacol.* **53**:456–457.

Elul, R., Brons, J., and Kravitz, K., 1975, Surface charge modifications associated with proliferation and differentiation in neuroblastoma cultures, *Nature (London)* **258**:616–617.

Engberg, I., and Marshall, K. C., 1971, Mechanism of noradrenaline hyperpolarization in spinal cord motoneurones of the cat, *Acta Physiol. Scand.* **83**:142–144.

Engberg, I., Flatman, J. A., and Kadzielawa, K., 1974, The hyperpolarization of motorneurones by electrophysiologically applied amines and other agents, *Acta. Physiol. Scand.* **91**:2A–4A.

Erlichman, J. R., Rosenfeld, R., and Rosen, O. M., 1974, Phosphorylation of a cyclic adenosine 3′,5′-monophosphate-dependent protein kinase from bovine cardiac muscle, *J. Biol. Chem.* **249**:5000–5003.

Erwin, V. G., 1969, Enhancement of brain glutamate dehydrogenase activity and glutamate oxidation by adenine nucleotides, *Mol. Pharmacol.* **5**:615–621.

Fain, J. N., 1973, Inhibition of adenosine cyclic 3′,5′-monophosphate accumulation in fat cells by adenosine, N^6-(phenylisopropyl) adenosine and related compounds, *Mol. Pharmacol.* **9**:595–604.

Farber, D. B., and Lolley, R. N., 1973, Proteins in the degenerative retina of C3H mice: Deficiency of a cyclic nucleotide phosphodiesterase and opsin. *J. Neurochem.* **21**:817–828.

Farber, D. B., and Lolley, R. N., 1974, Cyclic guanosine monophosphate: Elevation in degenerating photoreceptor cells of the C3H mouse retina, *Science* **186**:449–451.

Fernandez-Pol, J. A., and Hays, M. T., 1976, Effects of 8-bromo-cyclic GMP on cyclic AMP levels in urine and tissues of hypothyroid rats, *Life Sci.* **19**:35–40.

Ferrendelli, J. A., 1975, Role of cyclic GMP in the function of the central nervous system, in *Cyclic Nucleotides in Disease* (B. Weiss, ed.), pp. 377–390, University Park Press, Baltimore.

Ferrendelli, J. A., Chang, M. M., and Kinscherf, D. A., 1974, Elevation of cyclic GMP levels in central nervous system by excitatory and inhibitory amino acids, *J. Neurochem.* **22**:535–540.

Ferrendelli, J. A., Johnson, E. M., Jr., Chang, M.-M., and Needleman, P., 1973a, Inhibition of brain adenylate cyclase by ethacrynic acid and dithiobisnitrobenzoic acid, *Biochem. Pharmacol.* **22**:3133–3136.

Ferrendelli, J. A., Kinscherf, D. A., and Chang, M. M., 1973b, Regulation of levels of guanosine cycle 3′,5′-monophosphate in the central nervous system: Effects of depolarizing agents, *Mol. Pharmacol.* **9**:445–454.

Ferrendelli, J. A., Kinscherf, D. A., and Chang, M-M., 1975, Comparison of the effects of biogenic amines of cyclic GMP and cyclic AMP levels in mouse cerebellum *in vitro, Brain Res.* **84**:63–73.

Ferrendelli, J. A., Kinscherf, D. A., and Kipnis, D. M., 1972, Effects of amphetamine, chlorpromazine and reserpine on cyclic GMP and cyclic AMP levels in mouse cerebellum, *Biochem. Biophys. Res. Commun.* **46**:2114–2120.

Ferrendelli, J. A., Rubin, E. H., and Kinscherf, D. A., 1976, Influence of divalent cations on regulation of cyclic GMP and cyclic AMP levels in brain tissue, *J. Neurochem.* **26**:741–748.

Ferrendelli, J. A., Steiner, A. L., McDougal, D. B., Jr., and Kipnis, D. M., 1970, The effect of oxotremorine and atropine on cGMP and cAMP levels in mouse cerebral cortex and cerebellum, *Biochem. Biophys. Res. Commun.* **41**:1061–1067.

Fertel, R., and Weiss, B., 1974, A micro assay for guanosine 3′,5′-monophosphate phosphodiesterase activity, *Anal. Biochem.* **59**:386–398.

Florendo, N. T., Barrnett, R. J., and Greengard, P., 1971, Cyclic 3′,5′-nucleotide phosphodiesterase: Cytochemical localization in cerebral cortex, *Science* **173**:745–747.

Folbergrova, J., 1975, Cyclic 3′,5′-adenosine monophosphate in mouse cerebral cortex during homocysteine convulsions and their prevention by sodium phenobarbital, *Brain Res.* **92**:165–169.

Forn, J., and Krishna, G., 1971, Effect of norepinephrine, histamine and other drugs on cyclic 3′,5′-AMP formation in brain slices of various animal species, *Pharmacology* **5**:193–204.

Forn, J., and Valdecasas, F. G., 1971, Effects of lithium on brain adenyl cyclase activity, *Biochem. Pharmacol.* **20**:2773–2779.

Forn, J., Krueger, B. K., and Greengard, P., 1974, Adenosine 3′,5′-monophosphate content in rat caudate nucleus: Demonstration of dopaminergic and adrenergic receptors, *Science* **186**:1118–1120.

Forn, J., Tagliamonte, A., Tagliamonte, P., and Gessa, G. L., 1972, Stimulation by dibutyryl cyclic AMP of serotonin synthesis and tryptophan transport in brain slices, *Nature New Biol.* **237**:245–247.

Francis, D. L., Roy, A. C., and Collier, H. O. J., 1975, Morphine abstinence and quasi-abstinence effects after phosphodiesterase inhibitors and naloxone, *Life Sci.* **16**:1901–1906.

Frandsen, E. K., and Krishna, G., 1976, A simple ultrasensitive method for the assay of cyclic AMP and cyclic GMP in tissues, *Life Sci.* **18**:529–542.

Frank, R. N., and Bensinger, R. E., 1974, Rhodopsin and light-sensitive kinase activity in retinal outer segments, *Exp. Eye Res.* **18**:271–280.

Franks, D. J., Perrin, L. S., and Malamud, D., 1974, Calcium ion: A modulator of parotid adenylate cyclase activity, *FEBS Lett.* **42**:267–270.

Frazer, A., Pandey, G., Mendels, J., Neeley, S., Kane, M., and Hess, M. E., 1974, The effect of tri-iodothyronine in combination with imipramine on [³H]-cyclic AMP production in slices of rat cerebral cortex. *Neuropharmacology* **13**:1131–1140.

Frazier, W. A., Ohlendorf, C., Forrest, B., Aloe, L., Johnson, E. M., Ferrendelli, J. A., and Bradshaw, R. A., 1973, Mechanism of action of nerve growth factor and cyclic AMP on neurite outgrowth in embryonic chick sensory ganglia: Demonstration of independent pathways of stimulation, *Proc. Nat. Acad. Sci. USA* **70**:2448–2452.

Free, C. A., Paik, V. S., and Shada, J. D., 1974, Inhibition by phenothiazines of adenylate cyclase in adrenal and brain tissue, in *The Phenothiazines and Structurally Related Drugs,* (I. S. Forrest, C. J. Carr, and E. Usin, eds.) pp. 739–748, Raven Press, New York.

Freedman, R., and Hoffer, B. J., 1975, Phenothiazine antagonism of the noradrenergic inhibition of cerebellar Purkinje neurons, *J. Neurobiol.* **6**:277–288.

Freedman, R., Hoffer, B. J., and Woodward, D. J., 1975, A quantitative microiontophoretic analysis of the responses of central neurones to noradrenaline: Interactions with cobalt, manganese, verapamil and dichloroisoprenaline, *Brit. J. Pharmacol.* **54**:529–539.

French, S. W., and Palmer, D. S., 1973, Adrenergic supersensitivity during ethanol withdrawal in the rat, *Res. Commun. Chem. Pathol. Pharmacol.* **6**:651–662.

French, S. W., Reid, P. E., Palmer, D. S., Narod, M. E., and Ramey, C. W., 1974, Adrenergic subsensitivity of the rat brain during chronic ethanol ingestion, *Res. Commun. Chem. Pathol. Pharmacol.* **9**:575–578.

French, S. W., Palmer, D. S., and Narod, M. E., 1975a, Effect of withdrawal from chronic ethanol ingestion on the cAMP response of cerebral cortical slices using the agonists histamine, serotonin and other neurotransmitters, *Canad. J. Physiol. Pharmacol.* **53**:248–255.

French, S. W., Palmer, D. S., Narod, M. E., Reid, L. E., and Ramey, C. W., 1975b, Noradrenergic sensitivity of the cerebral cortex after chronic ethanol ingestion and withdrawal, *J. Pharmacol. Exp. Ther.* **194**:319–326.

Fuller, J. L., and Sjursen, F. H., 1967, Audiogenic seizures in eleven mouse strains, *J. Heredity* **58**:135–140.

Fumagalli, R., Bernareggi, V., Berti, F., and Trabucchi, M., 1971, Cyclic AMP formation in human brain: An *in vitro* stimulation by neurotransmitters, *Life Sci.* **10(I)**:1111–1115.

Furatani, V., Shimada, M., Hamada, M., Takeuchi, T., and Umezawa, H., 1975, Reticulol, an inhibitor of cyclic adenosine 3′,5′-monophosphate phosphodiesterase, *J. Antibiot.* **28**:558–560.

Furlanut, M., Carpenedo, F., and Ferrari, M., 1973, Effects of some isoquinoline compounds and certain derivatives on brain phosphodiesterase activity, *Biochem. Pharmacol.* **22**:2642–2644.

Furmanski, P., Silverman, D. J., and Lubin, M., 1971, Expression of differentiated functions in mouse neuroblastoma mediated by dibutyryl-cyclic adenosine monophosphate, *Nature (London)* **233**:413–415.

Fuxe, K., and Ungerstedt, U., 1974, Action of caffeine and theophyllamine on supersensitive dopamine receptors: Considerable enhancement of receptor response to treatment with dopa and dopamine receptor agonists, *Med. Biol.* **52**:48–54.

Gaballah, S., and Popoff, C., 1971a, Cyclic 3′,5′-nucleotide phosphodiesterase in nerve endings of developing rat brain, *Brain Res.* **25**:220–222.

Gaballah, S., and Popoff, C., 1971b, Localization of adenosine 3′,5′-monophosphate-dependent protein kinase in brain, *J. Neurochem.* **18**:1795–1797.

Gaballah, S., Popoff, C., and Sooknandan, G., 1971, Changes in cyclic 3′,5′-adenosine monophosphate-dependent protein kinase levels in brain development, *Brain Res.* **31**:229–232.

Gadd, R. E. A., Clayman, S., and Hebert, D., 1973, Inhibition of cyclic 3′,5′-nucleotide phosphodiesterase activity by diuretics and other agents, *Experientia* **29**:1217–1219.

Gahwiler, B. H., 1976, Inhibitory action of noradrenaline and cyclic AMP in explants of rat cerebellum, *Nature (London)* **259**:483–484.

Garbers, D. L., and Johnson, R. A., 1975, Metal and metal–ATP interactions with brain and cardiac adenylate cyclases, *J. Biol. Chem.* **250**:8449–8456.

Garelis, E., and Neff, N. H., 1974, Cyclic adenosine monophosphate: Selective increase in caudate nucleus after administration of L-dopa, *Science* **183**:532–533.

Gerhards, H. J., Carenzi, A., and Costa, E., 1974, Effect of nomifensine on motor activity, dopamine turnover rate and cyclic adenosine 3′,5′-monophosphate concentrations of rat striatum, *Naunyn-Schmiedeberg's Arch. Pharmacol.* **286**:49–64.

Gessa, G. L., and Tagliamonte, A., 1975, Effect of methadone and dextromoramide on dopamine metabolism: Comparison with haloperidol and amphetamine, *Neuropharmacol.* **14**:913–920.

Gessa, G. L., Krishna, G., Forn, J., Tagliamonte, A., and Brodie, B. B., 1970, Behavioral and vegetative effects produced by dibutyryl cyclic AMP injected into different areas of the brain, *Advan. Biochem. Psychopharmacol.* **3**:371–381.

Gibson, D. A., Reichlin, S., and Vernadakis, A., 1974, [³H] Uridine uptake and incorporation into RNA in the C-6 glial cells following dibutyryl cyclic AMP treatment, *Brain Res.* **81**:354–360.

Gill, G. N., and Kanstein, C. B., 1975, Guanosine 3′,5′-monophosphate receptor protein: Separation from adenosine 3′,5′-monophosphate receptor protein, *Biochem. Biophys. Res. Commun.* **63**:1113–1122.

Gillespie, E., 1971, Colchicine binding in tissue slices: Decrease by calcium and biphasic effect of adenosine 3′,5′-monophosphate, *J. Cell Biol.* **50**:544–549.

Gilman, A. G., and Minna, J. D., 1973, Expression of genes for metabolism of cyclic adenosine

3':5'-monophosphate in somatic cells. I. Responses to catecholamines in parental and hybrid cells, *J. Biol. Chem.* **248**:6610–6617.

Gilman, A. G., and Nirenberg, M., 1971a, Effect of catecholamines on the adenosine 3'-5'-cyclic monophosphate concentrations of clonal satellite cells of neurons, *Proc. Nat. Acad. Sci. USA* **68**:2165–2168.

Gilman, A. G., and Nirenberg, M., 1971b, Regulation of adenosine 3',5'-cyclic monophosphate metabolism in cultured neuroblastoma cells, *Nature (London)* **234**:356–358.

Gilman, A. G., and Schrier, B. K., 1972, Adenosine cyclic 3',5'-monophosphate in fetal rat brain cell cultures, *Mol. Pharmacol.* **8**:410–416.

Ginsborg, B. L., and Hirst, G. D., 1972, The effect of adenosine on the release of the transmitter from the phrenic nerve of the rat, *J. Physiol.* **224**:629–645.

Ginos, J., Cotzias, G., Tolosa, E., Tand, L. G., and Lo Monte, A., 1975, Cholinergic effects of molecular segments of apomorphine and dopaminergic effects of *N,N*-dialkylated dopamines, *J. Med. Chem.* **18**:1194–1200.

Glazer, R. I., and Schneider, F. H., 1975, Effects of adenosine 3',5'-monophosphate and related agents on ribonucleic acid syntheis and morphological differentiation in mouse neuroblastoma cells in culture, *J. Biol. Chem.* **250**:2745–2749.

Glick, N. B., and Quastel, J. H., 1972, Effects of cerebral stimuli on adenine incorporation into nucleotides and RNA in brain slices from the rat, *Canad. J. Biochem.* **50**:672–683.

Gnegy, M. E., Costa, E., and Uzunov, P., 1976a, Regulation of transsynaptically elicited increase of 3',5'-cyclic AMP by endogenous phosphodiesterase activator, *Proc. Nat. Acad. Sci. USA* **73**:352–355.

Gnegy, M. E., Costa, E., and Uzunov, P., 1976b, Release of phosphodiesterase activator (PDEA) from subcellular fractions of rat brain, *Fed. Proc.* **35**:609Abs.

Gnegy, M., Usunov, P., and Costa, E., 1976c, Drug-induced supersensitivity of dopamine receptors and membrane bound adenylate cyclase activator, *Pharmacologist* **18**:185 (Abs).

Godfraind, J. M., and Pumain, R., 1971, Cyclic adenosine monophosphate and norepineph rine: Effect on Purkinje cells in rat cerebellar cortex, *Science* **174**:1257–1258.

Godfraind, J. M., and Pumain, R., 1972, Cyclic-AMP and noradrenaline iontophoretic release on rat cerebellar Purkinje neurons, *Arch. Int. Pharmacodyn. Ther. Suppl.* **196**:131–132.

Godfraind, J. M., Krnejević, K., Maretic, H., and Pumain, R., 1973, Inhibition of cortical neurons by imidazole and some derivatives, *Canad. J. Physiol. Pharmacol.* **51**:790–797.

Godfraind, T., Koch, M-C., and Verbeke, N., 1974, The action of EGTA on the catecholamines stimulation of rat brain Na^+,-K^+-ATPase, *Biochem. Pharmacol.* **23**:3505–3511.

Goldberg, A. L., and Singer, J. J., 1969, Evidence for a role of cyclic AMP in neuromuscular transmission, *Proc. Nat. Acad. Sci. USA* **64**:134–141.

Goldberg, N. D., and O'Toole, A. G., 1969, The properties of glycogen synthetase and regulation of glycogen biosynthesis in rat brain, *J. Biol. Chem.* **244**:3053–3061.

Goldberg, N. D., Dietz, S. B., and O'Toole, A., 1969, Cyclic guanosine 3',5'-monophosphate in mammalian tissue and urine, *J. Biol. Chem.* **244**:4458–4466.

Goldberg, N. D., Haddox, M. K., Nicol, S. E., Glass, D. B., Sanford, C. H., Kuehl, F. A., Jr., and Estensen, R., 1975, Biologic regulation through opposing influences of cyclic GMP and cyclic AMP: The Yin Yang hypothesis, *Advan. Cyclic Nucleotide Res.* **5**:307–330.

Goldberg, N. D., Larner, J., Sasko, H., and O'Toole, A. G., 1967, Enzymatic analysis of cyclic 3',5'-AMP in mammalian tissues and urine, *Anal. Biochem.* **28**:523–544.

Goldberg, N. D., Lust, W. D., O'Dea, R. F., Wei, S., and O'Toole, A. G., 1970, A role of cyclic nucleotides in brain metabolism, *Advan. Biochem. Psychopharmacol.* **3**:67–87.

Goldberg, N. D., O'Dea, R. F., and Haddox, M. K., 1973, Cyclic GMP, *Advan. Cyclic Nucleotide Res.* **3**:155–223.

Goldfine, I. D., Perlman, R., and Roth, J., 1971, Inhibition of cyclic 3',5'-AMP phosphodiesterase in islet cells and other tissues by tolbutamide, *Nature (London)* **234**:295–296.

Goldstein, A., 1976, Opioid peptides (endorphins) in pituitary and brain, *Science* **193**:1081–1086.

Goldstein, G., Scheid, M. S., Hammerling, V., Boyse, E. A., Schlesinger, D. H., and Niall, H. D., 1975a, Isolation of a polypeptide that has lymphocyte-differentiating properties and is probably represented universally in living cells, *Proc. Nat. Acad. Sci. USA* **72**:11–15.

Goldstein, M., Ebstein, B., Bronaugh, R. L., and Roberge, C., 1975b, Stimulation of striatal tyrosine hydroxylase by cyclic AMP, in *Chemical Tools in Catecholamine Research* (O. Almgren, A. Carlsson, and J. Engel, eds.), Vol. II, pp. 257–264, North-Holland, Amsterdam.

Goldstein, M., Anagnoste, B., and Shirron, C., 1973, The effect of trivastal, haloperidol and dibutyryl cyclic AMP on [^{14}C]dopamine synthesis in rat striatum, *J. Pharm. Pharmacol.* **25**:348–351.

Goodman, D. B. P., Rasmussen, H., DiBella, F., and Guthrow, C. E., Jr., 1970, Cyclic adenosine 3′,5′-monophosphate-stimulated phosphorylation of isolated neurotubule subunits, *Proc. Nat. Acad. Sci. USA* **67**:652–659.

Goodman, R., Oesch, F., and Thoenen, H., 1974, Changes in enzyme patterns produced by high potassium concentrations and dibutyryl cyclic AMP in organ cultures of sympathetic ganglia, *J. Neurochem.* **23**:369–378.

Goridis, C., and Morgan, I. G., 1973, Guanyl cyclase in rat brain subcellular fractions, *FEBS Lett.* **34**:71–73.

Goridis, C., and Virmaux, N., 1974, Light-regulated guanosine 3′,5′-monophosphate phosphodiesterase of bovine retina, *Nature (London)* **248**:57–58.

Goridis, C., Massarelli, R., Sensenbrenner, M., and Mandel, P., 1974, Guanyl cyclase in chick embryo brain cell cultures: Evidence of neuronal localization, *J. Neurochem.* **23**:135–138.

Gourley, D. R. H., and Bechner, S. K., 1973, Antagonism of morphine analgesia by adenine, adenosine and adenine nucleotides, *Proc. Soc. Exp. Biol. Med.* **144**:774–778.

Govoni, S., Kumakura, K., Spano, P. F., Tonon, G. C., and Trabucchi, M., 1975, Interaction of narcotic analgesics with dopamine receptors in rat brain, *Pharmacol. Res. Commun.* **7**:95–100.

Green, A. R., Heal, D. J., and Grahame-Smith, D. G., 1975, Lack of change in the sensitivity of rat caudate nucleus adenyl cyclase to dopamine when thyrothrophin releasing hormone and cycloheximide produce opposite effects on the behavioral responses to certain centrally acting drugs, in *Chemical Tools in Catecholamine Research* (O. Almgren, A. Carlsson, and J. Engel, eds.), Vol. II, pp. 265–274, North-Holland, Amsterdam.

Greengard, P., 1976, Possible role for cyclic nucleotides and phosphorylated membrane proteins in postsynaptic actions of neurotransmitters, *Nature (London)* **260**:101–108.

Greengard, P., and Kebabian, J. W., 1974, Role of cyclic AMP in synaptic transmission in the mammalian peripheral nervous system, *Fed. Proc.* **33**:1059–1067.

Greengard, P., and Kuo, J. F., 1970, On the mechanism of action of cyclic AMP, *Advan. Biochem. Psychopharmacol.* **3**:287–306.

Greengard, P., McAfee, D. A., and Kebabian, J. W., 1972, On the mechanism of action of cyclic AMP and its role in synaptic transmission, *Advan. Cyclic Nucleotide Res.* **1**:337–355.

Guidotti, A., Biggio, G., and Costa, E., 1975, 3-Acetylpyridine: A tool to inhibit the tremor and increase of cGMP content in cerebellar cortex elicited by harmaline, *Brain Res.* **96**:201–205.

Guidotti, A., Cheney, D. L., Trabucchi, M., Doteuchi, M., Wang, C., and Hawkins, R. A., 1974, Focussed microwave radiation: A technique to minimize postmortem changes of cyclic nucleotides, dopa and choline and to preserve brain morphology, *Neuropharmacology* **13**:1115–1122.

Gullis, R. J., and Rowe, C. E., 1975a, The stimulation by synaptic transmitters of the incorporation of oleate into the phospholipid of synaptic membranes, *Biochem. J.* **148**:557–565.

Gullis, R. J., and Rowe, C. E., 1975b, The stimulation of phospholipase A2-acylation system of synaptic membranes of brain by cyclic nucleotides, *Biochem. J.* **148**:567–582.

Gullis, R. J., Traber, J., Fischer, K., Buchen, C., and Hamprecht, B., 1975a, Effects of cholinergic agents and sodium ions on the levels of guanosine and adenosine 3′,5′-cyclic monophosphates in neuroblastoma and neuroblastoma × glioma hybrids, *FEBS Lett.* **59**:74–79.

Gullis, R., Traber, J., and Hamprecht, B., 1975b, Morphine elevates levels of cyclic GMP in a neuroblastoma × glioma hybrid cell, *Nature (London)* **256**:57–58.

Gumulka, S. W., Dinnendahl, V., Peters, H. D. and Schonhofer, P. S., 1976, Effects of dopaminergic stimulants on cyclic nucleotide levels in mouse brain *in vivo, Naunyn-Schmiedeberg's Arch. Pharmacol.* **293**:75–80.

Gunaga, K. P., and Menon, K. M. J., 1973, Effect of catecholamines and ovarian hormones on cyclic AMP accumulation in rat hypothalamus, *Biochem. Biophys. Res. Commun.* **54**:440–448.

Gunaga, K. P., Kawano, A., and Menon, K. M. J., 1974, *In vivo* effect of estradiol benzoate on the accumulation of adenosine 3′,5′-cyclic monophosphate in the rat hypothalamus, *Neuroendocrinology* **16**:273–281.

Haas, D. C., Hier, D. B., Arnason, B. G. W., and Young, M., 1972, On a possible relationship of cyclic AMP to the mechanisms of action of nerve growth factor, *Proc. Soc. Exp. Biol. Med.* **140**:45–47.

Hamadah, K., Holmes, H., Barker, G. B., Hartman, G. C., and Parke, D. V. W., 1972, Effect of electric convulsion therapy on urinary excretion of 3′,5′-cyclic adenosine monophosphate, *Brit. Med. J.* **19**:439–441.

Hamprecht, B., and Schultz, J., 1973a, Stimulation of prostaglandin E₁ of adenosine 3′,5′-cyclic monophosphate formation in neuroblastoma cells in the presence of phosphodiesterase inhibitors, *FEBS Lett.* **34**:85–89.

Hamprecht, B., and Schultz, J., 1973b, Influence of norepinephrine, prostaglandin E₁ and inhibitors of phosphodiesterase activity on levels of adenosine 3′:5′-cyclic monophosphate in somatic cell hybrids, *Hoppe-Seylers Z. Physiol. Chem.* **354**:1633–1641.

Hamprecht, B., Traber, J., and Lamprecht, F., 1974, Dopamine β-hydroxylase activity in cholinergic neuroblastoma × glioma hybrid cells: Increase in activity by N^6,O^2-dibutyryl adenosine 3′,5′-cyclic monophosphate, *FEBS Lett.* **42**:211–226.

Hamprecht, B., Jaffe, B. M., and Philpott, G. W., 1973, Prostaglandin production by neuroblastoma, glioma and fibroblast cell lines, stimulation by $N^6,O^{2′}$-dibutyryl adenosine 3′,5′-cyclic monophosphate, *FEBS Lett.* **36**:193–198.

Hanbauer, I., Kopin, J., Guidotti, A., and Costa, E., 1975a, Induction of tyrosine hydroxylase elicited by beta adrenergic receptor agonists in normal and decentralized sympathetic ganglia: Role of cyclic 3′,5′-adenosine monophosphate, *J. Pharmacol. Exp. Ther.* **193**:95–104.

Hanbauer, I., Lovenberg, W., Guidotti., A., and Costa, E., 1975b, Role of cholinergic and glucocorticosteroid receptors in the tyrosine hydroxylase induction elicited by reserpine in superior cervical ganglion, *Brain Res.* **96**:197–200.

Hardman, J. G., and Sutherland, E. W., 1969, Guanyl cyclase, an enzyme catalyzing the formation of guanosine 3′,5′-monophosphate from guanosine triphosphate, *J. Biol. Chem.* **244**:6363–6370.

Harkins, J., Arsenault, M., Schlesinger, K., and Kates, J., 1972, Induction of neuronal functions: Acetylcholine-induced acetylcholinesterase activity in mouse neuroblastoma cells, *Proc. Nat. Acad. Sci. USA* **167**:3161–3164.

Harris, D. H., Chasin, M., Phillips, M. B., Goldenberg, H., Samaniego, S., and Hess, S. M., 1973, Effect of cyclic nucleotides on activity of cyclic 3′,5′-adenosine monophosphate phosphodiesterase, *Biochem. Pharmacol.* **22**:221–228.

Harris, J. E., 1976, β-Adrenergic receptor-mediated adenosine cyclic 3′,5′-monophosphate accumulation in the rat corpus striatum, *Mol. Pharmacol.* **12**:546–558.

Harris, J. E., Morgenroth, V. H., Roth, R. H., and Baldessarini, R. J., 1974, Regulation of catecholamine synthesis in rat brain *in vitro* by cyclic AMP, *Nature (London)* **252:**156–158.

Harris, J. E., Baldessarini, R. J., Morgenroth, V. H., and Roth, R. H., 1975, Activation by cyclic 3′,5′-adenosine monophosphate of tyrosine hydroxylase in the rat brain, *Proc. Nat. Acad. Sci. USA* **72:**789–793.

Haslam, R. J., and Rosson, G. M., 1975, Effects of adenosine on levels of adenosine cyclic 3′,5′-monophosphate in human blood platelets in relation to adenosine incorporation and platelet aggregation, *Mol. Pharmacol.* **11:**528–544.

Haulica, I., Ababei, L., Branisteanu, D., and Topolinceanu, F., 1973, Preliminary data on a possible hypnogenic role of adenosine, *J. Neurochem.* **21:**1019–1020.

Hayashi, S., Sakaguchi, T., and Ozawa, H., 1976, Studies on 3′,7′-dimethyl-1-(5-oxo-hexyl)-xanthine (BL 191): The inhibitory effect of BL 191 on PDE in various tissues of rats, *Jap. J. Pharmacol.* **26:**117–119.

Hedge, G. A., 1971, ACTH secretion due to hypothalamo-pituitary effects of adenosine 3′,5′-monophosphate and related substances, *Endocrinology* **89:**500–506.

Hegstrand, L. R., Kanof, P. D., and Greengard, P., 1976, Histamine-sensitive adenylate cyclase in mammalian brain, *Nature (London)* **260:**163–164.

Heikkinen, E. R., Myllyla, V. V., Vapaatalo, H., and Hokkanen, E., 1974, Urinary excretion and cerebrospinal fluid concentration of cyclic adenosine 3′,5′-monophosphate in various neurological diseases, *Eur. J. Neurol.* **11:**270–280.

Heikkinen, E. R., Simila, S., Myllyla, V. V., Hokkanen, E., and Vapaatalo, H., 1975, Adenosine 3′,5′-monophosphate concentration and enzyme activities of cerebrospinal fluid in meningitis of children, *Z. Kinderheilk.* **120:**243–250.

Heller, I. H., and McIlwain, H., 1973, Release of [^{14}C]adenine derivatives from isolated subsystems of the guinea pig brain: Actions of electrical stimulation and of papaverine, *Brain Res.* **53:**105–116.

Hendriks, T., DePont, J. J. H. M., Daemen, F. J. M., and Bonting, S. L., 1973, Biochemical aspects of the visual process. XXIV. Adenylate cyclase and photoreceptor membranes: A critical appraisal, *Biochim. Biophys. Acta* **330:**156–166.

Henion, W. F., Sutherland, E. W., and Posternak, T., 1967, Effects of derivatives of adenosine 3′,5′-phosphate on liver slices and intact animals, *Biochim. Biophys. Acta* **148:**106–113.

Herman, Z. S., 1973, Behavioral effects of dibutyryl cyclic 3′,5′-AMP, noradrenaline and cyclic 3′,5′-AMP in rats, *Neuropharmacology* **12:**705–709.

Hess, S. M., Chasin, M., Free, C. A., and Harris, D. N., 1975, Modulators of cyclic AMP systems, *Advan. Biochem. Psychopharmacol.* **14:**153–167.

Hetenyi, G., Jr., and Singhal, P. L., 1973, Effect of insulin on cerebral adenyl cyclase and phosphodiesterase, *Hormone Metab. Res.* **5:**139.

Hidaka, H., Shibuya, M., Asano, T., and Hara, F., 1975, Cyclic nucleotide phosphodiesterase of human cerebrospinal fluid, *J. Neurochem.* **25:**49–54.

Hier, D. B., Arnason, B. G. W., and Young, M., 1972, Studies on the mechanism of action of nerve growth factor, *Proc. Nat. Acad. Sci. USA* **69:**2268–2272.

Hier, D. B., Arnason, B. G. W., and Young, M., 1973, Nerve growth factor: Relationship to the cyclic AMP system of sensory ganglia, *Science* **182:**79–81.

Ho, I. K., Loh, H. H., and Way, E. L., 1972, Effect of cyclic AMP on morphine analgesia tolerance and physical dependence, *Nature (London)* **238:**397–398.

Ho, I. K., Loh, H. H., and Way, E. L., 1973a, Effects of cyclic 3′,5′-adenosine monophosphate on morphine tolerance and physical dependence, *J. Pharmacol. Exp. Ther.* **185:**347–357.

Ho, I. K., Loh, H.H., and Way, E. L., 1973b, Cyclic adenosine monophosphate antagonism of morphine analgesia, *J. Pharmacol. Exp. Ther.* **185:**336–346.

Ho, I. K., Loh, H. H., Bhargava, H. N., and Way, E. L., 1975a, Effect of cyclic nucleotides and phosphodiesterase inhibitors on morphine tolerance and physical dependence, *Life Sci.* **16**:1895–1900.

Ho, R. J., Russell, T. R., Asakawa, T., and Hucks, M. W., 1975b, Inhibition of cyclic nucleotide phosphodiesterase activity by an endogenous factor, *J. Cyclic Nucleotide Res.* **1**:81–88.

Ho, R. J., and Sutherland, E. W., 1971, Formation and release of a hormone antagonist by rat adipocytes, *J. Biol. Chem.* **216**:6822–6827.

Ho, R. J., and Sutherland, E. W., 1975, cAMP-mediated feedback regulation in target cells, *Advan. Cyclic Nucleotide Res.* **5**:533–548.

Hoffer, B. J., Siggins, G. R., and Bloom, F. E., 1969, Prostaglandins E_1 and E_2 antagonize norepinephrine effects on cerebellar Purkinje cells: Microelectrophoretic study, *Science* **166**:1418–1420.

Hoffer, B. J., Siggins, G. R., and Bloom, F. E., 1970, Possible cyclic AMP-mediated adrenergic synapses to rat cerebellar Purkinje cells: Combined structural, physiological, and pharmacological analyses, *Advan. Biochem. Psychopharmacol.* **3**:349–370.

Hoffer, B. J., Siggins, G. R., and Bloom, F. E., 1971a, Studies on norepinephrine-containing afferents of Purkinje cells of rat cerebellum. II. Sensitivity of Purkinje cells to norepinephrine and related substances administered by microiontophoresis, *Brain Res.* **25**:523–534.

Hoffer, B. J., Siggins, G. R., Oliver, A. P., and Bloom, F. E., 1971b, Cyclic AMP mediation of norepinephrine inhibition in rat cerebellar cortex: A unique class of synaptic responses, *Ann. N.Y. Acad. Sci.* **185**:531–549.

Hoffer, B. J., Siggins, G. R., Woodward, D. J., and Bloom, F. E., 1971c, Spontaneous discharge of Purkinje neurons after destruction of catecholamine-containing afferents by 6-hydroxydopamine, *Brain Res.* **30**:425–430.

Hoffer, B. J., Siggins, G. R., Oliver, A. P., and Bloom, F. E., 1972, Cyclic AMP-mediated adrenergic synapses to cerebellar Purkinje cells, *Advan. Cyclic Nucleotide Res.* **1**:411–423.

Hoffer, B. J., Freedman, R., Woodward, D. J., Daly, J. W., and Skolnick, P., 1976, β-Adrenergic control of cyclic AMP-generating systems in cerebellum: Pharmacological heterogeneity confirmed by destruction of interneurons, *Exp. Neurol.* **51**:653–667.

Hofmann, F., and Sold, G., 1972, A protein kinase activity from rat cerebellum stimulated by guanosine-3′:5′-monophosphate, *Biochem. Biophys. Res. Commun.* **49**:1100–1107.

Hommes, F. A., and Beere, A., 1971, The development of adenyl cyclase in rat liver, kidney, brain and skeletal muscle, *Biochim. Biophys. Acta* **237**:296–300.

Honda, F., and Imamura, H., 1968, Inhibition of cyclic 3′,5′-nucleotide phosphodiesterase by phenothiazine and reserpine derivatives, *Biochim. Biophys. Acta* **161**:267–269.

Horn, J. P., and McAfee, D. A., 1976, Peripheral nerve: Levels of cyclic nucleotides and their effect on excitability, *Fed. Proc.* **35**:424Abs.

Horn, A. S., and Phillipson, O. T., 1976, A noradrenaline-sensitive adenylate cyclase in the rat limbic forebrain: Preparation, properties, and effects of agonists, adrenolytics, and neuroleptic drugs, *Eur. J. Pharmacol.* **37**:1–11.

Horn, A. S., Cuello, A. C., and Miller, R. J., 1974, Dopamine in the mesolimbic system of the rat brain: Endogenous levels and the effects of drugs on the uptake mechanism and stimulation of adenylate cyclase activity, *J. Neurochem.* **22**:265–270.

Horn, A., Post, M., and Kennard, O., 1975, Dopamine receptor blockade and the neuroleptics, a crystallographic study, *J. Pharm. Pharmacol.* **27**:553–563.

Horovitz, Z. P., Beer, B., Clody, D. E., Vogel, J. R., and Chasin, M., 1972, Cyclic AMP and anxiety, *Psychosomatics* **13**:85–92.

Hsu, C. Y., and Brooker, G., 1976, Adrenergic agonists increase cyclic GMP in a rat glial cell line (C6-2B), *Fed. Proc.* **35**:295Abs.

Huang, M., and Daly, J. W., 1972, Accumulation of cyclic adenosine monophosphate in incubated slices of brain tissue. 1. Structure–activity relationships of agonists and antagonists of biogenic amines and of tricyclic tranquilizers and antidepressants, *J. Med. Chem.* **15**:458–462.

Huang, M., and Daly, J. W., 1974a, Adenosine-elicited accumulation of cyclic AMP in brain slices: Potentiation by agents which inhibit uptake of adenosine. *Life Sci.* **14**:489–503.

Huang, M., and Daly, J. W., 1974b, Interrelationships among levels of ATP, adenosine and cyclic AMP in incubated slices of guinea pig cerebral cortex: Effect of depolarizing agents, psychotropic drugs and metabolic inhibitors, *J. Neurochem.* **23**:393–404.

Huang, M., Shimizu, H., and Daly, J., 1971, Regulation of adenosine cyclic 3′,5′-phosphate formation in cerebral cortical slices: Interaction among norepinephrine, histamine, and serotonin, *Mol. Pharmacol.* **7**:155–162.

Huang, M., Shimizu, H., and Daly, J. W., 1972, Accumulation of cyclic adenosine monophosphate in incubated slices of brain tissue. 2. Effects of depolarizing agents, membrane stabilizers, phosphodiesterase inhibitors, and adenosine analogs, *J. Med. Chem.* **15**:462–466.

Huang, M., Gruenstein, E., and Daly, J. W., 1973a, Depolarization-evoked accumulation of cyclic AMP in brain slices: Inhibition by exogenous adenosine deaminase, *Biochim. Biophys. Acta* **329**:147–151.

Huang, M., Ho, A. K. S., and Daly, J. W., 1973b, Accumulation of adenosine cyclic 3′,5′-monophosphate in rat cerebral cortical slices: Stimulatory effect of alpha and beta adrenergic agents after treatment with 6-hydroxydopamine, 2,3,5-trihydroxyphenethylamine and dihydroxytryptamines, *Mol. Pharmacol.* **9**:711–717.

Hughes, J., Smith, T. W., Kosterlitz, H. W., Fothergill, L. A., Morgan, B. A., and Morris, H. R., 1975, Identification of two related pentapeptides from the brain with potent opiate agonist activity, *Nature (London)* **258**:577–579.

Hunt, W. A., Redos, J. D., and Catravas, G. N., 1976, Brain cyclic nucleotide levels after acute and chronic administration of ethanol, *Fed. Proc.* **35**:815Abs.

Hutchison, H. T. K., Werrbach, K., Vance, C., and Haber, B., 1973, Uptake of GABA by clonal astrocytoma and neuroblastoma cell lines in culture, *Trans. Amer. Soc. Neurochem.* **4**:136A.

Hynie, S., Cepelik, J., Cernohorsky, M., Kenerova, V., Skrivanova, J., and Wenke, M., 1975, 7-Oxa-13-prostynoic acid and polyphloretin phosphate as non-specific antagonists of the stimulatory effects of different agents on adenylate cyclase from various tissues, *Prostaglandins* **10**:971–982.

Inoue, Y., Yamamura, H., and Nishizuka, Y., 1973, Protamine kinase independent of adenosine 3′,5′-monophosphate from rat brain cytosol, *Biochem. Biophys. Res. Commun.* **50**:228–236.

Ishikawa, E., Ishikawa, S., Davis, J. W., and Sutherland, E. W., 1969, Determination of guanosine 3′,5′-monophosphate in tissues and of guanyl cyclase in rat intestine, *J. Biol. Chem.* **244**:6371–6376.

Israël, M. A., Kimura, H., and Kuriyama, K., 1972, Changes in activity and hormonal sensitivity of brain adenyl cyclase following chronic ethanol administration, *Experientia* **28**:1322–1323.

Iversen, L., 1975, Dopamine receptors in the brain: A dopamine-sensitive adenylate cyclase models synaptic receptors, illuminating antipsychotic drug action, *Science* **188**:1084–1085.

Iversen, L. L., Horn, A. S., and Miller, R. J., 1975a, Structure–activity relationships for agonist and antagonist drugs at pre- and postsynaptic dopamine receptor sites in rat brain, in *Pre- and Postsynaptic Receptors* (E. Usdin and W. E. Bunney, Jr., eds.), pp. 207–245, Marcel Dekker, New York.

Iversen, L. L., Horn, A. S., and Miller, R. J., 1975b, Actions of dopaminergic agonists on cyclic AMP production in rat brain homogenates, *Advan. Neurol.* **9**:197–212.

Iversen, L. L., Rogawski, M. A., and Miller, R. J., 1976, Comparison of the effects of neuroleptic drugs on pre- and postsynaptic dopaminergic mechanisms in the rat stratum, *Mol. Pharmacol.* **12**:251–262.

Iwangoff, P., and Enz, A., 1971, The effect of dihydroergotamine on the phosphodiesterase activity of cat grey matter, *Experientia* **27**:1258–1259.

Iwangoff, P., and Enz, A., 1972, The influence of various dihydroergotamine analogues on cyclic adenosine-3′,5′-monophosphate phosphodiesterase in the grey matter of cat brain *in vitro*, *Agents Actions* **2**:223–230.

Iwatsubo, K., and Clouet, D. H., 1975, Dopamine-sensitive adenylate cyclase of the caudate nucleus of rats treated with morphine or haloperidol, *Biochem. Pharmacol.* **24**:1499–1504.

Izumi, H., Oyama, H., and Ozawa, H., 1975a, The stimulatory effect of the boiled supernatant on cyclic AMP formation in synaptosomes from rat cerebral cortex, *Jap. J. Pharmacol.* **25**:375–382.

Izumi, H., Oyama, H., and Ozawa, H., 1975b, Endogenous inhibitor(s) in rat liver of dopamine β-hydroxylase, *Chem. Pharm. Bull.* **23**:2362–2368.

Jackson, D. M., Anden, N.-E., and Dahlstrom, A., 1975, A functional effect of dopamine in the nucleus accumbens and in some other dopamine-rich parts of the rat brain, *Psychopharmacologia* **45**:139–149.

Janiec, W., Trzeciak, H., and Herman, Z., 1970, The influence of adrenaline and optical isomers of INPEA on the adenyl cyclase activity in brain hemispheres of rats *in vitro*, *Arch. Int. Pharmacodyn. Ther.* **185**:254–258.

Jard, S., Premont, J., and Benda, P., 1972, Adenylate cyclase, phosphodiesterases and protein kinase of rat glial cells in culture, *FEBS Lett.* **26**:344–348.

Jastorff, B., and Bar, H.-B., 1973, Effects of 5′ amido analogues of adenosine 3′,5′-monophosphate and adenosine 3:5′-monophosphothioate on protein kinase, binding protein and phosphodiesterases, *Eur. J. Biochem.* **37**:497–504.

Jenner, F. A., Sampson, G. A., Thompson, E. A., Somerville, A. R., Beard, N. A., and Smith, A. A., 1972, Manic-depressive psychosis and urinary excretion of cyclic AMP, *Brit. J. Psychiat.* **121**:236–237.

Johnson, E. M., Maeno, H., and Greengard, P., 1971, Phosphorylation of endogenous protein of rat brain by a cyclic adenosine 3′, 5′-monophosphate-dependent protein kinase, *J. Biol. Chem.* **246**:7731–7739.

Johnson, E. M., Ueda, T., Maeno, H., and Greengard, P., 1972, Adenosine 3′,5-monophosphate-dependent phosphorylation of a specific protein in synaptic membrane fractions from rat cerebrum, *J. Biol. Chem.* **247**:5650–5652.

Johnson, G. A., Boukma, S. J., Lahti, R. A., and Mathews, J., 1973, Cyclic AMP and phosphodiesterase in synaptic vesicles from mouse brain, *J. Neurochem.* **20**:1387–1392.

Johnson, R. A., and Sutherland, E. W., 1973, Detergent-dispersed adenylate cyclase from rat brain: Effects of fluoride, cations and chelators, *J. Biol. Chem.* **248**:5114–5121.

Johnston, G. A. R., and Balcar, V. J., 1973, High affinity uptake of cyclic AMP in rat brain slices, *Brain Res.* **59**:451–453.

Jones, D. J., Medina, M., Ross, D. H., and Stavinoha, W. B., 1974, Rate of inactivation of adenyl cyclase and phosphodiesterase: Determinants of brain cyclic AMP, *Life Sci.* **14**:1577–1585.

Jones, E. R., Moscona, M., and Moscona, A. A., 1973a, Does cyclic-3′,5′-AMP induce glutamine synthetase in embryonic neural retina? *Biochem. Biophys. Res. Commun.* **51**:268–274.

Jones, G. H., Murthy, D. V. K., Tegg, D., Golling, R., and Moffatt, J. G., 1973b, Analogs of adenosine 3′,5′-cyclic phosphate. II. Synthesis and enzymatic activity of derivatives of 1, N^6-ethanoadenosine 3′,5′-cyclic phosphate, *Biochem. Biophys. Res. Commun.* **53**:1338–1343.

Joo, F., 1972, Effect of N^6, O^2-dibutyryl cyclic 3′,5′-adenosine monophosphate on the pinocytosis of brain capillaries of mice, *Experientia* **28**:1470–1471.

Joo, F., Rakonczay, Z., and Wollenmann, M., 1975a, cAMP-mediated regulation of the permeability in the brain capillaries, *Experientia* **3**:582–583.

Joo, F., Toth, I., and Jancso, G., 1975b, Brain adenylate cyclase: Its common occurrence in the capillaries and astrocytes, *Naturwissenschaften* **62**:397–398.

Jordan, L. M., Lake, N., and Phillis, J. W., 1972a, Mechanism of noradrenaline depression of cortical neurones: A species comparison, *Eur. J. Pharmacol.* **20**:381–384.

Jordan, L. M., Lake, N., and Phillis, J. W., 1972b, Noradrenaline excitation of cortical neurones: A reply, *J. Pharm. Pharmacol.* **24**:739–741.

Kakiuchi, S., and Rall, T. W., 1968a, Studies on adenosine $3',5'$-phosphate in rabbit cerebral cortex, *Mol. Pharmacol.* **4**:379–388.

Kakiuchi, S., and Rall, T. W., 1968b, The influence of chemical agents on the accumulation of adenosine $3',5'$-phosphate in slices of rabbit cerebellum, *Mol. Pharmacol.* **4**:367–378.

Kakiuchi, S., and Yamazaki, R., 1970a, Calcium dependent phosphodiesterase activity and its activating factor (PAF) from brain: Studies on cyclic $3',5'$-nucleotide phosphodiesterase, *Biochem. Biophys. Res. Commun.* **41**:1104–1110.

Kakuichi, S., and Yamazaki, R., 1970b, Properties of a heat-stable phosphodiesterase activating factor isolated from brain extract. II. Studies on cyclic $3',5'$ nucleotide phosphodiesterases, *Proc. Jap. Acad.* **46**:587–592.

Kakiuchi, S., and Yamazaki, R., 1970c, Stimulation of the activity of cyclic $3',5'$-nucleotide phosphodiesterase by calcium ion, *Proc. Jap. Acad.* **46**:387–392.

Kakiuchi, S., Rall, T. W., and McIlwain, H., 1969, The effect of electrical stimulation upon the accumulation of adenosine $3',5'$-phosphate in isolated cerebral tissue, *J. Neurochem.* **16**:485–491.

Kakiuchi, S., Yamazaki, R., and Teshima, Y., 1971, Cyclic $3',5'$-nucleotide phosphodiesterase. IV. Two enzymes with different properties from brain, *Biochem. Biophys. Res. Commun.* **42**:968–974.

Kakiuchi, S., Yamazaki, R., and Teshima, Y., 1972, Regulation of brain phosphodiesterase activity: Ca^{++} plus Mg^{++}-dependent phosphodiesterase and its activating factor from rat brain, *Advan. Cyclic Nucleotide Res.* **1**:455–477.

Kakiuchi, S., Yamazaki, R., Teshima, Y., and Uenishi, K., 1973, Regulation of nucleotide cyclic $3':5'$-monophosphate phosphodiesterase activity from rat brain by a modulator and Ca^{2+}, *Proc. Nat. Acad. Sci. USA* **70**:3526–3535.

Kakiuchi, S., Yamazaki, R., Teshima, Y., Uenishi, K., and Miyamoto, E., 1975a, Multiple cyclic nucleotide phosphodiesterase activities from rat tissues and occurrence of calcium plus magnesium-ion-dependent phosphodiesterase and its protein activator, *Biochem. J.* **146**:109–120.

Kakiuchi, S., Yamazaki, R., Teshima, Y., Uenishi, K., and Miyamoto, E., 1975b, Ca^{2+}/Mg^{2+}-Dependent cyclic nucleotide phosphodiesterase and its activator protein, *Advan. Cyclic Nucleotide Res.* **5**:163–178.

Kalisker, A., Rutledge, C. O., and Perkins, J. P., 1973, Effect of nerve degeneration by 6-hydroxydopamine on catecholamine-stimulated adenosine $3',5'$-monophosphate formation in rat cerebral cortex, *Mol Pharmacol.* **9**:619–629.

Kalix, P., and Roch, P., 1975, Effect of depolarizing agents on the adenosine $3',5'$-monophosphate content of the bovine superior cervical ganglion, *Naunyn-Schmiedeberg's Arch. Pharmacol.* **291**:131–137.

Kalix, P., McAfee, D., Schorderet, M., and Greengard, P., 1974, Pharmacological analysis of synaptically mediated increase in cyclic adenosine monophosphate in rabbit superior cervical ganglion, *J. Pharmacol. Exp. Ther.* **188**:676–687.

Karobath, M., 1974, Trizyklische antidepressive Substanzen and dopamine-sensitive Adenylcyclase ans dem Nucleus caudatus der Ratte, *Arzneimittelforschung* **24**:1019–1021.

Karobath, M. E., 1975, Tricyclic antidepressive drugs and dopamine-sensitive adenylate cyclase from rat brain striatum, *Eur. J. Pharmacol.* **30**:159–163.

Karobath, M., and Leitich, H., 1974, Antipsychotic drugs and dopamine-stimulated adenylate cyclase prepared from corpus striatum of rat brain, *Proc. Nat. Acad. Sci.* **71**:2915–2918.

Kato, G., and Somjen, G. G., 1969, Effects of micro-iontophoretic administration of calcium on neurones in the central nervous system of cats, *J. Neurobiol.* **1**:181–195.

Katz, S., and Tenenhouse, A., 1973a, The relationship of adenyl cyclase to the activity of other ATP utilizing enzymes and phosphodiesterase in preparations of rat brain, mechanism of stimulation of cyclic AMP accumulation by NaF, *Brit. J. Pharmacol.* **48**:505–515.

Katz, S., and Tenenhouse, A., 1973b, The relationship of adenyl cyclase to the activity of other ATP utilizing enzymes and phosphodiesterase in preparations of rat brain: Mechanism of stimulation of cyclic AMP accumulation by adrenaline, ouabain and Mg^{++}, *Brit. J. Pharmacol.* **48**:516–526.

Kauffman, F. C., Harkonen, M. H. A., and Johnson, E. C., 1972, Adenyl cyclase and phosphodiesterase activity in cerebral cortex of normal and undernourished neonatal rats, *Life Sci.* **11(II)**:613–621.

Keatinge, A. M. B., Sinanan, K., and Love, W. C., 1975, Effects of reserpine, chlorpromazine, imipramine and amitriptyline on urinary excretion of adenosine $3',5'$-cyclic monophosphate in rats, *Irish J. Med. Sci.* **144**:249–254.

Kebabian, J. W., and Greengard, P., 1971, Dopamine-sensitive adenyl cyclase: Possible role in synaptic transmission, *Science* **174**:1346–1349.

Kebabian, J. W., Petzold, G. L., and Greengard, P., 1972, Dopamine-sensitive adenylate cyclase in caudate nucleus of rat brain and its similarity to the "dopamine receptor," *Proc. Nat. Acad. Sci. USA* **69**:2145–2149.

Kebabian, J. W., Bloom, F. E., Steiner, A. L., and Greengard, P., 1975a, Neurotransmitters increase cyclic nucleotides in postganglionic neurons: Immunocytochemical demonstration, *Science* **190**:157–159.

Kebabian, J. W., Clement-Cormier, Y. C., Petzold, G. L., and Greengard, P., 1975b, Chemistry of dopamine receptors, *Advan. Neurol.* **9**:1–11.

Kebabian, J. W., Steiner, A. L., and Greengard, P., 1975c, Muscarinic cholinergic regulation of cyclic guanosine $3',5'$-monophosphate in autonomic ganglia: Possible role in synaptic transmission, *J. Pharmacol. Exp. Ther.* **193**:474–488.

Kebabian, J. W., Zatz, M., Romero, J. A., and Axelrod, J., 1975d, Rapid changes in rat pineal β-adrenergic receptor: Alterations in l-[^{3}H]alprenolol binding and adenylate cyclase, *Proc. Nat. Acad. Sci. USA* **72**:3735–3739.

Keen, P., and McLean, W. G., 1972a, Effect of dibutyryl cyclic-AMP on levels of dopamine-β-hydroxylase in isolated superior cervical ganglia, *Naunyn-Schmiedebergs Arch. Pharmacol.* **275**:465–469.

Keen, P., and McLean, W. G., 1972b, The effect of N^6, $O^{2'}$-dibutyryl adenosine $3':5'$-cyclic monophosphate on noradrenaline synthesis in isolated superior cervical ganglia, *Brit. J. Pharmacol.* **46**:529–530.

Keen, P., and McLean, W. G., 1974, Effect of dibutyryl-cyclic AMP and dexamethasone on noradrenaline synthesis in isolated superior cervical ganglia, *J. Neurochem.* **22**:5–10.

Keirns, J. J., Miki, N., Bitensky, M. W., and Keirns, M., 1975, A link between rhodopsin and disc membrane cyclic nucleotide phosphodiesterase. Action spectrum and sensitivity to illumination, *Biochemistry* **14**:2760–2766.

Khwaja, T. A., Boswell, K. H., Robins, R. K., and Miller, J. P., 1975, 8-Substituted derivatives of adenosine $3',5'$-cyclic phosphate require an unsubstituted $2'$-hydroxyl group in the ribo configuration for biological activity, *Biochemistry* **14**:4238–4244.

Kiessling, M., Lindl, T., and Cramer, H., 1975, Cyclic adenosine monophosphate in cerebrospinal fluid. Effects of theophylline, L-dopa and a dopamine receptor stimulant in rats, *Arch. Psychiatr. Nervenkr.* **230**:325–333.

Kimhi, Y., Palfrey, C., Spector, I., Barak, Y., and Littauer, U. Z., 1976, Maturation of neuroblastoma cells in the presence of dimethylsulfoxide, *Proc. Nat. Acad. Sci. USA* **73**:462–466.

Kimura, H., and Murad, F., 1974, Evidence for two different forms of guanylate cyclase in rat heart, *J. Biol. Chem.* **249**:6910–6916.

Kimura, H., and Murad, F., 1975a, Two forms of guanylate cyclase in mammalian tissues and possible mechanisms for their regulation, *Metabolism* **24**:439–445.

Kimura, H., and Murad, F., 1975b, Subcellular localization of guanylate cyclase, *Life Sci.* **17**:837–844.

Kimura, H., Mittal, C. K., and Murad, F., 1975, Increases in cyclic GMP levels in brain and liver with sodium azide an activator of guanylate cyclase, *Nature (London)* **257**:700–702.

Kimura, H., Thomas, F., and Murad, F., 1974, Effects of decapitation, ether and pentobarbital on guanosine 3',5'-phosphate and adenosine 3',5'-phosphate levels in rat tissues, *Biochim. Biophys. Acta* **343**:519–528.

Kinscherf, D. A., Chang, M. M., Rubin, E. H., Schneider, D. R., and Ferrendelli, J. A., 1976, Comparison of the effects of depolarizing agents and neurotransmitters on regional CNS cyclic GMP levels in various animals, *J. Neurochem.* **26**:527–530.

Kirkland, W. L., and Burton, P. R., 1972, Cyclic adenosine monophosphate-mediated stabilization of mouse neuroblastoma cell neurite microtubules exposed to low temperature, *Nature New Biol.* **240**:205–207.

Kish, V. M., and Kleinsmith, L. J., 1974, Nuclear protein kinases. Evidence for their heterogeneity, tissue specificity, substrate specificities and differential responses to cyclic adenosine 3', 5'-monophosphate, *J. Biol. Chem.* **249**:750–760.

Klainer, L. M., Chi, Y. -M., Freidberg, S. L., Rall, T. W., and Sutherland, E. W., 1962, The effects of neurohormones on the formation of adenosine 3',5'-phosphate by preparations from brain and other tissues, *J. Biol. Chem.* **237**:1239–1243.

Klawans, H. L., Moses, H., and Beaulieu, D. M., 1974, The influence of caffeine on *d*-amphetamine and apomorphine-induced stereotyped behavior, *Life Sci.* **14**:1493–1500.

Klee, W. A., Sharma, S. K., and Nirenberg, M., 1975, Opiate receptors as regulators of adenylate cyclase, *Life Sci.* **16**:1869–1874.

Klein, D. C., Yuwiler, A., Weller, J. L., and Plotkins, S., 1973, Postsynaptic adrenergic–cyclic AMP control of the serotonin content of cultured rat pineal glands, *J. Neurochem.* **21**:1261–1271.

Knopp, J., and Mitro, A., 1973, Effect of dibutyryl cyclic AMP injected into third ventricle on the thyroid ^{131}I-iodide accumulation, *Endokrinologie* **62**:237–238.

Kodama, T., Matsukado, Y., and Shimizu, H., 1973, The cyclic AMP system of human brain, *Brain Res.* **50**:135–146.

Kodama, T., Matsukado, Y., Suzuki, T., Tanaka, S., and Shimizu, H., 1971, Stimulated formation of adenosine 3',5'-monophosphate by desipramine in brain slices, *Biochim. Biophys. Acta* **252**:165–170.

Kohrman, A. F., 1973, Patterns of development of adenyl cyclase activity and norepinephrine responsiveness in the rat, *Pediat. Res.* **7**:575–581.

Koketsu, K., and Shirasawa, Y., 1974, 5-HT and the electrogenic sodium pump, *Experientia* **30**:1034–1035.

Koketsu, K., Shoji, T., and Nishi, S., 1973, Slow inhibitory postsynaptic potentials of bullfrog sympathetic ganglia in sodium-free media, *Life Sci.* **13**:453–458.

Koketsu, K., Shoji, T., and Yamamoto, K., 1974, Effects of GABA on presynaptic nerve terminals in bullfrog *(Rana catesbiana)* sympathetic ganglia, *Experientia* **30**:382–383.

Kostopoulos, G. K., Limacher, J. J., and Phillis, J. W., 1975, Action of various adenine derivatives on cerebellar Purkinje cells, *Brain Res.* **88**:162–165.

Kramer, S. G., 1971, Dopamine: A retinal neurotransmitter. I. Retinal uptake, storage and light stimulated release of H3-dopamine *in vivo*, *Invest. Ophthalmol.* **10**:438–452.

Krishna, G., and Krishnan, N., 1975, A rapid method for the assay of guanylate cyclase, *J. Cyclic Nucleotide Res.* **1**:293–302.

Krishna, G., Forn, J., Voight, K., Paul, M., and Gessa, G. L., 1970, Dynamic aspects of neurohormonal control of cyclic 3′,5′-AMP synthesis in brain, *Advan. Biochem. Psychopharmacol.* **3**:155–172.

Krishnan, N., and Krishna, G., 1976, A simple and sensitive assay for guanylate cyclase, *Anal. Biochem.* **70**:18–31.

Krivanek, J., 1976, Adenosine 3′,5′-monophosphate in rat cerebral cortex: Effect of potassium ions *in vivo* (cortical spreading depression), *J. Neurochem.* **26**:413–415.

Krueger, B. K., Forn, J., and Greengard, P., 1975, Dopamine-sensitive adenylate cyclase and protein phosphorylation in the rat caudate nucleus, in *Pre- and Postsynaptic Receptors* (E. Usdin and W. E. Bunney, Jr., eds.), pp. 123–147, Marcel Dekker, New York.

Krueger, B. K., Forn, J., Walters, J. R., Roth, R. H., and Greengard, P., 1976, Dopamine stimulation of adenosine 3′,5′-monophosphate formation in rat caudate nucleus: Effect of lesions of the nigro-neostriatal pathway, *Mol. Pharmacol.* **12**:639–648.

Kuehl, F. A., Jr., Humes, J. L., Cirillo, V. J., and Ham, E. A., 1972, Cyclic AMP and prostaglandins in hormone action, *Advan. Cyclic Nucleotide Res.* **1**:493–502.

Kuhn, H., Cook, J. H., and Dreyer, W. J., 1973, Phosphorylation in bovine photoreceptor membranes. A dark reaction after illumination, *Biochemistry* **12**:2495–2502.

Kumar, S., Becker, G., and Prasad, K. N., 1975, Cyclic adenosine 3′,5′-monophosphate phosphodiesterase activity in malignant and cyclic adenosine 3′,5′-monophosphate-induced "differentiated" neuroblastoma cells, *Cancer Res.* **35**:82–87.

Kuo, J. F., 1974, Guanosine 3′,5′-monophosphate-dependent protein kinases in mammalian tissue, *Proc. Nat. Acad. Sci. USA* **71**:4037–4041.

Kuo, J. F., 1975a, Changes in relative levels of guanosine-3′-5′-monophosphate-dependent and adenosine 3′-5′-monophosphate-dependent protein kinases in lung, heart and brain of developing guinea pigs, *Proc. Nat. Acad. Sci. USA* **72**:2256–2259.

Kuo, J. F., 1975b, Divergent actions of protein kinase modulator in regulating mammalian cyclic GMP-dependent and cyclic AMP-dependent protein kinases, *Metabolism* **24**:321–329.

Kuo, J. F., and Greengard, P., 1969a, Cyclic nucleotide-dependent protein kinases. IV. Widespread occurrence of adenosine 3′,5′-monophosphate dependent protein kinase in various tissues and phyla of the animal kingdom, *Proc. Nat. Acad. Sci. USA* **64**:1349–1355.

Kuo, J. F., and Greengard, P., 1969b, Adenosine 3′,5′-monophosphate-dependent protein kinase from brain, *Science* **165**:63–65.

Kuo, J. F., and Greengard, P., 1970a, Stimulation of adenosine 3′,5′-monophosphate-dependent and guanosine 3′,5′-monophosphate-dependent protein kinases by some analogs of adenosine 3′,5′-monophosphate, *Biochem. Biophys. Res. Commun.* **40**:1032–1038.

Kuo, J. F., and Greengard, P., 1970b, Cyclic nucleotide-dependent protein kinases. VII. Comparison of various histones as substrates for adenosine 3′,5′-monophosphate-dependent and guanosine 3′,5′-monophosphate-dependent protein kinases, *Biochim. Biophys. Acta* **212**:434–440.

Kuo, J. F., and Greengard, P., 1970c, Cyclic nucleotide-dependent protein kinase. VIII. An assay method for the measurement of adenosine 3′,5′-monophosphate in various tissues and a study of agents influencing its level in adipose cells, *J. Biol. Chem.* **245**:4067–4073.

Kuo, J. F., and Greengard, P., 1970d, Cyclic nucleotide-dependent protein kinases. VI. Isolation and partial purification of a protein kinase activated by guanosine 3′, 5′-monophosphate, *J. Biol. Chem.* **245**:2493–2498.

Kuo, J. F., Krueger, B. K., Sanes, J. R., and Greengard, P., 1970, Cyclic nucleotide-dependent protein kinases. V. Preparation and properties of adenosine 3′,5′-monophosphate-dependent protein kinase from various bovine tissues, *Biochim. Biophys. Acta* **212**:79–91.

Kuo, J. F., Lee, T.-P., Reyes, P. L., Walton, K. G., Donnelly, T. E., Jr., and Greengard, P., 1972, Cyclic nucleotide-dependent protein kinases. X. An assay method for the measurement of guanosine 3',5'-monophosphate in various biological materials and a study of agents regulating its levels in heart and brain, *J. Biol. Chem.* **247**:16–22.

Kuo, J. F., Miyamoto, E., and Reyes, P. L., 1974, Activation and dissociation of adenosine 3',5'-monophosphate-dependent and guanosine 3',5'-monophosphate-dependent protein kinases by various cyclic nucleotide analogs, *Biochem. Pharmacol.* **23**:2011–2021.

Kuo, W-M., Shoji, M., and Kuo, J. F., 1976a, Stimulatory modulator of guanosine 3',5'-monophosphate-dependent protein kinase from mammalian tissues, *Biochim. Biophys. Acta* **437**:142–149.

Kuo, W-M. Shoji, M., and Kuo, J. F., 1976b, Isolation of stimulatory modulator from rat brain and its specific effect on guanosine 3:5-monophosphate-dependent protein kinase from cerebellum and other tissues, *Biochem. Biophys. Res. Commun.* **70**:280–286.

Kurihara, K., 1972, Inhibition of cyclic 3',5'-nucleotide phosphodiesterase in bovine taste papillae by bitter taste stimuli, *FEBS Lett.* **27**:279–281.

Kurihara, K., and Koyama, N., 1972, High activity of adenyl cyclase in olfactory and gustatory organs, *Biochem. Biophys. Res. Commun.* **48**:30–34.

Kuriyama, K., and Isräel, M. A., 1973, Effect of ethanol administration on cyclic 3',5'-adenosine monophosphate metabolism in brain, *Biochem. Pharmacol.* **22**:2919–2922.

Kuroda, Y., and Kobayashi, K., 1975, Effects of adenosine and adenine nucleotides on the postsynaptic potential and on the formation of cyclic adenosine 3',5'-monophosphate from radioactive adenosine triphosphate in guinea pig olfactory cortex slices, *Proc. Jap. Acad.* **51**:495–500.

Kuroda, Y., and McIlwain, H., 1973, Subcellular localization of [14C]adenine derivatives newly-formed in cerebral tissues and the effects of electrical excitation, *J. Neurochem.* **21**:889–900.

Kuroda, Y., and McIlwain, H., 1974, Uptake and release of [14C]adenine derivatives at beds of mammalian cortical synaptosomes in a superfusion system, *J. Neurochem.* **22**:691–700.

Kuroda, Y., Saito, M., and Kobayashi, K., 1976, High concentrations of calcium prevent the inhibition of postsynaptic potentials and the accumulation of cyclic AMP induced by adenosine in brain slices, *Proc. Jap. Acad.* **52**:86–89.

Kurihara, T., and Tsukada, V., 1967, The regional and subcellular distribution of 2',3'-cyclic nucleotide 3'-phosphohydrolase in the central nervous system, *J. Neurochem.* **14**:1167–1174.

Kuschinsky, K., 1975, Dopamine receptor sensitivity after repeated morphine administrations to rats, *Life Sci.* **17**:43–48.

Laborit, H., and Thuret, F., 1974, Action de l'inosine et de l'inosine monophosphate cyclique seuls ou en association avec la 5-hydroxytryptamine sur trois étapes du métabolisme énergetique des coupes de cortex cérébral du rat, *Agressologie* **15**:377–380.

Laborit, H., Kunz, E., Lamothe, C., and Thuret, F., 1974, Sur quelques actions de la guanosine, combinée à l'acétylcholaine ou à l'insuline sur l'activité métabolique du cerveau et la glycémie, *Agressologie* **15**:239–245.

Laburn, H., Rosendorff, C., Willies, G., and Woolf, C., 1974, A role for noradrenaline and cyclic AMP in prostaglandin E$_1$ fever, *J. Physiol.* **240**:49P–50P.

Laduron, P., Verwimp, M., Janssen, P. F. M., and Leysen, J., 1976, Subcellular localization of dopamine-sensitive adenylate cyclase in rat brain striatum, *Life Sci.* **18**:433–440.

Lagnado, J., Tan, L. P., and Reddington, M., 1975, The *in situ* phosphorylation of microtubular protein in brain cortex slices and related studies on the phosphorylation of isolated brain tubulin preparations, *Ann. N.Y. Acad. Sci.,* **253**:577–597.

Lake, N., and Jordan, L. M., 1974, Failure to confirm cyclic-AMP as second messenger for norepinephrine in rat cerebellum, *Science* **183**:663–664.

Lake, N., Jordan, L. M., and Phillis, J. W., 1972, Mechanism of noradrenaline action in cat cerebral cortex, *Nature New Biol.* **240**:249–250.

Lake, N., Jordan, L. M., and Phillis, J. W., 1973, Evidence against cyclic adenosine 3',5'-

monophosphate (AMP) mediation of noradrenaline depression of cerebral cortical neurons, *Brain Res.* **60**:411–421.

Langan, T. A., 1970, Phosphorylation of histones *in vivo* under the control of cyclic AMP and hormones, *Advan. Biochem. Psychopharmacol.* **3**:307–323.

Laug, W. E., Jones, P. A., Nye, C. A., and Benedict, W. F., 1976, The effect of cyclic AMP and prostaglandins on the fibrinolytic activity of mouse neuroblastoma cells, *Biochem. Biophys. Res. Commun.* **68**:114–119.

Ledig, M., Ciesielski-Treska, J., Cam, Y., Montagnon, D., and Mandel, P., 1975, ATPase activity of neuroblastoma cells in culture, *J. Neurochem.* **25**:635–640.

Lee, C. -J., and Dubos, R., 1972, Lasting biological effects of early environmental influences. VII. Metabolism of adenosine 3′,5′-monophosphate in mice exposed to early environmental stress, *J. Exp. Med.* **135**:220–234.

Lee, T. -P., Kuo, J. F., and Greengard, P., 1972, Role of muscarinic cholinergic receptors in regulation of guanosine 3′,5′-cyclic monophosphate content in mammalian brain, heart muscle, and intestinal smooth muscle, *Proc. Nat. Acad. Sci. USA* **69**:3287–3291.

Lemay, A., and Jarett, L., 1975, Pitfalls in the use of lead nitrate for the histochemical demonstration of adenylate cyclase activity, *J. Cell Biol.* **65**:39–50.

Lentz, T. L., 1972, A role of cyclic AMP in a neurotrophic process, *Nature New Biol.* **238**:154–155.

Leonard, B. E., 1972, Effect of phentolamine on the increase in brain glycolysis following the intraventricular administration of dibutyryl-3,5′-cyclic adenosine monophosphate and sodium fluoride to mice, *Biochem. Pharmacol.* **21**:115–117.

Leonard, B. E., 1975a, The effect of 5-hydroxytryptamine and histamine on glycolyis in the mouse brain, *Z. Naturforsch.* **30c**:113–116.

Leonard, B. E., 1975b, A study of the neurohumoral control of glycolysis in the mouse brain *in vivo*. Role of noradrenaline and dopamine, *Z. Naturforsch.* **30c**:385–391.

Leonetti, J., and Seite, R., 1975, Effect of dibutyryl cyclic AMP and theophylline on the frequency of nuclear microtubules and microfilaments in sympathetic neurons, *C. R. Acad. Sci.* **281D**:423–428.

Lespagnol, A., Debaert, M., Mizon, J., and Mizon-Capron, C., 1970, Détermination de l'activité inhibitrice de quelques théophyllines substituées sur la phosphodiestérase spécifique de l'adénosine-3′,5′-monophosphate, *Thérapie* **25**:707–713.

Leterrier, J. F., Rappaport, L., and Nunez, J., 1974a, Phosphorylation and aggregation of neurotubulin and 'associated' protein-kinase, *Mol. Cell. Endocrinol.* **1**:65–76.

Leterrier, J. F., Rappaport, L., and Nunez, J., 1974b, Neurotubulin polymerization and phosphorylation reactions catalyzed by 'associated' protein kinase, *FEBS Lett.* **46**:285–288.

Levey, G. S., Lehotay, D. C., Canterbury, J. M., Bricker, L. A., and Meltz, G. J., 1975, Isolation of a unique peptide inhibitor of hormone-responsive adenylate cyclase, *J. Biol. Chem.* **250**:5730–5733.

Levin, R. M., and Weiss, B., 1976, Mechanism by which psychotropic drugs inhibit cyclic AMP phosphodiesterase of brain, *Mol. Pharmacol.* **12**:581–589.

Levine, R. A., 1970, Effects of exogenous adenosine 3′,5′-monophosphate in man. III. Increased response and tolerance to the dibutyryl derivative, *Clin. Pharmacol. Ther.* **11**:238–243.

Levitan, I. B., and Barondes, S. H., 1974, Octopamine- and serotonin-stimulated phosphorylation of specific protein in the abdominal ganglion of *Aplysia californica, Proc. Nat. Acad. Sci. USA* **71**:1145–1148.

Levitan, I. B., Madsen, C. J., and Barondes, S. H., 1974, Cyclic AMP and amine effects on phosphorylation of specific protein in abdominal ganglion of *Aplysia californica:* Localization and kinetic analysis, *J. Neurobiol.* **5**:511–525.

Lewin, E., Golden, T., and Walker, J. E., 1976, Stimulation of cyclic AMP accumulation by pentylenetetrazol, *Exp. Neurol.* **50**:422–426.

Liberman, E. A., Minina, S. V., and Golubtsov, K. V., 1975, The study of metabolic synapse. I. Effect of intracellular microinjection of 3',5'-AMP, *Biofizika* **20**:451–456.

Libet, B., and Kobayashi, H., 1969, Generation of adrenergic and cholinergic potentials in sympathetic ganglion cells, *Science* **164**:1530–1532.

Libet, B., and Tosaka, T., 1970, Dopamine as a synaptic transmitter and modulator in sympathetic ganglia. A different mode of synaptic action, *Proc. Nat. Acad. Sci. USA* **67**:667–673.

Libet, B., Kobayashi, H., and Tanaka, T., 1976, A dopamine-induced neuronal "memory trace," mediated by cyclic AMP and disruptable by cyclic GMP, *Fed Proc.* **35**:326Abs.

Lim, R., and Mitsunobu, K., 1972, Effect of dibutyryl cyclic AMP on nucleic acid and protein synthesis in neuronal and glial tumor cells, *Life Sci.* **11(II)**:1063–1070.

Lim, R., Mitsunobu, K., and Li, W. K. P., 1973, Maturation-stimulation effect of brain extract and dibutyryl cyclic AMP on dissociated embryonic brain cells in culture, *Exp. Cell. Res.* **79**:243–246.

Lin, Y. M., Liu, Y. P., and Cheung, W. Y., 1974, Cyclic 3',5'-nucleotide phosphodiesterase. Purification, characterization and active form of the protein activator from bovine brain, *J. Biol. Chem.* **249**:4943–4954.

Lin, Y. M., Liu, Y. P., and Cheung, W. Y., 1975, Cyclic 3',5'-nucleotide phosphodiesterase Ca^{++}-dependent formation of bovine brain enzyme-activator complex, *FEBS Lett.* **49**:356–360.

Lincoln, T. M., Hall, C. L., Park, C. R., and Corbin, J. D., 1976, Guanosine 3'-5' cyclic monophosphate binding proteins in rat tissues, *Proc. Nat. Acad. Sci. U.S.A* **73**:2559–2563.

Lindl, T., and Cramer, H., 1974, Formation, accumulation and release of adenosine 3',5'-monophosphate induced by histamine in the superior cervical ganglion of the rat *in vitro, Biochim. Biophys. Acta* **343**:182–191.

Lindl, T., and Cramer, H., 1975, Evidence against dopamine as the mediator of the rise of cyclic AMP in the superior cervical ganglion of the rat, *Biochem. Biophys. Res. Commun.* **65**:731–739.

Lindl, T., Behrendt, H., Heinl-Sawaja, M. C. B., Teufel, E., and Cramer, H., 1974, Effects of compound 40/80 on mast cells, histamine, and cyclic AMP in isolated superior cervical ganglia, *Naunyn-Schmiedeberg's Arch. Pharmacol.* **286**:283–296.

Lindl, T., Heinl-Sawaya, M. C. B., and Cramer, H., 1975, Compartmentation of an ATP substrate pool for histamine and adrenaline-sensitive adenylate cyclase in rat superior cervical ganglia, *Biochem. Pharmacol.* **24**:947–950.

Lindl, T., Heinl-Sawaya, M. C. B., and Cramer, H., 1976, Effects of compound 48/80, a histamine-releasing agent on accumulation and release of cyclic AMP in various regions of rat brain *in vitro, Res. Commun. Chem. Pathol. Pharmacol.* **13**:65–74.

Lippmann, W., Pugsley, T., and Merker, J., 1975, Effect of butaclamol and its enantiomers upon striatal homovanillic acid and adenyl cyclase of olfactory tubercle in rats, *Life Sci.* **16**:213–224.

Lipton, J. M., and Fossler, D. E., 1974, Fever produced in the squirrel monkey by intravenous and intracerebral endotoxin. *Amer. J. Physiol.* **226**:1022–1027.

Liu, Y. P., and Cheung, W. Y., 1976, Cyclic 3':5'-nucleotide phosphodiesterase. Ca^{2+} confers more helical conformation to the protein activator, *J. Biol. Chem.* **251**:4193–4198.

Lloyd, T., and Kaufman, S., 1975, Evidence for the lack of direct phosphorylation of bovine caudate tyrosine hydroxylase following activation by exposure to enzymatic phosphorylating conditions, *Biochem. Biophys. Res. Commun.* **66**:907–913.

Lolley, R. N., and Farber, D. B., 1975, Cyclic nucleotide phosphodiesterases in dystrophic rat retinas: Guanosine 3',5'-cyclic monophosphate anomalies during photoreceptor cell degeneration, *Exp. Eye Res.* **20**:585–598.

Lolley, R. N., Schmidt, S. Y., and Farber, D. B., 1974, Alterations in cyclic AMP metabolism associated with photoreceptor cell degeneration in the C3H mouse, *J. Neurochem.* **22**:701–707.

Lovenberg, W., and Bruckwick, E. A., 1975, Mechanisms of receptor mediated regulation of catecholamine synthesis in brain, in *Pre- and Postsynaptic Receptors* (E. Usdin and W. E. Bunney, Jr. eds.), pp. 149–169, Marcel Dekker, New York.

Lovenberg, W., Bruckwick, E. A., and Hanbauer, I., 1975, ATP, cyclic AMP and magnesium increase the affinity of rat striatal tyrosine hydroxylase for its cofactor, *Proc. Nat. Acad. Sci. USA* **72**:2955–2958.

Lust, W. D., and Passonneau, J. V., 1973, Cyclic adenosine monophosphate, metabolites, and phosphorylase in neural tissue: A comparison of methods of fixation, *Science* **181**:280–282.

Lust, W. D., and Passonneau, J. V., 1976, Cyclic nucleotides in murine brain: Effect of hypothermia on adenosine 3′,5′-monophosphate, glycogen phosphorylase, glycogen synthase and metabolites following maximal electroshock or decapitation, *J. Neurochem.* **26**:11–16.

Lust, W. D., Goldberg, N. D., and Passonneau, J. V., 1976, Cyclic nucleotides in murine brain: The temporal relationship of changes induced in adenosine 3′,5′-monophosphate and guanosine 3′,5′-monophosphate following maximal electroshock or decapitation, *J. Neurochem.* **26**:5–10.

Lust, W. D., Mrsulja, B. B., Mrsulja, B. J., Passonneau, J., and Klatzo, I., 1975, Putative neurotransmitters and cyclic nucleotides in prolonged ischemia of the cerebral cortex, *Brain Res.* **98**:394–399.

Lynch, T. J., Tallant, E. A., and Cheung, W. Y., 1976, Ca^{++}-Dependent formation of brain adenylate cyclase–protein activator complex, *Biochem. Biophys. Res. Commun.* **68**:616–625.

MacDonald, I. A., 1974, A convenient colorimetric method for routine assay of brain adenylate cyclase, *Experientia* **30**:1485–1486.

MacDonald, I. A., 1975, Differentiation of fluoride-stimulated and non-fluoride-stimulated components of beef brain cortex adenylate cyclase by calcium ions, EGTA and Triton X-100, *Biochim. Biophys. Acta.* **397**:244–253.

Machova, J., and Kristofova, A., 1973, The effect of dibutyryl cyclic AMP, dopamine and aminophylline on ganglionic surface potential and transmission, *Life Sci.* **13**:525–535.

MacIntyre, E. H., Wintersgill, C. J., Perkins, J. P., and Vatter, A. E., 1972, The responses in culture of human tumour astrocytes and neuroblasts to $N^6,O^{2'}$-dibutyryl adenosine 3′,5′-monophosphoric acid, *J. Cell Sci.* **11**:639–667.

Mackay, A. V. P., and Iversen, L. L., 1972a, Increased tyrosine hydroxylase activity of sympathetic ganglia cultured in the presence of dibutyryl cyclic AMP, *Brain Res.* **48**:424–426.

Mackay, A. V. P., and Iversen, L. L., 1972b, Trans-synaptic regultion of tyrosine hydroxylase activity in adrenergic neurones: Effect of potassium concentration on cultured sympathetic ganglia, *Naunyn-Schmiedeberg's Arch. Pharmacol.* **272**:225–229.

Maeno, H., and Greengard, P., 1972, Phosphoprotein phosphates from rat cerebral cortex, *J. Biol. Chem.* **247**:3269–3277.

Maeno, H., Johnson, E. M., and Greengard, P., 1971, Subcellular distribution of adenosine 3′,5′-monophosphate-dependent protein kinase in rat brain, *J. Biol. Chem.* **246**:134–142.

Maeno, H., Reyes, P. L., Ueda, T., Rudolph, S. A., and Greengard, P., 1974, Autophosphorylation of adenosine 3′,5′-monophosphate-dependent protein kinase from bovine brain, *Arch. Biochem. Biophys.* **164**:551–559.

Maeno, H., Ueda, T., and Greengard, P., 1975, Adenosine 3′,5′-monophosphate-dependent protein phosphatase activity in synaptic membrane fractions, *J. Cyclic Nucleotide Res.* **1**:37–48.

Maguire, M. E., Goldmann, P. H., and Gilman, A. G., 1974a, The reaction of

[³H]norepinephrine with particulate fractions of cells responsive to catecholamines, *Mol. Pharmacol.* **10**:563–581.

Maguire, M. E., Sturgill, T. W., Anderson, H. J., Minna, J. D., and Gilman, A. G., 1974b, Hormonal control of cyclic AMP metabolism in parental and hybrid somatic cells, *Advan. Cyclic Nucleotide Res.* **5**:699–718.

Maguire, M. E., Van Arsdale, P. M., and Gilman, A. G., 1976a, An agonist specific effect of guanine nucleotides on binding to the beta adrenergic receptor, *Mol. Pharmacol.* **12**:335–339.

Maguire, M. E., Wiklund, R. A., Anderson, H. J., and Gilman, A. G., 1976b, Binding of [¹²⁵I]iodohydroxybenzylpindolol to putative β-adrenergic receptors of rat glioma cells and other cell clones, *J. Biol. Chem.* **251**:1221–1231.

Mah, H. D., and Daly, J. W., 1975, Intracellular formation of analogs of cyclic AMP studies with brain slices labeled with radioactive derivatives of adenine and adenosine, *Biochim. Biophys. Acta.* **404**:49–56.

Mah, H. D., and Daly, J. W., 1976, Adenosine-dependent formation of cyclic AMP in brain slices, *Pharmacol. Res. Commun.* **8**:65–79.

Maitre, M., Ciesielski, L., Lehmann, P., Kempf, E., and Mandel, P., 1974, Protective effect of adenosine and nicotinamide against audiogenic seizure, *Biochem. Pharmacol.* **23**:2807–2816.

Makman, M. H., Brown, J. H., and Mishra, R. K., 1975a, Cyclic AMP in retina and caudate nucleus: Influence of dopamine and other agents, *Advan. Cyclic Nucleotide Res.* **5**:661–679.

Makman, M. H., Mishra, R. K., and Brown, J. H., 1975b, Drug interactions with dopamine-stimulated adenylate cyclases of caudate nucleus and retina: Direct agonist effect of a piridedil metabolite, *Advan. Neurol.* **9**:213–222.

Malkinson, A. M., 1975, Effect of calcium on cyclic AMP-dependent and cyclic GMP-dependent endogenous protein phosphorylation in mouse brain cytosol, *Biochem. Biophys. Res. Commun.* **67**:752–759.

Malkinson, A. M., Krueger, B. K., Rudolph, S. A., Casnellie, J. E., Haley, B. E., and Greengard, P., 1975, Widespread occurrence of a specific protein in vertebrate tissues and regulation by cyclic AMP of its endogenous phosphorylation and dephosphorylation, *Metabolism* **24**:331–341.

Mandel, L. R., 1971, Inhibition of cyclic 3′,5′-adenosine monophosphate phosphodiesterase by substituted imidazopyrazines, *Biochem. Pharmacol.* **20**:3413–3421.

Mandel, P., and Harth, S., 1961, Free nucleotides of the brain in various mammals, *J. Neurochem.* **8**:116–125.

Manthorpe, M., and McConnell, D. G., 1975, Cyclic nucleotide phosphodiesterases associated with bovine retinal outer-segment fragments, *Biochim. Biophys. Acta* **403**:438–445.

Mao, C. C., Guidotti, A., and Costa, E., 1974a, The regulation of cyclic guanosine monophosphate in rat cerebellum possible involvement of putative amino acid neurotransmitters, *Brain Res.* **79**:510–514.

Mao, C. C., Guidotti, A., and Costa, E., 1974b, Interactions between γ-aminobutyric acid and guanosine cyclic 3′,5′-monophosphate in rat cerebellum, *Mol. Pharmacol.* **10**:736–746.

Mao, C. C., Guidotti, A., and Costa, E., 1974c, Inhibition by diazepam of the tremor and the increase of cerebellar c-GMP content elicited by harmaline, *Brain Res.* **83**:516–519.

Mao, C. C., Guidotti, A., and Costa, E., 1975a, Evidence for involvement of GABA in the mediation of the cerebellar cGMP decrease and the anticonvulsant action of diazepam, *Naunyn-Schmiedeberg's Arch. Pharmacol.* **289**:369–378.

Mao, C. C., Guidotti, A., and Landis, S., 1975b, Cyclic GMP: Reduction of cerebellar concentrations in nervous mutant mice, *Brain Res.* **90**:335–339.

Markstein, R., and Wagner, H., 1975, The effect of dihydroergotoxin, phentolamine and pindolol on catecholamine-stimulated adenyl cyclase in rat cerebral cortex, *FEBS Lett.* **55**:275–277.

Marley, E., and Nistico, G., 1972, Effects of catecholamines and adenosine derivatives given into the brain of fowls, *Brit. J. Pharmacol.* **46**:619–636.

Martres, M. P., Baudry, M., and Schwartz, J. C., 1975, Subsensitivity of noradrenaline-stimulated cyclic AMP accumulation in brain slices of *d*-amphetamine-treated mice, *Nature (London)* **255**:731–733.

Matsuzawa, H., and Nirenberg, M., 1975, Receptor mediated shifts in cGMP and cAMP levels in neuroblastoma cells, *Proc. Nat. Acad. Sci. USA* **72**:3472–3476.

McAfee, D. A., and Greengard, P., 1972, Adenosine 3′,5′-monophosphate: Electrophysiological evidence for a role in synaptic transmission, *Science* **178**:310–312.

McAfee, D. A., Schorderet, M., and Greengard, P., 1971, Adenosine 3′,5′-monophosphate in nervous tissue: Increase associated with synaptic transmission, *Science* **171**:1156–1158.

McCune, R. W., Gill, T. H., Von Hungen, K., and Roberts, S., 1971, Catecholamine-sensitive adenyl cyclase in cell-free preparations from rat cerebral cortex, *Life Sci.* **10(II)**:433–450.

McIlwain, H., 1972, Regulatory significance of the release and action of adenine derivatives in cerebral systems, *Biochem. Soc. Symp.* **36**:69–85.

McIlwain, H., 1976, An extended messenger role in the brain for cyclic AMP, *FEBS Lett.* **64**:271–273.

McKelvy, J. F., 1975, Isolation of a cyclic AMP dependent protein kinase from bovine hypothalamus and its interaction with hypothalamic substituents, *Biochem. Biophys. Res. Commun.* **65**:54–62.

McKenzie, S. G., and Bar, H. P., 1973, On the mechanism of adenyl cyclase inhibition by adenosine, *Canad. J. Physiol. Pharmacol.* **51**:190–196.

McNeill, J. H., Lee, C.-Y., and Muschek, L. D., 1972, The effect of phentolamine and other drugs on rat brain phosphodiesterase, *Canad. J. Physiol. Pharmacol.* **50**:840–849.

McNiece, D. M., and Jacobs, R. S., 1976, Facilatory actions of 1-ethyl-4-(isopropylidene hydrazino)-1*H*-pyrazolo-(3,4-b)-pyridine-5-carboxylic acid, ethyl ester. HC1 (SQ 20,009) on neuromuscular transmission, *Fed. Proc.* **35**:696Abs.

Mehta, C. S., and Johnson, W. E., 1975, Possible role of cyclic AMP and dopamine in morphine tolerance and physical dependence, *Life Sci.* **16**:1883–1888.

Menon, K. M. J., Giese, S., and Jaffe, R. B., 1973, Hormone- and fluoride-sensitive adenylate cyclases in human fetal tissues, *Biochim. Biophys. Acta* **304**:203–209.

Merali, Z., Singhal, R. L., Hrdina, P. D., and Ling, G. M., 1975, Changes in brain cyclic AMP metabolism and acetylcholine and dopamine during narcotic dependence and withdrawal, *Life Sci.* **16**:1889–1894.

Meyer, R. B., and Miller, J. P., 1974, Analogs of cyclic AMP and cyclic GMP: General methods of synthesis and the relationships of structure to enzymic activity, *Life Sci.* **14**:1019–1040.

Meyer, R. B. Jr., Shuman, D. A., and Robins, R. K., 1974, A new purine ring closure and the synthesis of 2-substituted derivatives of adenosine cyclic 3′,5′-phosphate, *J. Amer. Chem. Soc.* **96**:4962–4966.

Meyer, R. B., Shuman, D. A., Robins, R. K., Bauer, R. J., Dimmitt, M. K., and Simon, L. N., 1972, Synthesis and biological activity of several 6-substituted 9-β-D-ribofuranosyl purine 3′,5′-cyclic phosphates, *Biochemistry* **11**:2704–2709.

Meyer, R. B., Shuman, D. A., Robins, R. K., Miller, J. P., and Simon, L. N., 1973, Synthesis and enzymic studies of 5′-aminoimidazole and N^1- and N^6-substituted adenine ribonucleotide cyclic 3′,5′-phosphates prepared from adenosine cyclic 3′,5′-phosphate, *J. Med. Chem.* **16**:1319–1323.

Meyer, R. B., Uno, H., Robins, R. K., Simon, L. N., and Miller, J. P., 1975a, 2-Substituted derivatives of adenosine and inosine cyclic 3′,5′-phosphates. Synthesis, enzymic activity, and analysis of the structural requirements of the binding locale of the 2-substituent on bovine brain protein kinase, *Biochemistry* **14**:3315–3321.

Meyer, R. B., Uno, H., Shuman, D., Robins, R., Simon, L., and Miller, J. P., 1975b, The synthesis of 2,6-disubstituted-9-β-D-ribofuranosylpurine cyclic 3′,5′-phosphates and the selectivity of cAMP and cGMP-specific enzymes to substituents in these positions, *J. Cyclic Nucleotide Res.* **1**:159–167.

Middlemiss, D., and Franklin, T., 1975, Preparation of a stable, highly active solubilized adenylate cyclase from rat cerebellum, *FEBS Lett.* **55**:225–228.

Miki, N., and Yoshida, H., 1972, Purification and properties of cyclic AMP phosphodiesterase from rat brain, *Biochim. Biophys. Acta* **268**:166–174.

Miki, N., Baraban, J. M., Keirns, J. J., Boyce, J. J., and Bitensky, M. W., 1975, Purification and properties of light-activated cyclic nucleotide phosphodiesterase of rod outer segments, *J. Biol. Chem.* **250**:6320–6327.

Miki, N., Keirns, J., Marcus, F. R., and Bitensky, M. W., 1974, Light regulation of adenosine 3′,5′-monophosphate levels in vertebrate photoreceptors, *Exp. Eye Res.* **18**:281–297.

Miki, N., Keirns, J. J. Marcus, F. R., Freeman, J., and Bitensky, M. W., 1973, Regulation of cyclic nucleotide concentrations in photoreceptors: An ATP-dependent stimulation of cyclic nucleotide phosphodiesterase by light, *Proc. Nat. Acad. Sci. USA* **70**:3820–3824.

Miller, R. J., 1976, Comparison of the inhibitory effects of neuroleptic drugs on adenylate cyclase in rat tissues stimulated by dopamine, noradrenaline and glucagon, *Biochem. Pharmacol.* **25**:537–541.

Miller, W. H., 1973, Cyclic nucleotides and photoreception, *Exp. Eye Res.* **16**:357–363.

Miller, C. A., and Levine, E. M., 1972, Neuroblastoma: Synchronization of neurite growth in cultures grown in collagen, *Science* **177**:799–801.

Miller, R. A., and Ruddle, F. H., 1974, Enucleated neuroblastoma cells form neurites when treated with dibutyryl cyclic AMP, *J. Cell Biology* **63**:295–299.

Miller, R. J., and Hiley, C. R., 1975, Antimuscarinic actions of neuroleptic drugs, *Advan. Neurol.* **9**:141–154.

Miller, R. J., and Hiley, C. R., 1976, Anti-dopaminergic and anti-muscarinic effects of dibenzodiazepines. Relationship to drug induced parkinsonism, *Naunyn-Schmiedeberg's Arch. Pharmacol.* **292**:289–294.

Miller, R. J., and Iversen, L. L., 1974a, Stimulation of a dopamine-sensitive adenylate cyclase in homogenates of rat striatum by a metabolite of piribedil (ET 495), *Naunyn-Schmiedeberg's Arch. Pharmacol.* **282**:213–216.

Miller, R. J., and Iversen, L. L., 1974b, Effect of psychoactive drugs on dopamine (3,4-dihydroxyphenethylamine)-sensitive adenylate cyclase activity in corpus striatum of rat brain, *Biochem. Soc. Trans.* **2**:256–259.

Miller, R. J., and Kelly, P. H., 1975, Dopamine-like effects of choleratoxin in the central nervous system, *Nature (London)* **255**:163–165.

Miller, J. P., Boswell, K. H., Muneyama, K., Simon, L. N., Robins, R. K., and Shuman, D. A., 1973a, Synthesis and biochemical studies of various 8-substituted derivatives of guanosine 3′,5′-cyclic phosphate, inosine 3′,5′-cyclic phosphate, and xanthosine 3′,5′-cyclic phosphate, *Biochemistry* **12**:5310–5319.

Miller, J. P., Boswell, K. H., Muneyama, K., Tolman, R. L., Scholten, M. B., Robins, R. K., Simon, L. N., and Shuman, D. A., 1973b, Activity of tubercidin-, toyocomycin-, and sangivamycin-3′,5′-cyclic phosphates and related compounds with some enzymes of adenosine-3′,5′-cyclic phosphate metabolism, *Biochem. Biophys. Res. Commun.* **55**:843–849.

Miller, J. P., Shuman, D. A., Scholten, M. B., Dimmitt, M. K., Stewart, C. M., Khwaja, T. A., Robins, R. K., and Simon, L. N., 1973c, Synthesis and biological activity of some 2′ derivatives of adenosine 3′,5′-cyclic phosphate, *Biochemistry* **12**:1010–1015.

Miller, J. P., Boswell, K. H., Mian, A. M., Meyer, R. B., Robins, R. K., and Khwaja, T. A., 1976a, 2′-Derivatives of guanosine and inosine cyclic 3′,5′-phosphates. Synthesis, enzymic activity and effect of 8-substituents, *Biochemistry* **15**:217–222.

Miller, R. J., Kelly, P. H., and Neumeyer, J. L., 1976b, Action of aporphine alkaloids on dopaminergic mechanisms in rat brain, *Eur. J. Pharmacol.* **35**:77–84.

Miller, R. J., Horn, A. S., and Iversen, L. L., 1974a, The action of neuroleptic drugs on dopamine-stimulated adenosine cyclic 3′,5′-monophosphate production in rat neostriatum and limbic forebrain, *Mol. Pharmacol.* **10**:759–766.

Miller, R., Horn, A., Iversen, L. L., and Pinder, R., 1974b, Effects of dopamine-like drugs on rat striatal adenyl cyclase have implications for CNS dopamine receptor topography, *Nature (London)* **250**:238–241.

Miller, R. J., Horn, A. S., and Iversen, L. L., 1975, Effect of butaclamol on dopamine-sensitive adenylate cyclase in the rat striatum, *J. Pharm. Pharmacol.* **27**:212–213.

Miller, W. H., Gorman, R. E., and Bitensky, M. W., 1971, Cyclic adenosine monophosphate: Function in photoreceptors, *Science* **174**:295–297.

Minna, J. D., and Gilman, A. G., 1973, Expression of genes for metabolism of cyclic adenosine 3′:5′-monophosphate in somatic cells. II. Effects of prostaglandin E_1 and theophylline on parental and hybrid cells, *J. Biol. Chem.* **248**:6618–6625.

Minneman, K. P., and Iversen, L. L., 1976a, Diurnal rhythm in rat pineal cyclic nucleotide phosphodiesterase activity, *Nature (London)* **260**:59–61.

Minneman, K. P., and Iversen, L. L., 1976b, Cholera toxin induces pineal enzymes in culture, *Science* **192**:803–805.

Mishra, R. K., Demirjian, C., Katzman, R., and Makman, M. H., 1975, A dopamine-sensitive adenylate cyclase in anterior limbic cortex and mesolimbic region of primate brain, *Brain Res.* **96**:395–399.

Mishra, R. K., Gardner, E. L., Katzman, R., and Makman, M. H., 1974, Enhancement of dopamine-stimulated adenylate cyclase activity in rat caudate after lesions in substantia nigra: Evidence for denervation supersensitivity, *Proc. Nat. Acad. Sci. USA* **71**:3883–3887.

Mittal, C. K., Kimura, H., and Murad, F., 1975, Requirement for a macromolecular factor for sodium azide activation of guanylate cyclase, *J. Cyclic Nucleotide Res.* **1**:261–269.

Miyake, M., Daly, J. W., and Creveling, C. R., 1976, Purification of phosphodiesterases from rat cerebrum by affinity chromatography on calcium-dependent activator protein-Sepharose, *Arch. Biochem. Biophys.*, in press.

Miyamoto, E., 1976, Phosphorylation of endogenous proteins in myelin of rat brain, *J. Neurochem.* **26**:573–577.

Miyamoto, T., 1975, Protein kinases in myelin of rat brain: Solubilization and characterization, *J. Neurochem.* **24**:503–512.

Miyamoto, E., and Kakiuchi, S., 1974, *In vitro* and *in vivo* phosphorylation of myelin basic protein by exogenous and endogenous adenosine 3′,5′-monophosphate-dependent protein kinases in brain, *J. Biol. Chem.* **249**:2769–2777.

Miyamoto, E., and Kakiuchi, S., 1975, Phosphoprotein phosphatases for myelin basic protein in myelin and cytosol fraction of brain, *Biochim. Biophys. Acta* **384**:458–465.

Miyamoto, M. D., and Breckenridge, B. M., 1974, A cyclic adenosine monophosphate link in the catecholamine enhancement of transmitter release at the neuromuscular junction, *J. Gen. Physiol.* **63**:609–624.

Miyamoto, E., Kuo, J. F., and Greengard, P., 1969a, Adenosine 3′,5′-monophosphate-dependent protein kinase from brain, *Science* **165**:63–65.

Miyamoto, E., Kuo, J. F., and Greengard, P., 1969b, Cyclic nucleotide-dependent protein kinases. I. Purification and properties of adenosine 3′,5′-monophosphate-dependent protein kinase from bovine brain, *J. Biol. Chem.* **244**:6395–6402.

Miyamoto, E., Petzold, G. L., Harris, J. S., and Greengard, P., 1971, Dissociation and concomitant activation of adenosine 3′,5′-monophosphate-dependent protein kinase by histone, *Biochem. Biophys. Res. Commun.* **44**:305–312.

Mizon, J., Shandrani, E., and Mizon, C., 1971, Détermination de l'activite inhibitrice de quelques nouvelles théophyllines substituées sur la phosphodiestérase spécifique des nucléotides cycliques, *Thérapie* **26**:911–917.

Monard, D., Solomon, F., Rentsch, M., and Gysin, R., 1973, Glia-induced morphological differentiation in neuroblastoma cells, *Proc. Nat. Acad. Sci. USA* **70**:1894–1897.

Monn, E., and Christiansen, R. O., 1971, Adenosine 3′,5′-monophosphate phosphate phosphodiesterases: Multiple molecular forms, *Science* **173**:540–541.

Montecucchi, P., 1976, Stimolazione della formazione di AMP ciclico nel cervello di ratto *in vitro* da parte della nicergolina, *Il Farmaco Ed. Pract.* **31**:10–17.

Moonen, G., Cam, Y., Sensenbrenner, M., and Mandel, P., 1975, Variability of the effects of serum-free medium, dibutyryl-cyclic AMP or theophylline on the morphology of cultured newborn rat astroblasts, *Cell Tissue Res.* **163**:365–372.

Moonen, G., Heinen, E., and Goessens, G., 1976, Comparative ultrastructural study of the effects of serum-free medium and dibutyryl-cyclic AMP on newborn rat astroblasts, *Cell Tissue Res.* **167**:221–228.

Morgan, J. L., and Seeds, N. W., 1975, Tubulin constancy during morphological differentiation of mouse neuroblastoma cells, *J. Cell Biol.* **67**:136–145.

Morgenroth, V., Hegstrand, L., Roth, R., and Greengard, P., 1975, Evidence for involvement of protein kinase in the activation by adenosine 3′,5′-monophosphate of brain tyrosine 3-monooxygenase, *J. Biol. Chem.* **250**:1946–1948.

Moyes, I. C. A., and Moyes, R. B., 1976, Further developments in the study of 3′,5′ cyclic adenosine monophosphate in relation to psychiatric illness, *Postgraduate Med. J.* **52** Suppl. 3)**:**110–115.

Mrsulja, B. B., 1972a, The influence of some biogenic amines and cyclic N-2-O-dibutyryl-adenosine-3′-5′-monophosphate on glycogen content in rat brain slices, *Experientia* **28**:1067.

Mrsulja, B. B., 1972b, The influence of propranolol and dibenzyline on glycogenolytic effects of some biogenic amines in rat brain slices, *Experientia* **28**:1072–1073.

Mrsulja, B. B., 1973, The influence of antistine on glycogenolytic effect of some biogenic amines in rat brain slices, *Experientia* **29**:76–77.

Mrsulja, B. B., 1974, Cyclic nucleotides and brain glycogen, *Experientia* **30**:66–67.

Munday, K. A., Poat, J. A., and Woodruff, G. N., 1974, Increase in the cyclic AMP content of rat striatum produced by a cyclic analogue of dopamine, *J. Physiol.* **241**:119P–120P.

Muneyama, K., Bauer, R. J., Shuman, D. A., Robins, R. K., and Simon, L. N., 1971, Chemical synthesis and biological activity of 8-substituted adenosine 3′,5′-cyclic monophosphate derivatives, *Biochemistry* **10**:2390–2395.

Muneyama, K., Shuman, D. A., Boswell, K. H., Robins, R. K., Simon, I. N., and Miller, J. P., 1974, Synthesis and biological activity of 8-halo-adenosine 3′,5′-cyclic phosphates, *J. Carbohyd. Nucleosides Nucleotides* **1**:55–60.

Murad, F., 1973, Clinical studies and applications of cyclic nucleotides, *Advan. Cyclic Nucleotide Res.* **3**:355–383.

Murad, F., Rall, T. W., and Vaughan, M., 1969, Conditions for the formation, partial purification and assay of an inhibitor of adenosine 3′,5′,-monophosphate, *Biochim. Biophys. Acta* **192**:430–455.

Murray, A. W., and Froscio, M., 1971, Cyclic adenosine 3′,5′-monophosphate and microtubule function: Specific interaction of the phosphorylated protein subunits with a soluble brain component, *Biochem. Biophys. Res. Commun.* **44**:1089–1095.

Myllyla, V. V., Heikkinen, E. R., Simila, S., Hokkanen, E., and Vapaatalo, H., 1974a, Cerebrospinal fluid concentration and urinary excretion of cyclic adenosine-3′,5′-monophosphate in various diseases of children. A preliminary study, *Z. Kinderheilk.* **118**:259–264.

Myllyla, V. V., Vapaatalo, H., Hokkanen, E., and Heikkinen, E. R., 1974b, Cerebrospinal fluid concentration of cyclic adenosine 3′,5′-monophosphate and pneumoencephalography, *Eur. Neurol.* **12**:28–32.

Myllyla, V. V., Heikkinen, E. R., Vapaatalo, H., and Hokkanen, E., 1975, Cyclic AMP concentration and enzyme activities of cerebrospinal fluid in patients with epilepsy or central nervous system damage, *Eur. Neurol.* **13**:123–130.

Nahorski, S. R., 1976, Association of high affinity stereospecific binding of ³H-propranolol to cerebral membranes with β-receptors, *Nature (London)* **259**:488–489.

Nahorski, S. R., and Rogers, K. J., 1973, The adenosine 3′,5′-monophosphate content of brain tissue obtained by an ultra-rapid freezing technique, *Brain Res.* **51**:332–336.

Nahorski, S. R., and Rogers, K. J., 1975, Altered sensitivity of β-adrenoceptor-mediated cyclic AMP formation in brain, *Brit. J. Pharmacol.* **55**:300P.

Nahorski, S. R., Rogers, K. J., and Pinns, J., 1973, Cerebral phosphodiesterase and dopamine receptor, *J. Pharm. Pharmacol.* **25**:912–913.

Nahorski, S. R., Rogers, K. J., and Smith, B. M., 1974, Histamine H₂-receptors and cyclic AMP in brain, *Life Sci.* **15**:1887–1894.

Nahorski, S. R., Rees, W., and Rogers, K. J., 1975a, Cyclic AMP in developing chick brain: Changes with ischaemia and catecholamine administration, *Brit. J. Pharmacol.* **54**:255P–256P.

Nahorski, S. R., Rogers, K. J., and Edwards, C., 1975b, Cerebral glycogenolysis and stimulation of β-adrenoreceptors and histamine H₂ receptors, *Brain Res.* **92**:529–533.

Nahorski, S. R., Rogers, K. J., Smith, B. M., and Auson, J., 1975c, Characterization of the adrenoreceptor mediating changes in cyclic adenosine 3′-5′monophosphate in chick cerebral hemispheres, *Naunyn-Schmiedeberg's Arch. Pharmacol.* **291**:101–110.

Nahorski, S. R., Patton, W., and Rogers, K. J., 1976, Developmental changes in the sensitivity of neurohormone-stimulated cyclic AMP formation in chick cerebral hemispheres, *Brit. J. Pharmacol.* **56**:380P–381P.

Naito, K., and Kuriyama, K., 1973, Effect of morphine administration on adenyl cyclase and 3′,5′-cyclic nucleotide phosphodiesterase activities in the brain, *Jap. J. Pharmacol.* **23**:274–276.

Nakamura, M., and Koketsu, K., 1972, The effect of adrenaline on sympathetic ganglion cells of bullfrogs, *Life Sci.* **11(I)**:1165–1173.

Nakazawa, K., and Sano, M., 1974, A new assay method for guanylate cyclase and properties of the cyclase from rat brain, *J. Biol. Chem.* **249**:4207–4211.

Nakazawa, K., Sano, M., and Saito, T., 1976, Subcellular distribution and properties of guanylate cyclase in rat cerebellum, *Biochem. Biophys. Acta* **444**:563–570.

Nathanson, J., and Bloom, F., 1975, Lead-induced inhibition of brain adenyl cyclase activity, *Nature (London)* **255**:419–420.

Nathanson, J. A., and Greengard, P., 1973, Octopamine-sensitive adenylate cyclase: Evidence for a biological role of octopamine in nervous tissue, *Science* **180**:308–310.

Nathanson, J. A., and Greengard, P., 1974, Serotonin-sensitive adenylate cyclase in neural tissue and its similarity to the serotonin receptor: A possible site of action of lysergic acid diethylamine, *Proc. Nat. Acad. Sci. USA* **71**:797–801.

Nathanson, J. A., Freedman, R., and Hoffer, B. J., 1976, Lanthanum inhibits brain adenylate cyclase and blocks noradrenergic depression of Purkinje cell discharge independent of calcium, *Nature* **261**:330–331.

Nesterova, M. V., Saschenko, L. P., Vasiliev, V. Y., and Sevfrin, E. S., 1975, Cyclic adenosine 3′,5′-monophosphate-dependent histone kinase from pig brain, Purification and some properties of the enzyme, *Biochim. Biophys. Acta* **377**:271–281.

Neufeld, A. H., Miller, W. H., and Bitensky, M. W., 1972, Calcium binding to retinal rod disc membranes, *Biochim. Biophys. Acta* **266**:67–71.

Newburgh, R. W., and Rosenberg, R. N., 1972, Effect of norepinephrine on glucose metabolism in glioblastoma and neuroblastoma cells in cell culture, *Proc. Nat. Acad. Sci. USA* **69**:1677–1680.

Nikodijevic, B., Nikodijevic, O., Wongyu, M. Y., Pollard, H., and Guroff, G., 1975, Effect of nerve growth factor on cyclic AMP levels in superior cervical ganglia of rat, *Proc. Nat. Acad. Sci. USA* **72**:4769–4771.

Nikodijevic, O., Nikodijevic, B., Zinder, O., Yi, M-. W., Guroff, G. and Pollard, H. B., 1976,

Control of adenylate cyclase from secretory vesicle membranes by β-adrenergic agents and nerve growth factor, *Proc. Nat. Acad. Sci. USA* **73**:771–774.

Nishi, S., and Koketsu, K., 1967, Origin of ganglionic inhibitory postsynaptic potential, *Life Sci.* **6**:2049–2055.

Nistico, G., Stephenson, J. D., and Preziosi, P., 1976, Behavioral, electrocortical and body temperature effects of cholera toxin, *Eur. J. Pharmacol.* **2**:459–462.

Obata, K., and Yoshida, M., 1973, Caudate-evoked inhibition and actions of GABA and other substances on cat pallidal neurons, *Brain Res.* **64**:455–459.

Oey, J., 1975, Noradrenaline induces morphological alterations in nucleated and enucleated rat C6 glioma cells, *Nature (London)* **257**:317–318.

Ohga, Y., and Daly, J. W., 1976a, The accumulation of cyclic AMP and cyclic GMP in guinea pig brain slices. Effect of calcium ions, norepinephrine and adenosine, *Biochim. Biophys. Acta*, submitted.

Ohga, Y., and Daly, J. W., 1976b, Calcium ion-elicited accumulations of cyclic GMP in guinea pig cerebellar slices, *Biochim. Biophys. Acta*, submitted.

Okada, Y., and Kuroda, Y., 1975, Inhibitory action of adenosine and adenine nucleotides on the postsynaptic potential of olfactory cortex slices of the guinea pig, *Proc. Jap. Acad.* **51**:491–494.

Oleshansky, M. A., and Neff, N. H., 1975, On the mechanism of tolerance to isoproterenol-induced accumulation of cAMP in rat pineal *in vivo, Life Sci.* **17**:1429–1432.

Oliverio, A., Castellano, C., and Messeri, P., 1972, Genetic analysis of avoidance, maze and wheel running behaviors in the mouse, *J. Comp. Physiological Psychol.* **79**:459–473.

Olson, D. R., Kon, C., and Breckenridge, B. M., 1976, Calcium ion effects on guanylate cyclase of brain, *Life Sci.* **18**:935–940.

Opler, L. A., and Makman, M. H., 1972, Mediation by cyclic AMP of hormone-stimulated glycogenolysis in cultured rat astrocytoma cells, *Biochem. Biophys. Res. Commun.* **46**:1140–1145.

Opmeer, F. A., Gumulka, S. W., Dinnendahl, V., and Schonhofer, P. S., 1976, Effects of stimulatory and depressant drugs on cyclic guanosine 3′,5′-monophosphate and adenosine 3′,5′-monophosphate levels in mouse brain, *Naunyn-Schmiedeberg's Arch. Pharmacol.* **292**:259–266.

Orenberg, E. K., Renson, J., Elliott, G. R., Barchas, J. D., and Kessler, S., 1975, Genetic determination of agressive behavior and brain cyclic AMP, *Psychopharmacol. Commun.* **1**:99–107.

Orenberg, E. K., Vandenberg, S. R., Barchas, J. D., and Herman, M. M., 1976, Neurochemical studies in a mouse teratoma with neuroepithelial differentiation. Presence of cyclic AMP, serotonin and enzymes of the serotonergic, adrenergic and cholinergic systems, *Brain Res.* **101**:273–281.

Otten, U., Mueller, R. A., Oesch, R., and Thoenen, H., 1974, Location of an isoproterenol-responsive cyclic AMP-pool in adrenergic nerve cell bodies and its relationship to tyrosine hydroxylase induction, *Proc. Nat. Acad. Sci. USA* **71**:2217–2221.

Otten, U., Oesch, F., and Thoenen, H., 1973, Dissociation between changes in cyclic AMP and subsequent induction of tyrosine hydroxylase in rat superior cervical ganglion and adrenal medulla, *Naunyn-Schmiedebergs Arch. Pharmacol.* **280**:129–140.

Ozawa, E., 1975, Activation of phosphorylase kinase from brain by small amounts of calcium ion, *J. Neurochem.* **20**:1487–1488.

Paalzow, G., and Paalzow, L., 1973, The effects of caffeine and theophylline on nociceptive stimulation in the rat, *Acta Pharm. Toxicol.* **32**:22–32.

Palmer, G. C., 1972, Increased cyclic AMP response to norepinephrine in the rat brain following 6-hydroxydopamine, *Neuropharmacology* **11**:145–149.

Palmer, G. C., 1973a, Adenyl cyclase in neuronal and glial-enriched fractions from rat and rabbit brain, *Res. Commun. Chem. Pathol. Pharmacol.* **5**:603–613.

Palmer, G. C., 1973b, Influence of amphetamines, protriptyline and pargyline on the time course of the norepinephrine-induced accumulation of cyclic AMP in rat brain, *Life Sci.* **12(II)**:345–355.

Palmer, G. C., 1976, Influence of tricyclic antidepressants on the adenylate cyclase-phosphodi-esterase system in rat cortex, *Neuropharmacology* **15**:1–17.

Palmer, G. C., and Burks, T. F., 1971, Central and peripheral adrenergic blocking actions of LSD and BOL, *Eur. J. Pharmacol.* **16**:113–116.

Palmer, G. C., and Duszynski, C., 1975, Regional cyclic GMP content in incubated tissue slices of rat brain, *Eur. J. Pharmacol.* **32**:375–379.

Palmer, G. C., and Evan, A. P., 1974, Effect of psychotropic drugs on the urinary excretion of cyclic AMP in the rat, *Proc. West. Pharmacol. Soc.* **17**:204–209.

Palmer, G. C., and Manian, A. A., 1974a, Inhibition of the catalytic site of adenylate cyclase in the central nervous system by phenothiazine derivatives, *Neuropharmacology* **13**:651–664.

Palmer, G. C., and Manian, A. A., 1974b, Modification of the receptor component of adenylate cyclase in the rat brain by phenothiazine derivatives, *Neuropharmacology* **13**:851–866.

Palmer, G. C., and Manian, A. A., 1974c, Effects of phenothiazines and phenothiazine metabolites on adenyl cyclase and the cyclic AMP response in the rat brain, in *The Phenothiazines and Structurally Related Drugs* (I. S. Forrest, C. J. Carr, and E. Usdin, eds.) pp. 749–767, Raven Press, New York.

Palmer, G. C., and Manian, A. A., 1976, Actions of phenothiazine analogues on dopamine-sensitive adenylate cyclase in neuronal and glial enriched fractions from rat brain, *Biochem. Pharmacol.* **25**:63–72.

Palmer, G. C., and Scott, H. R., 1974, The cyclic AMP response to noradrenalin in young adult rat brain following post-natal injections of 6-hydroxy-dopamine, *Experientia* **30**:520–521.

Palmer, G. C., Robison, G. A., and Sulser, F., 1971, Modification by psychotropic drugs of the cyclic adenosine monophosphate response to norepinephrine in rat brain, *Biochem. Pharmacol.* **20**:236–239.

Palmer, G. C., Robison, G. A., Manian, A. A., and Sulser, F., 1972a, Modification by psychotropic drugs of the cyclic AMP response to norepinephrine in the rat brain *in vitro, Psychopharmacologia* **23**:201–211.

Palmer, G. C., Schmidt, M. J., and Robison, G. A., 1972b, Development and characteristics of the histamine-induced accumulation of cyclic AMP in the rabbit cerebral cortex, *J. Neurochem.* **19**:2251–2256.

Palmer, G. C., Sulser, F., and Robison, G. A., 1973, Effects of neurohumoral and adrenergic agents on cyclic AMP levels in various areas of the rat brain *in vitro, Neuropharmacology* **12**:327–337.

Palmer, D. S., French, S. W., and Narod, M. E., 1976a, Noradrenergic subsensitivity and supersensitivity of the cerebral cortex after reserpine treatment, *J. Pharmacol. Exp. Ther.* **196**:167–171.

Palmer, G. C., Wagner, H. R., and Putnam, R. W., 1976b, Neuronal localization of the enhanced adenylate cyclase responsiveness to catecholamines in rat cerebral cortex following reserpine injections, *Neuropharmacology* **15**:695–702.

Panitz, N., Rieke, E., Morr, M., Wagner, K. G., Roeser, G., and Jastorff, B., 1975, The 3'-amido and 5'-amido analogues of adenosine 3',5'-monophosphate: Interaction with cAMP-specific proteins, *Eur. J. Biochem.* **55**:415–422.

Pannbacker, R. G., 1973, Control of guanylate cyclase activity in the rod outer segment, *Science* **182**:1138–1139.

Pannbacker, R. G., and Schoch, D. R., 1973, Protein kinases of the rod outer segment, *J. Gen. Physiol.* **261**:257–258Abs.

Pannbacker, R. G., Fleischman, D. E., and Reed, D. W., 1972, Cyclic nucleotide phosphodies-terase: High activity in a mammalian photoreceptor, *Science* **175**:757–758.

Patrick, R. L., and Barchas, J. D., 1976, Dopamine synthesis in rat brain striatal synapta-somes. II Dibutyryl cyclic adenosine 3',5'-monophosphoric acid and 6'methyltetrahydropterine-induced synthesis increases without an increase in endogenous dopamine release, *J. Pharmacol. Exp. Ther.* **197**:97–104.

Paul, M. I., Cramer, H., and Goodwin, F. K., 1970a, Urinary cyclic AMP in affective illness, *Lancet* **i**:996.

Paul, M. I., Ditzion, B. R., and Janowsky, D. S., 1970b, Affective illness and cyclic-AMP excretion, *Lancet* **i**:88.

Paul, M. I., Ditzion, B. R., Pauk, G. L., and Janowsky, D. S., 1970c, Urinary adenosine 3′,5′-monophosphate excretion in affective disorders, *Amer. J. Psychiat.* **126**:1493–1497.

Paul, M. I., Pauk, G. L., and Ditzion, B. R., 1970d, The effect of centrally acting drugs on the concentration of brain adenosine 3′,5′-monophosphate, *Pharmacology* **3**:148–154.

Paul, M. I., Cramer, H., and Bunney, W. E., Jr., 1971a, Urinary adenosine 3′,5′-monophosphate in the switch process from depression to mania, *Science* **171**:300–303.

Paul, M. I., Cramer, H., and Goodwin, F. K., 1971b, Urinary cyclic AMP excretion in depression and mania, *Arch. Gen. Psychiat.* **24**:327–333.

Penit, J., Huot, J., and Jard, S., 1976, Neuroblastoma cell adenylate cyclase: Direct activation by adenosine and prostaglandins, *J. Neurochem.* **26**:256–273.

Penit, J., Jard, S., and Benda, P., 1974, Probenecid sensitive 3′,5′-cyclic AMP secretion by isoproterenol stimulated glial cells in culture, *FEBS Lett.* **41**:156–160.

Perkins, J. P., 1973, Adenyl cyclase, *Advan. Cyclic Nucleotide Res.* **3**:1–64.

Perkins, J. P., 1975, Regulation of responsiveness of cells to catecholamines: Variable expression of the components of the second messenger system, in *Cyclic Nucleotides in Disease* (B. Weiss, ed.), pp. 351–376, University Park Press, Baltimore.

Perkins, J. P., and Moore, M. M., 1971, Adenyl cyclase of rat cerebral cortex: Activation by sodium fluoride and detergents, *J. Biol. Chem.* **246**:62–68.

Perkins, J. P., and Moore, M. M., 1973a, Characterization of the adrenergic receptors mediating a rise in cyclic 3′,5′-adenosine monophosphate in rat cerebral cortex, *J. Pharmacol. Exp. Ther.* **185**:371–378.

Perkins, J. P., and Moore, M., 1973b, Regulation of the adenosine cyclic 3′,5′-monophosphate content of rat cerebral cortex: Ontogenetic development of the responsiveness to catecholamines and adenosine, *Mol. Pharmacol.* **9**:774–782.

Perkins, J. P., Macintyre, E. H., Riley, W. D., and Clark, R. B., 1971, Adenyl cyclase, phosphodiesterase and cyclic AMP dependent protein kinase of malignant glial cells in culture, *Life Sci.* **10(I)**:1069–1080.

Perkins, J. P., Moore, M. M., Kalisker, A., and Su, Y-F., 1975, Regulation of cyclic AMP content in normal and malignant brain cells, *Advan. Cyclic Nucleotide Res.* **5**:641–660.

Perry, T. L., Hemmings, S., Drummond, G. I., Hansen, S., and Gjessing, L. R., 1973, Urinary cyclic AMP in periodic catatonia, *Amer. J. Psychiat.* **130**:927–929.

Phillipp-Dormston, W. K., and Siegert, R., 1975a, Adenosine 3′,5′-cyclic monophosphate in rabbit cerebrospinal fluid during fever induced by *E. coli* endotoxin, *Med. Microbiol. Immunol.* **161**:11–13.

Phillipp-Dormston, W. K., and Siegert, R., 1975b, Fever produced in rabbits by $N^6,O^{2'}$-dibutyryl adenosine 3′,5′-cyclic monophosphate, *Experientia* **31**:471–472.

Phillipson, O. T., and Sandler, M., 1975a, The influence of nerve growth factor potassium depolarization and dibutyryl (cyclic) adenosine 3′,5′-monophosphate on explant cultures of chick embryo sympathetic ganglia, *Brain Res.* **90**:273–281.

Phillipson, O. T., and Sandler, M., 1975b, The effect of hydrocortisone and adrenocorticotrophic hormone on monoamine oxidase and tyrosine hydroxylase in explant cultures of enbryonic chick sympathetic ganglia, *Brain Res.* **90**:283–296.

Phillis, J. W., 1974a, The role of calcium in the central effects of biogenic amines, *Life Sci.* **14**:1189–1201.

Phillis, J. W., 1974b, Neomycin and rhuthenium red antagonism of monoaminergic depression of cerebral cortical neurones, *Life Sci.* **15**:213–222.

Phillis, J. W., 1976, An involvement of calcium and Na^+,K^+-ATPase in the inhibitory actions of various compounds on central neurons, in *Taurine* (R. Huxtable and A. Barbeau, eds.), pp. 209–223, Raven Press, New York.

Phillis, J. W., and Kostopoulos, G. K., 1975, Adenosine as a putative transmitter in the cerebral cortex. Studies with potentiators and antagonists, *Life Sci.* **17**:1085–1094.

Phillis, J. W., and Limacher, J. J., 1974, Effects of some metallic cations on cerebral cortical neurones and their interactions with biogenic amines, *Canad. J. Physiol. Pharmacol.* **52**:566–574.

Phillis, J. W., Kostopoulos, G. K., and Limacher, J. J., 1974, Depression of corticospinal cells by various purines and pyrimidines, *Canad. J. Physiol. Pharmacol.* **52**:1226–1229.

Phillis, J. W., Kostopoulus, G. K., and Limacher, J. J., 1975a, A potent depressant action of adenine derivatives on cerebral cortical neurones, *Eur. J. Pharmacol* **30**:125–129.

Phillis, J. W., Kostopoulos, G. K., and Odutala, A., 1975b, On the specificity of histamine H₂-receptor antagonists in the rat cerebral cortex, *Canad. J. Physiol. Pharmacol.* **53**:1205–1208.

Phillis, J. W., Lake, N., and Yarbrough, G., 1973, Calcium mediation of the inhibitory effects of biogenic amines on cerebral cortical neurones, *Brain Res.* **53**:465–469.

Phillis, J. W., Tebecis, A. K., and York, D. H., 1968, Histamine and some antihistamines: Their actions on cerebral cortical neurones, *Brit. J. Pharmacol.* **33**:426–440.

Pichard, A.-L., Hanoune, J., and Kaplan, J.-C., 1972, Human brain and platelet cyclic adenosine 3′,5′-monophosphate phosphodiesterases: Different response to drugs, *Biochim. Biophys. Acta* **279**:217–220.

Pichichero, M., Beer, B., and Clody, D. E., 1973, Effects of dibutyryl cyclic AMP on restoration of function of damaged sciatic nerve in rats, *Science* **182**:724–725.

Pieri, L., Pieri, M., and Haefely, W., 1974, LSD as an agonist of dopamine receptors in the striatum, *Nature (London)* **252**:586–588.

Piras, M. M., and Piras, R., 1974, Phophorylation of vinblastine-isolated microtubules from chick-embryonic muscles, *Eur. J. Biochem.* **47**:443–452.

Pledger, W. J., Stangel, G. M., Thompson, W. J., and Strada, S. J., 1974, Separation of multiple forms of cyclic nucleotide phosphodiesterases from rat brain by isoelectrofocusing, *Biochim. Biophys. Acta* **370**:242–248.

Pledger, W. J., Thompson, W. J., and Strada, S. J., 1975, Isolation of an activator of multiple forms of cyclic nucleotide phosphodiesterase of rat cerebrum by isolectric focusing, *Biochim. Biophys. Acta* **391**:334–340.

Poech, G., and Kukovetz, W. R., 1971, Papaverine-induced inhibition of phosphodiesterase activity in various mammalian tissues, *Life Sci.* **10(I)**:133–144.

Pomerantz, A. H., Rudolph, S. A., Haley, B. E., and Greengard, P., 1975, Photoaffinity labeling of a protein kinase from bovine brain with 8-azidoadenosine 3′,5′-monophosphate, *Biochemistry* **14**:3858–3862.

Posner, J. B., Stern, R., and Krebs, E. G., 1965, Effects of electrical stimulation and epinephrine on muscle phosphorylase, phosphorylase b kinase and adenosine 3′,5′-phosphate, *J. Biol. Chem.* **240**:982–985.

Post, M. L., Kennard, O., and Horn, A. S., 1975, Stereoselective blockade of the dopamine receptor and the x-ray structures of α- and β-flupenthixol, *Nature (London)* **256**:342–343.

Prasad, K. N., 1972a, Neuroblastoma clone: Prostaglandin versus dibutyryl cyclic AMP, 8-benzylthio-cyclic AMP, phosphodiesterase inhibitors and x-rays, *Proc. Soc. Exp. Biol. Med.* **140**:126–129.

Prasad, K. N., 1972b, Morphological differentiation induced by prostaglandin in mouse neuroblastoma cells in culture, *Nature New Biol.* **236**:49–52.

Prasad, K. N., 1972c, Cyclic AMP-induced differentiated mouse neuroblastoma cells lose tumourgenic characteristics, *Cytobios* **6**:163–166.

Prasad, K. N., 1974, Manganese inhibits adenylate cyclase activity and stimulates phosphodiesterase activity in neuroblastoma cells: Its possible implication in manganese-poisoning, *Exp. Neurol.* **45**:554–557.

Prasad, K. N., 1975, Differentiation of neuroblastoma cells in culture, *Biol. Rev.* **50**:129–166.

Prasad, K. N., and Gilmer, K. N., 1974, Demonstration of dopamine-sensitive adenylate cyclase in malignant neuroblastoma cells and change in sensitivity of adenylate cyclase to catecholamines in "differentiated" cells, *Proc. Nat. Acad. Sci. USA* **71**:2525–2529.

Prasad, K. N., and Hsie, A. W., 1971, Morphologic differentiation of murine neuroblastoma cells induced *in vitro* by dibutyryl adenosine 3':5'-cyclic monophosphate, *Nature New Biol.* **233**:141–142.

Prasad, K. N., and Kumar, S., 1973, Cyclic 3',5'-phosphodiesterase activity during cyclic AMP-induced differentiation of neuroblastoma cells in culture, *Proc. Soc. Exp. Biol. Med.* **142**:406–409.

Prasad, K. N., and Kumar, S., 1974, Cyclic AMP and differentiation of neuroblastoma cells in culture in *Control of Proliferation in Animal Cells* (B. Clarkson and R. Baserga, eds.), pp. 581–594, Cold Spring Harbor Laboratory, Cold Spring Harbor.

Prasad, K. N., and Kumar, S., 1975, Role of cyclic AMP in differentiation of human neuroblastoma cells in culture, *Cancer* **36**:1338–1343.

Prasad, K. N., and Mandal, B., 1972, Catechol-*O*-methyl-transferase activity in dibutyryl cyclic AMP, prostaglandin and x-ray-induced differentiated neuroblastoma cell culture, *Exp. Cell Res.* **74**:532–534.

Prasad, K. N., and Mandal, B., 1973, Choline acetyltransferase level in cyclic AMP and X-ray induced morphologically differentiated neuroblastoma cells in culture, *Cytobios* **8**:75–80.

Prasad, K. N., and Sheppard, J. R., 1972a, Neuroblastoma cell culture: Membrane changes during cyclic AMP-induced morphological differentiation, *Proc. Soc. Exp. Biol. Med.* **141**:240–243.

Prasad, K. N., and Sheppard, J. R., 1972b, Inhibitors of cyclic-nucleotide phosphodiesterase induce morphological differentiation of mouse neuroblastoma cell culture, *Exp. Cell. Res.* **73**:436–440.

Prasad, K. N., and Vernadakis, A., 1972, Morphological and biochemical study in x-ray and dibutyryl cyclic AMP-induced differentiated neuroblastoma cells, *Exp. Cell Res.* **70**:27–32.

Prasad, K. N., Gilmer, K., and Kumar, S., 1973a, Morphologically "differentiated" mouse neuroblastoma cells induced by noncyclic AMP agents: Levels of cyclic AMP, nucleic acid and protein, *Proc. Soc. Exp. Biol. Med.* **143**:1168–1171.

Prasad, K. N., Kumar, S., Gilmer, K., and Vernadakis, A., 1973b, Cyclic AMP-induced differentiated neuroblastoma cells: Changes in total nucleic acid and protein contents, *Biochem. Biophys. Res. Commun.* **50**:973–977.

Prasad, K. N., Mandal, B., Waymire, J. C., Lees, G. J., Vernadakis, A., and Weiner, N., 1973c, Basal level of neutrotransmitter synthesizing enzymes and effect of cyclic AMP agents on the morphological differentiation of isolated neuroblastoma clones, *Nature New Biol.* **241**:117–119.

Prasad, K. N., Gilmer, K. N., and Sahu, S. K., 1974, Demonstration of acetyl-choline-sensitive adenyl cyclase in malignant neuroblastoma cells in culture, *Nature (London)* **249**:765–767.

Prasad, K. N., Becker, G., and Tripathy, K., 1975a, Differences and similarities between guanosine 3',5'-cyclic monophosphate phosphodiesterase and adenosine 3',5'-cyclic monophosphate phosphodiesterase activities in neuroblastoma cells in culture, *Proc. Soc. Exp. Biol. Med.* **149**:757–762.

Prasad, K. N., Bondy, S. C., and Purdy, J. L., 1975b, Polyadenylic acid-containing cytoplasmic RNA increases in adenosine 3',5'-cyclic monophosphate-induced "differentiated" neuroblastoma cells in culture, *Exp. Cell Res.* **94**:88–94.

Prasad, K. N., Gilmer, K. N., Sahu, S. K., and Becker, G., 1975c, Effect of neurotransmitters, guanosine triphosphate and divalent cations on the regulation of adenylate cyclase activity in malignant and adenosine cyclic 3',5'-monophosphate-induced "differentiated" neuroblastoma cells, *Cancer Res.* **35**:77–81.

Prasad, K. N., Kumar, S., Becker, G., and Sahu, S. K., 1975d, The role of cyclic nucleotides in differentiation of neuroblastoma cells in culture, in *Cyclic Nucleotides* in *Disease* (B. Weiss, ed.), pp. 45–66, University Park Press, Baltimore.

Prasad, K. N., Sinha, P. K., Sahu, S. K., and Brown, J. L., 1975e, Binding of cyclic nucleotides with soluble proteins increases in "differentiated" neuroblastoma cells in culture, *Biochem. Biophys. Res. Commun.* **66**:131–138.

Prasad, K. N., Fogleman, D., Gaschler, M., Sinha, P. K., and Brown, J. L., 1976, Cyclic nucleotide-dependent protein kinase activity in malignant and cyclic AMP-induced "differentiated" neuroblastoma cells in culture, *Biochem. Biophys. Res. Commun.* **68**:2148–2155.

Prasad, K. N., Waymire, J. C., and Weiner, N., 1972, A further study on the morphology and biochemistry of X-ray and dibutyryl cyclic AMP-induced differentiated neuroblastoma cells in culture, *Exp. Cell Res.* **74**:110–114.

Price, S., 1973, Phosphodiesterase in tongue epithelium: Activation by bitter taste stimuli, *Nature (London)* **241**:54–55.

Pull, I., and McIlwain, H., 1972a, Adenine derivatives as neurohumoral agents in the brain: The quantities liberated on excitation of superfused cerebral tissues, *Biochem. J.* **130**:975–981.

Pull, I., and McIlwain, H., 1972b, Metabolism of [^{14}C]adenine and derivatives by cerebral tissues, superfused and electrically stimulated, *Biochem. J.* **126**:965–973.

Pull, I., and McIlwain, H., 1973, Output of [^{14}C]adenine nucleotides and their derivatives from cerebral tissues: Tetrodotoxin-resistant and calcium ion-requiring components, *Biochem. J.* **136**:893–901.

Pull, I., and McIlwain, H., 1974, Rat cerebral cortex adenosine deaminase activity and its subcellular distribution, *Biochem. J.* **144**:37–41.

Pull, I., and McIlwain, H., 1975, Uptake of neurohumoral agents and cerebral metabolites on output of adenine derivatives from superfused tissues of the brain, *J. Neurochem.* **24**:695–700.

Pull, I., and McIlwain, H., 1976, Centrally-acting drugs and related compounds examined for action on output of adenosine derivatives from superfused tissues of the brain, *Biochem. Pharmacol.* **25**:293–298.

Puri, S. K., Cochin, J., and Volicer, L., 1975, Effect of morphine sulfate on adenylate cyclase and phosphodiesterase activities in rat corpus striatum, *Life Sci.* **16**:759–768.

Purpura, D. P., and Shoffer, R. J., 1972, Excitatory action of dibutyryl cyclic adenosine monophosphate on immature cerebral cortex, *Brain Res.* **38**:179–181.

Quinn, P. J., 1973, The association between phosphatidylinositol phosphodiesterase activity and a specific subunit of microtubular protein in rat brain, *Biochem. J.* **133**:273–281.

Racagni, G., and Carenzi, A., 1976, The anterior amygdala dopamine-sensitive adenylate cyclase: Point of action of antipsychotic drugs, *Pharmacol. Res. Commun.* **8**:149–158.

Racagni, G., Zsilla, G., Guidotti, A., and Costa, E., 1976, Accumulation of GMP in striatum of rats injected with narcotic analgesics: Antagonism by naltrexone, *J. Pharm. Pharmacol.* **28**:258–260.

Rall, T. W. and Gilman, A. G., 1970, The role of cyclic AMP in the nervous system, *Neuroscience Res. Prog. Bull.* **8**:221–317.

Rall, T. W., and Kakiuchi, S., 1966, The influence of certain neurohormones and drugs on the accumulation of cyclic AMP in brain tissue, in *Molecular Basis of Some Aspects of Mental Activity* (O. Walaas, ed), Vol. I, pp. 417–427. Academic Press, New York.

Rall, T. W., and Sattin, A., 1970, Factors influencing the accumulation of cyclic AMP in brain tissue, *Advan. Biochem. Psychopharmacol.* **3**:113–133.

Rappaport, L., Leterrier, J. F., and Nunez, J., 1972, Non phosphorylation *in vitro* of the 6S tubulin from brain and thyroid tissue, *FEBS Lett.* **26**:349–352.

Rappaport, L., Letterrier, J. F., and Nunez, J., 1975, Protein-kinase activity, *in vitro* phosphorylation and polymerization of purified tubulin, *Ann. N.Y. Acad. Sci.* **253**:611–629.

Rappaport, L., Leterrier, J. F., Virion, A., and Nunez, J., 1976, Phosphorylation of microtubule-associated proteins, *Eur. J. Biochem.* **62**:539–549.

Rasmussen, H., 1970, Cell communication, calcium ion, and cyclic adenosine monophosphate, *Science* **170**:404–412.

Rasmussen, H., and Goodman, D. B. P., 1975, Calcium and cAMP as interrelated intracellular messengers, *Ann. N. Y. Acad. Sci.* **253**:789–796.

Reddington, M., and Lagnado, J., 1973, The phosphorylation of cholchicine binding (microtubule) protein in respiring slices of guinea pig cerebral cortex, *FEBS Lett.* **30**:188–194.

Reddington, M., Rodnight, R., and Williams, M., 1973, Turnover of protein-bound serine phosphate in respiring slices of guinea-pig cerebral cortex, *Biochem. J.* **132**:475–482.

Reynolds, C. P., and Perez-Polo, J. R., 1975, Human neuroblastoma: Glial-induced morphological differentiation, *Neurosci. Lett.* **1**:91–98.

Richelson, E., 1973, Stimulation of tyrosine hydroxylase activity in an adrenergic clone of mouse neuroblastoma by dibutyryl cyclic AMP, *Nature New Biol.* **242**:175–176.

Rieke, E., Panitz, N., Eigel, A., and Wagner, K. G., 1975, On detachment of the regulatory unit of brain protein kinase from a cyclic AMP-polyacrylamide gel, *Hoppe-Seyler's Z. Physiol. Chem.* **356**:1177–1180.

Rigberg, M., Vacik, J. P., and Shelver, W. H., 1969, Utilization of radiometric analysis for measurement of activation of adenyl cyclase by sympathomimetic amines, *J. Pharmaceut. Sci.* **58**:358–359.

Rindi, G., Sciorelli, G., Poloni, M., and Acanfora, F., 1972, Induction of ingestive responses by cAMP applied into the rat hypothalamus, *Experientia* **28**:1047–1049.

Roberts, E., and Simonsen, D. G., 1970, Some properties of cyclic 3',5'-nucleotide phosphodiesterase of mouse brain: Effects of imidazole-4-acetic acid, chlorpromazine, cyclic 3',5'-GMP, and other substances *Brain Res.* **24**:91–111.

Robertson, H. A., and Steele, J. E., 1972, Activation of insect nerve cord phosphorylase by octopamine and adenosine 3',5'-monophosphate, *J. Neurochem.* **19**:1603–1606.

Robison, G. A., Copper, A. J., Whybrow, P. C., and Prange, A. J., 1970a, Cyclic AMP in affective disorders, *Lancet* **ii**:1028–1029.

Robison, G. A., Schmidt, M. J., and Sutherland, E. W., 1970b, On the development and properties of the brain adenyl cyclase system, *Advan. Biochem. Psychopharmacol.* **3**:11–30.

Roch, P., and Kalix, P., 1975a, Effects of biogenic amines on the concentration of adenosine 3',5'-monophosphate in bovine superior cervical ganglion, *Neuropharmacology* **14**:21–29.

Roch, P., and Kalix, P., 1975b, Adenosine 3',5'-monophosphate in bovine superior cervical ganglion: Effect of high extracellular potassium, *Biochem. Pharmacol.* **24**:1293–1296.

Rogers, M., Dismukes, K., and Daly, J. W., 1975, Histamine-elicited accumulations of cyclic adenosine 3',5'-monophosphate in guinea pig brain slices: Effect of H_1- and H_2-antagonists, *J. Neurochem.* **25**:531–534.

Roisen, F. J., and Murphy, R. A., 1973, Neurite development *in vitro.* II. The role of microfilaments and microtubules in dibutyryl adenosine 3',5'-cyclic monophosphate and nerve-growth-factor stimulated maturation, *J. Neurobiol.* **4**:397–412.

Roisen, F. J., Braden. W. G., and Friedman, J., 1975a, Neurite development *in vitro:* III. The effects of several derivatives of cyclic AMP, colchicine, and colcemid, *Ann. N.Y. Acad. Sci.* **253**:545–561.

Roisen, F. J., Murphy, R. A., and Braden, W. G., 1972b, Neurite development *in vitro.* I. The effects of adenosine 3',5'-cyclic monophosphate (cyclic AMP), *J. Neurobiol.* **4**:347–368.

Roisen, F. J., Murphy, R. A., and Braden, W. G., 1972c, Dibutyryl cyclic adenosine monophosphate stimulation of colcemid-inhibited axonal elongation, *Science* **177**:809–811.

Roisen, F. J., Murphy, R. A., and Braden, W. G., 1972d, Neurite development *in vitro.* I. The effects of adenosine 3'5'-cyclic monophosphate (cyclic AMP), *J. Neurobiol.* **3**:347–368.

Roisen, F. J., Murphy, R. A., Richichero, M. E., and Braden, W. G., 1972e, Cyclic adenosine monophosphate stimulation of axonal elongation, *Science* **175**:73–74.

Rojakovick, A. S., and March, R. B., 1972, The activation and inhibition of adenyl cyclase from the brain of the Madagascar cockroach *(Gromphadorhina portentosa)*, *Comp. Biochem. Physiol.* **43B**:209–215.

Rojakovick, A. S., and March, R. B., 1974, Characteristics of cyclic 3′,5′-nucleotide phosphodiesterase from the brain of the Madagascar cockroach *(Gromphadorhina portentosa)*, *Comp. Biochem. Physiol.* **47B**:189–199.

Romero, J. A., and Axelrod, J., 1975, Regulation of sensitivity to beta-adrenergic stimulation in induction of pineal *N*-acetyltransferase, *Proc. Nat. Acad. Sci. USA* **72**:1661–1665.

Romero, J. A., Zatz, M., and Axelrod, J., 1975, Beta-adrenergic stimulation of pineal *N*-acetyltransferase. Adenosine 3′-5′-cyclic monophosphate stimulates both RNA and protein synthesis, *Proc. Nat. Acad. Sci. USA* **72**:2107–2111.

Roth, R. H., Morgenroth, V. H., and Salzman, P. M., 1975, Tyrosine hydroxylase: Allosteric activation induced by stimulation of central noradrenergic neurons, *Naunyn-Schmiedeberg's Arch. Pharmacol.* **289**:327–343.

Rotrosen, J., Friedman, E., and Gershon, S., 1975, Striatal adenylate cyclase activity following reserpine and chronic chlorpromazine administration in rats, *Life Sci.* **17**:563–568.

Routtenberg, A., and Ehrlich, Y. H., 1975, Endogenous phosphorylation of four cerebral cortical membrane proteins: Role of cyclic nucleotides, ATP and divalent cations, *Brain Res.* **92**:415–430.

Routtenberg, A., Ehrlich, Y. H., and Rabjohns, R. R., 1975, Effect of a training experience on phosphorylation of a specific protein in neocortical and subcortical membrane preparations, *Fed. Proc.* **34**:293 (Abs.).

Roy, A. C., and Collier, H. O. J., 1975, Prostaglandins, cyclic AMP and the biochemical mechanisms of opiate agonist action, *Life Sci.* **16**:1857–1862.

Rubin, C. S., and Rosen, O. M., 1975, Protein phosphorylation, *Ann. Rev. Biochem.* **44**:831–887.

Rubin, E. H. and Ferrendelli, J. A., 1976, Quantitative localization of cyclic nucleotides in cerebellar folia, *J. Histochem. Cytochem.* **24**:964–966.

Rubio, R., Berne, R. M., Bockman, E. L., and Curnish, R. R., 1975, Relationship between adenosine concentration and oxygen supply in rat brain, *Amer. J. Physiol.* **228**:1896–1902.

Rudland, P. S., Seeley, M., and Seifert, W., 1974, Cyclic GMP and cyclic AMP levels in normal and transformed fibroblasts, *Nature (London)* **251**:417–419.

Russell, J. R., Thompson, W. J. Schneider, F. W., and Appleman, M. M., 1972, 3′:5′-Cyclic monophosphate phosphodiesterase: Negative cooperativity, *Proc. Nat. Acad. Sci. USA* **69**:1791–1795.

Sahu, S. K., and Prasad, K. N., 1975, Effect of neurotransmitters and prostaglandin E_1 on cyclic AMP levels in various clones of neuroblastoma cells in culture, *J. Neurochem.* **24**:1267–1270.

Salem, R., and De Vellis, J., 1976, Protein kinase (PK) activity and cAMP-dependent protein phosphorylation in subcellular fractions after norepinephrine (NE) treatment of glial cells, *Fed. Proc.* **35**:296Abs.

Sasaki, Y., Susuki, N., Sowa, T., Nozawa, R., and Yokota, T., 1976, Effects of 8-substituted adenosine 3′,5′-monophosphate derivatives on high K_m phosphodiesterase activity, *Biochemistry* **15**:1408–1413.

Sato, A., Onaya, T., Kotani, H., Harada, A., and Yamada, T., 1974, Effects of biogenic amines on the formation of adenosine 3′,5′-monophosphate in porcine cerebral cortex, hypothalamus and anterior pituitary slices, *Endocrinology* **94**:1311–1318.

Sattin, A., 1971, Increase in the content of adenosine 3′,5′-monophosphate in mouse forebrain during seizures and prevention of the increase by methylxanthines, *J. Neurochem.* **18**:1087–1096.

Sattin, A., 1975, Cyclic AMP accumulation in cerebral cortex tissue from inbred strains of mice, *Life Sci.* **16**:903–914.

Sattin, A., and Rall, T. W., 1970, The effect of adenosine and adenine nucleotides on the cyclic adenosine 3',5'-phosphate content of guinea pig cerebral cortex slices, *Mol. Pharmacol.* **6**:13–23.

Sattin, A., Rall, T. W., and Zanella, J., 1975, Regulation of cyclic adenosine 3',5'-monophosphate levels in guinea-pig cerebral cortex by interaction of alpha adenergic and adenosine receptor activity, *J. Pharmacol. Exp. Ther.* **192**:22–32.

Saxena, P. R., and Bahargava, K. P., 1974, Central beta-adrenoceptor sites and ouabain action, *Pharmacol. Res. Commun.* **6**:347–355.

Schimmer, B. P., 1971, Effects of catecholamines and monovalent cations on adenylate cyclase activity in cultured glial tumor cells, *Biochem. Biophys. Acta* **252**:567–573.

Schimmer, B. P., 1973, Influence of Li^+ on epinephrine-stimulated adenylate cyclase activity in cultured glial tumor cells, *Biochim. Biophys. Acta* **327**:186–192.

Schlaeger, E. J. and Köhler, G., 1976, External cyclic AMP-dependent protein kinase activity in rat C-6 glioma cells, *Nature (London)* **260**:705–707.

Schlegel, B., and Oey, J., 1975, Catecholamine-induced cyclic AMP and morphologic alterations in glioma cells, *Naturwissenshaften* **62**:534–535.

Schlesinger, D. H., Goldstein, G., and Niall, H. D., 1975, The complete amino acid sequence of ubiguitin, an adenylate cyclase stimulating polypeptide probably universal in living cells, *Biochemistry* **14**:2214–2218.

Schlesinger, K., Boggan, W. D., and Griek, B. J., 1968, Pharmacogenetic correlates of pentylenetetrazol and electroconvulsive seizure thresholds in mice, *Psychopharmacologia* **13**:181–188.

Schmidt, M. J., 1974, Effects of neonatal hyperthyroidism on activity of cyclic AMP-dependent microsomal protein kinase, *J. Neurochem.* **22**:469–471.

Schmidt, M. J., and Robison, G. A., 1971, The effect of norepinephrine on cyclic AMP levels in discrete regions of the developing rabbit brain, *Life Sci.* **10(I)**:459–464.

Schmidt, M. J., and Robison, G. A., 1972, The effect of neonatal thyroidectomy on the development of the adenosine 3',5'-monophosphate system in the rat brain, *J. Neurochem.* **19**:937–947.

Schmidt, M. J., and Sokoloff, L., 1973, Activity of cyclic AMP-dependent microsomal protein kinase and phosphorylation of ribosomal protein in rat brain during postnatal development, *J. Neurochem.* **21**:1193–1205.

Schmidt, M. J., Hopkins, J. T., Schmidt, D. E., and Robison, G. A., 1972, Cyclic AMP in brain areas: Effects of amphetamine and norepinephrine assessed through the use of microwave radiation as a means of tissue fixation, *Brain Res.* **42**:465–477.

Schmidt, M. J., Palmer, E. C., Dettbarn, W.-D., and Robison, G. A., 1970, Cyclic AMP and adenyl cyclase in the developing rat brain, *Develop. Psychobiol.* **3**:53–67.

Schmidt, M. J., Schmidt, D. E., and Robison, G. A., 1971, Cyclic adenosine monophosphate in brain areas: Microwave irradiation as a means of tissue fixation. *Science* **173**:1142–1143.

Schmidt, S. Y., and Lolley, R. N., 1973, Cyclic-nucleotide phosphodiesterase: An early defect in inherited retinal degeneration in C3H mice, *J. Cell Biol.* **57**:117–123.

Schorderet, M., 1974, AMP cyclique et systeme nerveux, *J. Physiol.* (Paris): **68**:471–505.

Schorderet, M., 1975, The effects of dopamine, piribedil (ET-495) and its metabolite S-584 on retinal adenylate cyclase, *Experientia* **31**:1325–1326.

Schousboe, A., Fosmark, H., and Hertz, L., 1975, High content of glutamate and of ATP in astrocytes cultured from rat brain hemispheres: Effect of serum withdrawal and of cyclic AMP, *J. Neurochem.* **25**:909–911.

Schrier, B. K., and Shapiro, D. L., 1973, Effects of N^6-monobutyryl-cyclic AMP on glutamate decarboxylase activity in fetal rat brain cells and glial tumor cells in culture, *Exp. Cell Res.* **80**:459–465.

Schubert, D., and Jacob, F., 1970, 5-Bromo-deoxyuridine-induced differentiation of a neuroblastoma, *Proc. Nat. Acad. Sci. USA* **67**:247–254.

Schubert, D., Heineman, S., Carlisle, N., Tarikas, H., Kimes, B., Patrick, J., Steinbach, J. H., Culp, W., and Brandt, B. L., 1974, Clonal lines from the rat central nervous system, *Nature (London)* **249**:224–227.

Schubert, D., Tarikas, H., and La Corbiere, M., 1976a, Neurotransmitter regulation of adenosine 3′,5′-monophosphate in clonal nerve, glia and muscle cell lines, *Science* **192**:471–472.

Schubert, P., Lee, K., West, M., Deadwyler, S. and Lynch, G., 1976b, Stimulation dependent release of ³H-adenosine derivatives from central axon terminals to target neurones, *Nature (London)* **260**:541–542.

Schubert, P., and Kreutzberg, G. W., 1975a, Axonal transport of adenosine and uridine derivatives and transfer to postsynaptic neurons, *Brain Res.* **90**:319–323.

Schubert, P., and Kreutzberg, G. W., 1975b, Parameters of dendritic transport, *Advan. Neurology* **12**:255–268.

Schultz, J., 1974a, Adenosine 3′,5′-monophosphate in guinea pig cerebral cortical slices: Effect of benzodiazepines, *J. Neurochem.,* **22**:685–690.

Schultz, J., 1974b, Inhibition of 3′,5′-nucleotide phosphodiesterase in guinea pig cerebral cortical slices, *Arch. Biochem. Biophys.* **163**:15–20.

Schultz, J., 1974c, Inhibition of phosphodiesterase activity in brain cortical slices from guinea pig and rat, *Pharmacol. Res. Commun.* **6**:335–341.

Schultz, J., 1975a, Cyclic adenosine 3′,5′-monophosphate in guinea-pig cerebral cortical slices: Studies on the role of adenosine, *J. Neurochem.* **24**:1237–1242.

Schultz, J., 1975b, Cyclic adenosine 3′,5′-monophosphate in guinea pig cerebral cortical slices: Possible regulation of phosphodiesterase activity by cyclic adenosine 3′,5′-monophosphate and calcium ions, *J. Neurochem.* **24**:495–501.

Schultz, J., 1976, Psychoactive drug effects on a system which generates cyclic AMP in brain, *Nature* **261**:417–418.

Schultz, J. and Daly, J. W., 1973a, Cyclic adenosine 3′,5′-monophosphate in guinea pig cerebral cortical slices. I. Formation of cyclic adenosine 3′,5′-monophosphate from endogenous adenosine triphosphate and from radioactive adenosine triphosphate formed during a prior incubation with radioactive adenine, *J. Biol. Chem.* **248**:843–852.

Schultz, J., and Daly, J. W., 1973b, Cyclic adenosine 3′,5′-monophosphate in guinea pig cerebral cortical slices. II. The role of phosphodiesterase activity in the regulation of levels of cyclic adenosine 3′,5′-monophosphate, *J. Biol. Chem.* **248**:853–859.

Schultz, J., and Daly, J. W., 1973c, Cyclic adenosine 3′,5′-monophosphate in guinea pig cerebral cortical slices. III. Formation, degradation, and reformation of cyclic adenosine 3′,5′-monophosphate during sequential stimulations by biogenic amines and adenosine, *J. Biol. Chem.* **248**:860–866.

Schultz, J., and Daly, J. W., 1973d, Adenosine 3′,5′-monophosphate in guinea pig cerebral cortical slices: Effects of α- and β-adrenergic agents, histamine, serotonin and adenosine, *J. Neurochem.* **21**:573–579.

Schultz, J., and Daly, J. W., 1973e, Accumulation of cyclic adenosine 3′,5′-monophosphate in cerebral cortical slices from rat and mouse stimulatory effect of α- and β-adrenergic agents and adenosine, *J. Neurochem.* **21**:1319–1326.

Schultz, J., and Hamprecht, B., 1973, Adenosine 3′,5′-monophosphate in cultured neuroblastoma cells: Effect of adenosine, phosphodiesterase inhibitors and benzazepines, *Naunyn-Schmiedebergs Arch. Pharmacol.* **278**:215–225.

Schultz, J., and Kleefeld, G., 1975, Stimulation of adenosine 3′,5′-monophosphate formation in guinea-pig cerebral cortical slices in a calcium free medium, *Naunyn-Schmiedeberg's Arch. Pharmacol.* **287**:289–296.

Schultz, J., Hamprecht, B., and Daly, J. W., 1972, Accumulation of adenosine 3′:5′-cyclic monophosphate in clonal glial cells: Labeling of intracellular adenine nucleotides with radioactive adenine, *Proc. Nat. Acad. Sci. USA* **69**:1266–1270.

Schwabe, U., and Daly, J. W., 1976, The role of calcium ions in accumulations of cyclic AMP elicited by α- and β-adrenergic agonists in rat brain slices, *J. Pharmacol. Exp. Ther.*, in press.

Schwabe, U., Miyake, M., Ohga, Y., and Daly, J. W., 1976a, 4-(3-Cyclopentyloxy-4-methoxy-phenyl)-2-pyrrolidone(ZK 62711): A potent inhibitor of cyclic AMP-phosphodiesterases in homogenates and tissue slices from rat brain, *Mol. Pharmacol.* **12**:900–910.

Schwabe, U., Ohga, Y., and Daly, J. W., 1976b, The role of calcium in the regulation of cyclic nucleotide levels in brain slices of rat and guinea pig, *Biochim. Biophys. Acta,* submitted.

Schwartz, J. P., and Passonneau, J. V., 1974, Cyclic AMP-mediated induction of the cyclic AMP phosphodiesterase of C-6 glioma cells, *Proc. Nat. Acad. Sci. USA* **71**:3844–3848.

Schwartz, J. P., Morris, N. R., and Breckenridge, B. M., 1973, Adenosine 3′,5′-monophosphate in glial tumor cells, *J. Biol. Chem.* **248**:2699–2704.

Sciorelli, G., Poloni, M., and Rindi, G., 1972, Evidence for cholinergic mediation of ingestive responses elicited by dibutyryl-adenosine-3′,5′-monophosphate in rat hypothalamus, *Brain Res.* **48**:427–431.

Seager, O. A., 1975, Effects of anesthetics on cyclic AMP levels in mouse neuroblastoma cells in culture, in *Molecular Mechanisms of Anesthesia* (B. R. Fink, ed.), Vol. I, pp. 471–481, Raven Press, New York.

Sebens, J. B., and Korf, J., 1975, Cyclic AMP in cerebrospinal fluid: Accumulation following probenecid and biogenic amines, *Exp. Neurol.* **46**:333–344.

Seeds, N. W., and Gilman, A. G., 1971, Norepinephrine stimulated increase of cyclic AMP levels in developing mouse brain cell cultures, *Science* **174**:292.

Segal, D. S., Geyer, M. A., and Weiner, B. E., 1975, Strain differences during intraventricular infusion of norepinephrine: Possible role of receptor sensitivity, *Science* **189**:301–303.

Segal, D. S., Kuczenski, R. T., and Mandell, A. J., 1972, Strain differences in behavior and brain tyrosine hydroxylase activity, *Behav. Biol.* **7**:75–81.

Segal, M., and Bloom, F. E., 1974a, The action of norepinephrine in the rat hippocampus. I. Ionotophoretic studies, *Brain Res.* **72**:79–97.

Segal, M., and Bloom, F. E., 1974b, The action of norepinephrine in the rat hippocampus. II. Activation of the input pathway, *Brain Res.* **72**:99–114.

Setchenska, M. S., Vassileva-Popova, J. G., and Russanov, E. M., 1975, Activations of glutamate dehydrogenase by 3′,5′-cyclic adenosine monophosphate, *FEBS Lett.* **60**:129.

Severin, E. S., Nesterova, M. V., Sashchenko, L. P., Rasumova, V. V., Tunitskaya, V. L., Kochetkov, S. N., and Gulyaev, N. N., 1975, Investigation of the adenosine 3′,5′-cyclic phosphate binding site of pig brain histone kinase with the aid of some analogues of adenosine 3′,5′-cyclic phosphate, *Biochim. Biophys. Acta* **384**:413–422.

Shanta, T. R., Woods, W. D., Waitzman, M. B., and Bourne, G. H., 1966, Histochemical method for localization of cyclic 3′,5′-nucleotide phosphodiesterase, *Histochemie* **7**:177–190.

Shapiro, D. L., 1973, Morphological and biochemical alterations in fetal rat brain cells cultured in the presence of monobutyryl cyclic AMP, *Nature (London)* **241**:203–204.

Sharma, S. K., Klee, W. A., and Nirenberg, M., 1975a, Dual regulation of adenylate cyclase accounts for narcotic dependence and tolerance, *Proc. Nat. Acad. Sci. USA* **72**:3092–3096.

Sharma, S. K., Nirenberg, M., and Klee, W. A., 1975b, Morphine receptors as regulators of adenylate cyclase activity, *Proc. Nat. Acad. Sci. USA* **72**:590–594.

Shashouva, V. E., 1971, Dibutyryl adenosine cyclic 3′:5′-monophosphate effects on goldfish behavior and brain RNA metabolism, *Proc. Nat. Acad. Sci. USA* **68**:2835–2838.

Sheppard, H., and Burghardt, C. R., 1974a, Effects of tetrahydroisoquinoline derivatives on the adenylate cyclases of the caudate nucleus (dopamine-type) and erythrocyte (β-type) of the rat, *Res. Commun. Chem. Pathol. Pharmacol.* **8**:527–534.

Sheppard, H., and Burghardt, C. R., 1974b, The dopamine-sensitive adenylate cyclase of rat caudate nucleus. I. Comparison with the isoproterenol-sensitive adenylate cyclase (beta receptor system) of rat erythrocytes in response of dopamine derivatives, *Mol. Pharmacol.* **10**:721–726.

Sheppard, J. R., and Prasad, K. N., 1973, Cyclic AMP levels and the morphological differentiation of mouse neuroblastoma cells, *Life Sci.* **12**:431–439.

Sheppard, H., and Wiggan, G., 1971, Different sensitivities of the phosphodiesterases (adenosine-3′,5′-cyclic phosphate 3′-phosphohydrolase) of dog cerebral cortex and erythrocytes to inhibition by synthetic agents and cold, *Biochem. Pharmacol.* **20**:2128–2130.

Sheppard, H., Wiggan, G., and Tsien, W. H., 1972, Structure–activity relationships for inhibitors of phosphodiesterase from erythrocytes and other tissues, *Advan. Cyclic Nucleotide Res.* **1**:103–112.

Shigekawa, B. L., and Olsen, R. W., 1975, Resolution of cyclic AMP-stimulated protein kinase from polymerization-purified brain microtubules. *Biochem. Biophys. Res. Commun.* **63**:455–462.

Shimizu, H., and Daly, J., 1970, Formation of cyclic adenosine 3′,5′-monophosphate from adenosine in brain slices, *Biochim. Biophys. Acta* **222**:465–473.

Shimizu, H., and Daly, J. W., 1972a, Methods for the measurement of cyclic AMP in brain, in *Methods in Neurochemistry* (R. Fried, ed.), Vol. 2, pp. 147–168, Marcel Dekker, New York.

Shimizu, H., and Daly, J. W., 1972b, Effect of depolarizing agents on accumulation of cyclic adenosine 3′,5′-monophosphate in cerebral cortical slices, *Eur. J. Pharmacol.* **17**:240–252.

Shimizu, H., and Okayama, H., 1973, An ATP pool associated with adenyl cyclase of brain tissue, *J. Neurochem.* **20**:1279–1283.

Shimizu, H., Creveling., C. R., and Daly, J., 1970a, Stimulated formation of adenosine 3′,5′-cyclic phosphate in cerebral cortex: Synergism between electrical activity and biogenic amines, *Proc. Nat. Acad. Sci. USA* **65**:1033–1040.

Shimizu, H., Creveling, C. R., and Daly, J. W., 1970b, Cyclic adenosine 3′,5′-monophosphate formation in brain slices: Stimulation by batrachotoxin, ouabain, veratridine, and potassium ions, *Mol. Pharmacol.* **6**:184–188.

Shimizu, H., Creveling, C. R., and Daly, J. W., 1970c, The effect of histamines and other compounds on the formation of adenosine 3′,5′-monophosphate in slices from cerebral cortex, *J. Neurochem.* **17**:441–444.

Shimizu, H., Creveling, C. R., and Daly, J. W., 1970d, Effect of membrane depolarization and biogenic amines on the formation of cyclic AMP in incubated brain slices, *Advan. Biochem. Psychopharmacol.* **3**:135–154.

Shimizu, H., Daly, J. W., and Creveling, C. R., 1969, A radioisotopic method for measuring the formation of adenosine 3′,5′-cyclic monophosphate in incubated slices of brain, *J. Neurochem.* **16**:1609–1619.

Shimizu, H., Ichishita, H., and Odagiri, H., 1974, Stimulated formation of cyclic adenosine 3′,5′-monophosphate by aspartate and glutamate in cerebral cortical slices of guinea pig, *J. Biol. Chem.* **249**:5955–5962.

Shimizu, H., Ichishita, H., and Miaokami, Y., 1975a, Stimulation of the cell-free adenylate cyclase from guinea pig cerebral cortex by acidic amino acids and veratridine, *J. Cyclic Nucleotide Res.* **1**:61–67.

Shimizu, H., Ichishita, H., Tateishi, M., and Umeda, I., 1975b, Characteristics of the amino acid receptor site mediating formation of cyclic adenosine 3′,5′-monophosphate in mammalian brains, *Mol. Pharmacol.* **11**:223–231.

Shimizu, H., Ichishita H., and Umeda, I., 1975c, Inhibition of glutamate-elicited accumulation of adenosine cyclic 3',5'-monophosphate in brain slices by α, ω-diaminocarboxylic acids, *Mol. Pharmacol.* **11**:866–873.

Shimizu, H., Takenoshita, M., Huang, M., and Daly, J. W., 1973, Accumulation of adenosine 3',5'-monophosphate in brain slices: Interaction of local anaesthetics and depolarizing agents, *J. Neurochem.* **20**:91–95.

Shimizu, H., Tanaka, S., and Kodama, T., 1972, Adenosine kinase of mammalian brain: Partial purification and its role for the uptake of adenosine, *J. Neurochem.* **19**:687–698.

Shimizu, H., Tanaka, S., Suzuki, T., and Matsukado, Y., 1971, The response of human cerebrum adenyl cyclase to biogenic amines, *J. Neurochem.* **18**:1157–1161.

Shoemaker, W. J., Balentine, L. T., Siggins, G. R., Hoffer, B. J., Henricksen, S. J., and Bloom, F. E., 1975, Characteristics of the release of adenosine 3',5'-monophosphate from micropipets by microiontrophoresis, *J. Cyclic Nucleotide Res.* **1**:97–106.

Shuman, D. A., Miller, J. D., Scholten, M. B., Simon, L. N., and Robins, R. K., 1973, Synthesis and biological activity of some purine 5'-thio-5'-deoxynucleoside 3',5'-cyclic phosphorothioates, *Biochemistry* **12**:2781–2791.

Shylapnikov, S. V., Arutyunyan, A. A., Kurochkin, S. N., Memelova, L. V., Nesterova, M. V., Sashchenko, L. P., and Severin, E. S., 1975, Investigation of the sites phosphorylated in lysine-rich histones by protein kinase from pig brain, *FEBS Lett.* **53**:316–319.

Siegel, R., Conforti, N., Feldman, S., and Chowers, I., 1974, Effects of neurogenic and systemic stresses on hypothalamic and adenohypophysial cAMP content, *Neuroendocrinology* **14**:24–33.

Siggins, G. R., and Henriksen, S. J., 1975, Analogs of cyclic adenosine monophosphate: Correlation of inhibition of Purkinje neurons with protein kinase activation, *Science* **189**:559–561.

Siggins, G. R., Battenberg, E. F., Hoffer, B. J., and Bloom, F. E., 1973, Noradrenergic stimulation of cyclic adenosine monophosphate in rat Purkinje neurons: An immunocyto-chemical study, *Science* **179**:585–588.

Siggins, G. R., Hoffer, B. J., and Bloom, F. E., 1969, Cyclic adenosine monophosphate: Possible mediator for norepinephrine effects on cerebellar Purkinje cells, *Science* **165**:1018–1020.

Siggins, G. R., Hoffer, B. J., and Bloom, F. E., 1971a, Cyclic adenosine monophosphate and norepinephrine: Effect on Purkinje cells in rat cerebellar cortex, *Science* **174**:1258–1259.

Siggins, G. R., Hoffer, B. J., and Bloom, F. E., 1971b, Studies on norepinephrine-containing afferents to Purkinje cells of rat cerebellum. III. Evidence for mediation of norepinephrine effects by cyclic 3',5'-adenosine monophosphate, *Brain Res.* **25**:535–553.

Siggins, G., Hoffer, B., and Bloom, F., 1971c, Prostaglandin-norepinephrine interactions in brain: Microelectrophoretic and histochemical correlates, *Ann. N.Y. Acad. Sci.* **180**:302–323.

Siggins, G. R., Hoffer, B. J., Oliver, A. P., and Bloom, F. E., 1971d, Activation of a central noradrenergic projection to cerebellum, *Nature (London)* **233**:481–483.

Siggins, G. R., Oliver, A. P., Hoffer, B. J., and Bloom, F. E., 1971e, Cyclic adenosine monophosphate and norepinephrine: Effects on transmembrane properties of cerebellar Purkinje cells, *Science* **171**:192–194.

Siggins, G. R., Hoffer, B. J., and Ungerstedt, U., 1974, Electrophysiological evidence for involvement of cyclic adenosine monophosphate in dopamine responses of caudate neurons, *Life Sci.* **15**:779–792.

Silberstein, S. D., Brimijoin, S., Molinoff, P. B., and Lemberger, L., 1972, Induction of dopamine-β-hydroxylase in rat superior ganglia in organ culture, *J. Neurochem.* **19**:919–921.

Simantov, R., and Sachs, L., 1972, Enzyme regulation in neuroblastoma cells: Selection of clones with low acetyl-cholinesterase activity and the independent control of acetylcholin-esterase and choline-*O*-acetyltransferase, *Eur. J. Biochem.* **30**:123–129.

Simantov, R., and Sachs, L., 1973, Regulation of acetylcholine receptors in relation to acetylcholinesterase in neuroblastoma cells, *Proc. Nat. Acad. Sci. USA* **70**:2902–2905.

Simantov, R. and Sachs, L., 1975a, Temperature sensitivity of cyclic adenosine 3',5'-monophosphate binding proteins and regulation of growth and differentiation in neuroblastoma cells, *J. Biol. Chem.* **250**:3236–3242.

Simantov, R., and Sachs, L., 1975b, Different mechanisms for the induction of acetylcholinesterase in neuroblastoma cells, *Devel. Biol.* **45**:382–385.

Simantov, R., and Sachs, L., 1975c, Temperature sensitivity of cyclic adenosine-3',5'-monophosphate-binding proteins, activity of protein kinases and regulation of cell growth, *Eur. J. Biochem.* **59**:89–96.

Simantov, R., Rutishauser, U., and Sachs, L., 1975, Reversible inhibition of cAMP-induced axon formation in neuroblastoma cells by concanavalin A and vinblastine. Relationship to microtubules and cytotoxicity, *Exp. Cell Res.* **95**:327–332.

Simon, L. N., Shuman, D. A., and Robins, R. K., 1973, The chemistry and biological properties of nucleotides related to nucleoside 3',5'-cyclic phosphates, *Advan. Cyclic Nucleotide Res.* **3**:225–353.

Sinanan, K., Keatinge, A. M. B., Beckett, P. G. S., and Love, W. C., 1975, Urinary cyclic AMP in endogenous and neurotic depression, *Brit. J. Psychiat.* **126**:49–55.

Sinanan, K., Love, W. C., and Keatinge, A. M. B., 1974, Urinary cyclic AMP and depression, *Brit. J. Psychiat.* **125**:609–610.

Singhal, R. L., Kacew, S., and Lafreniere, R., 1973a, Brain adenyl cyclase in methadone treatment of morphine dependency, *J. Pharm. Pharmacol.* **25**:1022–1024.

Singhal, R. L., Lafreniere, R., and Ling, G. M., 1973b, Cerebrocortical adenyl cyclase activity following neonatal thyroid hormone deficiency, *Int. J. Clin. Pharmacol. Ther. Toxicol.* **8**:1–4.

Skolnick, P., and Daly, J. W., 1974a, Norepinephrine-elicited accumulation of adenosine 3',5'-monophosphate in brain slices: Relationship to spontaneous behavioral activity and levels of brain tyrosine hydroxylase in several rat strains, *Science* **184**:175–177.

Skolnick, P., and Daly, J. W., 1974b, The accumulation of adenosine 3',5'-monophosphate in cerebral cortical slices of the quaking mouse, a neurologic mutant, *Brain Res.,* **73**:513–525.

Skolnick, P., and Daly, J. W., 1975a, Functional compartments of adenine nucleotides serving as precursors of adenosine 3',5'-monophosphate in mouse cerebral cortex, *J. Neurochem.* **24**:451–456.

Skolnick, P., and Daly, J. W., 1975b, Stimulation of adenosine 3',5'-monophosphate formation in rat cerebral cortical slices by methoxamine: Interaction with an alpha-adrenergic receptor, *J. Pharmacol. Exp. Ther.,* **193**:549–558.

Skolnick, P., and Daly, J. W., 1975c, Stimulation of adenosine 3',5'-monophosphate formation by alpha and beta adrenergic agonists in rat cerebral cortical slices: Effects of clonidine, *Mol. Pharmacol.* **11**:545–551.

Skolnick, P., and Daly, J. W., 1976a, Interaction of clonidine with pre- and post-synaptic adrenergic receptors of rat brain: Effects on cyclic AMP-generating systems, *Eur. J. Pharmacol.* **39**:11–21.

Skolnick, P., and Daly, J. W., 1976b, Regulation of cyclic AMP formation in brain tissue by putative neurotransmitters, in *Cyclic Nucleotides: Mechanisms of Action* (H. Cramer and J. Schultz, eds.), John Wiley and Sons Ltd., Sussex, England, in press.

Skolnick, P., and Daly, J. P., 1976c, Antagonism of α- and β-adrenergic-mediated accumulations of cyclic AMP in rat cerebral cortical slices by the β-antagonist, (-)alprenolol, *Life Sci.* **19**:497–504.

Skolnick, P., Daly, J. W., Freedman, R., and Hoffer, B. J., 1976, Interrelationship between catecholamine-stimulated formation of cyclic AMP in cerebellar slices and inhibitory effects on cerebellar Purkinje cells: Antagonism by neuroleptic compounds, *J. Pharmacol. Exp. Ther.* **197**:280–292.

Skolnick, P., Huang, M., Daly, J., and Hoffer, B., 1973, Accumulation of adenosine 3',5'-monophosphate in incubated slices from discrete regions of squirrel monkey cerebral cortex: Effect of norepinephrine, serotonin and adenosine, *J. Neurochem.* **21**:237–240.

Skolnick, P., Schultz, J., and Daly, J. W., 1975, Repetitive stimulation of cyclic adenosine 3',5'-monophosphate formation by adrenergic agonists in incubated slices from rat cerebral cortex, *J. Neurochem.,* **24**:1263–1265.

Sloboda, R. D., Rudolph, S. A., Rosenbaum, J. L., and Greengard, P., 1975, Cyclic AMP-dependent endogeneous phosphorylation of microtubule-associated protein, *Proc. Nat. Acad. Sci. USA* **72**:177–181.

Smoake, J. A., Song, S.-Y., and Cheung, W. Y., 1974, Cyclic 3',5'-nucleotide phosphodiesterase. Distribution and developmental changes of the enzyme and its protein activator in mammalian tissues and cells, *Biochim. Biophys. Acta* **341**:402–411.

Snyder, S. H., 1976, The dopamine hypothesis of schizophrenia: Focus on the dopamine receptor, *Amer. J. Psychiat.* **133**:197–202.

Soifer, D., 1975, Enzymatic activity in tubulin preparations: Cyclic-AMP dependent protein kinase activity of brain microtubule protein, *J. Neurochem.* **24**:21–33.

Soifer, D., Laszlo, A. H., and Scotto, J. M., 1972, Enzymatic activity in tubulin preparations. I. Intrinsic protein kinase activity in lyophilized preparations of tubulin from porcine brain, *Biochim. Biophys. Acta* **271**:182–192.

Soifer, D., Laszlo, A., Mack, K., Scotto, J., and Siconolfi, L., 1975, The association of a cyclic AMP-dependent protein kinase activity with microtubule protein, *Ann. N.Y. Acad. Sci.* **253**:598–610.

Sold, G., and Hofmann, F., 1974, Evidence for a guanosine-3',5'-monophosphate-binding protein from rat cerebellum, *Eur. J. Biochem.* **44**:143–149.

Solomon, F., Gysin, R., Rentsch, M. and Monard, D., 1976, Purification of tubulin from neuroblastoma cells: Absence of covalently bound phosphate in tubulin from normal and morphologically differentiated cells, *FEBS Lett.* **63**:316–319.

Somerville, A. R., 1973, Adenosine 3',5'-cyclic monophosphate and affective disorders, *Biochem. Soc. Spec. Publ.* **1**:127–132.

Somerville, A. R., and Smith, A. A., 1972, The effects of propranolol and electrical stimulation on the cyclic 3',5'-AMP content of isolated cerebral tissue, *J. Neurochem.* **19**:2003–2006.

Spano, P. F. and Trabucchi, M., 1976, On the cyclic nucleotides involvement in rat striatal function. *Pharmacol. Res. Commun.* **8**:143–148.

Spano, P. F., Kumakura, K., Govoni, S., and Trabucchi, M., 1975a, Post-natal development and regulation of cerebellar cyclic guanosine monophosphate system, *Pharmacol. Res. Commun.* **7**:223–237.

Spano, P. F., Kumakura, K., Tonon, G. C., Govoni, S., and Trabucchi, M., 1975b, LSD and dopamine-sensitive adenylate cyclase in various rat brain areas, *Brain Res.* **93**:164–167.

Spehlman, R., 1975, The effects of acetylcholine and dopamine on the caudate nucleus depleted of biogenic amines, *Brain Res.* **98**:219–230.

Spiker, M. D., Palmer, G. C., and Manian, A. A., 1976, Action of neuroleptic agents on histamine-sensitive adenylate cyclase in rabbit cerebral cortex, *Brain Res.* **104**:401–406.

Stalvey, L., Daly, J. W., and Dismukes, R. K., 1976, Behavioral activity and accumulation of cyclic AMP in brain slices of strains of mice, *Life Sci.,* in press.

Stefanovich, V., 1974, Concerning specificity of the influence of pentoxifyline on various cyclic AMP phosphodiesterases, *Res. Commun. Chem. Pathol. Pharmacol.* **8**673–680.

Stefanovich, V., and John, J. P., 1974, Increase of cyclic AMP in rat brain during anoxia, *Res. Commun. Chem. Pathol. Pharmacol.* **9**:591–593.

Stefanovich, V., Von Polnitz, M., and Reiser, M., 1974, Inhibition of various cyclic AMP phosphodiesterases by pentifylline and theophylline, *Arzneimittelforschung* **24**:1747–1751.

Steinbach, J. H., and Schubert, D., 1975, Multiple modes of dibutyryl cyclic AMP-induced process formation by clonal nerve and glial cells, *Exp. Cell Res.* **91**:449–453.

Steiner, A. L., Ferrendelli, J. A., and Kipnis, D. M., 1972, Radioimmunoassay for cyclic nucleotides. III. Effect of ischemia, changes during development and regional distribution of adenosine 3',5'-monophosphate and guanosine 3',5'-monophosphate in mouse brain, *J. Biol. Chem.* **247**:1121–1124.

Steiner, A. L., Parker, C. W., and Kipnis, D. M., 1970, The measurement of cyclic nucleotides by radioimmunoassay, *Advan. Biochem. Psychopharmacol.* **3**:89–112.

Steiner, F. A., and Felix, D., 1976, Antagonistic effects of GABA and benzodiazepines on vestibular and cerebellar neurones, *Nature (London)* **260**:346–347.

Stone, T. W., Taylor, D. A., and Bloom, F. E., 1975, Cyclic AMP and cyclic GMP may mediate opposite neuronal responses in the rat cerebral cortex, *Science* **187**:845–847.

Strada, S. J., and Pledger, W. J., 1975, The role of cyclic nucleotides in cell growth and development: Regulation and characterization of cyclic nucleotide phosphodiesterases in mammalian cells, in *Cyclic Nucleotides in Disease* (B. Weiss, ed.), pp. 3–34, University Park Press, Baltimore.

Strada, S. J., and Weiss, B., 1974, Increased response to catecholamines of the cyclic AMP system of rat pineal gland induced by decreased sympathetic activity, *Arch. Biochem. Biophys.* **160**:197–204.

Strada, S. J., Kirkegaard, L., and Thompson, W. J., 1976, Studies of rat pineal gland guanylate cyclase, *Neuropharmacology* **15**:261–266.

Strada, S. J., Uzunov, P., and Weiss, B., 1974, Ontogenetic development of a phosphodiesterase activator and the multiple forms of cyclic AMP phosphodiesterase of rat brain, *J. Neurochem.* **23**:1097–1104.

Straschill, M., and Perwein, J., 1969, The inhibition of retinal ganglion cells by catecholamines and γ-aminobutyric acid, *Pfluegers Arch.* **312**:45–54.

Sturgill, T. W., Schrier, M. B. K., and Gilman, A. G. 1975, Stimulation of cyclic AMP accumulation by 2-chloroadenosine: Lack of incorporation of nucleoside into cyclic nucleotides, *J. Cyclic Nucleotide Res.* **1**:21–30.

Sulakhe, P. V., and Phillis, J. W., 1975, The release of ^{3}H-adenosine and its derivatives from cat sensorimotor cortex, *Life Sci.* **17**:551–556.

Sun, M. -C., McIlwain, H., and Pull, I., 1976, The metabolism of adenine derivatives in different parts of the brain of the rat, and their release from hypothalamic preparations on excitation, *J. Neurobiol.* **7**:109–122.

Sundarraj, N., Schackner, M., and Pfeiffer, S. E., 1975, Biochemically differentiated mouse glial lines carrying a nervous system specific cell surface antigen, *Proc. Nat. Acad. Sci. USA* **72**:1927–1931.

Suria, A., 1976, Cyclic GMP modulates the intensity of post-tetanic potentiation in bullfrog sympathetic ganglia, *Neuropharmacology* **15**:11–16.

Suria, A., and Costa, E., 1973, Benzodiazepines and posttetanic potentiation in sympathetic ganglia of the bullfrog, *Brain Res.* **50**:235–239.

Suria, A., and Costa, E., 1974, Diazepam inhibition of post-tetanic potentiation in bullfrog sympathetic ganglia: possible role of prostaglandins, *J. Pharmacol. Exp. Ther.* **189**:690–696.

Suria, A., and Costa, E., 1975a, Action of diazepam, dibutyryl cGMP and GABA on presynaptic nerve terminals in bull frog sympathetic ganglia, *Brain Res.* **87**:102–106.

Suria, A., and Costa, E., 1975b, Evidence by GABA involvement in the action of diazepam on presynaptic nerve terminals in bullfrog sympathetic ganglia, *Advan. Biochemical Psychopharmacol.* **14**:103–112.

Sutherland, E. W., Rall, T. W., and Menon, T., 1962, Adenyl cyclase, I. Distribution preparation and properties, *J. Biol. Chem.* **237**:1220–1227.

Swislocki, N. I., and Tierney, J., 1973, Solubilization, stabilization, and partial purification of brain adenylate cyclase from rat, *Biochemistry* **12**:1862–1866.

Tagliamonte, A., Tagliamonte, P., Forn, J., Perez-Cruet, J., Krishna, G., and Gessa, G. L.,

1971a, Stimulation of brain serotonin synthesis by dibutyryl-cyclic AMP in rats, *J. Neurochem.* **18**:1191–1196.

Tagliamonte, A., Tagliamonte, P., Perez-Cruet, J., and Gessa, G. L., 1971b, Increase of brain tryptophan caused by drugs that stimulate serotonin synthesis, *Nature New Biol.* **229**:125–126.

Tagliamonte, A., Tagliamonte, P., Perez-Cruet, J., Stern, A., and Gessa, G. L., 1971c, Effect of psychotropic drugs on tryptophan concentration in the rat brain, *J. Pharmacol. Exp. Ther.* **177**:475–480.

Takagaki, G., 1972, Control of aerobic glycolysis in guinea-pig cerebral cortex slices, *J. Neurochem.* **19**:1737–1751.

Takahashi, T., Matsuzaki, S., and Nunez, J., 1975, Modifications in soluble protein kinase and cyclic-AMP binding capacity in developing rat brain, *J. Neurochem.* **24**:303–310.

Takai, Y., Nichiyama, K., Yamamura, H., and Nishizuka, Y., 1975, Guanosine 3′,5′-monophosphate-dependent protein kinase from bovine cerebellum. Purification and characterization, *J. Biol. Chem.* **250**:4690–4695.

Takamori, M., Ishii, M., and Mori, M., 1973, The role of cyclic 3′,5′-adenosine monophosphate in neuromuscular transmission, *Arch. Neurol.* **29**:420–422.

Taneda, M., Izumi, F., and Ika, M., 1974, Effect of dibutyryl adenosine 3′,5′-monophosphate on catecholamine synthesis in rat brain cortical slices and isolated vasa deferentia, *Jap. J. Pharmacol.* **24**:934–936.

Tang, L. C., Cotzias, G. C., and Dunn, M., 1974, Changing the actions of neuroactive drugs by charging brain protein synthesis, *Proc. Nat. Acad. Sci. USA* **71**:3350–3354.

Tell, G. P., Pasternak, G. W., and Cuatrecasas, P., 1975, Brain and caudate nucleus adenylate cyclase: Effects of dopamine, GTP, E prostaglandins and morphine, *FEBS Lett.* **51**:242–245.

Teshima, Y., and Kakiuchi, S., 1974, Mechanism of stimulation of Ca^{2+} plus Mg^{2+}-dependent phosphodiesterase from rat cerebral cortex by the modulator protein and Ca^{2+}, *Biochem. Biophys. Res. Commun.* **56**:489–495.

Teshima, Y., Yamazaki, R., and Kakiuchi, S., 1974, Effects of ATP on the activity of nucleoside 3′,5′-cyclic monophosphate phosphodiesterase from brain, *J. Neurochem.* **22**:789–791.

Thompson, W. J., and Appleman, M. M., 1971a, Characterizations of cyclic nucleotide phosphodiesterases of rat tissues, *J. Biol. Chem.* **246**:3145–3150.

Thompson, W. J., and Appleman, M. M., 1971b, Multiple cyclic nucleotide phosphodiesterase activities from rat brain, *Biochemistry* **10**:311–316.

Thompson, W. J., and Appleman, M. M., 1971c, Cyclic nucleotide phosphodiesterase and cyclic AMP, *Ann. N.Y. Acad. Sci.* **185**:36–41.

Thust, R., and Warzok, R., 1975, Differential morphological reaction of experimental CNS tumour clones *in vitro* to dibutyryl cyclic AMP or serum-free medium, resp., *Acta Neuropathol.* **33**:325–332.

Torda, C., 1972a, Cyclic AMP-dependent diphosphoinositide kinase, *Biochim. Biophys. Acta* **286**:389–395.

Torda, C., 1972b, Hyperpolarization by cyclic AMP (activation of diphosphoinositide kinase), *Experientia* **28**:1438–1439.

Torda, C., 1974, Restorative effect of cyclic AMP on the bioelectric processes of calcium deprived ganglia, *Experientia* **30**:1154–1155.

Traber, J., Fischer, K., Latzin, S., and Hamprecht, B., 1974, Morphine antagonizes the action of prostaglandin in neuroblastoma cells but not of prostaglandin and noradrenaline in glioma and glioma × fibroblast hybrid cells, *FEBS Lett.* **49**:260–263.

Traber, J., Fischer, K., Buchen, C., and Hamprecht, B., 1975a, Muscarinic response to acetylcholine in neuroblastoma × glioma hybrid cells, *Nature (London)* **255**:558–560.

Traber, J., Fischer, K., Latzin, S., and Hamprecht, B., 1975b, Morphine antagonizes action of prostaglandin in neuroblastoma and neuroblastoma × glioma hybrid cells, *Nature (London)* **253**:120–122.

Traber, J., Gullis, R., and Hamprecht, B., 1975c, Influence of opiates on the levels of adenosine 3',5'-cyclic monophosphate in neuroblastoma × glioma hybrid cells, *Life Sci.* **16**:1863–1868.

Traber, J., Reiser, G., Fischer, K., and Hamprecht, B., 1975d, Measurements of adenosine 3',5' cyclic monophosphate and membrane potential in neuroblastoma × glioma hybrid cells: Opiates and adrenergic agonists cause effects opposite to those of prostaglandin E_1, *FEBS Lett.* **52**:327–332.

Trams, E. G., and Lauter, C. J., 1975, Adenosine deaminase of cultured brain cells, *Biochem. J.* **152**:681–687.

Troyer, E. W., and Ferrendelli, J. A., 1976, Two forms of guanylate cyclase in cerebellum, *Fed. Proc.* **35**:456(Abs.).

Truding, R., Shelanski, M. L., Daniels, M. P., and Morell, P., 1974, Comparison of surface membranes isolated from cultured murine neuroblastoma cells in the differentiated or undifferentiated state, *J. Biol. Chem.* **249**:3973–3982.

Tsuzuki, J., and Newburgh, R. W., 1975, Inhibition of 5'-nucleotidase in rat brain by methylxanthines, *J. Neurochem.* **25**:895–896.

Ueda, T., Maeno, H., and Greengard, P., 1973, Regulation of endogenous phosphorylation of specific proteins in synaptic membrane fractions from rat brain by adenosine 3':5'-monophosphate, *J. Biol. Chem.* **248**:8295–8305.

Ueda, T., Rudolph, S. A., and Greengard, P., 1975, Solubilization of a phosphoprotein and its associated cyclic AMP-dependent protein kinase and phosphoprotein phosphatase from synaptic membrane fractions and some kinetic evidence for their existence as a complex, *Arch. Biochem. Biophys.* **170**:492–503.

Ungerstedt, U., Ljungberg, T., Hoffer, B., and Siggins, G., 1975, Dopaminergic supersensitivity in the striatum, *Advan. Neurol.* **9**:57–65.

Uno, H., Meyer, R. B., Shuman, D. A., Robins, R. K., Simon, L. N., and Miller, J. P., 1976a, Synthesis of some 1,8- and 2,8-disubstituted derivatives of adenosine cyclic 3',5'-phosphate and their interaction with some enzymes of cAMP metabolism, *J. Med. Chem.* **19**:419–422.

Uno, I., Ueda, T., and Greengard, P., 1976b, Differences in properties of cytosol and membrane-derived protein kinases, *J. Biol. Chem.* **251**:2192–2195.

Uzunov, P., and Weiss, B., 1971, Effects of phenothiazine tranquilizers on the cyclic 3',5'-adenosine monophosphate system of rat brain, *Neuropharmacology* **10**:697–708.

Uzunov, P., and Weiss, B., 1972a, Separation of multiple molecular forms of cyclic adenosine 3',5'-monophosphate phosphodiesterase in rat cerebellum by polyacrylamide gel electrophoresis, *Biochim. Biophys. Acta* **284**:220–226.

Uzunov, P., and Weiss, B., 1972b, Psychopharmacological agents and the cyclic AMP system in rat brain, *Advan. Cyclic Nucleotide Res.* **1**:435–453.

Uzunov, P., Revuelta, A., and Costa, E., 1975, A role for the endogenous activator of 3',5'-nucleotide phosphodiesterase in rat adrenal medulla, *Mol. Pharmacol.* **11**:506–510.

Uzunov, P., Shein, H. M., and Weiss, B., 1973, Cyclic AMP phosphodiesterase in cloned astrocytoma cells: Norepinephrine induces a specific enzyme form, *Science* **180**:304–306.

Uzunov, P., Shein, H. M., and Weiss, B., 1974, Multiple forms of cyclic 3',5'-AMP phosphodiesterase of rat cerebrum and cloned astrocytoma and neuroblastoma cells, *Neuropharmacology* **13**:377–392.

Van de Berg, J. S., 1974, Inhibitory effects of dibutyryl and cyclic AMP on the compound action potential in the frog *(Rana pipiens)* sciatic nerve, *Experientia* **30**:1025–1026.

Van Inwegen, R. G., Strada, S. J., and Robison, G. A., 1975, Effects of prostaglandins and morphine on brain adenyl cyclase, *Life Sci.* **16**:1875–1876.

Vapaatalo, H., 1974, Role of cyclic nucleotides in the nervous system, *Med. Biol. 52:*200–207.

Vapaatalo, H., and Anttila, P., 1972, Effects of some inhibitors of phosphodiesterase on neuromuscular transmission, *Naunyn-Schmiedeberg's Arch. Pharmacol.* **275:**227–232.

Varagic, V. M., and Beleslin, D. B., 1973, The effect of cyclic *N*-2-*O*-dibutyryladenosine-3′,5′-monophosphate, adenosine triphosphate and butyrate on the body temperatures of conscious cats, *Brain Res.* **57:**252–254.

Varagic, V. M., and Zugic, M., 1971, Interactions of xanthine derivatives, catecholamines and glucose-6-phosphate on the isolated phrenic nerve diaphragm preparation of the rat, *Pharmacology* **5:**275–286.

Varagic, V. M., and Zugic, M., 1973, The effect of N^6-2′-*O*-dibutyryl 3′,5′-cyclic adenosine monophosphate, imidazole and aminophylline on ganglionic transmission in the superior cervical ganglion of the cat, *Brit. J. Pharmacol.* **49:**407–414.

Varagic, V. M., Zugic, M., and Mrsulja, B. B., 1972, The effect of cyclic *N*-2-*O*-dibutyryl-adenosine-3′,5′-monophosphate on neuromuscular transmission and concentration of glycogen in the isolated phrenic nerve-diaphragm preparation of the rat, *Experientia* **28:**305–306.

Vargui, L., and Spano, P. F., 1971, Some central effects of a new derivative of cyclic 3′,5′-adenosine monophosphate, *Naunyn-Schmiedebergs Arch. Pharmacol.* **269:**410Abs.

Vedeckis, W. V., and Gilbert, L. I., 1973, Production of cyclic AMP and adenosine by the brain and prothoracic glands of *Manduca sexta, J. Insec. Physiol.* **19:**2445–2457.

Vernikos-Danellis, J., and Harris, C. G., III, 1968, The effect of *in vitro* and *in vivo* caffeine, theophylline and hydrocortisone on the phosphodiesterase activity of the pituitary, median eminence, heart and cerebral cortex of the rat, *Proc. Soc. Exp. Biol. Med.* **128:**1016–1021.

Vetulani, J., and Sulser, F., 1975, Action of various antidepressant treatments reduces reactivity of noradrenergic cyclic AMP-generating system in limbic forebrain, *Nature (London)* **257:**495–496.

Vetulani, J., Stawarz, R. J., Blumberg, J. B., and Sulser, F., 1975, Adaptive mechanisms in the norepinephrine (NE)-sensitive cyclic AMP generating system in the slices of the rat limbic forebrain (LFS). *Fed. Proc.* **34:**265Abs.

Virmaux, N., Nullans, G., and Goridis, C., 1976, Guanylate cyclase in vertebrate retina: Evidence for specific association with rod outer segments, *J. Neurochem.* **26:**233–235.

Volicer, L., and Gold, B. I., 1973, Effect of ethanol on cyclic AMP levels in the rat brain, *Life Sci.* **13:**269–280.

Volicer, L., Hurter, B. P., Williams, R., and Puri, S. K., 1976, Effects of acute and chronic ethanol administration and ethanol withdrawal on guanosine 3′,5′-monophosphate (cGMP) and gamma-aminobutyric acid (GABA) levels in the rat brain, *Fed. Proc.* **35:**467Abs.

Von Hungen, K., and Roberts, S., 1973a, Adenylate-cyclase receptors for adrenergic neuro-transmitters in rat cerebral cortex, *Eur. J. Biochem.* **36:**391–401.

Von Hungen, K., and Roberts, S., 1973b, Catecholamine and Ca^{2+} activation of adenylate cyclase systems in synaptosomal fractions from rat cerebral cortex, *Nature New Biol.* **242:**58–60.

Von Hungen, K. and Roberts, S., 1974, Neurotransmitter-sensitive adenylate cyclase systems in the brain, in *Reviews of Neuroscience* (S. Ehrenpreis, and I. J. Kopin, eds.), Vol. 1, pp. 231–281, Raven Press, New York.

Von Hungen, K., Roberts, S., and Hill, D. F., 1974, Developmental and regional variations in neurotransmitter-sensitive adenylate cyclase systems in cell-free preparations from rat brain, *J. Neurochem.* **22:**811–819.

Von Hungen, K., Roberts, S., and Hill, D. F., 1975a, Interactions between lysergic acid diethylamide and dopamine-sensitive adenylate cyclase systems in rat brain, *Brain Res.* **94:**57–66.

Von Hungen, K., Roberts, S., and Hill, D. F., 1975b, Serotonin-sensitive adenylate cyclase activity in immature rat brain, *Brain Res.* **84**:257–268.

Von Voigtlander, P. F., Boukma, S. J., and Johnson G. A., 1973, Dopaminergic denervation supersensitivity and dopamine stimulated adenyl cyclase activity, *Neuropharmacology* **12**:1081–1086.

Von Voightlander, P. F., Losey, E. G., and Triezenberg, H. S., 1975, Increased sensitivity to dopaminergic agents after chronic neuroleptic treatment, *J. Pharmacol. Exp. Ther.* **193**:88–94.

Wahlstrom, G., 1975, The effects of cyclic 3′,5′adenosine monophosphate on the acute tolerance induced by ethanol in male rats, *Life Sci.* **17**:1655–1662.

Wahn, H. L., Lightbody, L. E., Tchen, T. T., and Taylor, J. D., 1975a, Induction of neural differentiation in cultures of amphibian undetermined presumptive epidermis by cyclic AMP derivatives, *Science* **188**:366–369.

Wahn, H. L., Lightbody, L. E., Tchen, T. T., and Taylor, J. D., 1975b, Identification of neurons in cultures, *Science* **190**:490.

Waldeck, D., 1971, Some effects of caffeine and aminophylline on the turnover of catecholamines in the brain, *J. Pharm. Pharmacol.* **23**:824–830.

Waldeck, B., 1975, Effect of caffeine on locomotor activity and central catecholamine mechanisms: A study with special reference to drug interaction, *Acta Pharmacol. Toxicol.* **36**:4–23.

Walinder, O., 1972, Calf brain phosvitin kinase: Purification of the kinase associated with a phosphate-incorporating protein, *Biochim. Biophys. Acta* **258**:411–421.

Walinder, O., 1973, Calf brain phosvitin kinase. II. Purification and characterization of three different fractions of phosvitin kinase, *Biochim. Biophys. Acta* **293**:140–149.

Walker, J. B., 1974, The effect of lithium on hormone-sensitive adenylate cyclase from various regions of the rat brain, *Biol. Psychiat.* **8**:245–252.

Walker, J. B., and Walker, J. P., 1973a, Neurohumoral regulation of adenylate cyclase activity in rat striatum, *Brain Res.* **54**:386–390.

Walker, J. B., and Walker, J. P., 1973b, Properties of adenylate cyclase from senescent rat brain, *Brain Res.* **54**:391–396.

Walker, J. E., Lewin, E., and Moffit, B., 1974, Production of epileptiform discharges by application of agents which increase cyclic AMP levels in rat cortex, in *Epilepsy: Proceedings of the Hans Berger Centenary Symposium* (P. Harris and C. Mawdsley, eds.), pp. 30–36, Churchill Livingstone, New York.

Walker, J. E., Lewin, E., Sheppard, J. R., and Cromwell, R., 1973, Enzymatic regulation of adenosine 3′,5′-monophosphate (cyclic AMP) in the freezing epileptogenic lesion of rat brain and in homologous contralateral cortex, *J. Neurochem.* **21**:79–85.

Walland, A., 1975, cAMP as a second messenger in central blood pressue control, *Naunyn-Schmiedeberg's Arch. Pharmacol.* **290**:419–423.

Walsh, D. A., Ashby, C. D., Gonzalez, C., Calkins, D., Fischer, E. H., and Krebs, E. G., 1971, Purification and characterization of a protein inhibitor of adenosine 3′,5′-monophosphate-dependent protein kinases, *J. Biol. Chem.* **246**:1977–1985.

Wang, Y.-C., Pandey, G. N., Mendels, J., and Frazer, A., 1974, Platelet adenylate cyclase responses in depression: Implications for a receptor defect, *Psychopharmacologica* **36**:291–300.

Waris, J., Richard, L., and Waris, R., 1973, Differentiation of neuroblastoma cells induced by nerve growth factor, *Experientia* **29**:1128–1129.

Wasner, H. K., 1975, Regulation of protein kinase and phosphoprotein phosphatase by cyclic AMP and cyclic AMP antagonist, *FEBS Lett.* **57**:60–63.

Watanabe, H., and Ishii, S., 1976, The effect of brain ischemia on the levels of cyclic AMP and glycogen metabolism in gerbil brain *in vivo*, *Brain Res.* **102**:385–389.

Watanabe, H., and Passonneau, J. V., 1974, The effect of trauma on cerebral glycogen and related metabolites and enzymes, *Brain Res.* **66**:147–159.

Watanabe, H., and Passonneau, J. V., 1975, Cyclic adenosine monophosphate in cerebral cortex. Alterations following trauma, *Arch. Neurol.* **32**:181–184.

Watterson, D. M., Harrelson, W. G., Keller, P. M., Sharief, F., and Vanaman, T. C., 1976, Structural similarities between the Ca^{2+}-dependent regulatory proteins of 3':5'-cyclic nucleotide phosphodiesterase and actomyosin ATPase, *J. Biol. Chem.* **251**:4501–4513.

Waymire, J. C., Weiner, N., and Prasad, K. N., 1972, Regulation of tyrosine hydroxylase activity in cultured mouse neuroblastoma cells: Elevation induced by analogs of adenosine 3':5'-cyclic monophosphate, *Proc. Nat. Acad. Sci. USA* **69**:2241–2245.

Webb, J. G., Berv, K. R., and Kopin, I. J., 1975, Induction of dopamine-β-hydroxylase in superior cervical ganglia in organ culture, *Neuropharmacology* **14**:643–648.

Weight, F. F., Petzold, G., and Greengard, P., 1974, Guanosine 3',5'-monophosphate in sympathetic ganglia: Increase associated with synaptic transmission, *Science* **186**:942–944.

Weiner, M., and Olson, J. W., 1973, The behavioral effects of dibutyryl cyclic AMP in mice, *Life Sci.* **12**:345–356.

Weiner, M., and Olson, J. W., 1975, Comparative behavioral effects of dibutyryl cyclic AMP and prostaglandin E_1 in mice, *Prostaglandins* **9**:927–943.

Weinryb, I., Chasin, M., Free, C. A., Harris, D. N., Goldenberg, H., Michel, I. M., Paik, V. S., Phillips, M., Samaniego, S., and Hess, S. M., 1972, Effects of therapeutic agents on cyclic AMP metabolism *in vitro*, *J. Pharmaceut. Sci.* **61**:1556–1567.

Weiss, B., 1969, Effects of environmental lighting and chronic denervation on the activation of adenyl cyclase of rat pineal gland by norepinephrine and sodium flouride, *J. Pharmacol. Exp. Ther.* **168**:146–152.

Weiss, B., 1971, Ontogenetic development of adenyl cyclase and phosphodiesterase in rat brain, *J. Neurochem.* **18**:469–477.

Weiss, B., 1972, Psychopharmacological agents and the cyclic AMP system of rat brain, *Advan. Cyclic Nucleotide Res.* **1**:435–453.

Weiss, B., 1975, Differential activation and inhibition of multiple forms of cyclic nucleotide phosphodiesterase, *Advan. Cyclic Nucleotide Res.* **5**:195–211.

Weiss, B., and Costa, E., 1967, Adenyl cyclase activity in rat pineal gland: Effects of chronic denervation and norepinephrine, *Science* **156**:1750–1752.

Weiss, B., and Costa, E., 1968, Regional and subcellular distribution of adenyl cyclase and 3',5'-cyclic nucleotide phosphodiesterase in brain and pineal gland, *Biochem. Pharmacol.* **17**:2107–2116.

Weiss, B., and Greenberg, L. H., 1975, Cyclic AMP and Brain Function: Effects of psychopharmacologic agents on the cyclic AMP system, in *Cyclic Nucleotides in Disease* (B. Weiss, ed.), pp. 269–319, University Park Press, Baltimore.

Weiss, B., and Stiller, R. L., 1974, Dibutyrylcyclic adenosine 3',5'-monophosphate and brain lipid metabolism, *Lipids* **9**:514–519.

Weiss, B., and Strada, S. J., 1972, Neuroendocrine control of the cyclic AMP system of brain and pineal gland, *Advan. Cyclic Nucleotide Res.* **1**:357–374.

Weiss, B., and Strada, S. J., 1973, Adenosine 3',5'-monophosphate during fetal and postnatal development, in *Fetal Pharmacology,* (L. O. Borens, ed.), pp. 205–232, Raven Press, New York.

Weiss, B., Shein, H. M., and Snyder, R., 1971, Adenylate cyclase and phosphodiesterase activity of normal and SV_{40} virus transformed hamster astrocytes in cell culture, *Life Sci.* **10(I)**:1253–1260.

Weiss, B., Fertel, R., Figlin, R., and Uzunov, P., 1974, Selective alteration of the activity of the multiple forms of adenosine 3',5'-monophosphate phosphodiesterase of rat cerebrum, *Mol. Pharmacol.* **10**:615–625.

Weissman, B. A., and Skolnick, P., 1975, Stimulation of adenosine 3',5'-monophosphate formation in incubated rat hypothalamus by estrogenic compounds: Relationship to biologic potency and blockade by anti-estrogens, *Neuroendocrinology* **18**:27–34.

Weissman, B. A., Daly, J. W., and Skolnick, P., 1975, Diethylstilbestrol-elicited accumulation of cyclic AMP in incubated rat hypothalamus, *Endocrinology* **97**:1559–1566.

Welch, K. M. A., Meyer, J. S., and Chee, A. N. C., 1975, Evidence for disordered cyclic AMP metabolism in patients with cerebral infarction, *Eur. Neurol.* **13**:144–154.

Weller, M., and Morgan, I. G., 1976, Localization in the synaptic junction of the cyclic AMP stimulated intrinsic protein kinase activity of synaptasomal plasma membranes, *Biochim. Biophys. Acta* **433**:223–228.

Weller, M., and Rodnight, R., 1970, Stimulation by cyclic AMP of intrinsic protein kinase activity in ox brain membrane preparation, *Nature (London)* **225**:187–188.

Weller, M., and Rodnight, R., 1971, Turnover of protein-bound phosphorylserine in membrane preparations of ox brain catalyzed by intrinsic kinase and phosphatase activity, *Biochem. J.* **124**:393–406.

Weller, M., and Rodnight, R., 1973a, Protein kinase activity in membrane preparations from ox brain: Stimulation of intrinsic activity by adenosine 3′:5′-cyclic monophosphate, *Biochem. J.* **132**:483–492.

Weller, M., and Rodnight, R., 1973b, The state of phosphorylation *in vivo* of membrane-bound phosphoproteins in rat brain, *Biochem. J.* **133**:387–389.

Weller, M., and Rodnight, R., 1975a, Observations on the binding of adenosine 3′:5′-monophosphate to cell membrane fragments from ox cerebral cortex, *Biochim. Biophys. Acta* **389**:573–577.

Weller, M., and Rodnight, R., 1975b, Protein kinase activity stimulated by adenosine 3′:5′-cyclic monophosphate in synaptic-membrane fragments from ox brain, *Biochem. J.* **142**:605–609.

Weller, M., Rodnight, R., and Carrera, D., 1972, Determination of adenosine 3′,5′-cyclic monophosphate in cerebral tissues by saturation analysis: Assessment of a method using a binding protein from ox muscle, *Biochem. J.* **129**:113–121.

Weller, M., Goridis, C., Virmaux, N., and Mandel, P., 1975a, A hypothetical model for the possible involvement of rhodopsin phosphorylation in light and dark adaptation in the retina, *Exp. Eye Res.* **21**:405–408.

Weller, M., Virmaux, N., and Mandel, P., 1975b, Light stimulates phosphorylation of rhodopsin in the retina: The presence of a protein-kinase which is special for photobleached rhodopsin, *Proc. Nat. Acad. Sci. USA* **72**:381–385.

Weller, M., Virmaux, N., and Mandel, P., 1975c, The role of light and rhodopsin phosphorylation in the control of the permeability of retinal rod outer segment discs to Ca^{2+}, *Nature (London)* **256**:68–70.

Wellmann, W., and Schwabe, U., 1973, Effects of prostaglandins E_1, E_2 and $F_{2\alpha}$ on cyclic AMP levels in brain *in vivo*, *Brain Res.* **59**:371–378.

Werner, I., Peterson, G. R., and Shuster, L., 1971, Choline acetyltransferase and acetylcholine esterase in cultured brain cells from chick embryos, *J. Neurochem.* **18**:141–151.

Wexler, B., and Katzman, R., 1975, Effects of dibutyryl cyclic AMP on tyrosine uptake and metabolism in neuroblastoma cultures, *Exp. Cell Res.* **92**:291–298.

White, A. A., and Aurbach, G. D., 1969, Detection of guanyl cyclase in mammalian tissues, *Biochim. Biophys. Acta* **191**:686–697.

Wickson, R. D., Boudreau, R. J., and Drummond, G. I., 1975, Activation of 3′,5′-cyclic adenosine monophosphate phosphodiesterase by calcium ion and a protein activator *Biochemistry* **14**:669–675.

Wilkening, D., and Makman, M. H., 1975, 2-Chloroadenosine-dependent elevation of adenosine 3′,5′-monophosphate levels in rat caudate nucleus slices, *Brain Res.* **92**:522–528.

Williams, B. J., and Pirch, J. H., 1974, Correlation between brain adenyl cyclase activity and spontaneous motor activity in rats after chronic reserpine treatment, *Brain Res.* **68**:227–234.

Williams, M., and Rodnight, R., 1974, Evidence for a role for protein phosphorylation in synaptic function in the cerebral cortex mediated through a β-noradrenergic receptor, *Brain Res.* **77**:502–506.

Williams, M., and Rodnight, R., 1975, Stimulation of protein phosphorylation in brain slices by electrical pulses: Speed of response and evidence for net phosphorylation, *J. Neurochem.* **24**:601–603.

Williams, M., and Rodnight, R., 1976, Protein phosphorylation in respiring slices of guinea pig cerebral cortex. Evidence for a role for noradrenaline and adenosine 3':5'-cyclic monophosphate in the increased phosphorylation observed on application of electrical pulses, *Biochem. J.* **154**:163–170.

Williams, M., Pavlik, A., and Rodnight, R., 1974a, Cellular localization of phosphoproteins in guinea pig cerebral cortex slices sensitive to noradrenaline, histamine and 5-hydroxytryptamine, *Trans. Biochem. Soc.* **2**:259–261.

Williams, M., Pavlik, A., and Rodnight, R., 1974b, Turnover of protein phosphorus in respiring slices of guinea pig cerebral cortex: Cellular localization of phosphoprotein sensitive to electrical stimulation, *J. Neurochem.* **22**:373–376.

Williams, R. E., 1976, Phosphorylated sites in substrates of intracellular protein kinases: A common feature in amino acid sequences, *Science* **192**:473–474.

Williams, R. H., Little, S. A., Beug, A. G., and Ensinck, J. W., 1971, Cyclic nucleotide phosphodiesterase activity in man, monkey, and rat, *Metab. Clin. Exp.* **20**:743–748.

Williams, R. H., Little, S. A., and Ensinck, J. W., 1969, Adenyl cyclase and phosphodiesterase activities in brain areas of man, monkey and rat, *Amer. J. Med Sci.* **258**:190–202.

Williams, T. H., Black, A. C., Chiba, T., and Bhalla, R. C., 1975, Morphology and biochemistry of small, intensely fluorescent cells of sympathetic ganglia, *Nature (London)* **256**:315–317.

Willies, G. H., Woolf, C. J., and Rosendorff, C., 1976, The effect of sodium salicylate on dibutyryl cyclic AMP fever in the conscious rabbit, *Neuropharmacology* **15**:9–10.

Wilson, D. F., 1974, The effects of dibutyryl cyclic adenosine 3',5'-monophosphate, theophylline and aminophylline on neuromuscular transmission in the rat. *J. Pharmacol. Exp. Ther.* **188**:447–452.

Wintzerith, M., Ciesielski-Treska, J., Dierich, A., and Mandel, P., 1976, Comparative investigation of free nucleotides in two neuroblastoma clonal cell lines, *J. Neurochem.* **26**:205–207.

Witt, J. J., and Roskoski, R., 1975, Bovine brain adenosine 3',5'-monophosphate dependent protein kinase. Mechanism of regulatory subunit inhibition of the catalytic subunit, *Biochemistry* **14**:4503–4507.

Wolff, D. J., and Brostrom, C. O., 1974, Calcium-binding phosphoprotein from pig brain: Identification as a calcium-dependent regulator of brain cyclic nucleotide phosphodiesterase, *Arch. Biochem. Biophys.* **163**:349–358.

Wolff, D. J., and Brostrom, C. D., 1976, Calcium-dependent cyclic nucleotide phosphodiesterase from brain: Identification of phospholipids as calcium-independent activators, *Arch. Biochem. Biophys.* **173**:720–731.

Wolff, D. J., and Siegel, F., 1972, Purification of a calcium-binding phosphoprotein from pig brain, *J. Biol. Chem.* **247**:4180–4185.

Woolf, C. J., Willies, G. H., Laburn, H., and Rosendorff, C., 1975, Pyrogen and prostaglandin fever in the rabbit. I. Effects of salicylate and the role of cyclic AMP, *Neuropharmacology* **14**:397–404.

Woolf, C. J., Willies, G. H., and Rosendorff, C., 1976, Does cyclic AMP have a role in the pathogenesis of fever in the rabbit, *Naturwissenschaften* **63**:94–95.

Wong, P. C. L., and Henderson, J. F., 1972, Purine ribonucleotide biosynthesis intraconversion and catabolism in mouse brain *in vitro, Biochem. J.* **129**:1085–1094.

Woodward, D. J., Hoffer, B. J., and Altman, J., 1974, Physiological and pharmacological properties of Purkinje cells in rat cerebellum degranulated by postnatal X-irradiation, *J. Neurobiol.* **5**:283–304.

Woodward, D. J., Hoffer, B. J., Siggins, G. R., and Bloom, F. E., 1971, The ontogenetic development of synaptic junctions, synaptic activation and responsiveness to neurotransmitter substances, in rat cerebellar Purkinje cells, *Brain Res.* **34**:73–97.

Wooten, G. F., Thoa, N. B., Kopin, I. J., and Axelrod, J., 1973, Enhanced release of dopamine-β-hydroxylase and norepinephrine from sympathetic nerves by dibutyryl cyclic adenosine monophosphate and theophylline, *Mol. Pharmacol.* **9**:178–183.

Wulff, V. J., 1971, The effect of cyclic AMP on *Limulus* lateral eye retinular cells, *Vision Res.* **11**:1493–1495.

Yamamoto, M., and Massey, K. L., 1969, Cyclic 3',5'-nucleotide phosphodiesterase of fish *(Salmo gairdnerii)* brain, *Comp. Biochem. Physiol.* **30**:941–954.

Yamamoto, C., and Matsui, S., 1976, Effect of stimulation of excitatory nerve tract on release of glutamic acid from olfactory cortex slices *in vitro, J. Neurochem.* **26**:487–491.

Yarbrough, G. G., 1975, Supersensitivity of caudate neurones after repeated administration of haloperidol, *Eur. J. Pharmacol.* **31**:367–369.

Yarbrough, G. G., 1976, Ouabain antagonisms of noradrenaline inhibitions of cerebellar Purkinje cells and dopamine inhibitions of caudate neurones, *Neuropharmacology* **15**:335–338.

Yarbrough, G. G., Lake, N., and Phillis, J. W., 1974, Calcium antagonism and its effect on the inhibitory actions of biogenic amines on cerebral cortical neurones, *Brain Res.* **67**:77–88.

York, D. H., 1972, Dopamine receptor blockade: A central action of chlorpromazine on striatal neurones, *Brain Res.* **37**:91–99.

Yoshimura, K., 1973, Activation of Na-K activated ATPase in rat brain by catecholamine, *J. Biochem.* **74**:389–391.

Zanella, J., Jr., and Rall, T. W., 1973, Evaluation of electrical pulses and elevated levels of potassium ions as stimulants of adenosine 3',5'-monophosphate (cyclic AMP) accumulation in guinea-pig brain, *J. Pharmacol. Exp. Ther.* **186**:241–251.

Zavodskaya, I. S., Migas, E. A., and Bul'on, V. V., 1975, Effect of ethimizole on content of cyclic AMP in brain tissue, *Bull. Exp. Biol. Med.* **79**:274–276.

Zivkovic, B., Guidotti, A., and Costa, E., 1975, The regulation of the kinetic state of striatal tyrosine hydroxylase and the role of postsynaptic dopamine receptors, *Brain Res.* **92**:516–521.

Zivkovic, B., Guidotti, A., and Costa, E., 1976, Cyclic AMP and regulation of tyrosine-3-monoxygenase in rat striatum, *J. Cyclic Nucleotide Res.* **2**:1–10.

Zimmerman, I., and Berg, A., 1973, Levels of adenosine 3',5' cyclic monophosphate in the cerebral cortex of aging rats, *Mech. Ageing Devel.* **3**:33–36.

Zimmerman, I., and Isaacs, K., 1975, A possible effect of testosterone on the adenosine 3',5' cyclic monophosphate levels in rat cerebral cortex. A brief note, *Mech. Ageing Devel.* **4**:215–219.

Zor, U., Kaneko. T., Schneider, H. P. G., McCann, S. M., Lowe, I. P., Bloom, G., Borland, B., and Field, J. B., 1969, Stimulation of anterior pituitary adenyl cyclase activity and adenosine 3',5'-cyclic phosphate by hypothalamic extract and prostaglandin E_1, *Proc. Nat. Acad. Sci. USA* **63**:918–925.

Zornetzer, M. S., and Stein, G. S., 1975, Gene expression in mouse neuroblastoma cells: Properties of the genome, *Proc. Nat. Acad. Sci. USA* **72**:3119–3123.

Appendix

Structures of cyclic nucleotides and agonists and antagonists utilized for the study of cyclic nucleotide-generating systems in the nervous system.

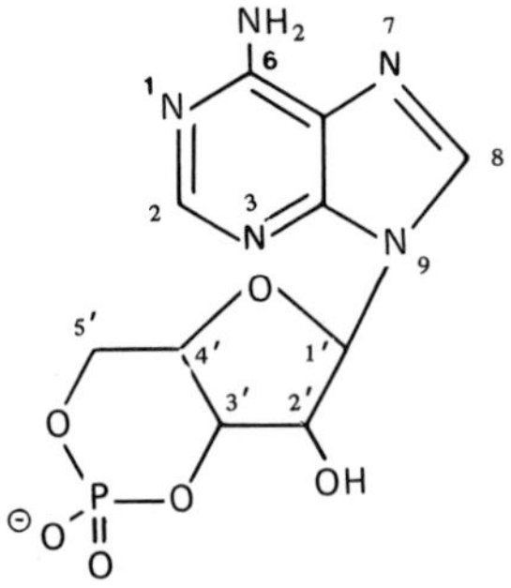

Cyclic AMP

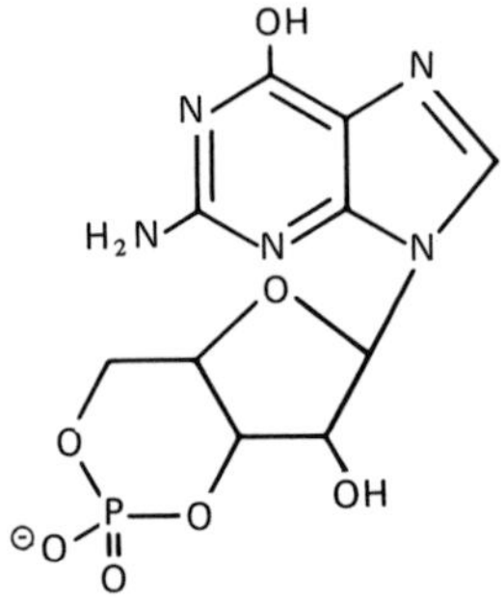

Cyclic GMP

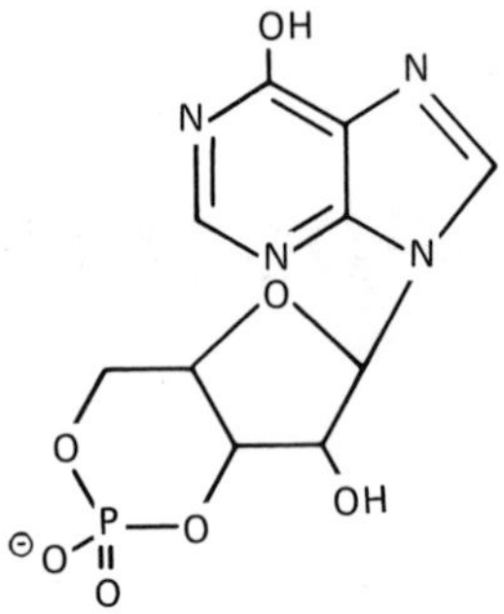

Cyclic IMP

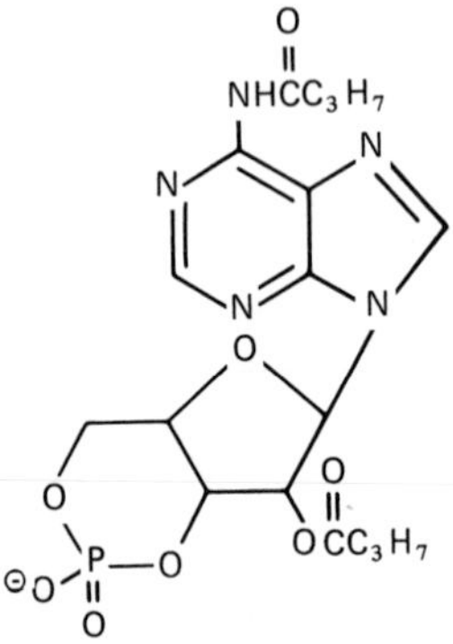

2′-O,N⁶-Dibutyryl Cyclic AMP

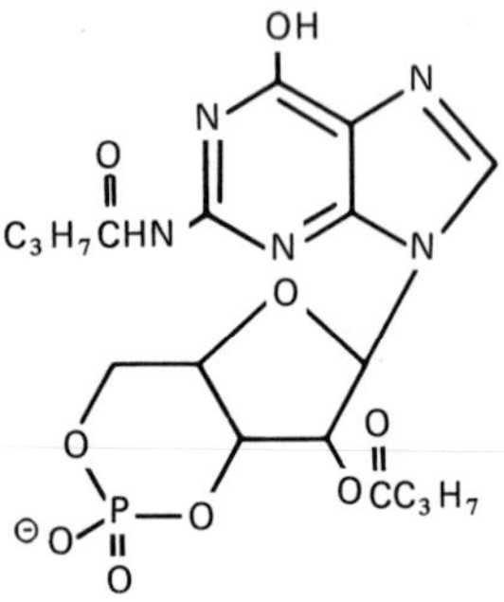

2′-O,N²-Dibutyryl Cyclic GMP

Plate I. Cyclic Nucleotides.

α-Agonists

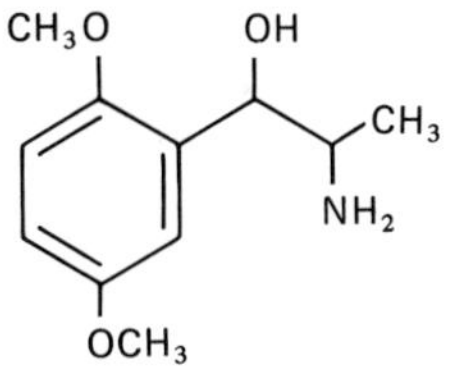

Methoxamine

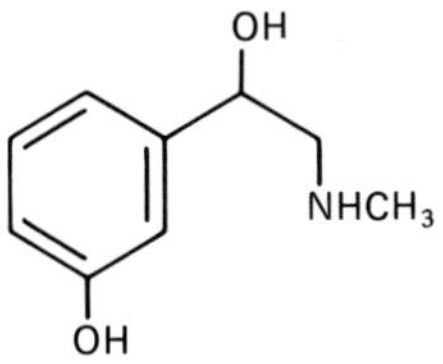

Phenylephrine

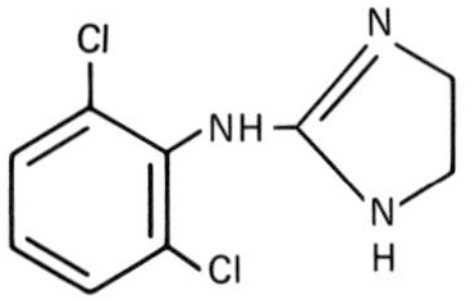

Clonidine

Mixed Agonists

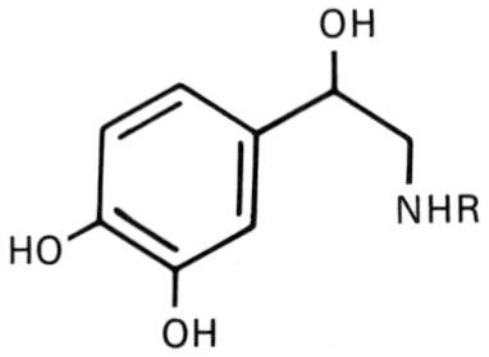

Norepinephrine
R = H
Epinephrine
R = CH$_3$

β-Agonists

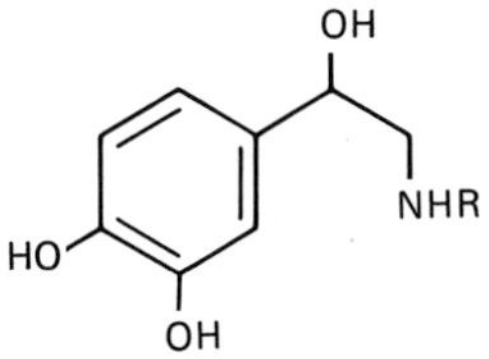

Isoproterenol
R = CH(CH$_3$)$_2$

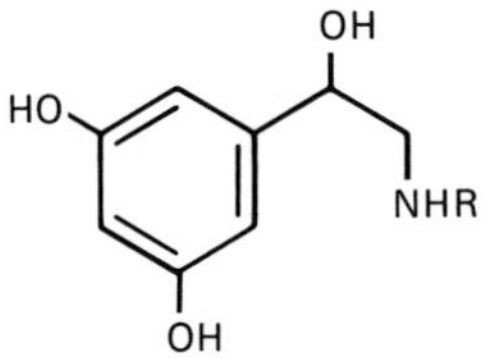

Metaproterenol
R = CH(CH$_3$)$_2$
Terbutaline (B$_2$)
R = CH(CH$_3$)$_3$

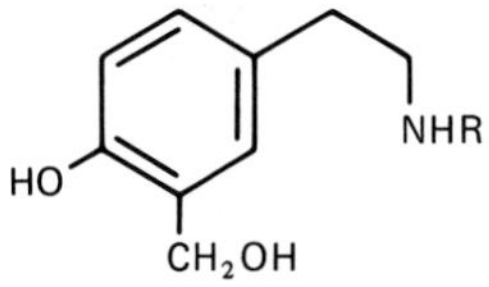

Salbutamol (B$_2$)
R = CH(CH$_3$)$_2$

Plate II. Noradrenergic Agonists.

Classical α-Antagonists

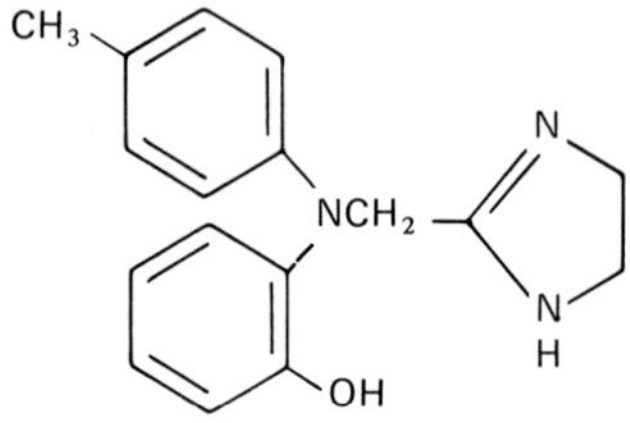

Phentolamine

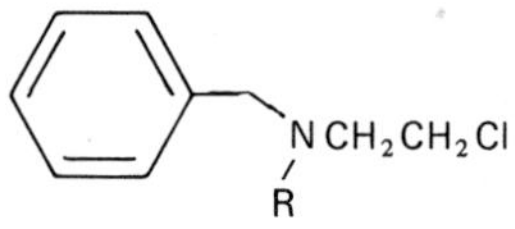

Phenoxy benzamine
R = − CHCH$_3$CH$_2$OC$_6$H$_5$
Dibenamine
R = − CH$_2$C$_6$H$_5$

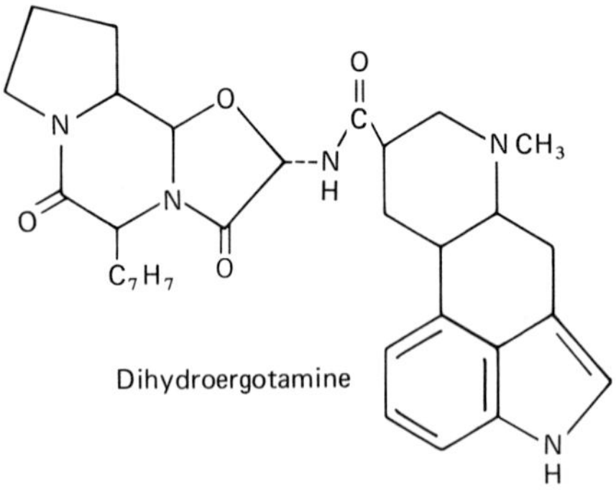

Dihydroergotamine

Antidepressants

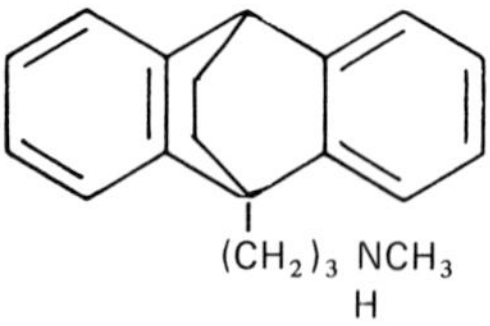

(CH$_2$)$_3$ NCH$_3$
                    H

Maprotiline

(CH$_2$)$_3$NCH$_3$ R

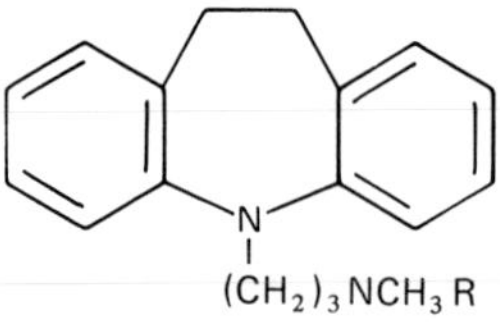

Imipramine
R = CH$_3$
Desipramine
R = H

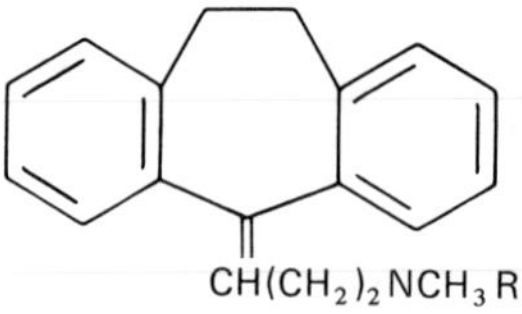

CH(CH$_2$)$_2$NCH$_3$ R

Amitriptyline
R = CH$_3$
Nortriptyline
R = H

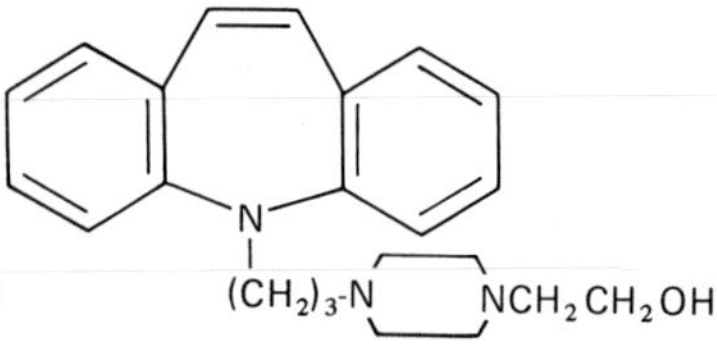

(CH$_2$)$_3$-N   NCH$_2$CH$_2$OH

Opipramol

Plate III. α-Adrenergic Antagonists.

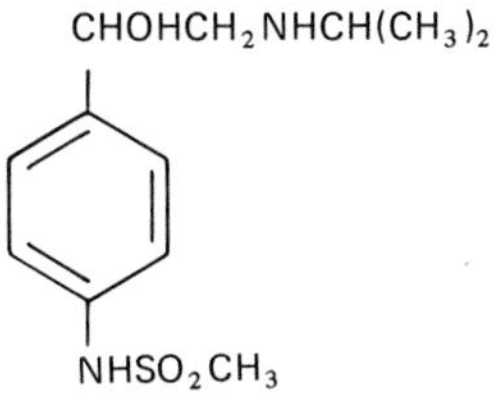

CHOHCH$_2$NHCH(CH$_3$)$_2$

NHSO$_2$CH$_3$

Sotalol

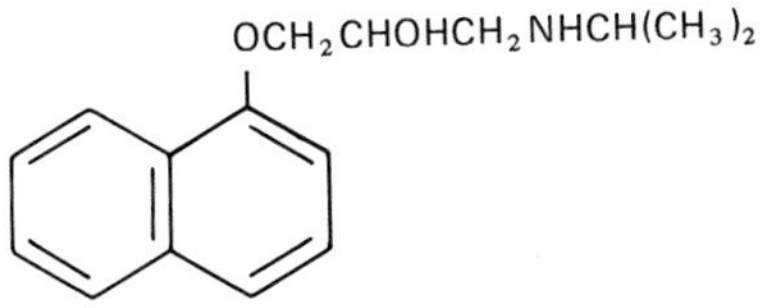

OCH$_2$CHOHCH$_2$NHCH(CH$_3$)$_2$

Propranolol

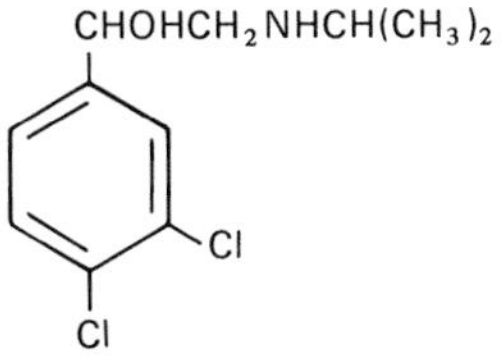

CHOHCH$_2$NHCH(CH$_3$)$_2$

Cl

Cl

Dichlorisoproterenol

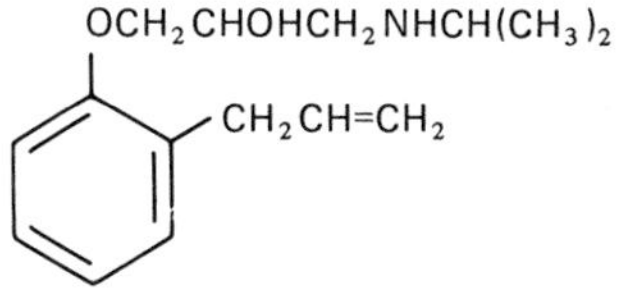

OCH$_2$CHOHCH$_2$NHCH(CH$_3$)$_2$

CH$_2$CH=CH$_2$

Alprenolol

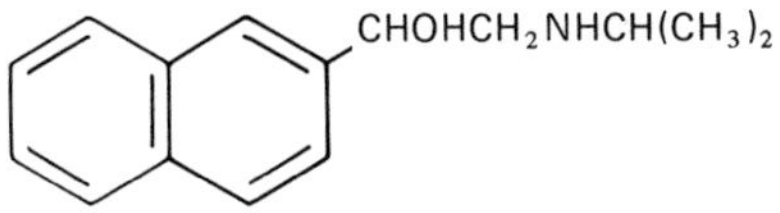

CHOHCH$_2$NHCH(CH$_3$)$_2$

Pronethalol

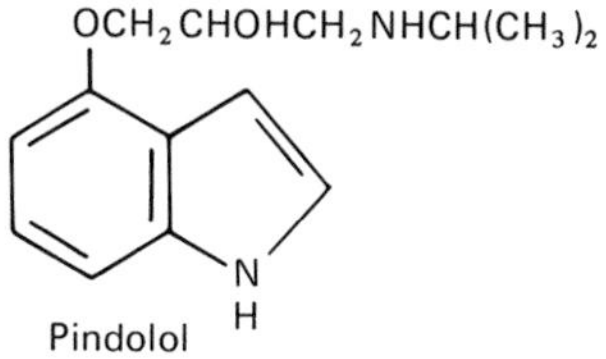

OCH$_2$CHOHCH$_2$NHCH(CH$_3$)$_2$

N
H

Pindolol

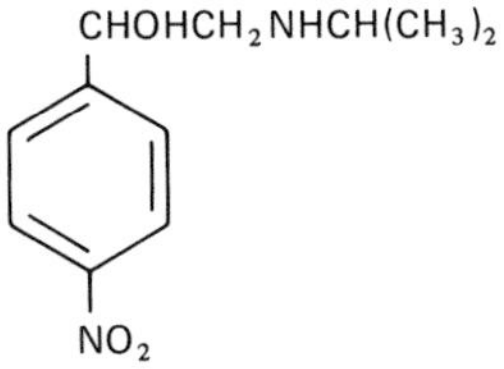

CHOHCH$_2$NHCH(CH$_3$)$_2$

NO$_2$

Nifenalol (IPNEA)

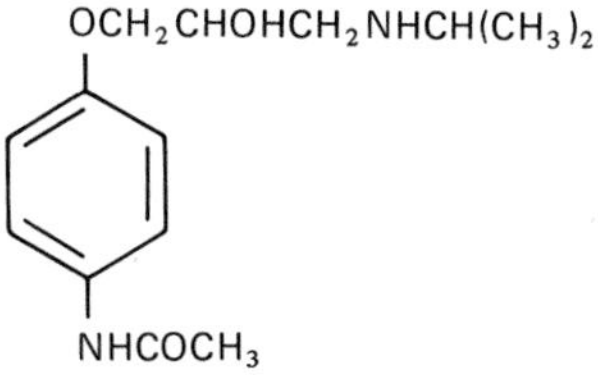

OCH$_2$CHOHCH$_2$NHCH(CH$_3$)$_2$

NHCOCH$_3$

Practolol (B$_1$)

Plate IV. β-Adrenergic Antagonists.

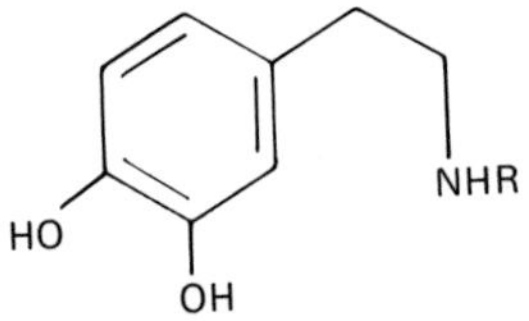

Dopamine
R—H
Epinine
R—CH₃

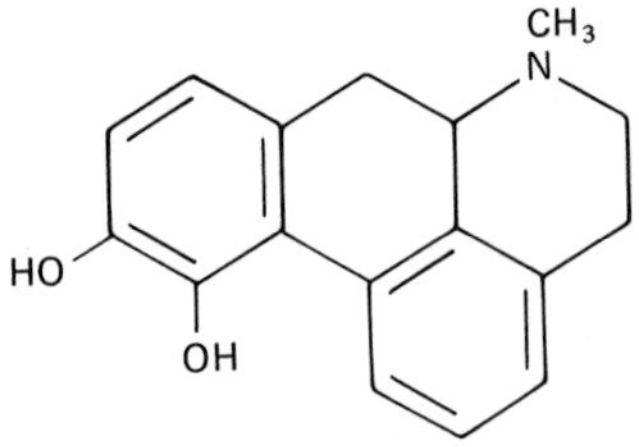

Apomorphine

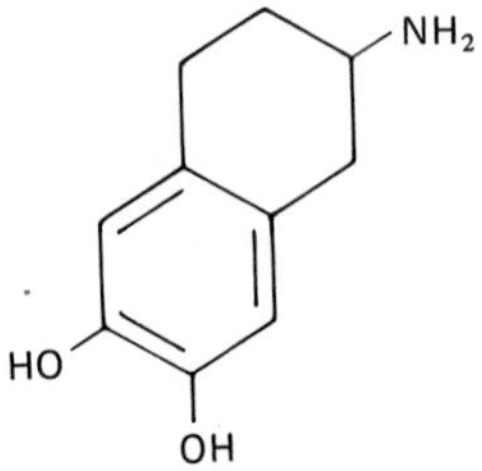

2-Amino-6,7-dihydroxy-
1,2,3,4-tetrahydro-
naphthalene

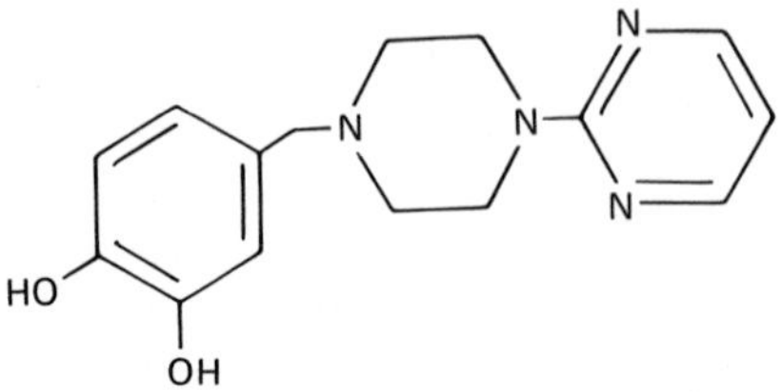

Catechol metabolite
of piribedil

Plate V. Dopaminergic Agonists.

Phenothiazines

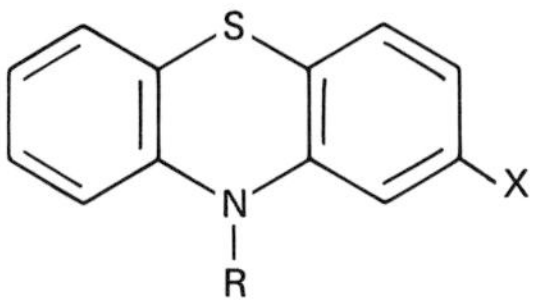
S
N
R
X

Fluphenazine

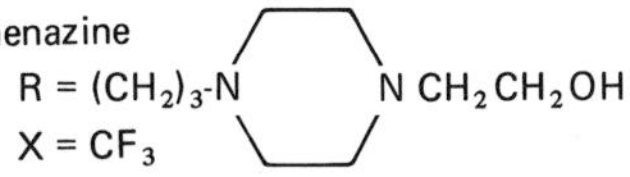
R = (CH2)3-N
N CH2CH2OH
X = CF3

Trifluoperazine

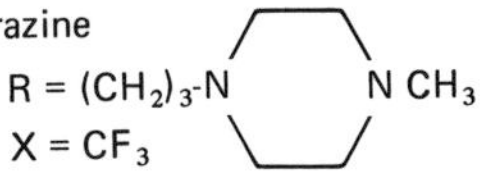
R = (CH2)3-N
N CH3
X = CF3

Chlorpromazine

$R = (CH_2)_3\text{-}N(CH_3)_2$

$X = Cl$

Prochlorperazine

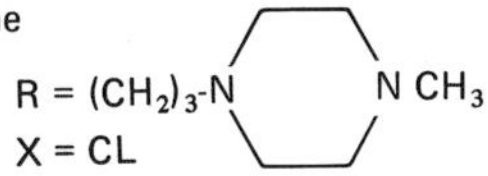
R = (CH2)3-N
N CH3
X = CL

Thioridazine

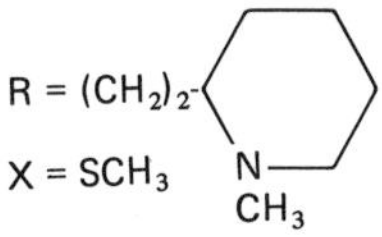
R = (CH2)2-
X = SCH3
N
CH3

Thioxanthenes

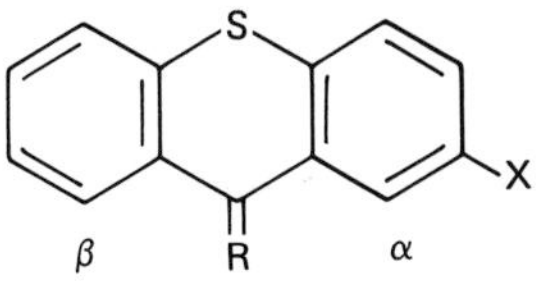
S
X
β
R
α

Flupenthixol (α or β)

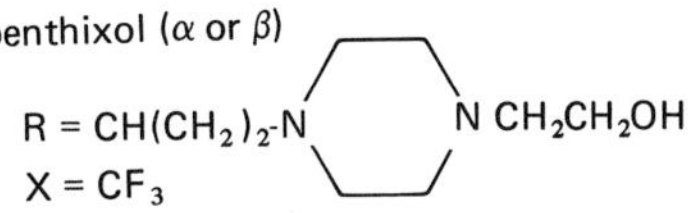
R = CH(CH2)2-N
N CH2CH2OH
X = CF3

Chlorprothixene (α or β)

$R = CH(CH_2)_2N(CH_3)_2$

$X = Cl$

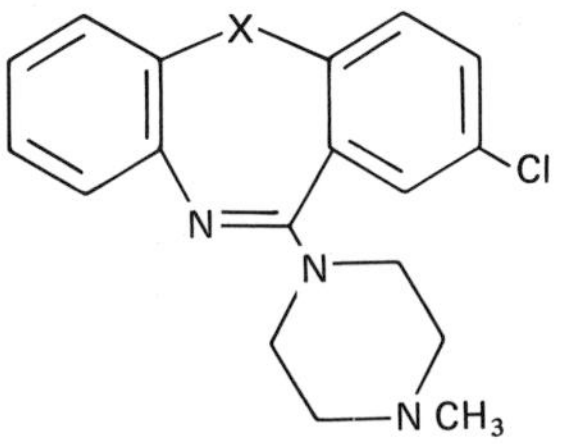
X
Cl
N
N
N CH3

Clothiapine $X = S$ Loxapine $X = O$

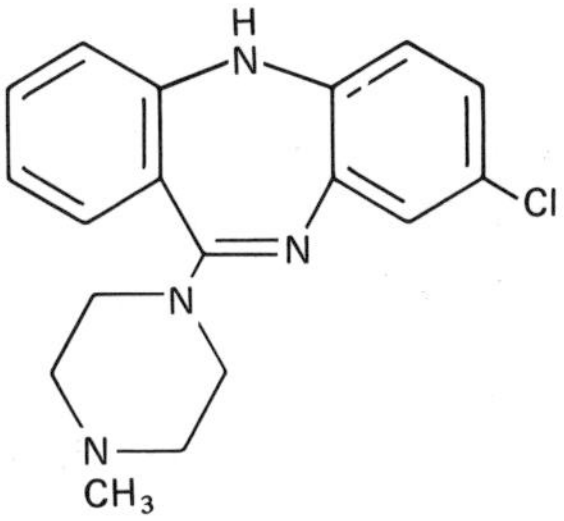
H
N
Cl
N
N
N
CH3

Clozapine

Plate VI. Dopaminergic Antagonists I.

Butyrophenones

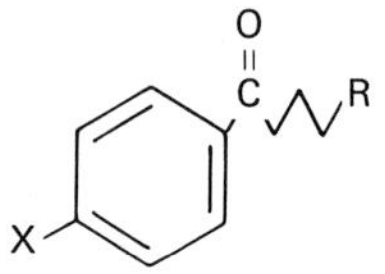

Haloperidol
R = N ... OH, C₆H₄Cl
X = F

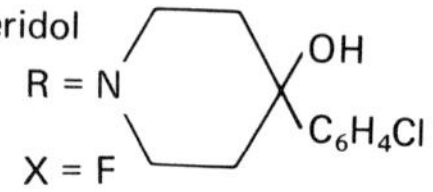

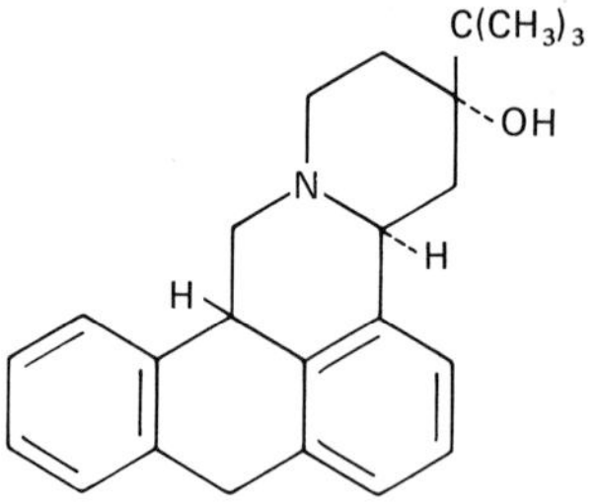

Butaclamol

Spiroperidol
R = N
X = H
C₆H₅

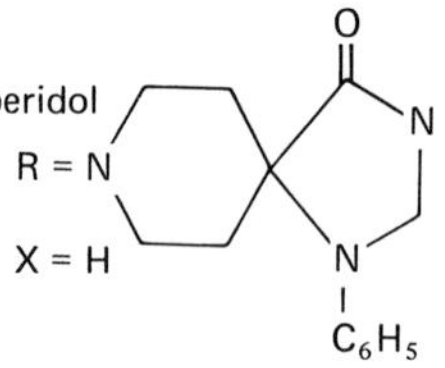

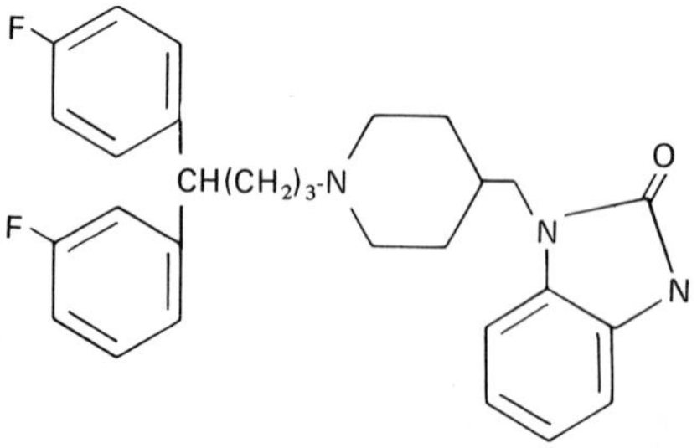

Pimozide

Droperidol
R = N
X = F

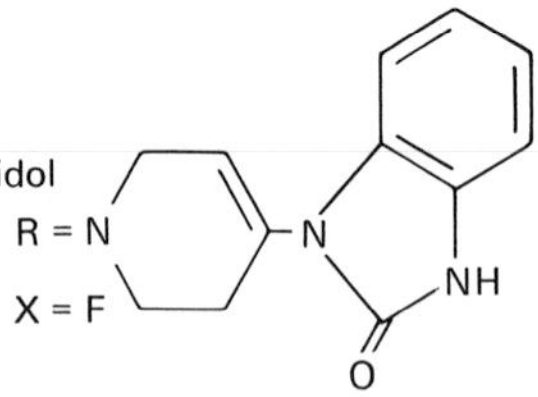

Plate VII. Dopaminergic Antagonists II.

Agonists

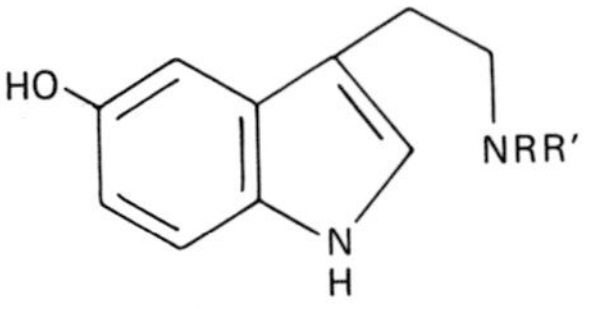

Serotonin
R,R′ = H
Bufotenine
R,R′ = CH$_3$

Antagonists

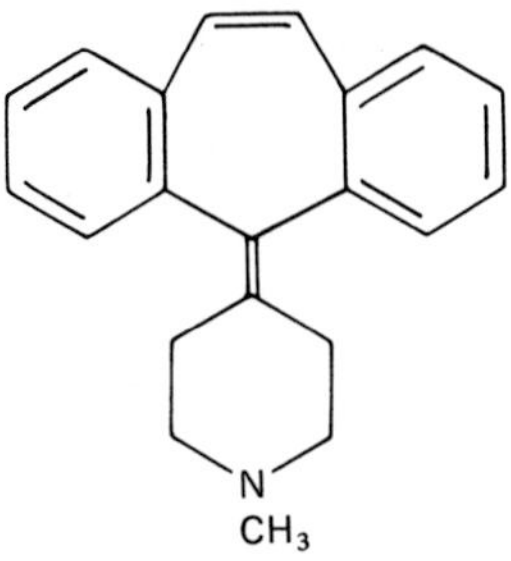

Cyproheptadine
(antihistamine)

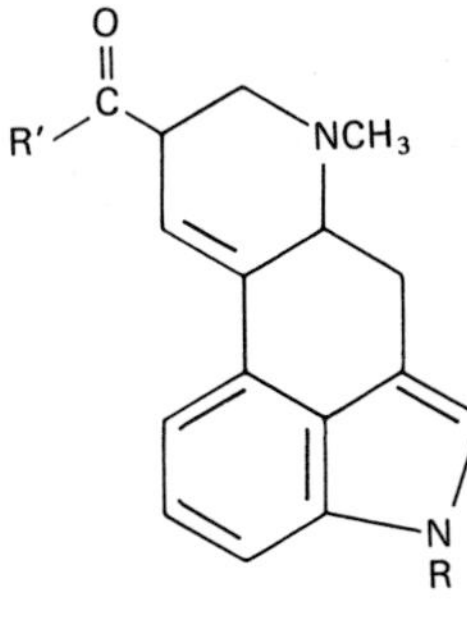

Lysergic and diethylamide
R = H, R′ = -N(C$_2$H$_5$)$_2$
Methysergide
R = CH$_3$, R′ = -NHCH(C$_2$H$_5$) (CH$_2$CH$_2$OH)

Plate VIII. Serotoninergic Agents.

H₁-agonists

S — N — NH₂

2-(2'-Aminoethyl)thiazole

Mixed-agonists

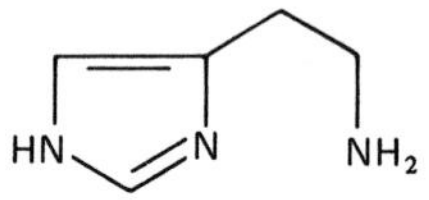

HN — N — NH₂

Histamine

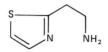

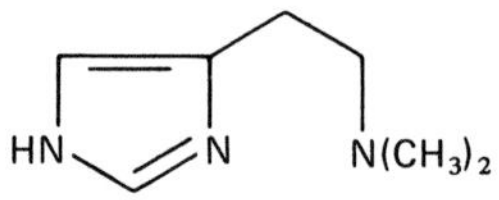

2-Methylhistamine

HN — N — N(CH₃)₂

ω-N,N-Dimethylhistamine

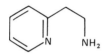

2-(2'-Aminoethyl)pyridine

N — HN — N — NH₂

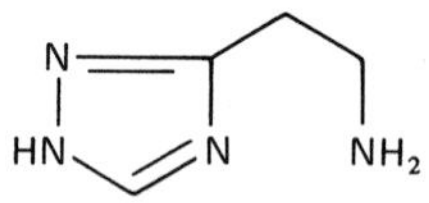

3-(2'-Aminoethyl)triazole

H₂-agonists

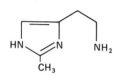

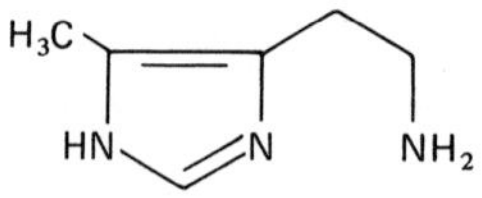

4-Methylhistamine

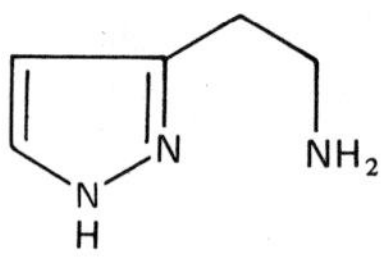

Betazole

Plate IX. Histaminergic Agonists.

H₁-Antagonists

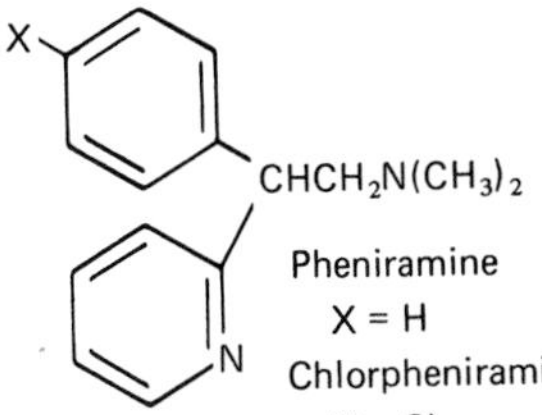

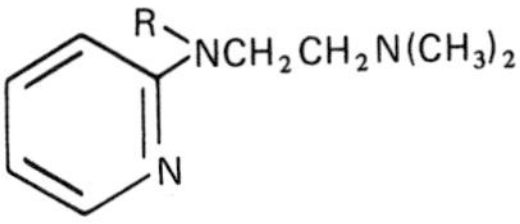

Pyrilamine
R = C₆H₄OCH₃
Tripellenamine
R = CH₂C₆H₅

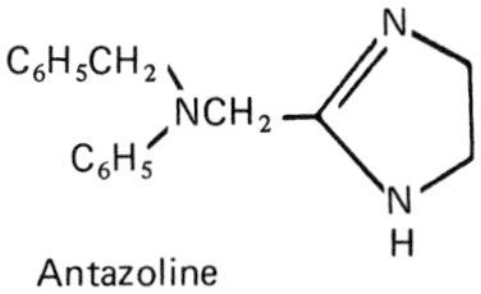

Pheniramine
X = H
Chlorpheniramine
X = Cl
Brompheniramine
X = Br

Antazoline

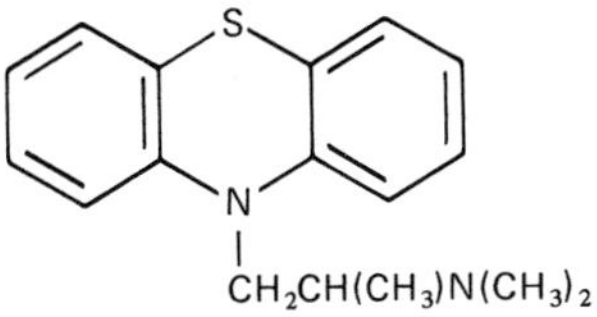

Promethazine

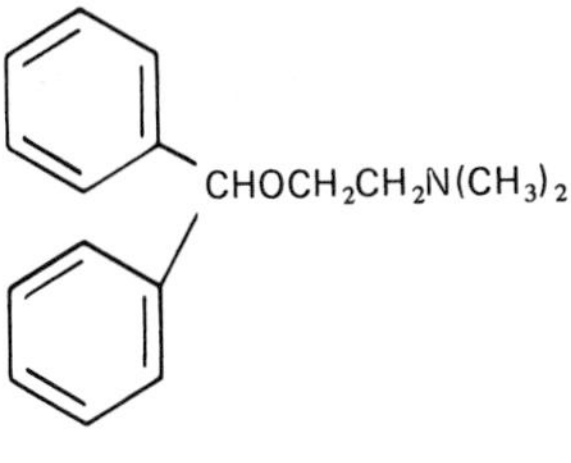

Diphenhydramine

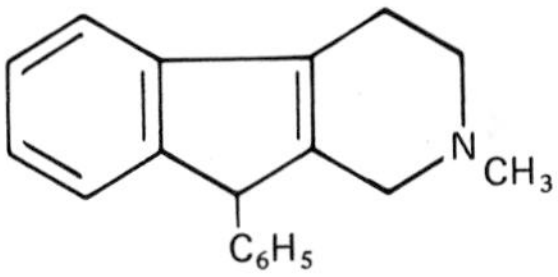

Phenindamine

H₂-Antagonists

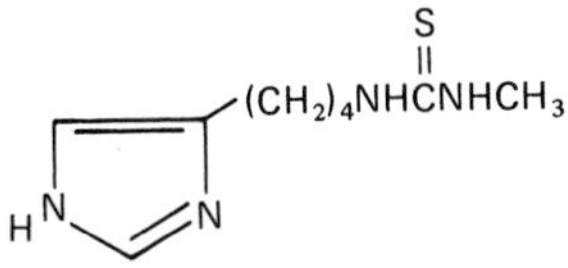

Burimamide

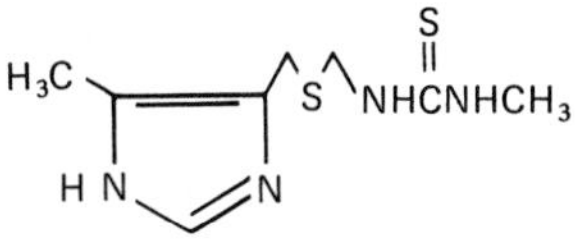

Metiamide

Plate X. Histaminergic Antagonists.

Nicotinic

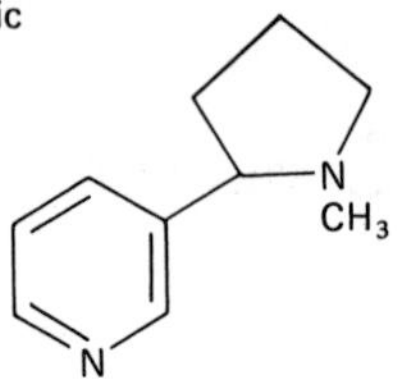

Nicotine

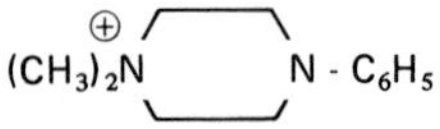

$(CH_3)_2\overset{\oplus}{N}$ ⟩—N - C_6H_5

Dimethylphenylpiperazinium

$\overset{\oplus}{N}(CH_3)_4$

Tetramethylammonium

Muscarinic

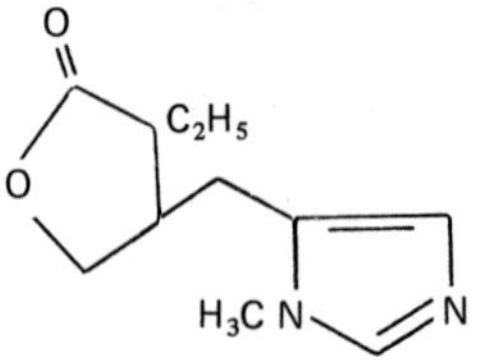

Pilocarpine

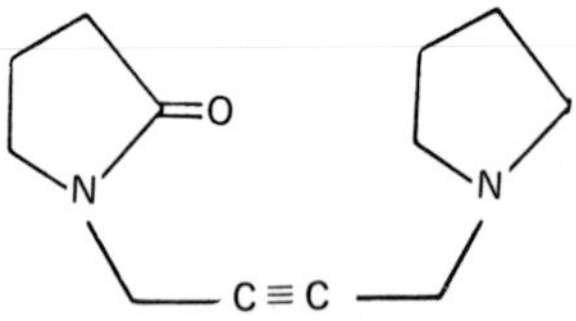

Oxotremorine

Mixed

$$\underset{RCOCH_2CH_2\overset{\oplus}{N}(CH_3)_3}{\overset{O}{\overset{\|}{}}}$$

Acetylcholine
R = CH_3
Carbamylcholine
R = NH_2

$$\underset{R\ COCHCH_2\overset{\oplus}{N}(CH_3)_2}{\overset{O\ CH_3}{\overset{\|\ |}{}}}$$

Methacholine
R = CH_3
Bethanechol
R = NH_2

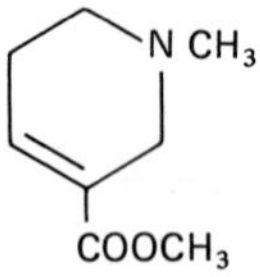

Arecoline

Plate XI. Cholinergic Agonists.

Nicotinic

$$(CH_3)_3\overset{\oplus}{N}(CH_2)_6\overset{\oplus}{N}(CH_3)_3$$

Hexamethonium

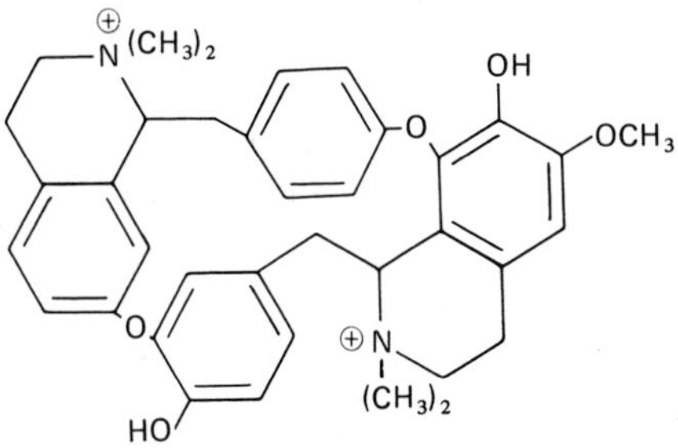

Muscarinic

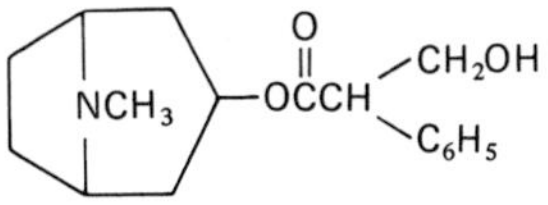

$NCH_3 \quad -O\overset{O}{\overset{\|}{C}}CH \overset{CH_2OH}{\underset{C_6H_5}{\big<}}$

Atropine

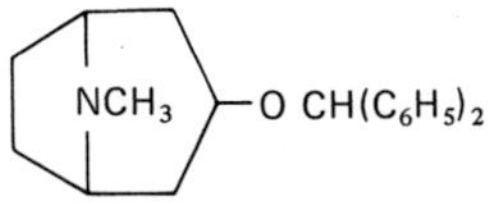

$-N^{\oplus}(CH_3)_2$ OH
O OCH_3

$NCH_3 \quad -O\ CH(C_6H_5)_2$

Benztropine
(antihistamine)

$\overset{\oplus}{N}(CH_3)_2$

HO

α - Tubocurarine

Ganglionic

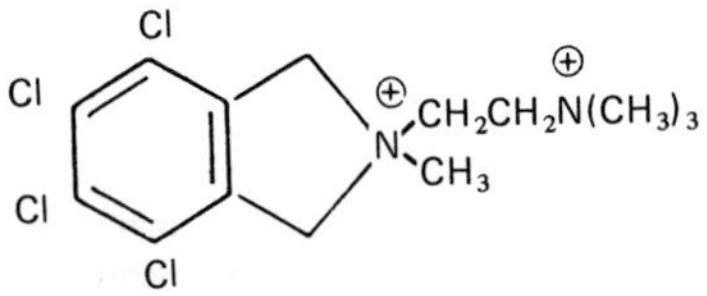

Cl
Cl
Cl
Cl

$\overset{\oplus}{N}$-CH_2CH_2$\overset{\oplus}{N}$(CH_3)_3
CH_3

Chlorisondamine

NH CH_3
CH_3
(CH_3)_2

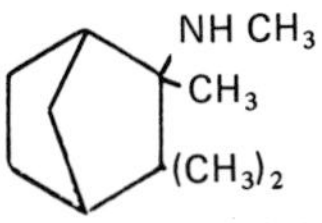

Mecamylamine

Plate XII. Cholinergic Antagonists.

Agonists

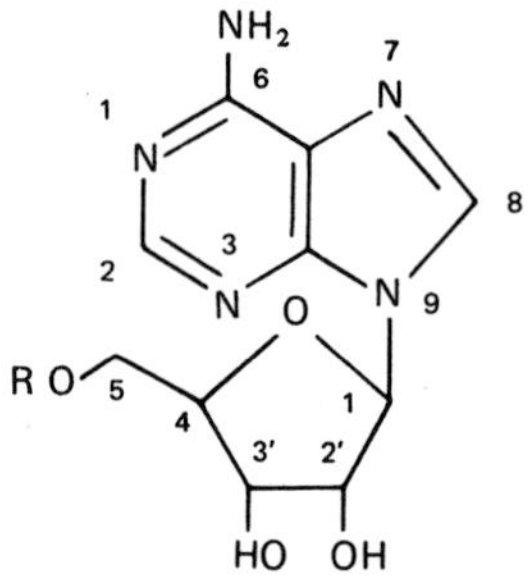

Antagonists

ATP

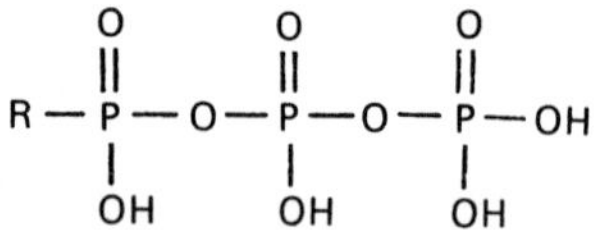

5'-AMP

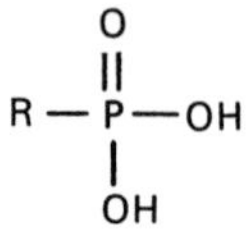

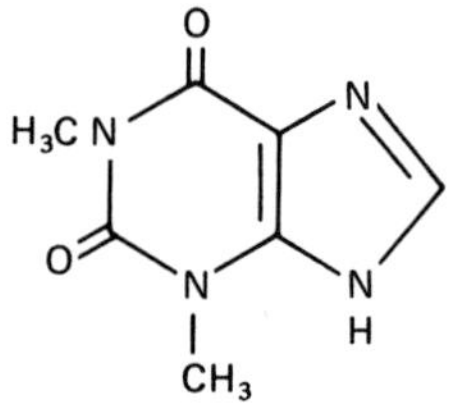

Theophylline

Caffeine

3-Isobutyl-1-methylxanthine

Adenosine   R = H

2 - Chloroadenosine
N^6 - Phenylisopropyladenosine

2' - Deoxyadenosine
3' - Deoxyadenosine

Plate XIII. Purinergic Agents.

Glutamate—Aspartate

Agonist   Antagonist

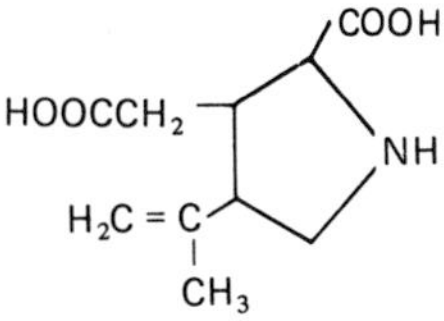

Kainic Acid

$C_2H_5OOCCH_2CH_2CHCOOC_2H_5$
$|$
NH_2

Diethylglutamate

γ - Amino Butyrate

Antagonists

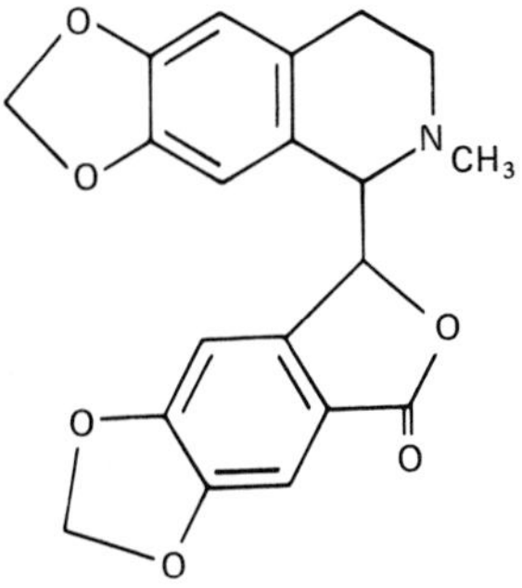

Biccuculine

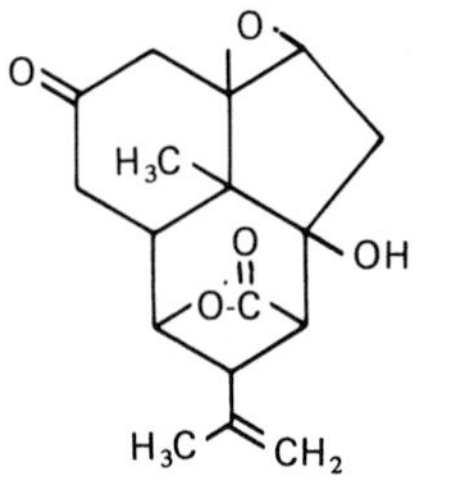

Picrotoxin

$\bullet\, C_{15}H_{18}O_7$

Glycine

Antagonist

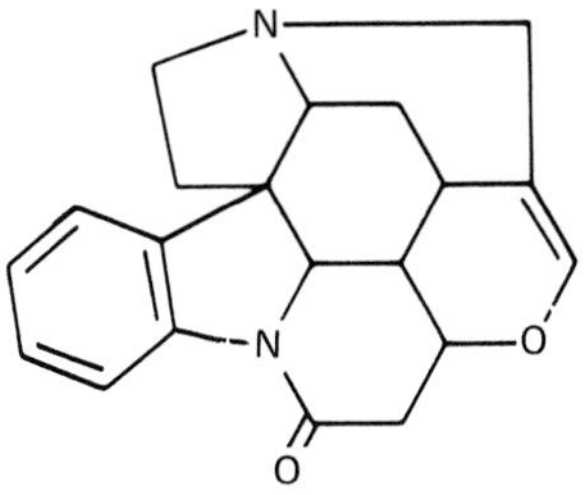

Strychnine

Plate XIV. Amino Acids and Antagonists.

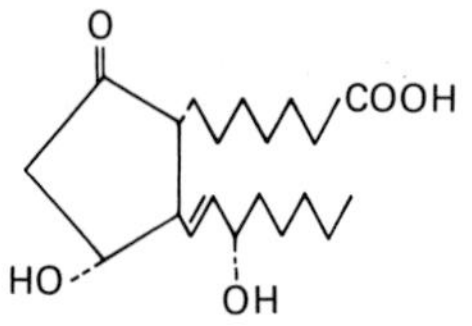

Prostaglandin E$_1$

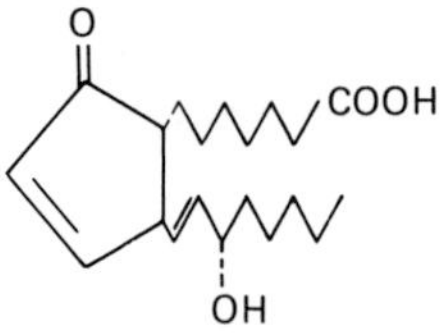

Prostaglandin A$_1$

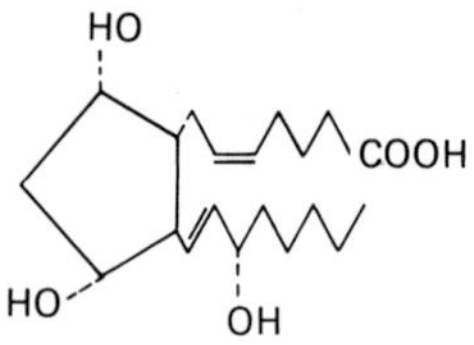

Prostaglandin F$_{2\alpha}$

Antagonists

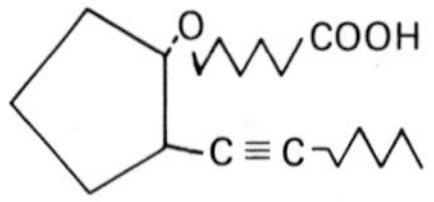

7-Oxa-13-prostynoic
acid

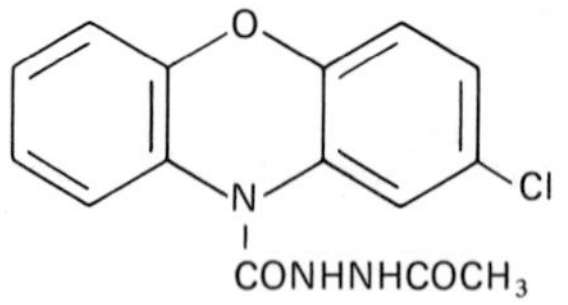

1-Acetyl-2-[8-chloro-10,11-dihydro-
benz (b,f)(1,4) oxazepine-10-
carbonyl] hydrazine
(SC 19220)

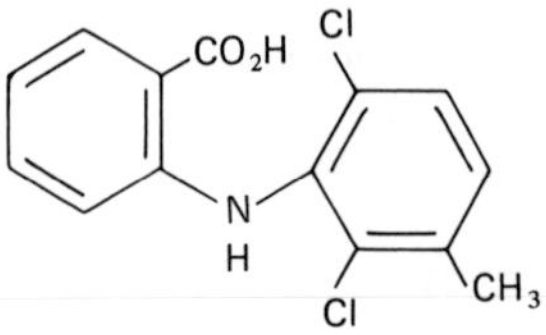

Meclofenamic acid

Plate XV. Prostaglandins and Antagonists.

Narcotic Analgesics

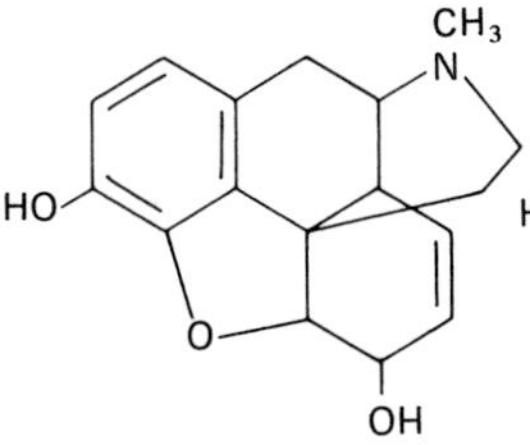

Morphine

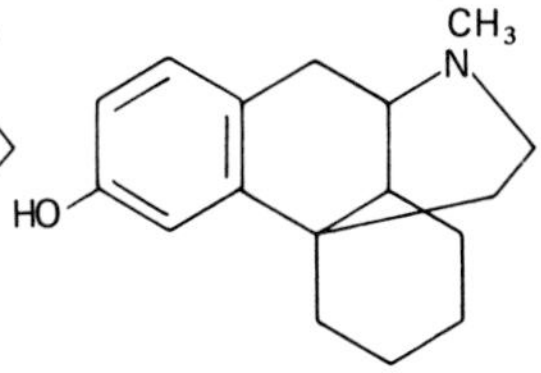

ℓ = Levorphan
d = Dextrophan
dℓ = Dromoran

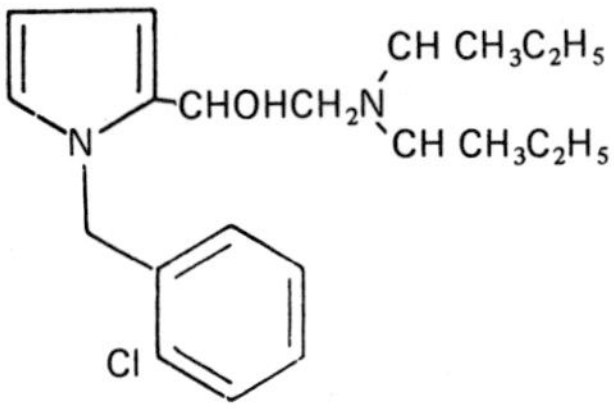

Viminol

Narcotic   Antagonists

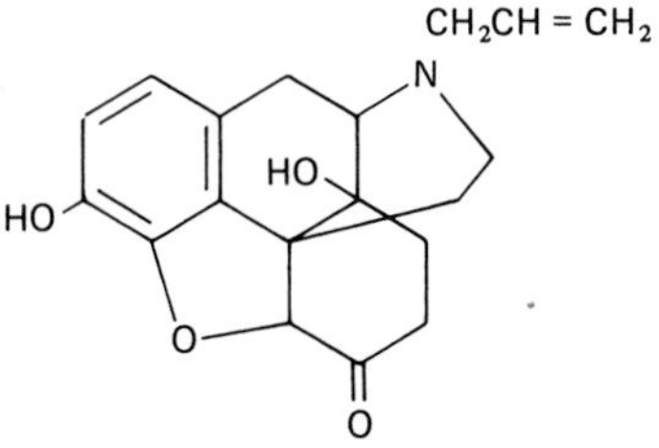

Naloxone

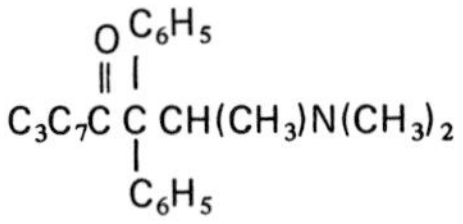

Methadone

Plate XVI. Prostaglandin "Antagonists."

Index

Italic entries are to structures of compounds.